LIVER TRANSPLANTATION – TECHNICAL ISSUES AND COMPLICATIONS

Edited by **Hesham Abdeldayem**
and **Naglaa Allam**

Liver Transplantation – Technical Issues and Complications
Edited by Hesham Abdeldayem and Naglaa Allam

Published by InTech
Janeza Trdine 9, 51000 Rijeka, Croatia

Notice
Statements and opinions expressed in the chapters are these of the individual contributors and not necessarily those of the editors or publisher. No responsibility is accepted for the accuracy of information contained in the published chapters. The publisher assumes no responsibility for any damage or injury to persons or property arising out of the use of any materials, instructions, methods or ideas contained in the book.

Publishing Process Manager Romana Vukelic

Technical Editor Teodora Smiljanic

Cover Designer InTech Design Team

Additional hard copies can be obtained from orders@intechopen.com

Liver Transplantation – Technical Issues and Complications,
Edited by Hesham Abdeldayem and Naglaa Allam
p. cm.
ISBN 978-953-51-0015-7

For EU product safety concerns:
IN TECH d.o.o., Prolaz Marije Krucifikse Kozulić 3, 51000 Rijeka, Croatia,
info@intechopen.com or visit our website at intechopen.com.

Meet the editors

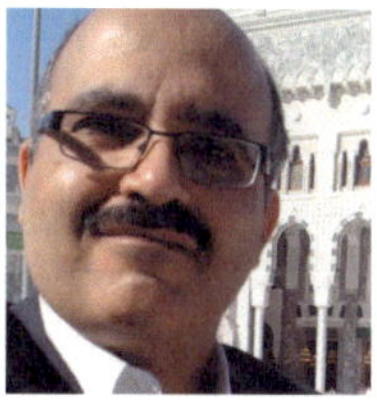

Dr Hesham Abdeldayem is a professor of surgery at the National Liver Institute, Menoufeyia University, in Egypt. He is a well known expert in the fields of hepatobiliary and pancreatic surgery and liver transplantation. He was trained at Starzl Transplantation Institute, University of Pittsburgh Medical Center, in USA. Dr Abdeldayem is a WHO-certified trainer in publishing medical journals. He is a reviewer in many medical journals, and published many papers and several books, both in English and Arabic, in the fields of liver transplantation and hepatobiliary and pancreatic surgery.

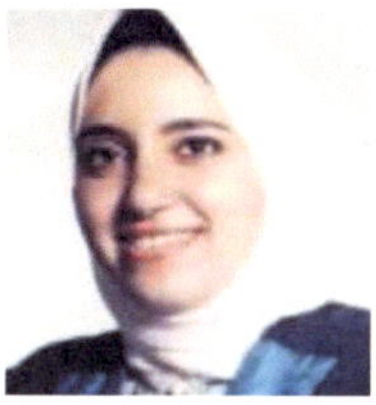

Dr Naglaa Allam is an associate professor of Hepatology at the National Liver Institute, Menoufeyia University, in Egypt. She was trained at the liver transplant unit at the Hospital of university of Pennsylvania in USA. Dr Allam has a number of international publications in the field of hepatology and liver transplantation. She is a reviewer in many journals and has also played an active role in editing books on liver transplantation.

Contents

Preface

Although the basic principles of liver transplantation have not changed, the field of liver transplantation is still young, evolving, and dynamic. In this book, the authors are pioneers in different aspects of liver transplantation and come from many centers across the world. The contributions resulted in a valuable reference to anyone interested in developing a global view on liver transplantation, including medical students, residents, fellows, nurses, and practicing physicians and surgeons, as well as researchers in the field of liver transplantation. This book covers a wide spectrum of topics including, but not limited to, the technical issues in living and deceased donor liver transplant procedures, cell and experimental liver transplantation, as well as the complications of liver transplantation. Some of the very important topics such as the arterial reconstruction in living donor liver transplantation, biliary complications, and the post-transplant-lymphoprolifrative disorders (PTLD), have been covered in more than one chapter.

As the editor, I wish to thank all of the authors for their co-operation and desire to share their precious experience with the medical community. On their behalf, I wish to express hope that our publication will facilitate access to the latest scientific achievements in the field of liver transplantation all across the world.

To all my colleagues at the National Liver Institute in Egypt who supported and embraced me with their warm feelings: I love you all. To all my professors who so generously guided me by their example, wisdom, and insights: thank you. Finally, to Ms. Romana Vukelic, the publishing manager, with whom editing this book was a real pleasure: thank you.

Hesham Abdeldayem, MD.
Professor of Surgery
National Liver Institute
Menoufeyia University
Egypt

Part 1

Living Donor Liver Transplantation

1

Living Donor Liver Transplantation

Hesham Abdeldayem
Professor of Surgery, National Liver Institute, Menoufeyia University, Egypt

"As to diseases, make a habit of two things: to help, or at least, to do no harm."

Hippocrates (460 - 377 BC)

1. Introduction

Living donor liver transplantation (LDLT) is probably the most high-profile of all surgical enterprises. At the same time, it is an amazing act of altruism. It requires hard work of dedicated multidisciplinary medical teams coupled with the courage of the patients and their families. The concept of LDLT is based on the following two factors: (1) the remarkable regenerative capacity of the liver, and (2) the shortage of cadaveric organs (Olthoff K, 2003). LDLT has become an acceptable alternative for patients in need of liver transplantation (LT) who are not likely to receive a deceased donor liver transplant (DDLT) in a timely fashion. This is seen especially in countries where cadaveric donation is limited by religious and cultural beliefs, as in Japan, Egypt, Korea, and India (Abdeldayem H, 2010).

This chapter outlines the advantages and disadvantages of LDLT, addresses the moral and ethical issues surrounding this procedure, reviews the evaluation process of the recipient and the donor candidates, highlights controversial indication for LDLT, outlines technical aspects of LDLT, and the middle hepatic vein controversy and reviews donor and recipient outcomes and complications. Where possible, emphasis is placed on the differences in LDLT compared to whole organ DDLT. At the end, the author addresses the issue of living donor mortality and highlights the importance of transparency in LDLT.

2. Historical perspective

Liver transplantation utilizing a partial-liver graft was theoretically proposed for children by Smith in 1969. On 8 December 1988, Raia et al. made the first attempt at LDLT in a four and a half-year-old girl suffering from biliary atresia. In July 1989, Strong et al. performed the first LDLT with long-term success in an 11-month-old boy using segments II and III graft. Broelsch et al. soon followed with publication of the first series of 20 successful cases of LDLT in children at the University of Chicago (Broelsch et al.,1991).

In 1991, Habib et al performed the first LDLT procedure in Africa and the Middle East at the National Liver Institute, in Egypt. They reported the success of their first case in 1993 (Habib et al, 1993). In the same year, Haberal et al. extended LDLT to adult recipients. In their series, they transplanted left-liver grafts to eight patients. In 1994, Yamaoka et al. reported unplanned adult-to-child LDLT using right liver .In this particular case, the operative procedure was changed from left hepatectomy to right hepatectomy because of unfavorable anatomy of the left hepatic artery.

3. Advantages and disadvantages

In LDLT, the waiting time is reduced, with the ability to perform transplantation when it is medically indicated and the recipient is in the most optimal condition. This ensures better outcome before serious decompensation, disease progression (e.g., hepatocellular carcinoma) or death occurs (Russo M et al., 2004).

LDLT is usually is scheduled on an elective basis, allowing time for completing pretransplant work-up of the recipient and donor. The entire surgical team is more rested since the surgery is planned electively. Extensive workup to exclude other diseases in the donor is made. Details of vascular and liver anatomy are known well before transplant. There will be an opportunity to treat, or at least control, viral hepatitis B or C infection prior to transplantation (in those who can tolerate the medication pretransplant). Bacteremia or sepsis, if present, can be cleared with appropriate antibiotic therapy prior to the procedure (Olthoff K, et al., 2005).

Since the graft is transported between adjacent operating rooms, the cold ischemia time is short. The complications associated with organ preservation are minimized, and primary nonfunction is rare. Another advantage may be related to avoiding the activation of the inflammatory cascade seen in cadaveric livers obtained from brain dead donors, which has been implicated in up-regulation of inflammatory cytokines, adhesion molecules, class II presentation and in affecting microcirculatory flow to the, liver with resultant hepatocellular damage and allograft dysfunction. The age of the living donor is usually young. This avoids the usage of organs procured from terminally ill patient with the possibility of end-organ damage. (Jassem W et al., 2003) In LDLT, there is a potential for better human leukocyte antigen (HLA) matching. Improved matching may have an immunological advantage similar to that observed in living donor kidney transplantation. However, this was not proved (Neumann U et al., 2003).

These advantages, though, need to be weighed against the fact that a healthy person is being exposed to an extensive abdominal surgery with its potential for morbidity and mortality. The incidence of biliary complications in the recipient are said to occur more frequently than in DDLT. LDLT recipients are also exposed to slightly higher risk of hepatic artery thrombosis. The so called "small-for-size syndrome", may occur if careful size-matching between the donor and the recipient is not made. Additionally the donor has to face financial and emotional consequences. The donation will limit the functionality of the donor for weeks or months after the surgery (Abdeldayem H et al., 2009).

4. Moral and ethical issues

Primum non nocere "First do no harm", a fundamental medical precept of Hippocrates, is an important philosophy believed in medicine. LDLT challenges this tenet, because a healthy individual undergoes a major operation for no physical benefit to himself or herself. Perhaps there is no greater ethical dilemma than to operate and remove an organ from a perfectly healthy individual to help another (Abdeldayem H et al., 2009). It seems that the general public strongly believes that it is the donor's sole right to donate an organ and this decision should rest with the donor. In liberal societies everyone has the right to participate in dangerous activities according to his or her will, but the transplant procedure involves an 'accomplice'; the transplant surgeon. Yet, for surgeons the principle according to the Hippocratic Oath is to 'do no harm'. Does a surgeon have an obligation to remove a person's organ upon request? (Mazaris E; Papalois V, 2006)

4.1 Donor's motivation

It is important that donors feel they are gaining something by donation so as to be sufficiently motivated and that their profit is of an emotional or moral nature (Sauer P et al., 2004). Donor motivation may be influenced by the type of relationship to the recipient and personal and religious beliefs and values. Donor motivations may include, a desire to help, a feeling of moral duty, a perception that donation is something that he or she is expected to do, and an increase in self-esteem from doing good deeds. Donors may imagine themselves in the recipient's situation, especially siblings, who are sure that the latter would act accordingly if they were in a similar state. That may be the case for parents as well. Spouses may be motivated by self-benefit from their companion's improved health and the improvement of the couple's quality of life (Lennerling A, et al, 2004). The reasons for donation must be thoroughly explored by the team and the donor. The social worker must assess whether the volunteer's decision is made freely without any undo pressure or coercion, and whether motivation is consistent with the donor's values and previous behaviors. Pressure may be more likely when the recipient's death is imminent without a transplant and when no other donor options exist (Lennerling A, et al, 2004).

4.2 Informed consent

Individuals considering living donation must be free to decide how much and what sort of risk is acceptable for them. Potential donors cannot make such decisions if they are not first provided with proper informed consent regarding the risks they are undertaking and potential implications their decision may have on the recipient. The person who consents to be a live donor should be competent, willing to donate, free from coercion, medically and psychosocially suitable, fully informed of the risks, benefits and alternative treatment available to the recipient. The professional who provides informed consent for donation should be a neutral third person. A transplant centre may have reasons for wanting an organ donation to go ahead: transplants are their source of income; they are able to increase their prestige and conduct research (Abdeldayem H. et al., 2009; Steiner R & Gert B 2000).

Issues to be fully explained to the potential donor include:

1. The technical elements of the evaluation process, surgery and recovery, short- and long-term follow-up care.
2. The risk for complications and death to both the donor and the recipient.
3. Medical uncertainties, including the potential for long-term donor complications.
4. Unforeseeable consequences that might change the donor's life, e.g. employment, and insurability, and expenses to be borne by the donor.

5. Expected outcome of transplantation for the recipient.
6. Any alternative therapies available to the recipient.
7. The specific experience and statistics of the transplant centre.

4.2.1 Informed understanding

The donor must demonstrate informed understanding. This is best achieved with written and verbal presentation of the necessary information in lay language and in accordance with the person's educational level. The potential donor must demonstrate their understanding of the essential elements of the donation process, particularly the risks of the procedure. Adequate time should be allowed for the potential donor to absorb the information, and ask questions. This may require several consultations. The donor's family/ loved ones are given the opportunity to discuss their concerns (Trotter J et al., 2007). The donor should be given a period of time to review the decision to donate (Abdullah K et al, 2005). It is very important to inform the prospective donor that he or she can choose not to proceed with the surgery without the risks of coercion or consequences. If the donor is not accepted, the reasons are kept confidential. Most transplant centers will inform the recipient that the donor is not suitable on medical grounds, even when the actual reason may be different. This is done to protect the donor and to avoid any deterioration in the relationship with the recipient (Trotter J et al., 2007). The team must establish that there is no donor monetary compensation and no coercion to donate by family or others. The potential donor's disclosure and consent process should be completely documented.

4.3 Donor advocate

In many transplant centers, a donor advocate evaluates the donor independent of the transplantation team. The advocate should not be in contact with the potential recipient and should not be influenced by the severity of the recipient's illness. The donor advocate could be a social worker, psychiatrist, or physician. The primary role of the donor advocate is to protect and promote the interests and well-being of the donor, and to help the donor through the entire process. The advocate should not pre-empt the donor's decision, since the donor continues to possess the ethical and legal right to decide to proceed with LDLT (Chen Y et al., 2003). The donor advocate should be able to answer the following questions. Is the donor adequately informed about the transplant procedure? Is consent truly informed? Is the donor vulnerable in any way to exploitation? Is the donor aware of alternative options for the recipient? Does the donor recognize the possibility of future health problems related to donation? (Trotter J 2000)

4.4 Relationship to the recipient

Reasons for donation are more understandable when there is a close bond between the pair. For genetically unrelated prospective living donors, questions must be tailored to the specific situation to fully understand why the individual wishes to donate.

4.4.1 Live unrelated donation

It has been well established that live genetically-unrelated emotionally-related donors such as spouses, partners or friends can be potential donors for LDLT. There are surgeons against spousal donation advising that since a good percentage of marriages end in divorce there is no guarantee of a long-lasting loving relationship as a motive for such donation. Friends have been accepted reluctantly as potential donors, despite the fact that they might feel less pressure to donate compared to a family member (Terasaki P. et al., 1997).

4.4.2 Donation by strangers and good samaritan donors

Occasionally, an unrelated (so-called "altruistic") donor may volunteer to be assessed for LDLT, but such a practice is best avoided if possible. The intrinsic reasons for such unreserved altruism, especially in the adult-to-adult LDLT setting, are usually ill-defined prior to the surgery, and may only surface afterward, leading to serious unforeseen problems (Choudhry et al., 2003). The majority of transplant centers disapprove living donation between strangers, expressing doubts about their motivation and commitment to donation, their understanding of the potential risks and their psychological stability.

Such donors may benefit from their act with increased self-esteem and may experience great satisfaction without being coerced by any sense of obligation. It has been proposed that in non-directed donation, the donor and recipient should remain anonymous to each other and probably meet only after the transplant, if they both agree. It has been suggested that true altruists do not need the name of those they help. Yet, the donors might want to see the results of their good deed, and the recipients might want to express their gratitude to the donor. It seems unethical to allow potential donors to specify particular characteristics of the recipient (e.g. sex, religion or race) (Levinsky N, 2000).

4.5 Commercialization of organ donation

It may be said that, living related donation involves a 'highly artificial altruism' according to which everyone is paid, including the transplant team as well as the recipient who gains an important benefit and only the donor is required to be altruistic. On the other hand, shortage of cadaveric organs has led to a worldwide black market for living-donor organs. Of course, it is unethical to sell human organs. A poor donor may be compelled by their financial status to donate, thus making the action non-voluntary. Yet, on the contrary, the donor may be choosing the best from a list of bad options, since it carries significantly less risk than working, for example, under harsh and dangerous conditions. Paid donors are, in their majority, poor and less educated, thus possibly unable to understand the risks involved (Choudhry et al., 2003).

4.6 Paired-exchange programs

A possible way to increase the live-donor pool is the paired exchange programs. In such programs, pairs of potential donors who are incompatible with their recipients donate eventually to each other's recipient. Some have suggested that strict confidentiality should be maintained for each donor-recipient pair because there is a possibility of frustration, anger or resentment between the two pairs, in case one recipient does not have such a good outcome as the other. It is also suggested that both procedures should be performed simultaneously in order to avoid the possibility of one donor refusing after the other donor procedure had already been performed (Park K et al, 1999). Psychological evaluation should be more meticulous to ensure that the donors are acting voluntarily. With the advances in immunosuppression and plasma-exchange techniques, such programs may be unnecessary, since ABO- incompatible transplants may be possible.

4.7 Orphan graft

The possibility of being unable to transplant a liver graft (orphan graft) into the intended recipient because of intraoperative death or other causes should be included in a prospective protocol at all institutions performing LDLT. Recommendations for handling an orphan liver graft include, (1) before donation, informed consent should be obtained from all donors indicating what the donor would want to have done with the orphan graft, (2) the sequence of steps in the operation should be structured to avoid removal of the donor graft until the recipient hepatectomy has been performed and the recipient's survival is likely, and (3) the orphan graft is allocated according to preestablished institutional guidelines (Siegler J et al., 2004). If the recipient dies intraoperatively and this possibility has not been covered in the preoperative consent discussion, the surgical team must obtain oral and written consent from the donor or the donor's family to reallocate the organ.

5. Evaluation and selection of the potential recipient

5.1 Selection of the potential recipient

Given the potential risks to the living donor, only recipients with a reasonably favorable post-transplant outcome should be considered for LDLT. Thus, before proceeding to work up any potential donor, the recipient candidate should first be deemed suitable for the LDLT operation both medically as well as surgically (Abdullah K et al, 2007).

All potential LDLT recipients must first be listed for DDLT. This ensures the following, (1) the recipient is an appropriate candidate for liver transplant and avoids LDLT being done in futile situations (e.g., inoperable hepatocellular carcinoma), (2) should there be any post-LDLT complications including poor- or nonfunctioning graft, the recipient can be immediately upgraded to a top priority status to obtain a DDLT, and (3) third-party payers may require listing for DDLT before approving a patient for LDLT (Tan et al., 2007).

It has been suggested that a MELD score of 18 may be a reasonably good cutoff level above which LDLT is indicated, because a patient with a MELD score above 18 has a greater than 10% risk of 90-day mortality without transplantation; this exceeds the 1-year mortality after LDLT (10%). On the other hand, for patients with a MELD score below 17, the risk of transplant surgery is said to outweigh the risk of death from liver disease (Li C et al, 2010).

Whether there is an upper limit for the MELD score above which LDLT may not be a viable option is unclear. Poorly decompensated patients have a comparatively poor prognosis and may not tolerate LDLT very well. It is thought that small grafts are unable to meet the needs of patients experiencing severe and prolonged illness. Some experts argue that a MELD score greater than 25 precludes LDLT, since a whole allograft, rather than a partial liver, is required to ensure adequate post-transplant recovery (Li C et al., 2010).

On the other hand, some of the patients with a low MELD score (below 18) may have other medically compelling reasons that prompt to consider LDLT (Li C et al., 2010; Trotter J et al., 2005). These cases may include:

1. Patients with HCC who may benefit from an expeditious LDLT before tumor progression occurs while on the waiting list (see later).
2. Patients with a low MELD score that does not truly reflect their illness e.g. those with cholestatic liver diseases such as primary biliary cirrhosis or primary sclerosing cholangitis. These patients may have significant refractory symptoms or complications, e.g. severe pruritus, intractable ascites, infections, or hepatic encephalopathy.
3. Patients with symptomatic benign hepatic masses, e.g. huge hemangioma, hemangioendothelioma, polycystic liver disease.
4. Patients with metabolic disorders, e.g. familial amyloidosis, hyperoxaluria, tyrosinemia, and glycogen storage disease.
5. Patients where LDLT can help prevent life-threatening complications, e.g. cholangiocarcinoma in primary sclerosing cholangitis.

5.2 Evaluation of the potential recipient

The evaluation of potential recipients for LDLT involves a multidisciplinary team approach which includes transplant surgeons, hepatologists, psychologists/psychiatrists, social workers, nurse coordinators, and other consultants (anesthesiologist, cardiologist, pulmonologist, infectious disease, neurologist, gynecologist, nutritionist, dentist, etc) (Abdullah K et al., 2005). Although the pretransplant workup varies with transplant centers, it should not differ from that of those accepted for DDLT. Most programs require a basic battery of laboratory tests, imaging studies, EKG, upper GI endoscopy and thorough evaluation of the general medical condition and fitness for major surgery (see Table 1).

5.2.1 Psychosocial evaluation of the potential recipient

The pretransplant period can be extremely stressful. Declining health, uncertainty about the possibility of LT, and inability to continue working and participating in daily activities all may increase the risk of depression and/or anxiety for the transplant candidate. Those patients who experience psychological distress prior to transplantation are likely to experience increased distress after transplantation, which may ultimately impact their recovery from transplantation (Walter M et al., 2002). Patients with chronic hepatitis C hepatitis have a greater incidence of depression and anxiety than patients with other forms of liver disease; thus, these patients in particular should be carefully screened and monitored. Patients who experience depression or anxiety are encouraged to seek psychiatric treatment prior to LT to improve their emotional and physical functioning. Some patients experience psychological distress or impairment that interferes with their health behavior to an extent that it may prevent them from adhering to medical directives. These patients should be required to pursue psychiatric services until their functioning is stable enough to be evaluated and satisfactorily listed for LT (Walter M et al., 2002).

5.2.2 Social support

Patients cannot and should not undergo stressful LT without considerable social support. Depending on the severity of the patient's illness at the time of LT evaluation, many family members and/or close friends may already have assumed care giving duties, including overseeing medication and dietary regimens and coordinating the patient's medical appointments. Specifically, the caregiver's relationship with the patient, current functioning, availability, and willingness to provide perioperative care should be assessed, as patients will rely heavily upon their caregivers during the perioperative period.

Laboratory tests
1. ABO blood grouping.
2. Complete blood count, serum electrolytes, BUN, creatinine, liver biochemistry, alpha-fetoprotein and coagulation panel.
3. Serology (hepatitis markers, RPR, HIV, CMV, EBV, etc).
4. Stool and urine analysis and cultures.
5. Others (serum alfa-1 antitrypsin, ferritin, ceruloplasmin, antinuclear antibody, antismooth muscle antibody etc.)

Imaging studies
1. Chest x-ray.
2. Abdominal ultrasound to assess the patency of hepatic vasculature, presence of ascites, and to exclude focal lesions.
3. Abdominal CT/MRI to exclude HCC, and to clarify abnormalities seen in ultrasound.

EKG

Endoscopy: Upper GI endoscopy to evaluate and treat varices.

For selected patients
1. Mammography, pap smear and pregnancy tests for female patients.
2. Dental and dermatology evaluation.
3. Cardiac stress test if EKG is abnormal.
4. Coronary angiogram if cardiac stress test is positive.
5. Carotid duplex.
6. Pulmonary function tests and arterial blood gas.
7. Bone scan and bone density.
8. Liver biopsy.
9. ERCP.
10. Colonoscopy.
11. PPD skin test.

Table 1. list of investigations required for evaluation of a potential LDLT recipient

5.2.3 Readiness for transplantation

Certain patients may be in denial regarding the severity of their liver disease. It is important to ensure that patients possess a good understanding of the transplant process. When assessing readiness for transplantation, patients are reminded of the importance of continued adherence to all medical directives.

5.3 Contraindications for recipient listing for LDLT

Contraindications to LDLT are becoming fewer. Absolute contraindications for LDLT are similar to those for DDLT and include multisystem organ failure, severe and uncontrolled sepsis, irreversible brain damage, extrahepatic malignancy, advanced cardiopulmonary disease, active substance abuse, and medical noncompliance. Common relative contraindications include thrombosis of multiple visceral veins, multiple significan abdominal surgeries, morbid obesity, uncontrolled diabetes, HIV, adverse psychosocial factors, and advanced age. Budd-Chiari syndrome and portal vein thrombosis are not usually deemed to be absolute contraindications (Trotter J et al., 2005).

6. Controversial indication for LDLT

6.1 Hepatitis C infection

At present, patients with HCV should not be denied live donor transplants. Large number of studies has been published supporting differing views including that LDLT for patients with hepatitis C yields worse results, equivalent results, and even better results than those of DDLT. The majority of studies, however, have suggested the outcome is not different for HCV-positive recipients undergoing LDLT (Gallegos-Orozco J 2009). The benefits of LDLT in HCV-positive patients include: younger donors, less cold ischemia time, and the possibility of successfully treating patients with antiviral therapy prior to transplantation. It is not certain whether the regeneration of a partial liver graft, particularly in small-for-size grafts may stimulate and increase the rate of reactivation of the latent infection. Previous concerns about a higher frequency of cholestatic hepatitis or more aggressive fibrogenesis with live donors have not turned out to be true (Kuo A; Terrault NA 2009.).

6.2 Hepatocellular carcinoma (HCC)

Success in treating HCC with transplantation has been complicated by the supply and demand issues. LDLT was developed as a solution to this imbalance between cadaveric donor graft availability and the growing number of potential recipients. Changes in organ allocation systems giving priority to specific HCC patients have raised questions to the use of LDLT as a treatment for HCC. From an operative standpoint, the HCC patient is an ideal LDLT recipient, because the MELD priority points assigned to HCC patients mean that they have a much lower calculated MELD score. HCC patients generally have preserved liver function and less portal hypertension, and they are better able to tolerate implantation of a relatively undersized graft (Takada Y et al., 2010).

6.2.1 Indications for LDLT for patients with HCC

6.2.1.1 Long time on the waiting-list for DDLT

A main indication for LDLT in HCC is when the patient will not likely receive a deceased donor organ in a timely fashion with the resulting potential for tumor progression to an untransplantable state. Therefore, in regions where cadaveric donation is limited by religious and cultural beliefs or there is a prolonged waiting time for deceased organs, the use of LDLT to curb tumor progression and increase survival is indicated. Even in areas where the waiting time is moderate, LDLT may still be valuable, if it can be determined that tumor progression is accelerated. Independent predictors of tumor progression may be useful to define aggressive tumors that are more sensitive to waiting list time. Thus, in those patients with large and multiple tumors, and those with high AFP levels, LDLT may still be indicated in those settings with short to moderate waiting time (Bhangui P et al., 2011).

6.2.1.2 HCC exceeding the Milan criteria

A second potential indication for LDLT in HCC patients is the presence of tumors exceeding the Milan Criteria. There is evidence to suggest, that Milan criteria may be too restrictive, and that there may be patients with potentially curable tumors that go untreated because of their exclusion from DDLT listing. The idea of using LDLT to transplant those patients with HCC exceeding the Milan Criteria requires a reasonable possibility of long-term survival (Shirabe K et al., 2011).

6.2.2 Impact of LDLT on HCC recurrence

Some centers have noted an increase in the recurrence of HCC when examined on a stage-for-stage basis in those patients who have had their transplant waiting time shortened by using expanded donor options (LDLT, split liver transplants, domino liver transplants). In contrast, other centers have described no difference in recurrence rates between LDLT and cadaveric transplant for HCC. The explanations offered by the groups that report a higher rate of recurrence are: (1) the release of growth factors and cytokines that induce hepatic regeneration in LDLT. These factors have tumor-promoting effects (2) the biological aggressiveness of the tumor. Prolonged waiting time allows a tumor to declare its biological aggressiveness. Using LDLT to shorten the time on the waiting list may result in transplanting very aggressive tumors that have already metastasized on a microscopic level but are not yet apparent. A short waitlist time may prevent identification of these aggressive tumors, so that LDLT may result in transplanting those patients that are likely to have recurrent HCC. Preoperative microdissection genotyping of the HCC, with measurements of DCP levels, may identify HCC with a high certainty of recurrence and allow judicious use of LDLT minimizing recurrence attributed to "fast-tracking." (Kaido T et al., 2011)

6.2.3 Ethical concerns

Because the donor safety is the paramount concern in LDLT, it is important to consider ethical issues related to LDLT specific to HCC. The potential risks and complications to the donor mean that LDLT should only take place when there is an acceptable survival. However, some will argue that survival outcomes for LDLT for HCC should be compared to nonsurgical/no-treatment outcomes rather than compared to outcomes from transplanting non-HCC patients (Mazzaferro V et al, 2008).

LDLT is ethically justified in those cases where waiting time is disproportionately long and the prolonged waitlist increases the risk of the HCC progression to a nontransplantable state. The risk to the donor can be justified because acceptable survival results can be expected. On the other hand, when LDLT is performed for HCC that exceeds the Milan Criteria it is ethically less clear, because the LDLT is being done due the recipient's exclusion from a possible cadaveric transplant. It is difficult to justify the potential risks to the donor in such a situation where the society prohibits a transplant because it is unlikely to be of benefit. As stated above, there is accumulating evidence, however, that slightly exceeding the Milan Criteria can still yield acceptable survival and for this situation LDLT may be ethically acceptable. Beyond this, there is poor survival, and it is not acceptable to expose the donor to the risks in this situation. Normally if a graft acutely fails, it requires an urgent retransplant (Shirabe K et al., 2011). If LDLT were used in a situation where a cadaveric donor is contraindicated, such as exceeding the Milan Criteria, the urgent retransplant would require a cadaveric organ, even though the patient was originally contraindicated. In these situations, the patient should not be retransplanted (Takada Y et al., 2010).

6.3 Acute liver failure

Patients with fulminant hepatic failure (FHF) rarely recover spontaneously, and there is a limited interval between the onset and irreversible complications and death. Despite advances in medical management, including hemodiafiltration and plasma exchange, the survival rate of patients with FHF under these treatments is low. Liver transplantation is the only available effective treatment for this group of patients. Timely access to an organ is paramount, to ensure reversibility of the condition. Although the outcomes of LDLT are fairly acceptable despite severe general conditions and emergent transplant settings, the use of LDLT for patients with FHF is a matter of controversy and raises significant ethical issues. The major advantage of LDLT for FHF is the timely availability of a liver graft. This has beneficial effects on the neurological outcomes (Matsui Y et al., 2008).

But LDLT also has major disadvantages. The donor needs to be selected in a timely fashion, under medical and social pressures. In addition, there is the possibility of acquiring an extra small graft, which cannot support the metabolic demand of a recipient. Some physicians have expressed concern that the expedited evaluation in the setting of acute liver failure potentially could preclude the potential donor from making a careful reasoned decision about donation. Because of these concerns, some centers have elected to exclude acute liver failure as an indication for LDLT (Rudow D et al, 2003).

In countries where DD transplants are limited, LDLT is the only chance to rescue patients suffering from highly urgent conditions like FHF, with satisfactory overall patient and graft survival rates. On the other hand, in countries where DDLT is available, such patients are listed as high priority and thus have a good chance to receive a DDLT in a short time. However, even programs with good access to DDLT, LDLT should be kept as a viable option in emergency situations, when any wait increases the risk to the potential recipient.

6.3.1 Ethical concerns

The emergency nature of FHF could preclude the potential donor from making a careful decision about donation. The process of informed consent by the donor could also be influenced by coercion from family members or from the medical team. Autocoercion is also a strong possibility. In the context of extending elective LDLT to the more urgent situation of FHF, transplant programs must pay special attention to the autonomy of the potential donor and must ensure truly informed consent (Rudow D et al., 2003).

7. Donor evaluation

Donor evaluation consists of comprehensive examinations evaluating medical suitability for major surgery, psychological suitability, and liver-related suitability. The two fundamental purposes of the donor evaluation are to ensure (1) donor safety and (2) that the donor is able to yield a suitable graft for the recipient. Members of the evaluation team should include hepatologist, surgeon, psychologist, social worker, and transplant coordinator (Marcos A et al., 2000).

Guidelines for evaluating potential living liver donors are not standardized. There is a great deal of variability among individual centers regarding components of their living donor evaluation protocols. Variability exists in the performance of some diagnostic studies, such as liver biopsy, hepatic angiography, and cholangiography (Totter J et al., 2002). The most frequently used model is a process that involves phases that are progressively more invasive and expensive (see table 2). In principle, one should try to limit the number of invasive investigations and reserve them for the later part of the evaluation. In an effort to limit the cost, more expensive tests are generally performed later in the evaluation process (Abdullah K et al., 2007). Another advantage of such a process includes several opportunities for the donor candidate to re-evaluate and reaffirm the decision to donate. The entire process usually takes a period of 1 to 2 months. In emergent situations, it can be shortened to less than 24 hours.

The initial phase is designed to determine that the potential donor meets all the appropriate inclusion criteria for donation: appropriate blood type, age, body size, and relationship to the recipient. The initial screening history may be performed by an experienced transplant coordinator, or the donor is asked to fill out an information sheet. Questions regarding age; height; weight; blood type (if known); past and current medical, surgical, or psychosocial problems (including a history of alcohol use); and current medication use are included in the questionnaire (Totter J et al., 2002). The lower limit of age for donation is determined by the ability to give legal consent. The potential donor must be between the ages of 18 and 55 years. However, some extend the upper limit to 60 years. Most centers require that the potential donor should show a significant long-term relationship with the recipient. Body size compatibility between the donor and recipient is an important preliminary consideration in the donor evaluation. The potential donor should have an identical or compatible blood type and no significant medical problems. Surgical history is documented, along with current medications. Serum electrolyte levels, blood count, liver function tests, and hepatitis serological tests are performed. Relative contraindications for donor evaluation are discovered frequently in this phase and include, previous significant abdominal surgery, hypertension, hypercholesterolemia, and obesity (Chen Y et al., 2003).

The next phase, involves a thorough history and physical examination to determine eligibility for the operation. Female potential donors of reproductive age should undergo a pregnancy test. The use of oral contraceptive pills or hormonal devices indicates perioperative deep vein thrombosis prophylaxis by subcutaneous heparin in addition to physical means. This phase involves evaluation of the donor liver. This can be subdivided into three components, which include assessment of the (1) hepatic parenchyma, (2) liver volume, and (3) vascular and biliary anatomy (Bradhagen D, et al., 2003).

7.1 Evaluation of hepatic parenchyma

The presence of chronic liver disease and steatosis could have potential implications for both the donor and recipient. This begins with liver biochemistry tests, including aspartate aminotransferase, alanine aminotransferase, bilirubin, alkaline phosphatase, albumin, and international normalized ratio (Chen Y et al., 2003). Blood tests to exclude chronic liver disease often are performed early in the course of the evaluation. These tests include serum transferrin saturation, ferritin, ceruloplasmin, alfa-1-antitrypsin phenotype, antinuclear antibody, smooth muscle antibody, antimitochondrial antibody, and hepatitis serological

Phase 1

The potential donor should satisfy the following before proceeding to the next phases

1. Clinical evaluation:
   - Age: between 18 and 55 years.
   - Identical or compatible blood type with recipient.
   - Body weight, height and Body mass index.
   - Absence of previous significant abdominal surgery and/or medical problems.
   - Significant long-term relationship with recipient.
2. Normal liver function test results, serum electrolyte levels, complete blood count with differential cell count, and negative hepatitis B surface antigen and hepatitis C antibody results.
3. Informed consent (for testing and surgery).

Phase 2

1. Complete and thorough medical history and physical examination.
2. Laboratory tests:
   - Serology: hepatitis A, B and C (surface antigen, core antibody, surface antibody), rapid plasmin reagin, cytomegalovirus antibody (immunoglobulin G), Epstein-Barr virus antibody (immunoglobulin G), antinuclear antibody, human immunodeficiency antibody, toxicology/substance abuse screen.
   - Serum ferritin, iron, transferrin, ceruloplasmin, alpha-1-antitrypsin, transferring, alpha fetoprotein, carcinoembryonic antigen.
   - Urinalysis.
   - Coagulation profile; protein C; antithrombin III; factor V, VII, and VIII.
   - C-reactive protein.
   - Thyroid function tests .
   - Pregnancy test for female donors.
3. Imaging studies:
   - Chest X-ray.
   - Abdominal ultrasound scan.
   - CT scan and magnetic resonance imaging to assess the liver volume, the biliary system, and vascular anatomy.
4. Electrocardiogram.

Phase 3

1. Psychological evaluation, and informed consent.
2. Other tests or consultations to clarify any potential problems uncovered during evaluation: e.g., endoscopic retrograde cholangiopancreatography, hepatic angiogram, liver biopsy, echocardiogram, and stress echocardiogram (some centers routinely perform some or all of these tests as part of the donor evaluation).

Step 4

1. Planning of OR date and availability of intensive care unit facilities.
2. Blood bank: autologous blood donation.
3. Second informed consent (for blood and surgery).

Table 2. Suggested protocol for living donor evaluation

tests (hepatitis B surface antigen and antibody, hepatitis B core antibody, and hepatitis C antibody). Donors with evidence of underlying chronic liver disease or a positive hepatitis C antibody or, hepatitis B surface antigen result are excluded from further consideration. There is no consensus on the use of donors who are alfa-1-antitrypsin phenotype MZ or hemochromatosis C282Y heterozygotes. (Bradhagen D, et al., 2003)

7.1.1 Steatosis

Hepatic steatosis can be characterized histologically as microvesicular or macrovesicular. In general, macrovesicular steatosis is regarded as a benign lesion and often is asymptomatic, whereas microvesicular steatosis often is more serious. Hepatic steatosis can adversely affect both of the recipient and the donor. Steatotic livers may not function well because they are more susceptible to injury from general anesthesia and ischemia-reperfusion. In addition, steatosis has been shown to increase cold ischemic injury and impair hepatic regeneration. Several studies have shown that the risk for primary allograft nonfunction increases with increasing severity of steatosis. Because steatosis reduces functional hepatic mass, some advocate subtracting the percentage of steatosis from the estimated liver mass before calculating the final mass of the hepatic allograft and remnant (Bradhagen D, et al., 2003).

There is currently no agreed cutoff value on the percentage of steatosis that is safe for performance of LDLT. The maximal acceptable amount of steatosis in the donor liver varies among LDLT programs and ranges from 10% to 30%. Several studies have shown that livers from deceased donors with less than 30% steatosis can be transplanted with results similar to organs without fat. Additional studies are needed to better define the acceptable amount of steatosis in the donor liver that will ensure a safe and successful operation for both the donor and recipient. There are some data to suggest that steatosis identified on a predonation biopsy can be reversed with a program of dieting and exercise, and rebiopsy in this situation may show the potential donor to be suitable (Chen Y et al., 2003).

7.1.1.1 Liver biochemistry tests

Liver biochemistry tests are not sensitive or specific and may even show normal results in those with advanced hepatic fibrosis. Other methods, such as body topography and lipid levels, have shown a weak correlation with hepatic steatosis. Of all biochemical parameters, serum triglyceride level appears to have the strongest correlation.

7.1.1.2 Anthropometric measures

Waist-hip ratio seems to be a good predictor of steatosis. An increased waist-hip ratio, which is present more commonly in men, is associated with a greater risk for hepatic steatosis. Of all noninvasive methods for assessment of hepatic steatosis, body mass index (BMI) may have the greatest utility. Several studies have shown a correlation between hepatic steatosis and increasing BMI. In addition, obese patients are more likely to have comorbid conditions (hypertension, hypercholesterolemia, and diabetes), which could increase the risk for postoperative complications after donor hepatectomy. Studies from the general surgery literature, suggest an increased incidence of surgical complications such as bleeding and wound problems in obese individuals. Obesity is also a risk factor for underlying cardiovascular problems, which could lead to an increased chance for medical complications posttransplant. Because of these risk factors, most obese donors will not be suitable donors. In general, obese individuals (BMI > 28 kg/m2) are unsuitable for donation. Certainly a BMI of > 35 would be a contraindication. Many centers exclude donors with BMI > 30, but others will selectively evaluate these donors and perform a liver biopsy to rule out the possibility of liver steatosis (Bradhagen D, et al., 2003).

7.1.1.3 Abdominal imaging

Ultrasound, CT, and MRI, may detect the presence of hepatic steatosis. Their sensitivity and specificity are technique and operator dependent and also may vary based on degree of steatosis. The imaging modalities are not able to quantify the amount of steatosis or distinguish between simple steatosis and steatohepatitis. Iwasaki and colleagues (2004) have demonstrated that liver-to-spleen CT alternation values ratios using noncontrast CT scan are useful to detect appreciable hepatic macrovesicular steatosis. Newer imaging modalities, such as dual-echo and gradient-echo MR sequences, may provide increasing accuracy for the detection and quantification of hepatic steatosis. At present, the available abdominal imaging studies do not appear to be sufficiently sensitive or specific to replace liver biopsy in most situations (Iwasaki et al, 2004) .

7.1.1.4 Liver biopsy

Liver biopsy is the gold standard for the assessment of hepatic parenchymal disease, including steatosis. In general, liver biopsy is a safe procedure with a low risk for serious complications. Liver biopsy also is useful in excluding occult chronic liver disease. The appropriate use of liver biopsy in the evaluation of living donor candidates is an area of continuing controversy (Bradhagen D, et al., 2003). The role of liver biopsy in the donor evaluation process varies greatly from center to center. Some centers perform liver biopsy on all potential donors, whereas others perform liver biopsy based only on clinical findings that suggest some degree of concern e.g., significant history of alcohol intake, BMI greater than 28 kg/m2, elevated serum ferritin level, presence of steatosis on imaging studies, and so on. Liver biopsy may be avoided is patients with a BMI less than 25 who do not have diabetes, hypertension, or a history of excess alcohol consumption. In addition, they also should have normal liver test results and lipid levels and undergo tests to exclude chronic liver disease and hepatic imaging studies. Liver biopsy results that would preclude donation include fibrosis, nonalcoholic steatohepatitis (NASH), steatosis > 30% and histologic abnormalities such as inflammatory changes (Nadalin S et al, 2005).

7.2 Volumetric assessment

Donor safety is of primary concern, and the smallest resection that provides adequate actual and functional mass for the recipient is selected. Determination of adequate hepatic mass is critical for successful outcomes for both donor and recipient. Height and weight of the donor and recipient pair can be useful in excluding a very small donor when the intended recipient is large, but is not accurate enough in most other situations. Volumetric assessment of the hepatic segments can be performed using either CT or MRI. In general, hepatic mass estimated by volumetric imaging correlates well with actual hepatic mass determined at the time of hepatectomy. It is helpful for the surgeon to work with the radiologist in making the planned line of liver transection and to provide the most accurate assessment of graft volume (Hill MJ, et al., 2009).

Two formulas are used to assess graft size adequacy: (1) graft-recipient body weight ratio (GRBWR) and (2) graft weight as a percentage of standard liver mass. There is an excellent linear correlation between the two, and either is acceptable. It probably is reasonable to correct the GRBWR for steatosis by subtracting the percentage of steatosis noted on liver biopsy from the functional hepatic mass (Hill MJ, et al., 2009).

Resection should not exceed 70% of the total liver volume; that is, the donor should be left with at least 30% of the measured total liver volume. Liver failure has been reported postdonation, with at least one donor requiring an urgent liver transplant because of liver failure after donation. As a result, LDLT has limited applicability in large patients because of the inability to identify a suitable donor (Nadalin S et al, 2004).

A GRBWR of 1% is approximately equal to 50% of standard liver mass. The consensus is that the GRBWR should be equal or greater than 0.8 % (equivalent to about 40 % of the standard liver volume). It should be stressed, however, that these values are based upon LDLT performed in noncritically ill patients. Patients with significant decompensation of chronic liver disease will have excessive metabolic demands and require the maximum liver volume available. On the other hand, some authorities (Selzner et al, 2009) suggest that, patients with Child's class A cirrhosis or those without portal hypertension could receive an allograft with a GRBWR greater than 0.6%. Marcos A (2000) summarized the issue of hepatic mass by stating, "Neither the minimum transplantable hepatic mass nor the optimal mass have been accurately determined. In all likelihood, these values are dependent on both donor- and recipient-specific characteristics and could never be determined with precision".

For physically large recipients greater than 100 kg, the likelihood of finding a donor physically large enough to yield a sufficiently large graft is small. For a pediatric recipient, the main issue is not usually whether the liver volume may be too small; rather the issue is whether it may be too large; this may lead to problems with closure of the abdomen in the recipient. Usually the GRBWR should not exceed 5%(Bradhagen D, et al., 2003).

7.3 Donor liver anatomy

Variations in vascular and biliary anatomy can be quite common. Preoperative knowledge of the anatomical variations is important for planning the operative procedure and for maximizing the chances of a safe and successful operation for both donor and recipient. Preoperative imaging studies include MR angiography and cholangiography, CT angiography, ERCP, and mesenteric angiography. The choice of the imaging modalities is dependent on institutional experience and expertise. Most centers have abandoned the use of invasive tests such as angiogram, and routinely use CT or MRI with 3-D reconstructions (Tsang Let al, 2008).

Common arterial variations include replaced right and left hepatic arteries with and without the presence of proper, right, and left hepatic arteries. These variations are usually detectable by CT or MR angiography. A replaced left hepatic artery increases donor safety because the artery is away from the surgical field and less prone to injury during right hepatectomy (Takatsuki M et al,2006). A completely replaced right hepatic artery is a favorable situation for both donor and recipient. It is longer than a right hepatic artery, remote from the left liver arterial in-flow, and more amenable to dissection from surrounding tissue. The presence of both replaced and standard right hepatic arteries introduces more complexity. Reconstruction before implantation is possible with a bifurcated recipient proper hepatic artery graft, or the arteries can be sewn separately to the recipient right and left hepatic arteries. Nevertheless, the presence of two arteries increases the risk for thrombosis. Occasionally, a right hepatic branch may arise from the left hepatic artery or a left hepatic branch may arise from the right hepatic artery; both situations may preclude donation (Sugawara Y, et al. 2003).

The most common portal venous variation is separate right anterior and posterior portal venous trunks which may require reconstruction before implantation (most commonly with a bifurcated venous graft) or separate anastomoses during implantation to the recipient right and left portal veins. A sizable left portal branch arising from the right portal system or a right branch from the left system may preclude donation (Xu M, et al, 2008).

Hepatic venous anatomy is also variable. Most commonly, there are two tributaries to the middle hepatic vein (MHV) within the anterior segments of the right liver, segments V and VIII. The need for reconstruction of these tributaries in the recipient remains controversial. Some centers routinely reconstruct both veins, others reconstruct them when large, and others never do (see later). Large caudate veins also are common. Most centers reimplant caudate veins larger than 0.5 cm. Intraoperative ultrasonography is helpful, as well (Radtke A et al., 2010).

The biliary anatomy may be difficult to evaluate accurately preoperatively. Some centers routinely perform MRCP or ERCP as part of the evaluation process. The latter is an invasive test, whereas the former may not provide the degree of accuracy and clarity required to be of value. As a result many centers choose to perform an intraoperative cholangiogram, rather than preoperative biliary imaging. However, ongoing improvements in imaging modalities may soon allow for preoperative noninvasive imaging that is equivalent to the intraoperative cholangiogram with regards to its detail and clarity. The most common variations are multiple right hepatic ducts that require separate anastomoses in the recipient, but. Occasionally, a left duct arises from the right system, but these ducts usually are small and can be safely divided during right hepatectomy (Limanond P et al, 2004).

7.4 Evaluation for thrombophilia

Deep venous thrombosis with subsequent pulmonary embolism represents a serious postoperative complication to the living donor. Several cases of pulmonary embolism have been reported with at least one donor mortality due to this complication. Known risk factors for thromboembolic complications include obesity, use of oral hormone therapy, old age, smoking, positive family history, and an identified underlying procoagulation disorder. These risk factors should be addressed during the evaluation process, including screening tests to identify a procoagulation disorder. Tests include, protein C and S and alfa-1-antitrypsin deficiency, checking for factor VIII elevation, evaluating for the presence of antiphospholipid or anticardiolipin antibodies, and screening for the factor V Leiden and prothrombin gene mutations (Ogawa H, et al., 2011).

7.5 Psychosocial evaluation

This part of the evaluation assesses the donor's mental fitness and willingness to donate, ensuring that consent is obtained in a voluntary manner with the absence of coercion. A trained transplant psychiatrist, psychologist, clinical social worker, and psychiatric nurse perform this psychological assessment. The professional(s) responsible for psychological assessment should be part of the transplant team and must be experienced in the assessment of liver transplant recipients, so that they understand the particular context and unique psychological demands of liver transplants (Walter M, et al, 2002).

No strict guidelines exist for psychological assessment of prospective donor. However, most transplant centers have adopted formal psychological assessment as an integral part of their donor evaluation. There are several components to this part of the evaluation, but basically the following issues should be addressed: (1) mental, psychological, emotional, and social stability, (2) motivation for donation including a careful assessment to ensure that there is no coercion or inducement involved and competency to give informed consent, and (3) full understanding of, the donation process, the surgery involved, the potential complications, and the recovery involved (Walter M, et al, 2002).

The presence of underlying mental illness, cognitive impairments, aberrant personality traits, or other factors that may interfere with the potential donor's ability to make a reasoned decision may preclude donation. A history of anxiety, depression, or other concerns are discussed to determine whether donation could exacerbate underlying symptoms. Present and past behaviors are explored because they may be predictors to coping with potential donor outcomes. Donors must understand how donation could impact on their mental health (Noma et al., 2010).

The clinical psychologist makes an independent recommendation as to whether the donor is suitable to undergo donation. Informed consent to proceed with the necessary tests and surgery is discussed in detail with the prospective donor. After all the donor candidate's questions are answered to his or her satisfaction, written consent is obtained, and a copy of the consent form is given to the candidate to keep; this is separate from a second written informed consent, which is obtained prior to the LDLT surgery itself. Upon completion of this step, a decision regarding donor acceptability needs to be made by a multidisciplinary committee, which takes into consideration both the medical and ethical aspects of each case.

8. Hepatitis B virus core antibody positive donors

The presence of antibody to hepatitis B core antigen (anti-HBc) in the absence of hepatitis B surface antigen (HBsAg) signifies past exposure to hepatitis B virus (HBV) and may represent a state of resolved infection with immunity or recent clearance of HbsAg and yet persistent low-grade hepatitis activity. The use of live donors who are anti-HBc positive involves consideration of two factors: risk to the donor and potential risk of transmission to the recipient. With regard to the recipient, the issues are no different from those for a deceased donor who is core positive (Suehiro T et al., 2005).

8.1 Risks to the recipient

Experience with the use of anti-HBc-positive livers from deceased donors indicated that the risk of HBV reactivation varies with the recipient's HBV serology status. A variety of terms such as *de novo* hepatitis B, recurrent hepatitis B, transmission of hepatitis B, or reactivation of hepatitis B have been used to describe HBV infection in this setting. The presence of anti-HBs in the recipient has been reported to protect against reactivation. Anti-HBc seropositivity has also been shown to be associated with a lower risk of HBV reactivation. On the other hand, the concomitant presence of anti-HBs in the donor's serum does not offer any protective effect. Other factors as the Child-Pugh score and the type of immunosuppressive therapy, have been suggested to affect the rate of HBV reactivation through its effect on the host immune response (Munoz S, 2002).

8.1.1 Strategies to minimize the risks to the recipient

a. **Matching:** In DDLT. anti-HBc-positive liver graft from a deceased donor is usually allocated first to HBsAg-positive recipients who would in any case need prophylaxis against recurrence. Unfortunately, a matching policy has little role in the practice of LDLT. A living donor is evaluated for the possibility of donation to a specific recipient (Fontana R & Merion R, 2003).
b. **Prophylaxis against HBV reactivation:** Strategies including hepatitis- B-immune globulin (HBIG) and/or lamivudine to prevent recurrent hepatitis B in HBsAg-negative recipients have been used (Suehiro T et al., 2005).

8.2 Risks to the donor

Theoretically, the potential problems in anti-HBc-positive donors include, (1) the underlying hepatitis infection may delay the recovery and regeneration of the liver remnant. (2) reactivation of integrated HBV virus in the postoperative period, (3) on the long-term, the occult hepatitis infection may progress to the development of cirrhosis or HCC and the previous hepatic resection for liver donation may compromise the prospects for appropriate treatment (Suehiro T et al., 2005). Whether the risk is significant in patients with biochemically and histologically normal liver is controversial. Transplant centers that accept living donors positive for anti-HBc are obliged to continue lifelong follow-up of these donors in order to assess these potential long-term sequels.

8.3 Recommendations

a. Detailed preoperative assessment is mandatory for both the donor and the recipient.
b. Donors with ongoing chronic hepatitis and viremia as indicated by abnormal liver biochemistry and positive serum HBV DNA should be excluded.
c. A routine preoperative liver biopsy is mandatory in the HB c antibody-positive donor. The presence of hepatic fibrosis would preclude donor hepatectomy.
d. Donors seronegative for anti-HBs should receive HBV vaccination to protect against the risk of future HBV reactivation.
e. For the HBsAg-positive recipients, there is no need for any adjustment to the appropriate prophylaxis against HBV recurrence.
f. All HBsAg-negative recipients should receive prophylactic treatment with lamivudine alone or in combination with HBIG after transplantation.
g. Both the donor and the recipient should receive regular and lifelong follow-up. Any episode of liver dysfunction should be investigated for HBV reactivation with serological and virological testing. (Suehiro T et al., 2005; Fontana R; Merion R, 2003)

9. Technical aspects of LDLT

Timing of the donor procedure in relation to the recipient procedure is very important. Recipients with nonmalignant disorders are usually brought to the operating room after the anatomy in the donor has been assessed and found to be suitable for donation. Recipients with potentially malignant lesions should be explored through a relatively small right subcostal incision before the donor is anesthetized. If enlarged lymph nodes are found, biopsies are sent for frozen section (Henrik P et al., 2009; Polak W et al., 2009).

9.1 Recipient hepatectomy

A generous bilateral subcostal incision and upward midline extension is made. Native hepatectomy with caval flow preservation is performed in a standard fashion except for vascular and biliary management. Hilar dissection is made to free the right and left hepatic artery, the common hepatic duct, the right and left portal vein and its main trunk. The tissue around the common hepatic duct is preserved as far as possible in order to retain its blood supply (Soejima Y, et al., 2008). It is then divided close to the liver hilum so as to retain enough length for subsequent duct-to-duct anastomosis. The left and right portal veins must be free for the full length (Kim B et al., 2009). The portal vein is not divided until the liver graft is available. Then, the main portal vein is clamped and the right and left portal veins are divided close to the liver hilum. The hepatic veins are clamped and divided. The hepatic vein stump intended for venous outflow reconstruction is slit open to fashion a triangular venotomy opening that matches in size and shape with the hepatic vein opening of the liver graft (Henrik P et al., 2009; Polak W et al., 2009).

9.2 Donor right hepatectomy

9.2.1 Access

Access is gained through a bilateral subcostal incision with upper midline extension. The ligamentum teres is ligated and divided, and the falciform ligament severed toward the suprahepatic vena cava to reveal the border between the RHV and the MHV. The right liver is then mobilized by dissection of the triangular ligament (Cipe G, et al., 2011).

9.2.2 Intraoperative cholangiogram and Doppler ultrasound

Cholecystectomy is performed and a tube for cholangiogram is inserted through the cystic duct. Cholangiogram can be postponed until the right hepatic duct is roughly dissected and marked with a clip. Intraoperative Doppler ultrasound is performed to map the position and direction of the MHV. The route of the MHV can be drawn on the anterior surface of the liver with electrocautery (Haberal M et al,2011).

9.2.3 Mobilization

The liver is rotated to expose the retrohepatic cava. Tiny, short hepatic veins are meticulously divided. Posterior hepatic veins with a diameter larger than 0.5 cm should be eventually reanastomosed to the cava of the recipient. The caval side of the vein is oversewn, and the venous stump is temporarily clipped. The IVC ligament just below the RHV usually contains vessels of significant caliber and should be oversewn after transection. The RHV is fully exposed and encircled. The extent of the dissection of the retrohepatic-cava plane can be pictured as a longitudinal line drawn from the space between RHV and MHV to the midportion of the process of the caudate lobe. It usually corresponds to half to two thirds of the anterior surface of the IVC (Cipe G, et al., 2011).

9.2.4 Hilar time

Hilar dissection is started from the right side of the CBD. The RHA is identified first, followed by the portal vein. The RHA is dissected from its origin to the liver parenchyma. All large branches to segment IV should be spared. The posterior aspect of the RPV is then exposed with division of caudate lobe branches, if necessary. The RPV and RHA are temporarily clamped, with a noncrushing vascular clip, to visualize the demarcation line of the liver. The space between the right hepatic artery and the right hepatic duct should not be disrupted in order to preserve the blood supply of the latter (Soejima Y, et al., 2008).

9.2.5 Parenchymal transection

No matter whether CUSA, Water Jet Dissector, Monopolar and Bipolar Coagulator, Tissue Link or Staple Devices are used, the ultimate goal is to transect the parenchyma with the minimal blood loss possible, respecting the anatomical structures vital to the graft and to the donor. Individual preferences dictate the level of comfort in relying on the aforementioned devices (Cipe G, et al., 2011). Under a low central venous pressure and complete muscle relaxation, bleeding during liver transection would not be excessive. The plane of transection is dictated by the position of the MHV and whether it will be taken with the graft or not. (Humar A et al., 2006; Tanaka K et al., 2010; Belghiti J; R Kianmanesh 2003).

The control and transection of the posterior plane above the vena cava can be facilitated by passing the umbilical tape between the hilar structures and the space between the RHV and MHV and pulling it by both ends *"the hanging maneuver"*. In this way the liver is lifted upward and the resection is greatly facilitated.. To include the MHV in the graft during the hanging maneuver, the origin of the MHV is rounded and a tape is passed to the space between the LHV and MHV (Ogata S, 2007; Cipe G, et al., 2011).

Some surgeons routinely give heparin before vascular clamping. The RHA, RPV, and RHV in sequence are separately clamped and divided, and the liver segment is immediately removed. The vascular stumps are oversewn with Prolene sutures. The donor side of the bile duct is closed after the graft is removed and the vascular stumps are oversewn (Henrik P et al., 2009; Polak W et al., 2009; Humar A et al., 2006).

To shorten the cold ischemic time, the graft is not delivered until the recipient is almost ready for graft implantation. Precise communication between the two teams is vital in this regard (Cipe G, et al., 2011).

9.2.6 Back-table procedure

Once delivered, the graft is flushed with cold preservative solution either, University of Wisconsin (UW) (Via Span, Duramed Pharmaceuticals) or histidine-tryptophane-ketoglutarate (HTK; Custodial, Odyssey Pharmaceuticals). The flushing is continued through the portal vein until the effluent from the hepatic vein is completely clear. This usually requires 3 mL/g of liver weight (Henrik P et al., 2009; Polak W et al., 2009; Humar A et al., 2006; Tanaka K et al., 2010).

Back-table reconstruction may be required as follows:

a. Tributaries of the donor MHV may require extensions with an autologous vein grafts.
b. The RHV may require a venoplasty using an autologous (portal) vein graft. If two right hepatic veins are present, and if they are not too far apart, they can be sewn together.
c. If two portal vein orifices are present, and are not too far apart, they can be sewn together; alternatively, a venous Y-graft (of autologous portal vein branches from the recipient's resected native liver) can be used.
d. The orifices of the bile duct(s), if they are not too far apart, are sewn together; they can also be incised to create a larger anastomosis.
e. The liver's cut surface is inspected. Leaks identified during flushing are oversewn.

9.3 Right liver implantation

The liver graft is placed in a natural position. The implantation starts with *the hepatic vein anastomosis* performed in a triangular fashion using 5-0 Prolene. Attention should be paid to prevent inversion, especially of the posterior wall. There should be no tension on the suture (Polak W et al., 2009; Humar A et al., 2006; Tan H et al., 2007; Tanaka K et al., 2010).

Portal vein anastomosis is completed using running 6-0 sutures to the RPV, portal bifurcation, or portal trunk of the recipient, depending on its diameter and distance. The running sutures are taken on the anterior wall from the medial to the lateral aspects of the recipient and donor portal veins. The suture is tied at the lateral side with incorporation of a "growth factor." to prevent portal vein narrowing at the anastomotic site itself (Starzl TE et al., 1984; Xu MQ et al., 2008).

The vascular clamp is removed from the recipient portal vein and the liver is reperfused. About 500 mL of blood are vented through the (untied) medial aspect of the vena cava anastomosis. The portal vein is clamped again, and the running suture of the medial aspect of the caval anastomosis is tied to the corner stitch. The clamps on the vena cava and the portal vein are now removed, and the liver graft is reperfused (Humar A et al., 2006; Tan H et al., 2007; Tanaka K et al., 2010). The surgeon assesses the quality of liver perfusion and stops any significant bleeding with suture ligation. Usually, the liver pinks up immediately. If the MHV was not included in the graft or if venous tributaries were not reconstructed, the medial aspects of segments 5 and 8 (right anterior or paramedian segments) may be dusky-blue and are frequently swollen. The cut surface is assessed for bleeding and hemostasis is obtained (Henrik P et al., 2009; Polak W et al., 2009; Tan H 2007; Tanaka K et al., 2010).

The arterial anastomosis is usually tedious because of its small size. The arterial anastomosis is usually performed end-to-end with 7-0 or 8-0 nonabsorbable sutures in interrupted fashion and the use of surgical loop magnification. Alternatively, an operating microscope can be used. After revascularization is complete, flow velocity and signal patterns are checked by Doppler ultrasonography (Henrik P et al., 2009; Polak W et al., 2009).

Biliary reconstruction is technically demanding because of the small diameter and short length. More frequently, multiple small ducts are cut flush in the donor's hilar plate are present. As a consequence, the incidence of technical complications, such as leaks and strictures, is significantly higher with LDDT (vs. DDLT). The requirements are a tension-free anastomosis and preserving periductal connective tissue to maintain the bile ducts' ascending axial vascular circulation (which originates from the RHA and the superior posterior pancreaticoduodenal artery). Biliary reconstruction is by direct anastomosis or hepaticojejunostomy (Kim B et al., 2009). Direct duct-to-duct anastomosis is now increasingly performed. In general, a duct-to-duct anastomosis is advantageous because it reduces operative time, represents a simpler biliary anastomosis, preserves physiologic bilioenteric and bowel continuity, preserves the physiologic sphincter mechanism with a decreased risk of ascending or reflux cholangitis, eliminates the need for bowel manipulation with a decreased risk of intraabdominal contamination and of postoperative ileus, results in earlier return of gastrointestinal function, allows easy radiologic access to the biliary tract. The decision to stent the biliary anastomosis is controversia (Kim B et al., 2009).

Possible options if more than one duct orifice is encountered (Haberal M et al., 2011):

a. If the ducts are in close proximity or share a common wall, they can be joined together and only 1 anastomosis needs to be done.
b. If the distance between the bile ducts is > 1 cm, two enterotomies may need to be made.
c. Multiple orifices can be anastomosed to RHD, LHD, or the cystic duct of the recipient.
d. If only one recipient bile duct is available for anastomosis, the remaining ducts require construction of a Roux-en-Y loop.
e. Very small (< 1mm), distant biliary orifices are sometimes sacrificed and oversewn.

9.4 Donor left hepatectomy

Donor left hepatectomy consists of either full left, or left lateral hepatectomy depending on the relative donor–recipient size ratio(Humar A et al., 2006; Tanaka K et al., 2010).

9.4.1 Exposure

The abdomen is entered through a bilateral subcostal incision and a midline extension. After division of the round and falciform ligament, the LHV and MHV are exposed to their insertion to the IVC. The left triangular and coronary ligaments are excised to reveal the left surface of the LHV. Any accessory or replaced left hepatic artery from the left gastric artery is carefully preserved as the gastrohepatic ligament is divided (Humar A et al., 2006).

9.4.2 Intraoperative cholangiography and Doppler ultrasound

Intraoperative ultrasonography is performed to study the anatomy of the MHV and the LHV. Doppler study is also performed to locate the site of hepatic artery. Cholecystectomy is then performed and the cystic duct cannulated for operative cholangiography. The location of the proposed division of the left hepatic duct is marked by a large size metal clip (Henrik P et al., 2009; Polak W et al., 2009; Humar A et al., 2006).

9.4.3 Mobilization

The retrohepatic cava is defined after incising the overlying peritoneum along its lateral aspect, exposing the cava up to the LHV junction. Smaller draining veins are ligated or clipped as the entire left lobe and caudate lobe are retracted to the LHV, MHV and RHV are isolated as they drain into the cava (Humar A et al., 2006; Tanaka K et al., 2010).

9.4.4 Hilar time

Hilar dissection is confined to the left side to free the LHA and LPV. Attention should be paid to the caudate branches of the LPV when moved back to its origin. The LPV is usually longer than the right, and a reasonable segment is isolated and looped. Some surgeons advocate preserving the caudate lobe and its dominant vein draining into the vena cava. If a large branch of the LHA arising from the left gastric artery is encountered, it must be preserved for subsequent reconstruction if needed (Soejima Y, et al., 2008).

9.4.5 Parenchymal transection

The Cantlie line is marked at the anterior surface of the liver by diathermy at a plane demarcated after temporary occlusion of the LHA and LPV. At the inferior surface of the liver, the division plane deviates to the left side of gallbladder fossa to meet the proposed dividing line of the LHD. The transection plane is angled to the left after identification of tributaries to the MHV. The LHD is cut sharply and the donor side is oversewn (Tan H et al., 2007 & Tanaka K et al., 2010). Further transection of the parenchyma is performed along the plane of the ligamentum venosus. Once parenchymal transection is complete, hemostasis and absence of bile leak are confirmed on both surfaces. The LHA, LPV, and LHV in sequence are separately clamped and divided, and the liver segment is immediately removed. Some surgeons routinely give heparin before vascular clamping. The vascular stumps are oversewn with Prolene sutures and the donor side of the bile duct is closed (Henrik P et al., 2009; Polak W et al., 2009).

9.4.6 Left-sided liver implantation

The implantation starts with the hepatic vein anastomosis performed in a triangular fashion using 5-0 Prolene. Attention should be paid to prevent inversion, especially of the posterior wall. There should be no tension on the suture. Depending on its length and diameter, the graft portal vein is anastomosed with the LPV, the portal bifurcation, or the portal trunk of the recipient, using running 6-0 sutures. At this point, the hepatic vein and portal vein are declamped. Arterial anastomosis is performed using interrupted 8-0 sutures . Sharp edges, adequate removal of surrounding tissue, and absence of tension or kinks in the anastomosis contribute to the success of this procedure. When two significant arteries are present within the graft, a good back flow in the second one after the reperfusion of the major one can be a good reason to ligate the second one. After revascularization is complete, flow velocity and signal patterns are checked by Doppler ultrasonography. Biliary reconstruction is by duct-to-duct anastomosis or hepaticojejunostomy. Previously, hepatico-jejunostomy was thought to be the only reconstruction method for left-liver graft. Recently, more and more surgeons perform duct-to-duct anastomosis (Kim B et al., 2009).

The liver graft is fixed by suturing the falciform ligament to the anterior abdominal wall to prevent rotation into the right subphrenic cavity. The latter may lead to graft congestion (as a result of MHV kinking) or poor vascular inflow (as a result of folding of the portal vein) and ultimately graft failure (Henrik P et al., 2009; Humar A et al., 2006).

10. The middle hepatic vein controversy

The construction of an optimal venous outflow determines the outcome of LDLT. The routine anastomosis of the accessory inferior hepatic veins with a diameter larger than 0.5 cm was accepted by almost all centers. However, there are no defined standards for the reconstruction of MHV or its tributaries (Chan SC et al, 2011).

The MHV is responsible for the drainage segment 4 together with variable part of the anterior sector of the right liver (segments 5 and 8) in the great majority of the cases. Transection of the drainage territory of the MHV at the time of procurement leads to venous congestion of "marginal zones" in both graft and donor remnant (Radtke A et al., 2010).

Poor venous outflow has been associated with increased sinusoidal pressure, disruption of sinusoidal epithelium, hepatic artery thrombosis, impaired liver regeneration, and dismal outcome. Such physiologic harm can be particularly detrimental in recipients with relatively small grafts and significant portal hypertension, in whom an underlying SFSS situation can turn into graft failure or at least lead to severe biliary and/or vascular complications. A triangular interrelationship between inflow, outflow, and GRBW ratio has been proposed to determine the fate of the graft (Humar A et al., 2006; Tan H et al., 2007).

When the MHV is not taken with the graft, a variable portion of the anterior sector of the right liver remains congested. The relief of the congestion may occur either through intraparenchymal communication between the venous outflow of the anterior sector and the posterior sector drained by the RHV or by reversal of flow in the anterior branch of the portal vein into the posterior branch. The percentage of the congested portion relative to the overall volume of the graft, the GRBWR, the presence and the degree of portal hypertension, and the compliance of the liver determine the magnitude of graft malfunction after transplantation. If the functional mass of the right-lobe graft is adequate without the MHV (high GRWR), some degree of congestion may be tolerated early posttransplant, until the graft has regenerated or the anterior sector drainage is rerouted (Chan SC et al, 2011).

10.1 Available options for the surgical management of the MHV

(1) Exclusion of the MHV from the graft: The rationale is that not all right grafts present with congestion after reperfusion, and simple RHV anastomosis is sufficient in many cases. Obviously, if venous drainage from segments 5 and 8 is predominately via the RHV, including the MHV with the right-lobe graft is unnecessary. With the donor MHV clamped and reversal of flow in the anterior branch of the portal vein detected by Doppler, the temporary occlusion of the right hepatic artery will determine the portion of right liver affected by congestion (Chan SC et al, 2011).

(2) Inclusion of the MHV with the right-lobe graft: This guarantees the most complete drainage of the anterior sector of the right graft. Contraindications are a small predicted residual liver volume (< 30%) in the donor as this may pose the donor at a higher risk of postoperative complications because the regeneration of segment 4 is stunned by the lack of adequate venous drainage (Radtke A et al., 2010).

(3) Inclusion of the distal part of the MHV with the right-lobe graft (leaving the proximal remnant in the donor): This technique preserves large segment 4a venous tributaries into the

MHV in its most proximal portion. Inclusion of the distal MHV improves segment V drainage but not that of segment VIII (Chan SC et al, 2011).

(4) Anastomosing the major tributaries draining the anterior sector of the right liver into the MHV to the vena cava leaving the MHV with the donor rest liver. Doppler waveform characteristics may identify tributaries that could benefit from separate anastomosis. Reversed flow in the MHV tributaries may indicate that reconstruction is not required. Reconstructing MHV tributaries according to diameter (> 5 mm) has also been recommended. The tributaries from segments 5 and 8 are anastomosed to venous conduits of various origins that serve as jump grafts. This has been accomplished with the donor inferior mesenteric vein, iliac vein, ovarian vein, cryopreserved iliac vein, recipient saphenous vein, umbilical vein, LPV, superficial femoral vein, and internal jugular vein. Reconstruction of interposition grafts is, preferably, done on the back table; it can also be done after restoration of portal flow, in order to first assess the degree of venous congestion.

Reconstruction of these branches with interposition grafts results in a more complex operation, longer operating time, and longer warm ischemia time. Also, a relatively long segment of interposition graft makes it more prone to thrombosis (Radtke A et al., 2010).

Whether one technical approach is sounder than the other is probably not possible to decide. Thus, individualized planning is mandatory for the optimal outcome of both donors and recipients in the setting of the high degree of variability of MHV, RHV, and IHV drainage. A selective approach based on GRBWR, greater or less than 1; graft/recipient standard liver, greater or less than 50%; and size of the MHV tributaries, greater or less than 5 mm in diameter; is used by the some groups to decide whether the graft will be harvested with or without the middle hepatic vein (Chan SC et al, 2011).

11. Double liver transplant

If the donor has a large right lobe (> 70% of total liver volume), the remaining left lobe will be small (< 30% of total liver volume) and thus will threaten donor safety. An alternative is to simultaneously transplant two small liver grafts (left lobe or left lateral segment) from two different donors; that is, a double or dual-graft transplant, to solve graft-size insufficiency and provide donor safety. The recipient and two donor operations are started simultaneously. The first graft is orthotopically positioned in the original left position. The second graft is heterotopically positioned to the right-upper-quadrant fossa, rotating it 180°, so that the graft's hilar structures are at the same level as the recipient's right hilar structures (Lu Q, et al., 2010).

12. Retransplantation

The only therapeutic option for failing hepatic allograft is a liver retransplant. The most common causes are chronic rejection, chronic cholangitis, and vascular complications, small for size graft and primary nonfunction. In Re-LDLTs, ethical problems and the timing of the retransplant are controversial. Furthermore, availability of LDLT and DDLT for retransplants differs in each country or region. Donor selection for Re-LDLTs is difficult. The probability of retransplants (with either DDLT or LDLT) is low because of the lack of donors. Thus, serious posttransplant complications after LDLT often lead to death, with no chance of a retransplant. During the procedure, surgeons encounter difficulty in dissecting surrounding tissues and identifying the important vessels due to the relatively small size and short length of vessels in LDLT grafts (Lerner S et al., 2005).

13. Recipient outcomes and complications of LDLT

The spectrum of posttransplant complications is not different for LDLT versus DDLT. However, the incidence of biliary, and vascular complications may be more common and severe in nature than in DDLT. In addition, new problems such as small-for-size syndrome have been introduced (Soin A et al., 2010).

13.1 Hepatic artery complications

13.1.1 Hepatic artery thrombosis (HAT)

Risk Factors include, recipients body weight < 10 kg or age < 3 years, reconstructing arteries with diameters < 3 mm, ABO incompatibility, excessive intraoperative fresh frozen plasma transfusion, and elevated hematocrite levels. Doppler ultrasonography has high sensitivity for the diagnosis of HAT. By performing serial examinations at frequent intervals during the first 1 to 2 weeks posttransplant, HAT can be detected before it becomes clinically obvious. Early diagnosis permits immediate thrombectomy and revascularization before the patient deteriorates. If there is suspicion for HAT, one can choose to delineate the anatomy with angiography or proceed urgent re-exploration. Angiography offers nonoperative method to diagnose and potentially treat with balloon angioplasty (Steinbrück K, et al., 2011).

Management depends on the timing and the clinical condition . Early HAT, once diagnosed by ultrasound, the patient is immediately taken to the operating room. The anastomosis is taken down. The vessel is cleared of all clot, inspected for intimal injury, and assessed for adequate inflow. If good inflow is present, a primary anastomosis is attempted. If adequate inflow is not provided, an arterial conduit is anastomosed to the aorta. Postoperatively, the patient is closely watched with frequent Doppler. Systemic heparinization is used according to coagulation parameters (Steinbrück K, et al., 2011).

If there is a delay in the diagnosis, or if ultrasound is questionable, selective arteriography may be employed to diagnose the site of thrombosis and to begin therapeutic thrombolysis. Decisions on retransplantation are made based on the clinical condition, patency of the vessels, and appearance of late complications as biliary stricture (Steinbrück K et al., 2011).

Late HAT is often asymptomatic because of the development of a rich collateral network. Attempts at operative revision should not be undertaken, as a large majority survive with normal allograft function, and any operative procedure carries the risk of destroying the graft-sustaining collaterals. Significant late allograft dysfunction needs careful monitoring for septic complications, biloma and cholangitis. Attempts at graft salvage in this population are universally unsuccessful (Henrik P et al., 2009; Polak W et al., 2009).

13.1.2 Hepatic Artery Stenosis (HAS)

HAS, although usually asymptomatic, will eventually progress to HAT. Frequently, patients develop biliary strictures and bile leaks. HAS may be detected on surveillance Doppler. Dampened waveforms with decreased resistive indices (RI) and slow peak velocities suggest HAS. Stenosis should be suspected when the RI is <0.5 or the systolic ascending time (SAT) is >10 msec. The diagnosis should be confirmed by angiography. If diagnosed in the immediate postoperative period, planned exploration and revision of the arterial anastomosis should be undertaken. Although conventional treatment is either surgical repair or a retransplant, percutaneous transluminal angioplasty (PTA) or stent placement is becoming predominant (Polak W et al., 2009; Humar A et al., 2006; Tanaka K et al., 2010).

13.2 Biliary complications

Biliary complications remain the most common cause of postoperative morbidity and the most challenging complications in LDLT recipients, and occasionally graft loss and death. Risk factors include, small size or multiple bile duct anastomoses, delayed arterial revascularization, HAT, extensive periductal dissection and biliary leaks from the cut-surface of liver tissue., cytomegalovirus infection, and rejection (Yuan Y & Gotoh M, 2010).

13.2.1 Biliary leaks

The sources of biliary leaks could be from (1) The cut surface of the liver, (2) The site of the biliary anastomosis, (3) The site of the intestinal anastomosis, and (4) The exit site of a T tube (or other types of external stents). Anastomotic leaks are caused either by ischemic necrosis of the end of the bile duct or by a technically unsatisfactory anastomosis. Leaks can manifest as sudden onset of biliary drainage from the abdominal drain, or they may present by intraabdominal collection, referred to as "biloma". Biloma can be detected by ultrasonography or CT scan before the recipient becomes symptomatic (Khalaf H et al., 2011).

Leaks from the cut-surface can be managed expectantly as long as it is adequately drained. Leaks from the anastomosis also can be successfully managed with nonsurgical treatment if they are small and localized. Stenting with percutaneous transhepatic cholangiography (PTC) or ERCP at the anastomotic site can resolve minor leaks. If the anastomosis is seriously disrupted, surgical revision is the safest approach (Kohler S et al. 2009).

For bilomas, percutaneous drainage is performed. Once the patient is stabilized, ERCP or PTC is performed, and a stent is placed to bypass the flow of bile through the leak. If excessive leak is diagnosed in the immediate post operative period, operative exploration, drainage, and revision of the anastomosis may be warranted (Khalaf H et al., 2011).

13.2.2 Biliary strictures

Risk factors include, CMV infection, hepatic artery complications, ABO incompatible transplantation, and prior anastomotic leak. The patient may present with asymptomatic elevation of cholestatic liver enzymes or may present with manifestations of cholangitis: fever, jaundice abdominal pain. Ultrasound scan is the initial imaging technique, however, ductal dilatation is often late. Direct cholangiogram is the gold-standard for diagnosing biliary strictures. Any patient with biliary stenosis, especially with multiple strictures, should be evaluated for HAT (Kohler S et al. 2009). Early strictures are often amenable to endoscopic or transhepatic intervention with good long-term results. Operative treatment is indicated for complications of percutaneous therapies and intractable strictures. Patients with strictures associated with HAT should continue to undergo percutaneous treatment. Operative exploration should be avoided, as it disrupts the arterial collaterals supplying the graft. Evaluation for retransplantation should occur if the strictures affect graft function, associated with bilomas and frequent bouts of cholangitis (Yuan Y and Gotoh M, 2010).

13.3 Portal vein thrombosis (PVT)

Risk factors include, native PVT, the use of interposition grafts, extensive collaterals, portosystemic shunts and splenectomy. The patient may present with ascites, elevated LFTs, and splenomegaly, and gastrointestinal hemorrhage. Diagnosis is made with Doppler and confirmed by venography. Early PVT is treated with surgical thrombectomy and revision of the anastomosis. Late PVT may require surgical shunting to decompress the portal system as treatment of the complications of portal hypertension (Kyoden Y, et al., 2008).

13.4 Hepatic venous outflow block (HVOB)

Risk factors include, technical causes, graft rotation and kinking of the anastomosis and graft regeneration with subsequent rotation. HVOB is occasionally diagnosed during transplant surgery on the basis of swelling and congestion of the graft. The diagnosis is confirmed if intraoperative ultrasonography detects a flat waveform in the hepatic vein. Postoperatively, the clinical presentation includes ascites, elevated liver function test results, splenomegaly, variceal bleeding, lower-extremity edema, and kidney dysfunction. A persistent monophasic wave pattern from the hepatic vein on Doppler ultrasonography suggests substantial stenosis. Subsequent angiography with direct contrast can confirm the diagnosis; the pressure gradient across the stenosis is typically > 3 to 10 mm Hg. Management is by percutaneous balloon venoplasty. Multiple procedures are often required. Stent placement may be required for cases that do not respond to simple dilatation. In severe cases, HVOB may cause graft dysfunction or failure, requiring a retransplantion (Ikeda O, et al., 2010).

13.5 Abdominal compartment syndrome

Causes include, oversized allograft as in adult to pediatric LDLT, closure with considerable intra-abdominal tension, and intestinal edema due to prolonged portal vein clamping. The patient presents with, respiratory compromise, renal insufficiency, hemodynamic instability, and allograft thrombosis because of excessive pressure and positional kinking of the graft.

13.6 The 'small for size' liver graft syndrome (SFSS)

SFSS is a clinical syndrome, which occurs in the presence of a reduced mass of liver insufficient to maintain normal liver function. It is characterized by a combination of early postoperative progressive cholestasis, persistent portal hypertension, ascites, kidney failure, and coagulopathy. Microscopic features include cholestasis with hepatocyte ballooning, vacuolar degeneration, sinusoidal disruption, steatosis, and centrilobular necrosis. SFSS reduces the graft survival rate and increases the mortality rate (Selvaggi G& Tzakis A, 2009).

13.6.1 Pathophysiology

A partial liver graft transplanted into an adult recipient is, by definition, a small-for-size graft. Such a graft is, however, well tolerated when it is not under a critical size. The pathogenesis of the syndrome is primarily tied to graft volume, but three other factors have been proved to contribute to its occurrence, (1) functional liver mass (graft volume, steatosis, donor age), (2) recipient status and the severity of hepatic disease at the time of the transplant, and (3) graft perfusion (portal hypertension, impaired venous outflow, and immune-mediated cellular infiltration) (Dahm F et al., 2005).

Reduced intrahepatic vascular bed with higher portal flow per gram of remnant liver results in increased portal pressure. Following reperfusion, portal vein flow (PVF) is inversely related to graft size, while hepatic artery flow is reduced proportionately to graft size. Impaired HA flow is results from increased PVF. Enhanced PVF induces shear stress and endothelial injury with progressive alterations of hepatic microcirculation. Shear stress is responsible for up-and-down regulation of vasoregulatory genes, alteration of tissue repair mechanisms, and imbalance of intracellular homeostasis. Liver regeneration may be hindered by increased hepatic portal resistance (Selvaggi G & Tzakis A, 2009).

13.6.2 Prevention and treatment

Different strategies have been proposed (Selvaggi G& Tzakis A, 2009; Dahm F et al., 2005):

a. Pharmacologic approach aiming to reduce the portal pressure.
b. Ischemic preconditioning of the liver to protect the parenchyma against prolonged ischemic periods.
c. Extracorporeal liver support to enhance of liver regeneration.
d. Surgical techniques to control high PVF and PVP after graft reperfusion:
   - Splenic artery ligation (SAL) with or without splenectomy.
   - Meso-caval shunt with downstream ligation of the superior mesenteric vein.
   - Graded porto-caval shunt, portal vein band, or porto-mesenteric disconnection.
e. Retransplantation

14. Donor outcomes and complications

14.1 Recovery of the liver function after donor hepatectomy

Early aminotransferase elevation is common after donor hepatectomy. Liver enzymes peak early, in the first 48 hours, whereas bilirubin tends to peak later, approximately postoperative day 3. Exaggerated enzyme leak in the absence of synthetic dysfunction suggests focal ischemia, which can occur for example with a devascularized segment 4 following lateral segmentectomy. Prolonged or exaggerated cholestasis in the absence of a biliary complication suggests ischemia or a small residual volume. Unusual clinical patterns of liver function should be investigated with ultrasound scanning, duplex sonography and/or computed tomography (Dindo D et al., 2004).

14.2 Donor complications

In worldwide reports donor morbidity ranged between 0% and 67%, depending on the individual definition and recognition of morbidity. Donor morbidity is influenced by variables including center experience, extent and technique of hepatic resection, anatomic factors, and general health of the donor (Fernandes R, et al., 2010). The lack of a standardized assessment of perioperative complications is a limitation to the analysis of donor-related morbidity. A universally accepted classification system for living donor complications would be ideal. This would allow accurate comparisons and help establish trends in the assessment of morbidity. In this regard, modifications of the Clavien scale for LDLT is gaining acceptance as the standard for reporting surgical morbidity. This system consists of four grades of severity (Clavien P et al. 1994; Dindo D et al., 2004).

Grade I consists of complications that are not life threatening and do not result in any significant morbidity, such as superficial wound infections or transient bile leaks.

Grade II includes complications that have the potential to be life threatening or those requiring drug therapy or <1 foreign blood unit, but does not require therapeutic invasive therapy and does not result in residual disability. An example is any infectious sequelae requiring antimicrobial treatment, postoperative bleeding without requiring relaparotomy and local controlled deep venous thrombosis without thrombembolic complications.

Grade III complications are potentially life threatening, requiring invasive intervention, blood transfusions and/or leads to readmission into the ICU, but does not lead to residual disability. For example, postoperative bleeding requiring relaparotomy, bile leak requiring endoscopic or surgical procedures, deep wound infections requiring relaparotomy or interventional drainage and deep venous thrombosis with pulmonary embolism

Grade IV includes any complication with residual or lasting disability or that leads to death. Examples include liver failure requiring liver transplantation.

The majority of donor morbidity are Grades I and II, with Grade III complications less frequent. The most commonly reported complications are listed in Table 3.

Medical complications

1. Transient cholestasis
2. Pulmonary complications: atelectasis, pneumonia, pleural effusion, and pneumothorax
3. Hypophosphatemia
4. Thrombocytopenia
5. Psychiatric complications
6. Urinary infection

General Surgical complications

1. Wound infection
2. Postoperative bleeding
3. Deep vein thrombosis and pulmonary embolism
4. Incisional hernia
5. Nerve palsy
6. Bowel obstruction, ileus

Hepatectomy related complications

1. Aborted donation
2. Portal vein thrombosis
3. Biliary tract complications: leaks, biloma, strictures
4. Liver failure, hepatic encephalopathy

Table 3. The most commonly reported complications in living donors

14.2.1 Biliary complications

Biliary leaks after left lateral segment donation range from 5% to 10%, with a higher rate (up to 13%) in right hepatectomy. The source of leaks are typically the cut surface of the liver, however, the stump of the bile duct could be the source. Most leaks are diagnosed in the early postoperative period during the initial hospitalization by assessment of postoperative drain fluid, though late leaks are also reported. For most cases, observation and simple external drainage of the otherwise asymptomatic patient will be sufficient to avoid sepsis until the leak spontaneously resolves. More severe leaks require an interventional radiology procedure, endoscopic biliary, or reoperation (Yuan Y & Gotoh M. 2010).

Strictures are reported less commonly but will more likely require invasive intervention. Bile duct strictures result from injury to the right, left or common hepatic duct during hepatectomy. Bile duct strictures may increase the lifetime risk of the donor for developing secondary biliary cirrhosis (Yuan Y, & Gotoh M. 2010).

14.2.2 Acute liver failure

Early postoperative acute liver failure suggests a vascular event like portal vein or arterial thrombosis, or acute outflow obstruction. Although acute vascular events can be reversible with immediate intervention (usually surgical), the patient should be listed for transplantation because survival in acute liver failure is directly related to the timing of liver replacement before the development of multiorgan failure or neurological injury (Fernandes R, et al, 2010; Dindo D et al., 2004).

14.2.3 Small-for-size remnant liver

Liver failure in the absence of an early technical complication like arterial or portal venous thrombosis is likely to be caused by a small-for-size remnant liver. Remnant liver volumes less than 30%, especially if there is underlying steatosis have been associated with prolonged cholestasis, portal hypertension, and normal or near enzymes and synthetic function after hepatectomy ("small-for size-syndrome"), especially in the presence of moderate steatosis. Outcome data for small for size syndrome in donors are sparse. The presence of a concomitant complication like bile leak, infection, or bleeding may exacerbate the poor recovery in a small-for-size liver. Treatment of small-for-size syndrome is supportive care and avoidance of further injury to the remnant (Fernandes R et al., 2010).

15. Living donor mortality

Liver donation puts the donor at risk of medical and surgical complications and even death. Unfortunately, the actual risk of death after a donor hepatectomy is unknown, because of the absence of sufficient database to allow an accurate determination of this infrequent but devastating outcome. When death occurs in a healthy donor, there are exceptional consequences. A donor death will have a devastating effect not only on the families and friends of the donor and recipient but also on all the clinical staff involved in the procedure. The impact of death may spread to other potential donors and recipients, and brings negative publicity and potential economic damage to the transplant center (Trotter J, 2006; Hashikura Y et al., 2009).

Placing a healthy individual at risk of death for a procedure that does not directly benefit him or her needs to be balanced by the autonomy and the psychological benefit to the donor. If a donor gives informed consent and if the transplant team is prepared to undertake the procedure, where is the problem?(Akabayashi A et al., 2004; B Ringe & R Strong 2008)

The estimated donor mortality rate is 0.5%. The causes of death include, pulmonary embolism, pulmonary infection due to uncommon pathogen, emphysematous gastritis, liver failure due to congenital lipodystrophy and non-alcoholic steatohepatitis, acute pancreatitis and cerebral hemorrhage. Donor suicide was also reported. The exact number of live liver donor mortality in the world is not available because no central reporting agency exists. Current estimates of donor death rates are derived from either survey data or single-center reports. The use of survey data (in which transplant programs are retrospectively queried regarding clinical outcomes) is inexact because of incomplete follow-up of all donor outcomes and bias toward reporting favorable results (Trotter, J. et al., 2006). Single-center reports are likely to provide more complete follow-up data but, may be biased and are limited by the relatively small numbers of cases. In the absence of a definitive means to record all donor deaths, the medical literature has included reports of deaths that in many cases are based on verbal communications, circular references, or frankly unsubstantiated outcomes. As a result, the actual number of donor deaths after LDLT is difficult to ascertain and is a subject of considerable speculation (Trotter J 2006; Akabayashi A et al., 2004)

The first donor death reported in the world was related to a fatal pulmonary embolus occurring in an adult-to-child living donor liver transplantation and was reported in the literature in detail. The first reported death in the United States was related to anaphylaxis secondary to medication, also in a left lateral segment donor (Trotter J 2006 B Ringe &R Strong 2008). The first death reported from Asia occurred in Kyoto, Japan (Akabayashi A et al., 2004). The donor was a mother in her late forties donated the right lobe of her liver to her daughter with biliary atresia. The mother fell into liver failure and underwent an unsuccessful domino liver transplant from a donor with a metabolic disease. Histological examination of the donor liver revealed that she had nonalcoholic steatohepatitis (NASH).

In Egypt, the number of LDLT procedures performed annually has increased rapidly in the past few years (Abdeldayem H et al., 2008 & 2009). In January, 2010, the number of LDLT procedures performed in Egypt topped out to more than one thousand procedures, done in 11 centers. The case number 1000 had been performed at the National Liver Institute in Menoufeyia. Although the author is aware of at least 6 deaths among living donors in Egypt. the reported deaths were only two. While one case has apparently been fully reported in the literature, the second death was reported in brief in the proceedings of the international congress of organ transplantation, in November 2008 (Abdeldayem H et al., 2008) The first death was a 45 year-old male who donated the right hepatic lobe to his brother and died of sepsis from bile leak 1 month after donation (El-Meteini M et al., 2010). The second donor was a 22 year-old male who donated his right lobe to his father, suffered from massive intraoperative bleeding from the stump of the portal vein and died of multisystem organ failure after 10 days (Abdeldayem H et al., 2009).

15.1 What is the acceptable risk of mortality to the donor?

The main issue is what the acceptable risk of mortality to the donor is and, who should determine if this risk is acceptable? ? Donors may be willing to accept high rates of mortality if the life of a loved one is in jeopardy. But what mortality rate is acceptable when the donor understands the risks and coercion has been excluded? There has to be a balance between the risk incurred by the donor and what is acceptable to the recipient, the society, and. the medical community (Trotter J 2006; Hashikura Y et al., 2009; Akabayashi A et al., 2004; B Ringe & R Strong 2008; Abdeldayem H et al., 2008 & 2010, Abdullah K et al., 2005, 2007)

16. Transparency and LDLT

Many, including the author, believe that, the true death, and complication rates among both the donors and the recipients in LDLT are underestimated. As clinicians involved in the evaluation of LDLT, we strive to present accurate information on the risks of the procedure. Because of the discrepancy found between published and unpublished data, the dilemma between reporting rumor vs. reporting facts currently prevails. The reluctance to publish any death or serious complication, although understandable in a fraught medicolegal environment, is not good for patient care or the procedure of LDLT itself. Potential liver transplant donors and recipients are best served by accurate information derived from *genuine transparency*. To maintain truly informed consent, it is imperative that all serious complications and deaths be reported. Transplant centers must be fully aware of their own responsibility: being *honest to themselves and their patients. Secrecy is unacceptable,* as it leads to gossip and speculation by others. If the mortality of this surgery is truly as high as reported by some editorialists, a very different message needs to be conveyed to the patients (Ringe & R Strong 2008; Abdeldayem H et al., 2008, 2009 &2010; Abdullah K et al., 2005& 2007). *To be "transparent" or not to be?* That's the question!, … and the answer is clear.

17. Conclusions

LDLT will continue to play an important role for many patients who have no chance of receiving an organ from a deceased donor in timely fashion. This procedure demands technical expertise in both hepatobiliary surgery and whole-liver transplantation and hard work of multidisciplinary medical team. Every step requires attention and should be planned and performed meticulously. The main drawback with LDLT is the potential for donor morbidity and mortality. In order to promote living donation, absolute transparency about the risks and benefits of this procedure is mandatory.

18. Acknowledgement

The author is grateful to the members of the Department of Surgery at the National Liver Institute in Egypt.

19. References

Abdeldayem H, Allam N, Adawy N, Salah E, Aziz A, Kashkoush S, Gad H, Helmy A. (2009). Moral and Ethical Issues in Liver Transplantation in Egypt. *Exp Clin Transplant.* 1: 18-24.

Abdeldayem H, Bahaa M, Allam N, Salah E, Helmy A, (2008) Present Status and Prospects of Living Donor Liver Transplantation in Egypt: 1268, *Transplantation:* 86 (2S) : 429-30.

Abdeldayem H. (2010). Transparency and living donor liver transplantation in Egypt. *Nile Liver Journal* 1(1):7-13.

Abdullah K, Abdeldayem H, Hali WO, Sakran A, Yassen K, Abdulkareem A. (2005). Twenty cases of adult-to-adult living-related liver transplantation: single-center experience in Saudi Arabia., *Transplant Proc.* 37(7):3144-6

Abdullah K, Abdeldayem H, Salaama IA, Badah K, Al-Somali B, Abdulkareem A., (2007). Retrospective analysis of the causes of rejection of potential donors for living related liver transplantation., *Hepatol Int.*;1(4):431-6.

Akabayashi A, Slingsby BT, Fujita M. (2004). The first donor death after living-related liver transplantation in Japan. *Transplantation* 27; 77(4):634.

Belghiti J & Kianmanesh R (2003). Surgical Techniques Used in Adult Living Donor Liver Transplantation *Liver Transplantation*, Vol 9, No 10, Suppl 2: pp S29-S34

Bhangui P, Vibert E, Majno P, Salloum C, Andreani P, Zocrato J, Ichai P, Saliba F, Adam R, Castaing D, Azoulay D. (2011). Intention-to-treat analysis of liver transplantation for hepatocellular carcinoma: living versus deceased donor transplantation. *Hepatology.* 53(5):1570-9. doi: 10.1002/hep.24231

Brandhagen D, Fidler J, Rosen C (2003) Evaluation of the Donor Liver for Living Donor Liver Transplantation, Liver *Transplantation,* Vol 9, No 10, Suppl 2 S16-28

Broelsch C E, Whitington P F, Emond J C, Heffron T G, Thistlethwaite J R, Stevens L, Piper J, Whitington S H, Lichtor J L. (1991). Liver transplantation in children from living related donors. Surgical techniques and results. *Ann Surg*; 214(4):428.

Chan SC, Lo CM, Ng KK, Ng IO, Yong BH, Fan ST. (2011) Portal inflow and pressure changes in right liver living donor liver transplantation including the middle hepatic vein. *Liver Transpl.* 17(2):115-21. doi: 10.1002/lt.22034.

Chen YS, Cheng YF, De Villa VH, Wang CC, Lin CC, Huang TL, Jawan B, Chen CL. (2003) Evaluation of living liver donors. *Transplantation.* 15;75(3 Suppl):S16–S19

Choudhry S, Daar AS, Radcliffe Richards J, Guttmann RD, Hoffenberg R, Lock M, (2003). Unrelated living organ donation: ULTRAneeds to go. *J. Med. Ethics.* 29(3):169–70.

Cipe G, Tuzuner A, Genc V, Orozakunov E, Ozgencil E, Yılmaz AA, Can OS, Cakmak A, Karayalcin K, Ersoz S, Hazinedaroglu SM. (2011) Living-donor hepatectomy. *Transplant Proc.* 43(3):888-91.

Clavien PA, Camargo CA Jr, Croxford (1994). Defi nition and classification of negative outcomes in solid organ transplantation: application in liver transplantation. *Ann Surg*. 220:109–120.

Dahm F, Georgiev P, Clavien P-A. (2005) Small-for-size syndrome after partial liver transplantation: definition, mechanisms of disease and clinical implications. *Am J Transpl* 5:2605–2610.

Dindo D, Demartines N, Clavien P. (2004) Classification of surgical complications: a new proposal with evaluation in a cohort of 6,336 patients and results of a survey. *Ann. Surg.*;240:205–13.

El-Meteini M, Hamza A, Abdalaal A, Fathy M, Bahaa M, Mukhtar A, Abouelfetouh F, Mostafa I, Shaker M, Abdelwahab S, El-Dorry A, El-Monayeri M, Hobballah A, Sabry H. (2010). Biliary complications including single-donor mortality: experience of 207 adult-to-adult living donor liver transplantations with right liver grafts. *HPB (Oxford).* 12 (2):109-14 20495654

Fernandes R, Pacheco-Moreira L, Enne M, Steinbrück K, Alves J, Filho G, Gouvêa G, Martinho J. (2010) Surgical complications in 100 donor hepatectomies for living donor liver transplantation in a single Brazilian center. *Transplant Proc.* 42(2):421-3.

Fontana RJ, Merion RM. (2003) Are we ready for marginal hepatitis B core antibody-positive living liver donors? *Liver Transpl* 9:833–836.

Gallegos-Orozco JF, Yosephy A, Noble B, Aqel BA, Byrne TJ, Carey EJ, Douglas DD, Mulligan D, Moss A, de Petris G, Williams JW, Rakela J, Vargas HE. (2009) Natural history of post-liver transplantation hepatitis C: A review of factors that may influence its course. *Liver Transpl.* 15(12):1872-81.

Haberal M, Bilgin N, Velidedeoglu E, Turan M. (1993) Living-donor organ transplantation at our centre. *Transplant. Proc* 25:3147–8

Haberal M, Karakayali H, Atiq A, Sevmis S, Moray G, Ozcay F, Boyvat F. (2011) Duct-to-duct biliary reconstruction without a stent in pediatric living-donor liver transplantation. Transplant Proc. 43(2):595-7.

Habib NA, Higgs BD, Marman I, El-Masry R, Helmi A, Saifi T, Abbas A, Abdel-Wohab F, Abaza A, Koensa H, Hamouda A, Saleh M, Abdel-Ghaffar Y. (1993). Living-related liver transplantation in Africa. *International Surgery*;78:121-123.

Hashikura Y, Ichida T, Umeshita K, Kawasaki S, Mizokami M, Mochida S, Yanaga K, Monden M, Kiyosawa K; (2009) Japanese Liver Transplantation Society., Donor complications associated with living donor liver transplantation in Japan. *Transplantation* 15;88(1):110-4.

Henrik P, B Ronald, (2009) Evolving Surgical Approaches in Liver Transplantation. Seminars in Liver Disease. *Liver Transplantation.* 29(1):121-133.

Hill M, Hughes M, Jie T, Cohen M, Lake J, Payne W (2009) Humar A. Graft weight/recipient weight ratio: how well does it predict outcome after partial liver transplants? *Liver Transpl.* 15(9):1056-62.

Humar A, Matas A, Payne W, (2006) Atlas of Organ Transplantation Springer-Verlag London

Ikeda O, Tamura Y, Nakasone Y, Yamashita Y, Okajima H, Asonuma K, Inomata Y. (2010) Percutaneous transluminal venoplasty after venous pressure measurement in patients with hepatic venous outflow obstruction after living donor liver transplantation. *Jpn J Radiol.* 28(7):520-6.

Iwasaki M, Takada Y, Hayashi M, (2004) Noninvasive evaluation of graft steatosis in living donor liver transplantation. *Transplantation* 78(10):1501 –5.

Jassem W, Koo DD, Cerundolo L. (2003) Cadaveric versus living-donor livers: differences in infl ammatory markers after transplantation. *Transplantation* 76(11):1599–1603.

Kaido T, Mori A, Ogura Y, Hata K, Yoshizawa A, Iida T, Uemoto S. (2011) Recurrence of hepatocellular carcinoma after living donor liver transplantation: what is the current optimal approach to prevent recurrence? *World J Surg.* 35(6):1355-9.

Khalaf H, Alawi K, Alsuhaibani H, Hegab B, Kamel Y, Azzam A, Albahili H, Alsofayan M, Al Sebayel M. (2011) Surgical management of biliary complications following living donor liver transplantation. *Clin Transplant.* 25(3):504-10. doi: 10.1111/j.1399-0012.2010.01338.x.

Kim B, Bae B, Lee J, Won J, Park Y, Xu W, Wang H, Kim M. (2009) Duct-to-duct biliary reconstructions and complications in 100 living donor liver transplantations. *Transplant Proc.* 41(5):1749-55

Kohler S, Pascher A, Mittler J, Neumann U, Neuhaus P, Pratschke J. (2009) Management of biliary complications following living donor liver transplantation--a single center experience. *Langenbecks Arch Surg.* 394(6):1025-31. Epub 2009 May 27.

Kuo A, Terrault NA. (2009) Is recurrent hepatitis C worse with living donors? *Curr Opin Organ Transplant.* 14(3):240-4.

Kyoden Y, Tamura S, Sugawara Y, Matsui Y, Togashi J, Kaneko J, Kokudo N, Makuuchi M. (2008) Portal vein complications after adult-to-adult living donor liver transplantation. *Transpl Int.* 21(12):1136-44. Epub 2008 Sep 1.

Lennerling A, Forsberg A, Meyer K, Nyberg G. Motives for becoming a living kidney donor. *Nephrol. Dial. Transplant* 2004;19(6):1600–5.

Lerner SM, Markmann J, Jurim O (2005) Retransplantation. In: Busuttil RW, Klintmalm GB, eds. *Transplantation of the Liver,* 2nd ed. Philadelphia: WB Saunders; 767.

Levinsky NG. Organ donation by unrelated donors. *N Engl J Med* 2000;343:430–432.

Li C, Wen T, Yan L, Li B, Wang W, Xu M, Yang J, We i Y. (2010) Does model for end-stage liver disease score predict the short-term outcome of living donor liver transplantation? *Transplant Proc.* 42(9):3620-3.

Limanond P, Raman SS, Ghobrial RM (2004) The utility of MRCP in preoperative mapping of biliary anatomy in adult-to-adult living related liver transplant donors. *J Magn Reson Imaging* 19(2):209- 15.

Lu Q, Wu H, Yan L, Chen Z, Fan Y, Luo Y. (2010) Living donor liver transplantation using dual grafts: ultrasonographic evaluation. *World J Gastroenterol.* 21;16(31):3979-83.

Marcos A, Fisher R, Ham J, Olzinski A, Shiffman M, Sanyal A, (2000) Selection and outcome of living donors for adult to adult right lobe transplantation. *Transplantation* 69: 2410-2415.

Matsui Y, Sugawara Y, Yamashiki N, Kaneko J, Tamura S, Togashi J, Makuuchi M, Kokudo N. (2008) Living donor liver transplantation for fulminant hepatic failure. *Hepatol Res.* 38(10):987-96. Epub 2008 Jun 28.

Mazaris E, Papalois VE. (2006) Ethical issues in living donor kidney transplantation. *Exp Clin Transplant.* 4(2):485-97.

Munoz SJ. (2002) Use of hepatitis B core antibody-positive donors for liver transplantation. *Liver Transpl* 8:S82–S87.

Nadalin S, Malago M, Valentin-Gamazo C (2005) Preoperative donor liver biopsy for adult living donor liver transplantation: risks and benefits. *Liver Transpl.* 11;(8):980–986

Neumann UP, Guckelberger O, Langrehr JM, (2003) Impact of human leukocyte antigen matching in liver transplantation. *Transplantation* 75(1):132–137

Noma S, Hayashi A, Uehara M, Uemoto S, Murai T. (2010) Comparison between psychosocial long-term outcomes of recipients and donors after adult-to-adult living donor liver transplantation. *Clin Transplant.* doi: 10.1111/j.1399-0012.2010.01337.x.

Ogata S., Belghiti J., Varma D. (2007) Two hundred liver hanging maneuvers for major hepatectomy: a single-center experience. *Ann Surg* 245. 31-35.

Olthoff KM, Merion RM, Ghobrial RM. (2005) Outcomes of 385 adult-to-adult living-donor liver transplant recipients: a report from the A2ALL consortium. Ann Surg; 242:314–325.

Olthoff KM.(2003). Hepatic regeneration in living donor liver transplantation. *Liver Transplant;* 9 (Suppl 2) S35–41.

Park K, Moon JI, Kim SI, Kim YS. (1999) Exchange donor program in kidney transplantation. *Transplantation*;67(2):336–8.

Polak W, P Peeters, M Slooff, (2009) The evolution of surgical techniques in clinical liver transplantation. A review, *Clin Transplant* DOI: 10.1111/j.1399-0012.2009.

Radtke A, Sgourakis G, Sotiropoulos GC, Beckebaum S, Molmenti EP, Saner FH, Schroeder T, Nadalin S, Schenk A, Lang H, Malagó M, Broelsch CE. (2010) Donor/recipient algorithm for management of the middle hepatic vein in right graft live donor liver transplantation. *Am J Surg*.199(5):708-15.

Raia S, Nery J, Mies S. (1989). Liver transplantation from live donors. *Lancet* 2: 497.

Ringe B & Strong R, (2008). The Dilemma of Living Liver Donor Death: to Report or not to Report? *Transplantation* 85: 790–79.

Rudow DL, Russo MW, Hafliger S, Emond JC, Brown RS Jr. (2003) Clinical and ethnic differences in candidates listed for liver transplantation with and without potential living donors. *Liver Transpl*;9:254-259.

Russo MW, LaPointe-Rudow D, Kinkhabwala M, Emond J, Brown RS, Jr. (2004) Impact of adult living-donor liver transplantation on waiting time survival in candidates listed for liver transplantation. *Am J Transplant*; 4(3):427.

Sauer P, Schemmer P, Uhl W, Ecke J. (2004) Living-donor liver transplantation: evaluation of donor and recipient. *Nephrol Dial Transplant* 19(Suppl 4):iv11–iv15.

Selvaggi G, Tzakis A. (2009) Surgical considerations in liver transplantation: small for size syndrome. Review. *Panminerva Med.* 51(4):227-33.

Selzner M, Kashfi A, Cattral MS, Selzner N, Greig PD, Lilly L, McGilvray ID, Therapondos G, Adcock LE, Ghanekar A, Levy GA, Renner EL, Grant DR. (2009) A graft to body weight ratio less than 0.8 does not exclude adult-to-adult right-lobe living donor liver transplantation. *Liver Transpl.* 15(12):1776-82.

Shirabe K, Taketomi A, Morita K, Soejima Y, Uchiyama H, Kayashima H, Ninomiya M, Toshima T, Maehara Y. (2011) Comparative evaluation of expanded criteria for patients with hepatocellular carcinoma beyond the Milan criteria undergoing living-related donor liver transplantation. *Clin Transplant.* doi: 10.1111/j.1399-0012.2011.01463.x.

Siegler J, Siegler M, Cronin DC 2nd. (2004) Recipient death during a live donor liver transplantation: who gets the "orphan" graft? *Transplantation.* 78(9):1241-1244.

Smith B. (1969). Segmental liver transplantation from a living donor. *J Pediatr Surg;* 4: 126–32.

Soejima Y, Fukuhara T, Morita K, Yoshizumi T, Ikegami T, Yamashita Y, Sugimachi K, Taketomi A, Maehara Y. (2008) A simple hilar dissection technique preserving maximum blood supply to the bile duct in living donor liver transplantation. *Transplantation.* 27;86(10):1468-9.

Soin AS, Kumaran V, Rastogi AN, Mohanka R, Mehta N, Saigal S, Saraf N, Mohan N, Nundy S. (2010) Evolution of a reliable biliary reconstructive technique in 400 consecutive living donor liver transplants. *J Am Coll Surg.* 211(1):24-32.

Starzl TE, Iwatsuki S, Shaw BW Jr. A growth factor in fine vascular anastomoses. (1984) *Surg Gynecol Obstet.* 159: 164

Steinbrück K, Enne M, Fernandes R, Martinho JM, Balbi E, Agoglia L, Roma J, Pacheco-Moreira LF. (2011) Vascular complications after living donor liver transplantation: a Brazilian, single-center experience. *Transplant Proc.* 43(1):196-8.

Steiner RW, Gert B. (2000) Ethical selection of living kidney donors. *Am. J. Kidney Dis.* 36(4):677–86.

Suehiro T, Shimada M, Kishikawa K, Shimura T, Soejima Y, Yoshizumi T, Hashimoto K, Mochida Y, Maehara Y, Kuwano H. (2005) Prevention of hepatitis B virus infection from hepatitis B core antibody-positive donor graft using hepatitis B immune globulin and lamivudine in living donor liver transplantation. *Liver Int.* 25(6):1169-74.

Sugawara Y, Kaneko J, Akamatsu N, (2003) Arterial anatomy unsuitable for a right liver donation. *Liver Transpl* 9:1116.

Takada Y, Uemoto S. (2010) Liver transplantation for hepatocellular carcinoma: the Kyoto experience.*J Hepatobiliary Pancreat Sci.* 17(5):527-32..

Takatsuki M, Chiang Y, Lin T, Wang C, Concejero A, Lin CC, Huang TL, Cheng YF, Chen CL. (2006) Anatomical and technical aspects of hepatic artery reconstruction in living donor liver transplantation. *Surgery.* 140(5):824-8; discussion 829.

Takatsuki M, Eguchi S, Yamanouchi K, Tokai H, Hidaka M, Soyama A, Miyazaki K, Hamasaki K, Tajima Y, Kanematsu T. (2009) Two-surgeon technique using saline-linked electric cautery and ultrasonic surgical aspirator in living donor hepatectomy: its safety and efficacy. *Am J Surg.* 197(2):e25-7.

Taketomi A, Morita K, Toshima T, Takeishi K, Kayashima H, Ninomiya M, Uchiyama H, SoejimaY, ShirabeK, MaeharaY (2010) Living donor liver hepatectomies with procedures to prevent biliary complications. *J Am Coll Surg.* 211(4):456-64.

Tan H, Marcos A, Shapiro R, *Living Donor Transplantation,* Thomas E. Starzl Transplantation Institute Pittsburgh, Pennsylvania, USA,Informa Healthcare USA, Inc., 2007

Tan H, Patel-Tom K, Marcos A. (2005) Adult living donor liver transplantation: who is the ideal donor and recipient? *J Hepatol* 43:13–17.

Tanaka K, T Kiuchi, MDc, S Kaihara, (2004) Living related liver donor transplantation: techniques and caution . *Surg Clin N Am* 84 481–493

Terasaki PI, Cecka JM, Gjertson DW, Cho YW. (1997) Spousal and other living renal donor transplants. *Clin. Transpl.* 269–84.

Trotter JF, Hayashi PH, Kam I. (2005) Donor and recipient evaluation and selection for adult-to-adult right hepatic lobe liver transplantation. In: Busuttil RW, Klintmalm GB, eds. *Transplantation of the Liver*. Philadelphia: Elsevier :655–674.

Trotter JF, Wachs M, Everson GT, Kam I. (2002) Adult-to-adult transplantation of the right hepatic lobe from a living donor. *N Engl J Med;*346:1074-1082.

Trotter JF, Wisniewski KA, Terrault NA, Everhart JE, Kinkhabwala M, Weinrieb RM, Fair JH, Fisher RA, Koffron AJ, Saab S, Merion RM; A2ALL Study Group. (2007) Outcomes of donor evaluation in adult-to-adult living donor liver transplantation. *Hepatology.* 46(5):1476-84.

Trotter JF. Selection of donors and recipients for living donor liver transplantation. (2000) *Liver Transpl.* 6(6 Suppl 2):S52–S58.

Trotter, J.F., Adam, R., Lo, C.M. & Kenison, J. (2006) Documented deaths of hepatic lobe donors for living donor liver transplantation. *Liver Transpl* Vol. 12(No. 10): 1485-1488.

Tsang LL, Chen CL, Huang TL, Chen TY, Wang CC, Ou HY, Lin LH, Cheng YF. (2008) Preoperative imaging evaluation of potential living liver donors: reasons for exclusion from donation in adult living donor liver transplantation. *Transplant Proc.* 40(8):2460-2.

Walter M, Bronner E, Steinmuller T, Klapp B, Danzer G. (2002). Psychosocial data of potential living donors before living donation liver transplantation. *Clin Transpl* 16:55-59.

Xu MQ, Yan LN, Li B, Zeng Y, Wen TF, Zhao JC, Wang WT, Yang JY, Ma YK, Cheng ZY. (2008) Surgical procedures for management of right portal venous branching in right lobe living donor liver transplantation. *Transplant Proc.* 40(5):1529-33.

Yuan Y & Gotoh M. Biliary complications in living liver donors. (2010). *Surg Today.* 40(5): 411-7.

2

Arterial Anastomosis in Living Donor Liver Transplantation

Mirela Patricia Sirbu Boeti, Vladislav Brašoveanu, Sadiq Shoaib and Irinel Popescu
Fundeni Clinical Institute, Department of General Surgery and Liver Transplantation Romania

1. Introduction

Since the first successful operation in 1989, living donor liver transplantation (LDLT) for children with end-stage liver diseases has emerged as an alternative to cadaveric liver transplantation. (Strong et al., 1990) The applicability of LDLT was extended to adult patients in 1994. (Kiuchi et al., 1999) Justification of LDLT has evolved from increased organ-waiting times, wait-list morbidity and mortality of transplant candidates. (Renz & Busuttil, 2000) The left lobe or the left lateral segment of an adult liver is most often of adequate size for donation to a child recipient. However in the adult, the right hepatic lobe transplantation is usually the procedure of choice to provide adequate liver volume to the recipient. (Nakamura et al., 2002)

By having a thorough and accurate knowledge of vascular variants, the transplant surgeon can adopt the optimal techniques for vascular reconstruction, with the intent to provide an adequate inflow and outflow through liver parenchyma and to avoid postoperative vascular complications.

The present chapter reviews the surgical anatomy of the hepatic artery (HA), arterial reconstruction techniques as applied to LDLT, and postoperative arterial complications.

2. Preoperative assessment of hepatic arterial anatomy

Hepatic arterial anomalies are present in almost half of the living donors. (Macdonald et al., 2005) To accomplish a successful and uncomplicated operation, preoperative assessment of anatomy of hepatic vasculature is of paramount importance for both donor and recipient. Preoperative work-up may involve computed tomography (CT), ultrasonography (US) including Doppler imaging, magnetic resonance (MR) imaging, and catheter angiography.

Conventional angiography was substituted by three-dimensional computer tomography (3D CT) angiography which is a safer, more convenient, cheaper, and better-tolerated procedure for determination of hepatic arterial anatomy. (Winter et al., 1995; Coskun et al., 2005)

CT has progressed from dual slice CT to 64-Multidetector Computed Tomography (MDCT) (Johnson & Fishman, 2006), which represents a non-invasive technological advance that permits high-speed and high-resolution helical imaging of the entire liver volume during a single breath-hold. (Johnson & Fishman, 2006)

CT angiography has become a key component of state-of-the-art imaging. The reconstruction of CT angiographic data sets obtained on 16- and 64-section scanners may result in 1000–5000 images per examination. The large size of the data set makes it impractical to extract all the information present by using standard two-dimensional techniques and makes clear the importance of volume imaging and 3D image display. (Fishman et al., 2006) The 3D high-quality reconstruction images are easy for post editing, and make possible to observe the origin, flow pattern and branches of the hepatic artery in fine anatomic details, from multiple angles, positions and layers, as well as adjacent structures. (Huang et al., 2009) Although 2D data sets show small arteries to better advantage than 3D multidetector CT angiography (MDCTA), the 3D MDCT angiograms provide a useful overview of hepatic anatomy. (Stemmler et al., 2004)

Radiologists now have workstations that provide capabilities for evaluation of these data sets by using a range of software programs and processing tools. Although different systems have unique capabilities and functionality, all provide the options of volume rendering (VR) and maximum intensity projection (MIP) for image display and analysis. In the MIP technique, only the pixel of highest intensity is used to calculate each line of pixel data through the viewed object and about 90% of data is discarded. A cine loop of multiple MIP images can be incorporated to facilitate determination of the vascular interrelations. In contrast, in the VR technique, all the helical CT data set is used for image reconstruction, thus multiple overlapping vessels, spatial relations between the arteries and the viscera, and arteries with small diameters can be displayed. (Fishman et al., 2006)

MDCT is a valuable evaluation of potential living liver donors because it provides an excellent pre-operative mapping of the hepatic arterial, hepatic, and portal venous systems of the potential donors prior LDLT, a comprehensive assessment of the liver parenchyma (e.g. fatty infiltration) and of many other intra-abdominal diseases or abnormalities, an accurate measurement of graft and remnant liver volume, and an excellent defining of the curved virtual hepatectomy plane that provides sufficient volume to satisfy the metabolic demands of both donors and recipients. (Alonso-Torres et al., 2005; Stemmler et al., 2004)

The most critical aspect of imaging potential liver donors is the accurate depiction of the origin and course of the artery to segment IV. Unlike currently available conventional helical scanners, MDCTA results in 1.25-mm resolution. If the acquisition parameters and timing of the contrast bolus are optimized, this resolution allows even a tiny artery to be viewed with minor interruption in adjacent slices or with no interruption in 3D models.

MR volumetry, venography, angiography, and cholangiography with 3D reconstruction is considered by some authors to be sufficient for all major imaging evaluation for LDLT. (Cheng et al., 2001, Sahani et al., 2004)

With the advantage of advanced imaging techniques used pretransplant, now it is possible to identify the anatomical type of hepatic artery (HA) according to Michels classification (Tabel 1).

There was no significant difference observed in the overall incidence of arterial complications between grafts with normal and abnormal anatomy. (Soin et al., 1996) Anomalies of hepatic arterial vasculature occur in one-third of all livers and do not compromise graft outcome unless multiple anastomoses or direct anastomosis to the recipient aorta are required for arterial reconstruction. (Soin et al., 1996)

Type	Description
I	Entire hepatic trunk arising from CHA
II	Replaced LHA arising from LGA
III	Replaced RHA arising from SMA
IV	Replaced LHA and replaced RHA
V	Accessory LHA arising from LGA
VI	Accessory RHA arising from SMA
VII	Accessory LHA and accessory RHA
VIII	Replaced RHA and accessory LHA or replaced LHA and accessory RHA
IX	Entire hepatic trunk arising from SMA
X	Entire hepatic trunk arising from LGA

Table 1. Michels classification of the anatomical types of hepatic artery. (Michels, 1955 as cited in Coskun et al., 2005)

Hepatic arterial branching patterns do not correlate well with the presence of anomalous biliary drainage. In patients with normal hepatic vascular anatomy, biliary anomalies are more frequent than in those with anomalous vascular anatomy (50% versus 30%). (Macdonald et al., 2005) Arterial blood supply to the left lobe often shows variations such as multiple branches, aberrant left hepatic artery (Sakamoto et al., 2002), whereas the right hepatic artery is often unique. (Kishi et al., 2004) Anatomic variations in graft hepatic arteries are classified by Takatsuki et al. into 3 types (Figure 1): Type I, single pedicle with (Ia) or without (Ib) aberrant artery (left hepatic artery (HA) from the left gastric artery or right HA from the superior mesenteric artery); Type II, double pedicles with (2a) or without (2b) aberrant artery; and Type III, equal to or more than three pedicles. (Takatsuki et al., 2006) The arterial reconstruction is anticipated based on this classification. Type I of arterial vasculature will allow the reconstruction of only one artery. Type II and III will necessitate a very careful intraoperative assessment of the arterial flow and an elaborated decision for the arterial reconstruction.

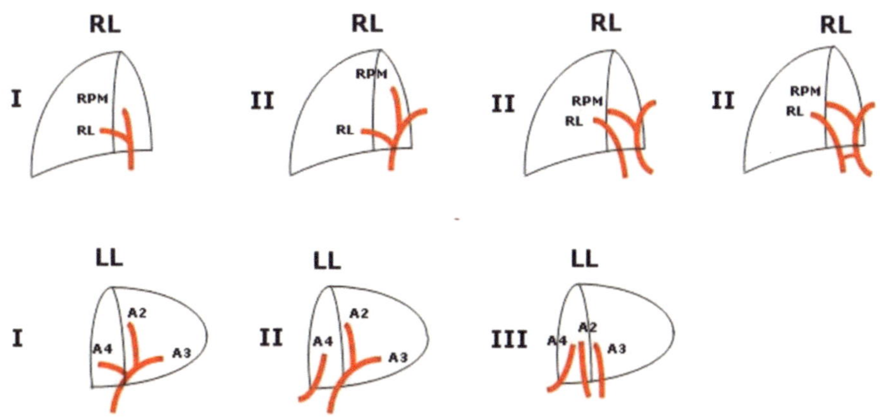

Fig. 1. Type I, single pedicle; Type II, double pedicles; and Type III, equal to or more than three pedicles. RL – right lobe, LL – left liver (modified after Takatsuki et al., 2006)

A rare anatomical variant is worth mentioning. In Fig. 2 it is depicted a communication between a normal right medial arterial branch emerging from proper hepatic artery and a replaced right lateral arterial branch emerging from superior mesenteric artery. This communication is favorable by avoiding the reconstruction of both branches. Both branches are cut proximal to the interconnection. Only the larger donor's artery is used to perform the arterial anastomosis with the receptor's proper hepatic artery.

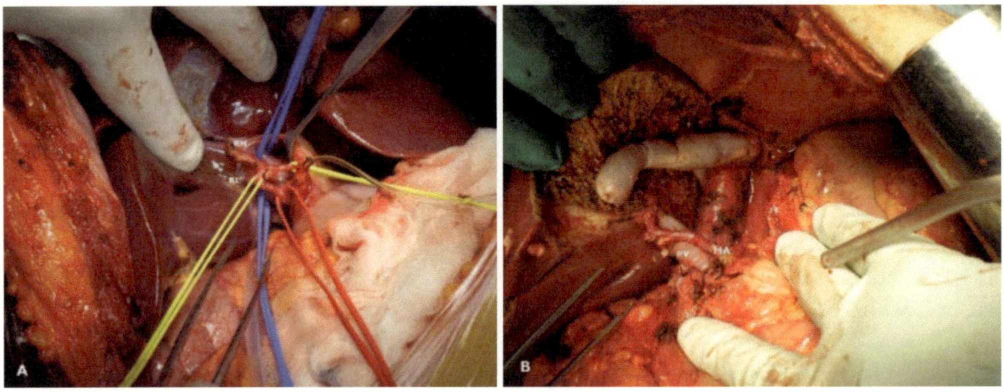

Fig. 2. A) Dissection of hepatic hilum with the identification of a communication between a normal right medial arterial branch emerging from proper hepatic artery and a replaced right lateral arterial branch emerging from superior mesenteric artery. B) Arterial anastomosis is completed between the donor's hepatic branch from superior mesenteric artery and recipient's proper hepatic artery

3. Reconstruction techniques of the liver arterial vasculature

During hilar dissection in donor operation, the HA and portal vein of the donor are individually exposed and carefully divided. In left grafts, the proper HA is exposed up to the bifurcation of the left (or middle) HA and the right HA. In right grafts, the right HA is identified and isolated to the right side of the hepatic duct. The division point of HA is determined by the length and size of the artery, its relationship with the cutting plane of the liver, and the position of the arteries. (Takatsuki et al., 2006) Division of the donor vessels at a point further distal to the main trunk than would be considered ideal for donor protection. Anastomosis of first- or second-order vascular branches is a requirement of LDLT. (Marcos et al., 2001)

The reconstruction technique of the liver arterial vasculature is selected by the surgeon based on the anatomical arterial variants, differences in vessel caliber, length and quality of recipient HA (i.e. aneurysm, stenosis, intimal dissection, inflammation of the porta hepatis, inadvertent injury of donor or recipient HA).

In the recipient, HA reconstruction is carried out after reconstructing of both hepatic and portal veins followed by the reperfusion of the implanted graft. In liver transplantation arterial reconstruction is essential to ensure a good blood inflow for proper graft function. The absence of an adequate hepatic arterial supply usually results in graft loss due to biliary ischemia and parenchymal complications. Hepatic arterial reconstruction in LDLT is technically more difficult and troublesome than in orthotopic liver transplantation (OLT), mainly because of the need to reconstruct thin, short, and/or multiple arterial branches in limited surgical fields. Moreover the hilar structures lie in a different plane than native vessels, and optimal realignment for anastomosis is sometimes impossible to achieve. Reconstruction under these circumstances requires an unusual degree of precision. (Marcos et al., 2001)

Microsurgical reconstruction of the liver vasculature in LDLT rises significant challenges to the surgeon. There are various aspects to be addressed: (1) difficulty in obtaining a good operative field and a sufficient view through the microscope due to the deep location of the liver in the abdominal cavity; (2) the respiratory movement and heart pulsation; (3) vessel-size discrepancy between the graft and recipient hepatic arterial stumps; (4) possible intimal dissection and atheromatosis, small caliber, and/or short stalk of the donor hepatic artery/arteries.

Longer microsurgical instruments are required to get an easier access. One or two soft suction tubes are placed at both sides of the HA to provide a bloodless operative field. When an operating microscope is used, it is draped with a sterile plastic bag and adjusted as the operator stand at the patient's right side and the assistant stand at patient's left side. HA in LDLT can also be safely reconstructed with microsurgical techniques without microscope using, with 6x loupe magnification. (Enne et al., 2010; Guarrera et al., 2004) To provide a wide anastomosis and consecutively to avoid microscope usage, native and graft hepatic arteries can be spatulated from both the anterior and posterior walls. (Haberal et al., 2007)

To overcome large movement caused by respiration, the suturing of the hepatic arteries should be synchronized according to the rhythmic chest wall up-and-down movement. If this has not the expected result, a decrease of the tidal volume to 300–400 mL/min may help. An alternative stabilization of the operative field is to use smooth manual bagging technique instead of mechanical ventilation.

In most cases the caliber discrepancy is dealt with simple methods such as gently dilatation of the vessel edge, enlargement of the circumference of the smaller lumen by cutting artery obliquely or in fish-mouth, making a longitudinal side-cut, funnelization, suturing with wider bites on the larger vessel. (Inomoto et al., 1996) When the size mismatch is greater than 1:3, the alternatives are: the interposition of an arterial graft (e.g. superior rectal artery, ovarian artery, radial artery (Kamei et al., 2006)) or venous conduct, the construction of an end-to-side anastomosis or anastomosis with a side branch of the larger vessel. When a discrepancy in the thickness of the vessel walls is encountered, full bites of the thinner vessel and only inner layers of the thicker vessel should be taken in the sutures.

Multiple arterial tributaries in right liver graft procurement are rare. Due to its anatomic characteristics RHA anastomosis is relatively straightforward (Marcos et al., 2000) with no complications and is often aided only by loupe magnification, sometimes using an artifice. (Di Benedetto et al., 2004) In case of a very short right arterial stump in the graft, there are two options: (1) the use of microsurgical techniques with double needle threads; (2) the interposition technique proposed as a reversed extension graft. Harvesting an arterial graft for interposition will subject either the donors or recipients to an additional incision or more extensive dissection and prolonged operation time with consecutive increased risk of thrombosis in the recipient. Thus the arterial conduct interposition should be avoided as much as possible.

It is still debated in LDLT whether all arterial stumps should be anastomosed. However a simple method of only one anastomosis is sufficient if backflow from another tributary is confirmed, indicating that a compensation of arterial perfusion exists in both left (Ikegami et al., 1996) and right liver grafts (Kishi et al., 2004). When backflow from the second tributary is absent, this artery should be reconstructed. (Marcos et al., 2001)

Different from the right lobe, multiple arteries to the left lobe are rather common, and care must be taken when harvesting the graft in such cases. Incidence of HA thrombosis was showed to be four times higher in the grafts with multiple arteries than those with a single artery. When encountering dual arteries during donor surgery, there are three options to be considered: (1) division of both arteries and reconstruction of only one; (2) division and reconstruction of both arteries; (3) 2-in-1 segmental resection followed by donor HA reconstruction.

The arterial reconstruction is sometimes needed in the donor when a 2-in-1 segmental resection is performed and, as in the recipient, it is of paramount concern. The incidence of arterial occlusion after reconstruction in the donor HA must be lower than in the recipient in order to address the most important ethical issue of LDLT - donor safety.

The average diameters of the stump of the graft and recipient's arteries are 2.5-0.5 mm and the average of these caliber differences are 0.3-0.5 mm. The end-to-end arterial anastomosis is the choice whenever possible. Depending on the diameter of the vessels, the surgeon has to choose between loupe and microscope. The use of microvascular techniques has revolutionized reconstruction and expanded the range of options for reconstructing small and incongruent arteries. Microsurgery is complex and technically demanding, but with careful preparation and proper execution, it has been proved beneficial to the patient and rewarding to the surgeon. (Inomoto et al., 1996)

Arterial anastomoses in the left lobe and left lateral segment living donor transplantation incur a relative frequent complication rate when performed by loupe magnification but a significant lower incidence of these when microvascular techniques are used. By using the microscope, a fine hepatic artery less than 2 mm in diameter is no longer regarded as a contraindication for LDLT due to the potential arterial complications. (Inomoto et al., 1995)

The graft should be prepared in such a way that only one arterial anastomosis is performed in order to avoid the risk of thrombosis. The single independent arterial anastomosis technique is most commonly used for arterial anastomosis in LVLT.

After preparing the graft for anastomosis, the fitness of each arterial branch should be assess for microvascular reconstruction. In this assessment the quality of the recipient hepatic artery should be inspected carefully using the high power of microscope. The interior of vessel should be observed for signs of intimal irregularity such as separation from the media due to preexisting conditions (e.g. atherosclerosis, previous surgical trauma). Any sign of damage indicates the need for further debridement. After adequate debridement, there should be a strong pulsatile flow from the recipient artery. After assessment of quality of arteries, the length and caliber matching should be carefully observed.

The difficulty related to correct match of vessels diameter is present mostly in pediatric LDLA cases where the caliber of the graft artery is smaller than that of the recipient hepatic artery. In most cases the caliber difference is dealt with simple methods such as gently dilatation of the vessel edge, oblique cutting of the graft artery, fish-mouth method, and short longitudinal incision. Funnelization is an appropriate method to accommodate a much wider size disparity by enlarging the circumference of the smaller lumen.

In LDLT graft HAs are usually reconstructed with a recipient HA branch (anatomical HA reconstruction). Surgeons often encounter difficulties in extra-anatomical HA reconstruction, when a recipient artery other than a HA branch must be used. When biliary reconstruction is chosen to be performed by duct-to-duct anastomosis, recipient's left HAs should be selected for HA reconstruction in right liver LDLT in order to decrease the rate of septic and biliary complication. (Uchiyama et al., 2010) In extra-anatomical HA reconstructions, the arteries used are right gastroepiplooic artery, gastric artery, gastroduodenal artery, left gastric artery, splenic artery, cystic artery (Lee et al., 2008), and infrarenal abdominal aorta (Uchiyama et al., 2010).

The single independent arterial anastomosis can be performed with or without interposition graft depending on the condition of arteries that are to be anastomosed. When the intimal condition, length, and diameter of the recipient and donor artery are appropriate to each other then the single independent arterial anastomosis without interposition graft is performed in an end-to-end fashion in LDLT.

In almost all the situations vessel anastomosis in recipient is performed in end-to-end fashion using interrupted sutures. For a HA with a diameter of at least 3.0 mm, 8-0 suture is indicated. For a HA with a diameter less than 3.0 mm, 9-0 suture is indicated (Okochi M et al., 2010). The monofilament suture can be nylon (Ethilon; Ehicon Inc, Somerville, NJ) or polypropylene (Prolene; Ehicon Inc, Somerville, NJ). Less frequently, arterial anastomoses are performed using continuous suturing. The reason to avoid continuous suturing is to minimize narrowing of the arterial lumen. Some authors describe the placement of continuous suture on the posterior wall and interrupted sutures on the anterior wall. (Okochi M et al., 2010)

An alternative surgical technique that avoids interpositional vessel grafts or tension on the connection is successfully used by some authors. An end-to-side anastomosis is performed between allograft hepatic vein and recipient inferior vena cava in a more caudate location. The level of venotomy on the recipient vena cava is decided according to the pre-anastomotic placement of the allograft in the recipient hepatectomy site with sufficient width to have a hepatic artery anastomosis without tension or need for an interposition graft during hepatic artery and portal vein anastomoses. (Ersozet et al., 2003)

There are various techniques applicable for hepatic arterial reconstruction.

1. The double clip-fixation technique is feasible when the donor arterial stump is long enough to allow to turn over the vessels after the completion of the anterior wall of the anastomosis. The double micro-clamp is applied first to the donor HA then the recipient HA and a silastic background is placed behind the hepatic vessels.
2. The two stay suture technique is performed without using a double clip. Two stay sutures are placed 180° apart at the center of the anterior and posterior walls, left untied,

3. and retracted gently to keep the anastomotic site in the best position. Some sutures are placed on one lateral side between the stay sutures, and left untied to ensure precise placement of the sutures in the direct view of the lumen. After all these side sutures are placed, they are tied. Next, the two stay sutures are turned over 180° and retracted in the opposite direction, and the other lateral side sutures are placed in the same manner. The anastomosis is completed by tying the stay sutures.
4. The doubly-armed microsuture technique or back wall support suture technique is recommended to avoid the twisting during suturing and thus to overcome the drawbacks of the conventional method performed in a deep abdominal cavity and/or on a short hepatic artery with no possibility for turning of the microclamps. (Ikegamiet et al., 2000) Microvascular anastomosis without turning over the clamp is considered by some authors superior to the conventional method in terms of reducing intimal damage to the vessels. (Yamamoto et al., 1999) Back wall-first approach should be favored especially when dealing with a fragile HA due to age, liver disease, atherosclerosis or post-transcatheter interventions such as arterial embolization in hepatocellular carcinoma before transplant. (Takatsuki et al, 2006) The recipient and graft arteries are clamped with single microclamps. The first double needle 9-0 monofilament microsuture is placed at the most difficult point (usually at the middle of the posterior wall) in the artery to be visualized through the microscope. Each stitch is always placed from the inner side of the arterial wall to the outer side. The posterior stitch is tied pulling toward the back. The subsequent sutures are advanced anteriorly on either side adjacent to the previous suture. The anterior vessel wall is sutured with a regular microsuture with a single needle. (Miyagi et al, 2008)
5. The branch patch anastomosis for hepatic arteries uses the bifurcation of hepatic arterial branches. The bifurcation of the arteries are cut longitudinally and then the plasty is performed to make a patch. To create a large orifice for the arterial anastomosis, the short part of the patch is wrapped with a long flap of the arteries from the other side. Cystic artery bifurcation from right hepatic artery can also be used to prepare a patch to be anastomosed to the recipient right branch of the hepatic artery. (Di Benedetto et al., 2004) During the procedure, a small vascular catheter can be used as a guide inside the gastroduodenal artery (GDA) which then is removed at the end of the anastomosis, as the GDA itself is sutured.
6. The technique of the ex situ reconstruction with a Y-extension graft is suited for the complex situation of double hepatic arteries. In the case of a donor graft with two arteries, the Y-extension graft procedure appears to be necessary. (Marcos et al., 2001, 2003) The recipient's HA is dissected well beyond both the right and left hepatic arteries which are transected to obtain the Y-extension graft. The artery is transected just distal to the takeoff of the gastroduodenal artery while the recipient liver continues to be perfused by portal blood flow during ex situ reconstruction of the arteries. Because arterial inflow to the recipient common bile duct may be sacrificed, duct-to-duct biliary reconstruction is contraindicated.

   On back table the right and left hepatic arteries are anastomosed with interrupted sutures to the dual arterial system on the donor right lobe under loupe magnification. The patency and integrity of the anastomoses are reassessed through the free end of the vascular conduit before engraftment. The free end of the Y-extension graft (proper hepatic artery) is sutured in situ to the recipient hepatic artery branched cuff of the common hepatic artery and gastroduodenal artery. The wide lumen created by branch patching usually allows for running anastomosis with 5-0 or 6-0 prolene suture (Figure 3). (Marcos et al., 2001)

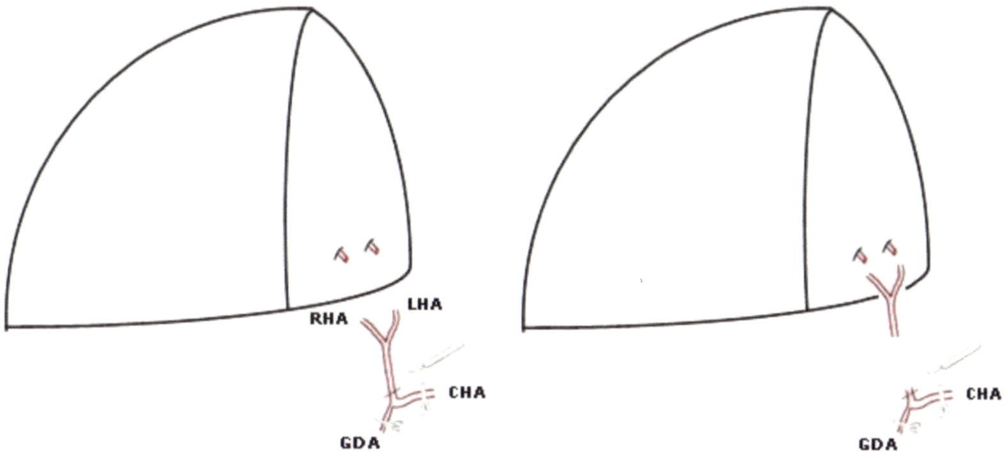

(a) (b)

Fig. 3. Reconstruction of two right hepatic branches. A. Recipient' s right, left, and proper hepatic arteries are sectioned to obtain a Y-vascular graft. The level of section of proper hepatic artery is at the takeoff of gastroduodenal artery. B. The arterial branches of the hepatic graft are anastomosed on table using the bifurcation of Y-graft. The free end of the Y-graft is anastomosed at the bifurcation of common hepatic artery

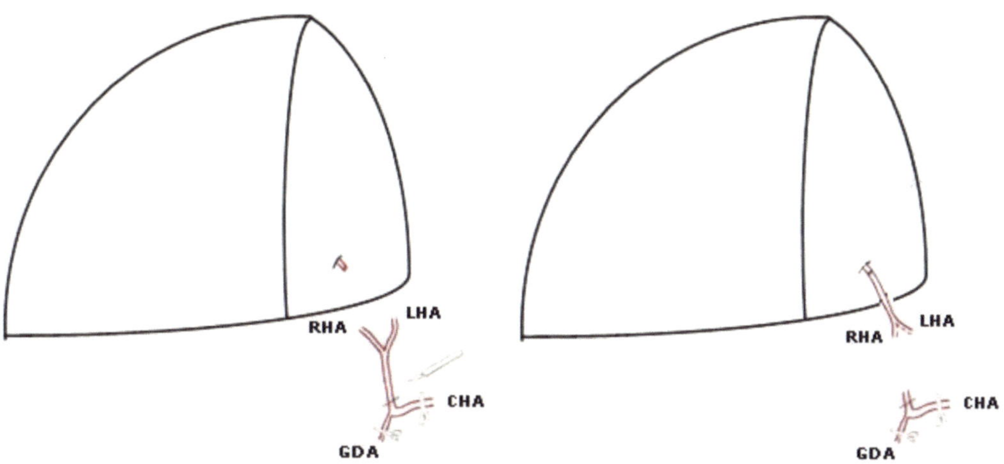

(a) (b)

Fig. 4. Reconstruction of a short right hepatic artery. A. Right, left, and proper hepatic arteries are sectioned to obtain a Y-vascular graft. The level of section of proper hepatic artery is at the takeoff of gastroduodenal artery. B. The free end of Y-graft is anastomosed with the right hepatic artery of the graft on back table. The branches of Y-graft are cut at the bifurcation to obtain a larger lumen that will be anastomosed with the bifurcation of recipient's common hepatic artery

7. The reversed extension bifurcated graft technique is a standard technique for single arterial anastomosis in the recipients. The modification begins with the dissection of the recipient hepatic artery well beyond the bifurcation of the RHA and LHA.
   The proper hepatic artery is transected just distal to the takeoff of the gastroduodenal artery from the common hepatic artery while the recipient liver continues to receive portal perfusion. The bifurcation of the RHA and LHA is opened to create a wider bifurcated cuff. Then the arterial segment is reversed so that the once-proximal end of the PHA is sutured to the donor graft RHA under direct vision ex situ, and tension free, with interrupted 7-0 prolene. The reversed bifurcated (RHA/LHA) graft, with its new arterial extension, is then anastomosed to the larger branched cuff of the CHA and GDA using standard branch-patch technique (Figure 4). (Marcos et al., 2003)
8. The ex situ graft extension is another feasible and alternative technique for reconstruction of hepatic artery in LDLT if there are issues regarding length, size discrepancy or reconstruction of more than one artery. (Marcos et al., 2003) From cadaveric grafts it can be used internal and external iliac artery, splenic artery, reversed saphenous vein, and superior mesenteric artery. The SMA has proved particularly useful to overcome large size discrepancies and also reconstruct multiple arteries into a single vessel. Splenic artery can be ligated because the short gastrosplenic vessels and the left gastric artery maintain the vascularization of the spleen. However the risk of splenic infarction exists especially in case of a large spleen. (Lehar et al., 1990) The right gastroepiplooic artery can be dissected free from the greater curvature of the stomach and the surrounding tissue without causing ischemia of the stomach. An end-to-end anastomosis between this artery and the donor hepatic artery can be performed. The major disadvantage of any interpositional graft is that it needs two anastomosis to be performed which may lead toward increased risk of HAT. Anastomosis to the recipient's common hepatic artery resulted in a high incidence of thrombosis, whereas anastomosis to the infrarenal aorta nearly always remained patent, regardless of the length of the interposition of the saphenous vein. The inferior mesenteric vein can also be used for the arterial reconstruction. (Margreiter et al., 2008) There is a high risk for the inferior mesenteric vein to become ectatic when exposed to arterial pressure, which causes turbulence, and thrombosis may result. (Broelsch et al., 1999)
9. The superior mesenteric artery branch of Roux-en-Y limb technique is an alternative when porta hepatis inflammation makes difficult to use the hepatic, gastroduodenal or right gastroepiplooic artery for hepatic arterial reconstruction, or when a subintimal dissection or atheromatosis extends to all tributaries of the celiac arterial trunk. (Kasahara et al., 2005) A jejunal arterial arcade of Roux-en-Y limb mobilized for biliary reconstruction is anastomosed to the donor hepatic artery in end-to-end fashion. (Ikegami, et al., 2008) The arterial reconstruction in Roux-en-Y hepaticojejunostomy technique is performed before biliary reconstruction (Figure 5).
10. When multiple graft arteries are encountered, the dominant artery is reconstructed first. The dominant HA in grafts with multiple hepatic arteries can be determined by comparing arterial flows during intraoperative DUS after temporary occlusion of each artery using microvascular clips in the donor operation. This is followed by careful check-up on back-bleeding from the other arteries. If back-bleeding is insufficient both arteries must be reconstructed. Despite the fact that complex HA reconstructions are needed in such circumstances, with technical advancement, HA-related complications can be avoided in most cases. (Uchiyama et al., 2010) If back-bleeding is sufficient, the

unreconstructed arteries can be ligated. The blood flow through the vessel anastomosis is verified by color flow DUS.

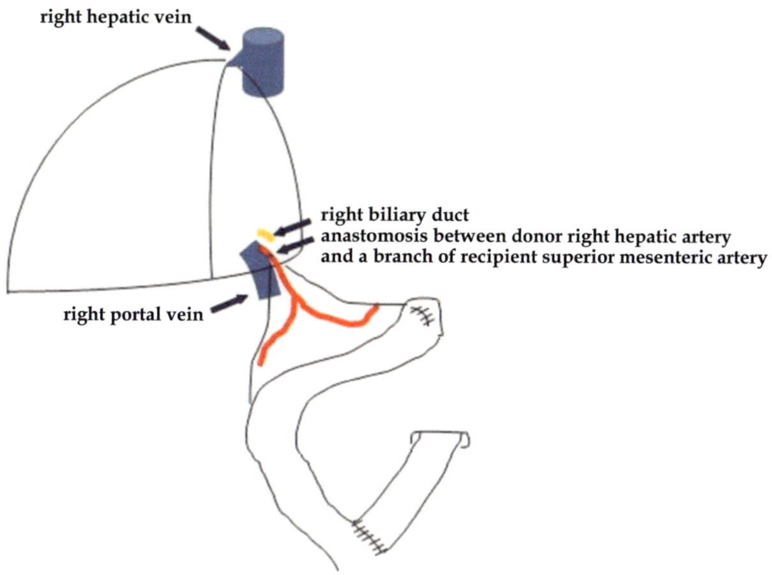

Fig. 5. A segment of jejunum is mobilized. An arterial branch of superior mesenteric artery of Roux-en-Y limb is anastomosed with the arterial stump of the liver graft. Biliary anastomosis is performed after arterial reconstructions

In rare case of right graft dual arterial supply the anastomosis of the larger branch is made first, then the backflow is checked from the smaller branch. If not good, the smaller branch must be reconstructed. The cystic artery can be used as a conduit for the reconstruction. The length of cystic artery is preserved as long as possible. The cystic arterial stump is anastomosed to the stump of the posterior branch the of RHA under microscopic guidance on the back table. Patency is checked through the stump of the anterior branch of the RHA. With this technique, only one orifice, the stump of right anterior hepatic artery, is used for hepatic artery reconstruction. (Lee et al., 2008)

In case of left graft dual arterial supply Douard et al. use a two-step strategy for the development of flow-induced enlargement of a small diameter artery. The smaller arterial branch is ligated during a laparoscopic first-step procedure to induce a 30% enlargement of the remaining branch. The second-step donor hepatectomy is performed one week later using a larger artery for successful vascular anastomosis. (Douard et al., 2002) It is worth underlining the importance of preoperative imaging for the identification of anatomic vascular variants which can be addressed in two-step strategy. The same authors reported a case with angiographic revealed celiac trunk compression by the median arcuate ligament and reverse vascularization of the middle hepatic artery via the gastroduodenal artery, a proper hepatic artery 2 mm in diameter irrigating the left lateral segment exclusively, and a right hepatic artery irrigating the right lobe and segment IV. First-step division of the median arcuate ligament and gastroduodenal artery ligation was followed by a repeat angiography at the third week showing a 50% enlargement of the middle hepatic artery (3 mm) and the second-step left lobectomy performed at the fifth week. (Douard et al., 2002)

Upon completion of the arterial anastomosis the distal clamp is released first and any major leaks should be dealt with by reapplying the clamp, irrigating, and inserting additional sutures.

4. Posttransplant arterial complications

In the early days of LDLT, the primary cause of postsurgical hepatic ischemia and failure used to be acute thrombosis of the HA with consecutive ischemia of the bile ducts and patch necrosis of the graft. Later, anastomotic stenosis of the HA has also been recognized as an important cause of posttransplant liver ischemia. An additional cause of graft ischemia is arterial steal syndrome, in which liver ischemia is caused by reduced blood flow through the HA rather than by obstruction. Other arterial complications are arterio-venous fistulas, anastomotic leakage, and intimal dissection.

Multivariate analysis of cases revealed that microsurgical experience was the only significant factor in reducing the incidence of HA complications in LDLT. (Matsuda et al., 2006)

In the face of donor organ shortage and high mortality related to liver re-transplantation, earlier detection of arterial complications using various imaging techniques followed by prompt revascularization as an alternative to re-transplant is very important.

4.1 Hepatic artery thrombosis (HAT)

Hepatic artery thrombosis (HAT) still remains the most devastating event that may occur in patients after LDLT, with a higher incidence than in patients with OLT. HAT most commonly occurs within the first postoperative week. There are three clinical presentations of the patient with HAT. The first one is fulminant hepatic necrosis with rapid clinical deterioration. In this situation HAT is the primary concern and the diagnosis should be actively pursued even when the US finding is negative. If focal parenchymal alterations such as infarcts or abscesses are seen with US, the diagnosis is certain in 90% cases. This is invariably fatal without transplantation. The second clinical presentation is the development of a delayed bile leak due to ischemic necrosis of the bile duct, a direct result of the HAT. Subhepatic fluid collections, frank bile peritonitis, bacteremia, and sepsis may occur. In milder cases, episodes of cholangitis, bile duct strictures, or segmental biliary dilatation are encountered. The third clinical presentation consists in relapsing bacteremia, gastrointestinal bleeding, fever of unknown origin, coagulopathy, or unexplained increase in liver enzymes.

When compared to adults, children have been reported to be at greater risk for HAT after pediatric LDLT due to small arterial size, nonuse of intraoperative microscope, and postoperative hypercoagulable state. LT recipients diagnosed with HAT have a relative risk of 90% for developing biliary complications. Up to 50% of patients with HAT may require retransplantation.

Surgical technique remains the primary cause for HAT, especially if thrombosis occurs within 2 months since transplantation. Surgical risk factors include small volume of graft or small arterial size in donor and/or recipient [specifically small recipient (< 10 kg or < 15 kg) or recipient artery (< 3 mm)], disparity in hepatic artery diameter between donor and recipient, the use of interposition, and tight anastomosis. In this category are also mentioned changes in hepatic arterial flow caused by tension, twisting, kinking, or compression of the vascular pedicle. Incriminated non-surgical causes for HAT are ABO-incompatible graft, anticardiolipin antibody in the recipient, cigarette smoking, prolonged cold ischemic time, acute rejection episodes, excessive intraoperative transfusion of clotting factor, coagulation abnormalities including heritable thrombophilia, absence of postoperative prophylactic anticoagulation, over-transfusion of fresh frozen plasma, high hematocrit levels, low donor/recipient age ratio, re-transplantation, and CMV infection.

The incidence of HAT has been reduced not only with the use of new and innovative surgical and microsurgical techniques (Aramaki et al., 2006) (Uchiyama et al., 2002), but also with posttransplantation administration of heparin, aspirin, alprostadil (PGE) (Heffron, et al., 2003), and/or gabexate mesilate (Miyagi et al., 2010). Overtransfusion of fresh-frozen plasma in high-risk patients (ABO incompatible) may be a critical factor in the development of HAT in LDLT. (Hatano et al., 1997) Although HA thrombosis is not always due to technical causes, some authors believe that when anastomosis is done correctly, no additional medication is necessary. (Takatsuki et al., 2006)

A proposed administration regime for heparin is 200 U/ kg of body weight per day for a period of 14 days. Administration of single dose of aspirin as low as 3 mg/kg will inactivate circulating platelets by acetylating the enzyme cyclooxigenase present in platelet wall and has a beneficial effect on anastomosis patency. Some authors proved that anticoagulation utilizing ASA and alprostadil is sufficient to avoid HAT in pediatric recepients. (Heffron et al., 2003) Dextran can be administered as 500 mL over 5 to 6 hours once daily for 3 to 5 days or 500 mL slowly over a 24 hour period. The allergic reactions can be avoided by administration of dextran 1 instead of dextran 40. When gabexate mesilate was administered as full-dose of 40 mg/kg/day no HAT occured. (Miyagi et al., 2010)

Doppler ultrasound (DUS) has been accepted as the best diagnostic tool for HAT and has surpassed angiography, which is invasive and time-consuming. Upon the completion of arterial anastomosis in LDLT an immediate intraoperative ultrasonography (IOUS) with 8-12-MHz linear transducer is mandatory both on gray-scale and Doppler study. HA anastomosis is identified on gray-scale US, and the diameter and percentage of stenosis of the anastomosis is measured. The HA is also evaluated to detect thrombus or dissection in the region of anastomosis. Doppler study of the graft HA is performed to search for the abnormal parameters (e.g. peak systolic velocity < 30 cm/s or > 2 m/s, resistive index (RI) < 0.5, and systolic acceleration time > 80 msec). (Mun et al., 2010) Intraoperative identification of arterial complication may impose arterial reanastomosis (Figure 6).

The sonographist must know the details of arterial anastomosis. In patients making an uneventful recovery, the arterial velocity tended to increase and the resistive index to decrease during the first postoperative week. (Stell et al., 2004) The peak systolic velocities, end-diastolic velocities, and resistive indices are associated with the length and caliber of the type of hepatic artery anastomosis used. End-to-end anastomoses are short and have a uniform small caliber; aortohepatic bypasses are longer and have a progressively by smaller caliber. (De Candia et al., 2002)

The normal hepatic artery shows a hepatopedal flow, with a systolic flow maximum greater than 30 cm/sec (Broering et al., 2004), a rapid systolic upstroke with an acceleration time

(time from end diastole to the first systolic peak) of less than 100 msec, and a continuous flow through diastole with a resistive index between 0.5 and 0.7 (Muradali & Wilson, 2005) (Figure 7).

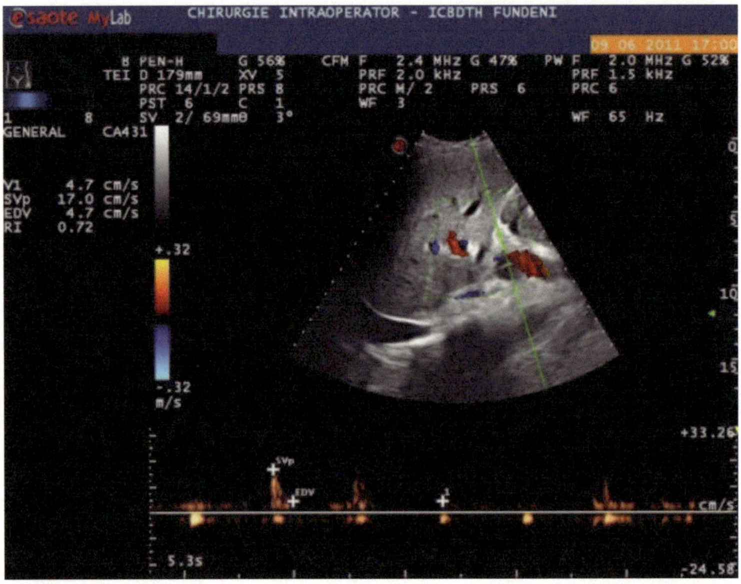

Fig. 6. IOUS with Doppler study. Resistive index (RI) 0.72 indicates stenosis of hepatic arterial anastomosis on a patient with right hepatic lobe transplantation. The intraoperator correction of arterial anastomosis was performed

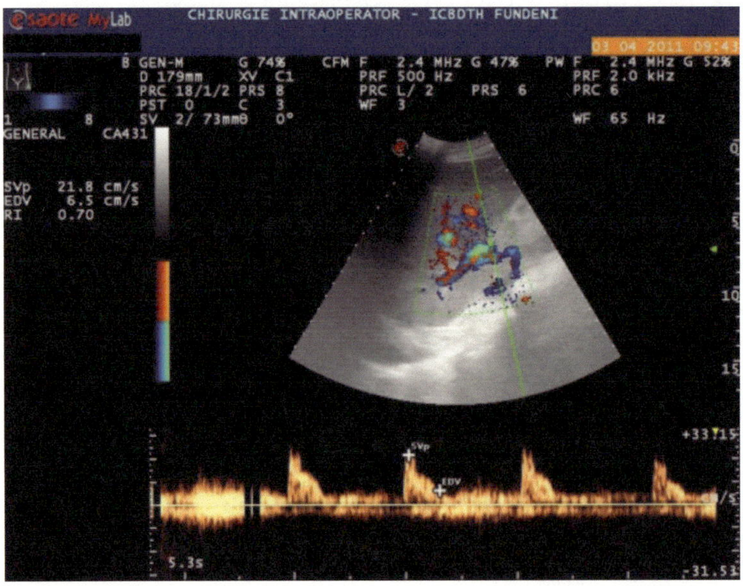

Fig. 7. Percutaneous DUS performed on a patient with right hepatic lobe transplantation on the third postoperative day shows a resistive index (RI) of hepatic artery at the upper limit of the normal. The outcome was favorable after i.v. infusion of Iloprost (Ilomedin®)

DUS has become the best diagnostic tool for HAT, thus surpassing angiography, which is invasive and time-consuming. Ultrasound can detect the absence of flow up to 92% of cases of hepatic artery thrombosis. Occasionally, a blunted waveform (tardus parvus arterial waveform) with resistive index < 0.5 and acceleration time > 100 ms may be obtained within the hepatic parenchyma. (Muradali & Wilson, 2005) This waveform is produced by collateral arterial vessels, which may develop as early as two weeks posttransplant. A false positive diagnostic of HAT may occur with severe hepatic edema, systemic hypotension, and high-grade hepatic artery stenosis. A diminished resistance index is an indication for an arteriogram.

Percutaneous DUS follow-up is scheduled daily during the first 2 weeks posttransplant, every other day on the third week, and twice a week thereafter until discharge. After discharge DUS should be done at intervals between 6 and 12 months. A diagnosis of vessel obstruction or thrombosis made by DUS (Figure 8) had to be confirmed by 3D CT angiography (Figure 9). (Okochi et al., 2010) In donors who underwent 2-in-1 segmental resection of the hepatic arteries, DUS is carried out on the second postoperative day and before discharge.

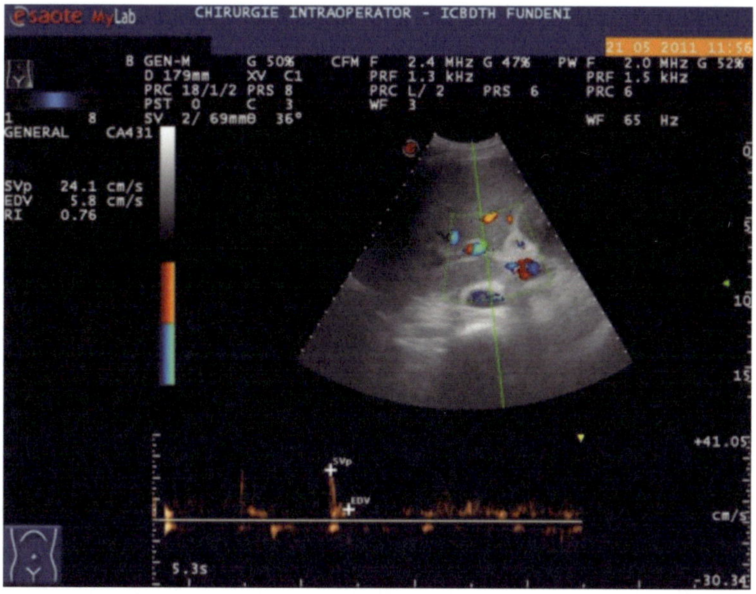

Fig. 8. Percutaneous DUS performed on a patient with right liver transplantation shows RI of 0.76 which is higher than normal suggesting HAT

DUS criteria for HAT include the following features: total absence of hepatic artery signal, absence of extrahepatic signal with intrahepatic low amplitude, delayed upstroke signal suggesting thrombosis with collateralization, direct visualization of abrupt loss of arterial signal in the extrahepatic arterial branches, visualization of arterial collaterals in the porta hepatis. Ancillary ultrasound findings that suggest HAT include parenchymal infarcts, intrahepatic bilomas or abscesses, or multifocal biliary dilatation.

Angiographic confirmation of HAT is needed if DUS diagnosis is equivocal.

Early detection of HAT by DUS with no suggestion of underlying clinical or biological factors is an indication for emergency revascularization with thrombectomy, which has

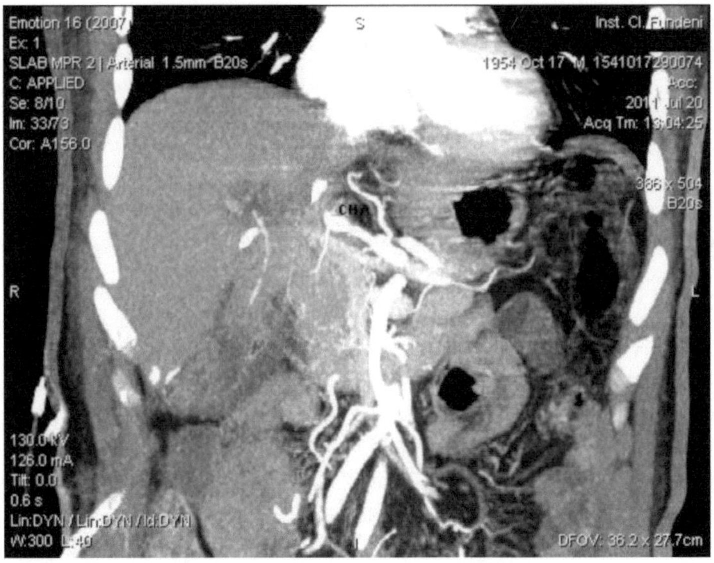

Fig. 9. 3D CT angiography confirmed complete stenosis of hepatic artery on a patient with right hepatic lobe transplantation

replaced retransplantation as the first treatment strategy for early HAT, with good rates of graft salvage and patient survival. (Nishida et al., 2002; Sakamoto et al., 1999) If recipient HA cannot be reanastomosed to the graft hepatic artery, other revascularization methods should be contemplated (e.g. anastomosis of hepatic artery with right gastroepiplooic artery (Tannuri et al., 2006), usage of a vein graft from the common iliac artery (Asakura et al., 2000) or recipient sigmoid artery (Inomoto et al., 1995).

In the past, early HAT after undergoing LT was considered uniformly fatal if the patient did not undergo urgent re-transplantation. Recently, the importance of urgent thrombectomy and revascularization has been reported. However, biliary complications, graft loss and late re-transplantation have tempered enthusiasm for this approach. The success of urgent revascularization clearly depends on early diagnosis and prompt intervention before the development of irreversible hepatic or biliary ischemia. The optimum treatment modality depends mostly on the condition of the patient, viability of the liver, availability of specific medical expertise, and availability of organ for re-transplantation, surgical revascularization, thrombolytic treatment, thrombectomy, and percutaneous transluminal balloon angioplasty with stent placement.

4.2 Hepatic arterial stenosis

Hepatic arterial stenosis (HAS) is the second most common arterial complication that occurs between few days to several months posttransplant. Critical hepatic artery stenosis (HAS) is considered mainly as a result of technical error and is characterized by 30% reduction in the diameter of the HA. HAS frequently progresses to thrombosis. In most cases it is caused by a technical failure. The incidence of HAS after LTx is reported to be 3 - 11%, although the introduction of microsurgery has significantly lowered the incidence of hepatic artery complications in the field of LDLT (Ulusal et al., 2006). More than 50% of HAS involve arterial anastomosis or graft artery (donor), while recipient artery stenosis is extremely rare.

The etiological factors for HAS are poor surgical technique, inappropriate angulation at the anastomotic site, clamp injury, excessive removal of the adventitia, intimal dissection, allograft rejection, or preservation injury, or the result of underlying liver disease. The risk factors for the development of HAS are a recipient weighing less than 10 kg, a long cold ischemic time, an insufficient inflow, a small diameter of the artery lumen, anatomic arterial variant, or repeated anastomosis.

The diagnostic procedure for HAS is DUS. Direct evidence of HAS involves identifying and localizing a hemodynamically significant narrowing within vessel. If the stenosis is significant, peak systolic velocities will be greater than 2-3 m/sec), with associated turbulent flow distally. Indirect evidence of HAS includes a tardus parvus waveform anywhere within the HA (resistive index < 0.5, acceleration time > 100 msec) and is more common seen in clinical practice. (Muradali & Wilson, 2005)

Angiographic confirmation is needed if DUS shows signs of HAS because therapy for HAS depends mainly on the location and length of the stenotic segment. Angiography is also needed if clinic suspicion of HAS is high despite a normal Doppler study.

Early diagnosis of HAS with deliberated follow-up of graft arterial circulation using DUS contributes to graft salvage by preventing graft infarction or devastating biliary ischemia, and thus the compensatory growth of abundant collateral arterial flow into the liver effects better outcome of the patient, even if the HA is stenosed. Angiographic confirmation is needed in cases where DUS screening shows signs of HAS. Management of HAS depends mainly on the location and length of the stenotic segment. The initial therapy for HAS should be medical treatment with anti-coagulants, vasodilators, hyperbaric oxygen administration and correction of dehydration until collateral vessels grow in the graft. If conservative treatment fails, an interventional procedure should be considered. In the first few days posttransplant, direct surgical re-anastomosis of the HA is occasionally possible. After the first postoperative week surgical reanastomosis is often difficult and unsuccessful because of fragile artery wall tissue. A substitute for surgery in relatively short HAS is percutaneous transluminal angioplasty (PTA) and stenting. Interventional radiology can be safely and successfully applied to the treatment of vascular complications using balloon dilatation (Tanaka et al., 1993) and/or stent placement techniques before graft dysfunction becomes irreversible. (Egawa, 2004) However major complications can occur (e.g. dehiscence of the surgical anastomoses if an inappropriate size of balloon catheter is used). Moreover the long-term results remain to be evaluated in the future with such approach of treatment.

Untreated HAS carries a high morbidity rate. HA PTA have better patency rates than those associated with hepatic artery stent placement. (Saad et al., 2005) If the treatment with PTA is ineffective or stenosis is extensive, surgical revision should be performed. Retransplantation is the last resort and is indicated if there are biliary complications.

4.3 Pseudoaneurysm of hepatic artery

Pseudoaneurysm of hepatic artery is seldom encountered, but when occurs, it may lead to serious life threatening complications of liver transplant, especially when it ruptures. It usually develops at the site of the arterial anastomosis as result of a technical error or bacterial or fungal infection. If located intrahepatic, it indicates a relation to a needle biopsy of the transplanted liver. The rupture of an intrahepatic false aneurysm may lead toward the formation of an arterio-portal fistula with subsequent development of hyperkinetic portal hypertension. If a pseudoaneurysm perforates into the bile ducts, it can cause hematobilia, severe shock, or even death. Consequently, bacterial and fungal infections are also a serious threat. Diagnosis of pseudoaneurysm of hepatic artery requires a high degree of suspicion. On gray-scale ultrasound, pseudoaneurysm appears as a cystic (anechoic) periportal structure, with intense swirling flow on DUS and a disorganized spectral waveform. DUS and CT may miss the diagnosis. (Tobben et al., 1988) Any suspicion of a hepatic aneurysm mandates arteriography during which a stent placement or transcatheter arterial coil embolization of the aneurysm can be performed. (Maleux et al., 2005)

The surgical therapeutic options include: (1) resection of the pseudoaneurysm and ligation of the hepatic artery, as long as sufficient collateral circulation into the graft within 1 month after transplantation can be anticipated; (2) reconstruction of the hepatic artery using autograft interposition or bypass (e.g. cadaveric iliac artery conduit between the donor hepatic artery and the recipient aorta) (Jarzembowski et al., 2008) only if the perioperative site is not contaminated; (3) retransplantation. In anticipation of such unpredictable complication, it might be useful to preserve both hepatic arteries of the recipient in adequate length and shape.

4.4 Arterial steal syndrome

Arterial steal syndrome is a significant problem after liver transplantation and is characterized by arterial hypoperfusion of the graft, which is caused by a shift in blood flow into other arteries that originate from the same trunk. Most cases of steal syndrome are associated with the splenic artery which has been reported in 3.2-4% of patients. The onset of the splenic artery steal syndrome, which varies among patients, may occur either during the first few hours after liver transplantation or as late as several weeks after transplantation. If the hyperdynamic state does not improve immediately after liver transplantation, reduced splenic arterial resistance and increased splenic arterial flow may divert celiac blood flow into the spleen. In some patients, swelling of the liver develops as a result of preservation injury, which usually causes increased intrahepatic arterial resistance and further diversion of blood flow away from the hepatic artery into the splenic artery. In other patients it may be more related to the progressive increase in splenic arterial flow caused by the pre-surgical hyperdynamic state, with or without the development of clinical hypersplenism. Development of splenic artery steal syndrome might also be related to pre-surgical increased splenic arterial flow that is not clinically significant at the time of transplantation but is exacerbated by the rejection of the graft or by viral hepatitis. Cases of gastroduodenal artery steal syndrome have also been reported.

Dramatic recovery of the graft and LFTs after cessation of the steal makes it mandatory to consider this condition in the differential diagnosis of postoperative hepatic dysfunction.

Arterial steal syndrome is suggested by elevated levels of liver enzymes and the results of DUS and computed tomographic angiography. In steal syndrome hepatic artery is patent but characterized by sluggish flow. The filling of the intrahepatic arterial branches by contrast material is delayed in comparison with the filling of other branches of the celiac trunk. Poor peripheral hepatic parenchymal perfusion is associated with early and abundant filling of the splenic or left gastric artery, which also shows increased size and flow. The diagnosis is confirmed by angiography.

Angiography offers the possibility of therapy by transcatheter splenic or left gastric artery occlusion with metallic coils or by placement of an endoluminal narrowing stent. The result is checked by angiography. In each patient, vital signs should be monitored, LFTs reassessed, and DUS scheduled twice a day for 2 days and then once a day for 1 week. Significant recovery of the graft and LFTs after cessation of the steal syndrome makes mandatory to consider it in the differential diagnosis of postoperative hepatic dysfunction.

5. Conclusions

Anatomical variability is the rule rather than the exception in liver transplantation. Hepatic arterial reconstruction is one of the most difficult procedures in LDLT. HA reconstruction in LDLT is more complex in left grafts when compared with right grafts due to a higher incidence of multiple arteries in the former. This problem is surmounted by meticulous perioperative planning, intraoperative surgical innovations, and postoperative close follow-up. Currently, dynamic contrast material–enhanced CT and MR imaging have replaced other imaging tests for preoperative evaluation. Surgeons who perform hepatic arterial reconstruction in LDLT should be highly trained in microvascular techniques. In LDLT with right lobe microvascular arterial anastomosis is not necessary, and vascular complications should be infrequent. In LDLT with left liver microsurgical techniques are a requisite that enables the reconstruction of arteries with reduced diameter or caliber difference, and thus decreases arterial complications. With the implementation of broadly applicable, practical, surgical techniques for arterial reconstruction, LDLT would be less laborious and with more consistent results and no contraindication for LDLT should be affirmed based on anatomical variants of arterial vasculature of the liver. Close surveillance of the vascular anastomoses and multidisciplinary approach to the treatment of vascular complication after LRLT considerably reduces graft loss and patient mortality. Gray-scale sonography coupled with color Doppler is the best first intention screening examination to be performed after hepatic transplantation. Arteriography not only remains the key examination for the diagnosis and evaluation of these complications but also has proved to be a graft-saving approach in the treatment of arterial complications.

6. References

Cheng, Y.F.; Chen, C.L.; Huang, T.L.; Chen, T.Y.; Lee, T.Y.; Chen, Y.S.; Wang, C.C.; de, Villa, V., Goto, S.; Chiang, Y.C.; Eng, H.L.; Jawan, B. & Cheung, H.K. Single imaging modality evaluation of living donors in liver transplantation: magnetic resonance imaging. *Transplantation*, Vol.72, No.9 , (November 2001), pp:1527-1533, ISSN 1534-0608

Coskun, M.; Kayahan, E.M.; Ozbek, O.; Cakir, B.; Dalgic, A. & Haberal, M. Imaging of hepatic arterial anatomy for depicting vascular variations in living related liver transplant donor candidates with multidetector computed tomography: comparison with conventional angiography. *Transplant Proc*, Vol.37, No.2, (March 2005), pp:1070-1073, ISSN 0041-1345

De Candia, A.; Como, G.; Tedeschi, L.; Zanardi, R.; Vergendo, M.; Rositani, P. & Bazzocchi, M. Color Doppler sonography of hepatic artery reconstruction in liver transplantation. *Journal Clinical Ultrasound*, Vol.30, No.1, (January 2002), pp:12-17, ISSN 1097-0096

Di Benedetto, F.; Lauro, A.; Masetti, M.; Cautero, N.; Quintini, C.; Dazzi, A.; Ramacciato, G.; Risaliti, A.; Miller, C.M. & Pinna, A.D. Use of a branch patch with the cystic artery in living-related liver transplantation. *Clin Transplant*, Vol.18, No.4, (August 2004), pp:480-483, ISSN 1399-0012

Egawa H. [Application of interventional radiology for stenosis of vascular anastomosis in living-donor liver transplantation]. *Nippon Geka Gakkai Zasshi*, Vol.105, No.6, (June 2004), pp:364-368, ISSN 0301-4894

Enne, M.; Pacheco-Moreira, L.; Balbi, E.; Cerqueira, A.; Alves, J.; Valladares, M.A.; Santalucia, G. & Martinho, J.M. Hepatic artery reconstruction in pediatric living donor liver transplantation under 10 kg, without microscope use. *Pediatr Transplant*, Vol.14, No.1, (February 2010), pp:48-51, ISSN 1399-3046

Ersoz, S.; Tuzuner, A.; Hazinedaroglu, S.; Karayalcin, K.; Yerdel, M.A. & Anadol, E. Could the use of interposition grafts for arterial reconstruction be avoided by more caudate graft placement in living donor liver transplantation? *Transplant Proc*, Vol.35, No.4, (June 2003), pp:1427-1429, ISSN 0041-1345

Guarrera, J.V.; Sinha, P.; Lobritto, S.J.; Brown, R.S. Jr., Kinkhabwala, M. & Emond, J.C. Microvascular hepatic artery anastomosis in pediatric segmental liver transplantation: microscope vs loupe. *Transpl Int*, Vol.17, No. 10, (November 2004), pp:585-588, ISSN 1432-2277

Haberal, M.; Sevmis, S.; Karakayali, H.; Moray, G.; Yilmaz, U.; Ozcay, F.; Torgay, A.; Aydogan, C. & Arslan, G. A novel technique for hepatic arterial reconstruction in living-donor liver transplant. *Exp Clin Transplant*, Vol.5, No. 1, (June 2007), pp:585-589, ISSN 1304-0855

Heffron, T.G.; Pillen, T.; Welch, D.; Smallwood, G.A.; Redd, D. & Romero, R. Hepatic artery thrombosis in pediatric liver transplantation. *Transplant Proc*, Vol.35, No.4, 2003, (June 2003), pp:1447-1448, ISSN 0041-1345

Ikegami, T.; Masuda, Y.; Ohno, Y.; Urata, K.; Nakazawa, Y.; Miwa, S.; Hashikura, Y. & Miyagawa, S. Arterial reconstruction in a case of subintimal dissection of celiac arterial tributaries in living donor liver transplantation: a case report. *Transplant Proc*, Vol.40, No.10, (December 2008); pp:3794-3796, ISSN 0041-1345

Inomoto, T.; Nishizawa, F.; Sasaki, H.; Terajima, H.; Shirakata, Y.; Miyamoto, S.; Nagata, I.; Fujimoto, M.; Moriyasu, F.; Tanaka, K. & Yamaoka, Y. Experiences of 120 microsurgical reconstructions of hepatic artery in living related liver transplantation. *Surgery*, Vol.119, No.1, (January 1996), pp:20-26, ISSN 0039-6060

Inomoto, T.; Nishizawa, F.; Terajima, H.; Shirakata, Y.; Yamamoto, Y.; Miyamoto, S.; Fujimoto, M.; Tanaka, K. & Yamaoka, Y. The use of the recipient sigmoid artery for a revision of hepatic arterial reconstruction after thrombosis in living related liver transplantation. *Transplantation*, Vol:60, No.8, (Octomber 1995), pp:881-882, ISSN 0041-1337

Jarzembowski, T.M.; Sankary, H.N.; Bogetti, D.; Manzelli, A.; Ong, E.; Oberholzer, J.; Benedetti, E. & Testa, G. Living donor liver graft salvage after rupture of hepatic artery pseudoaneurysm. *Int Surg*, Vol.93, No.5, (September 2008), pp:300-303, ISSN 0020-8868

Johnson, P.T. & Fishman, E.K. IV contrast selection for MDCT: current thoughts and practice. *AJR Am J Roentgenol*, Vol.186, No.2, (February 2006), pp:406-415, ISSN 031-803X

Kamei, H.; Fujimoto, Y.; Yamamoto, H.; Nagai, S.; Kamei, Y. & Kiuchi T. The use of radial artery interpositional graft between recipient splenic artery and graft artery in living donor liver transplantation. *Transpl Int*, Vol.19, No. 11, (November 2006), pp:945-946, ISSN 1432-2277

Kasahara, M.; Sakamoto, S.; Ogawa, K.; Uryuhara, K.; Matsuoka, J.; Uchida, Y.; Ito, T.; Ueda, M. &Tanaka K. The use of a mesenteric artery of Roux-en-Y limb for hepatic arterial reconstruction after living-donor liver transplantation. *Transplantation,* Vol.80, No.4, (August 2005), pp:538, ISSN 1543-0608

Lee, C.C.; Jeng, L.B.; Li, P.C.; Yang, H.R.; Lu, C.W.; Chen, T.H.; Cheng, H.T.; Chang, S.C.; Lin, M.S.; Poon, K.S.; Chen, Y.F. & Ho, Y.J. Innovative technique to reconstruct two branches of the right hepatic artery in living donor liver transplantation. *Transplant Proc,* Vol.40, No.8, (October 2008), pp:2525-2526, ISSN 0041-1345

Lehar, S.C.; Zajko, A.B.; Koneru, B.; Stevenson, W. & Sumkin J. Splenic infarction complicating pediatric liver transplantation: incidence and CT appearance. *J Comput Assist Tomogr,* Vol.14, No.3, (May 1990), pp:362-365, ISSN 1532-3145

Macdonald, D.B.; Haider, M.A.; Khalili, K.; Kim, T.K.; O'Malley, M.; Greig, P.D.; Grant, D.R.; Lockwood, G. & Cattral MS. Relation between vascular and biliary anatomy in living liver donors. *AJR Am J Roentgenol,* Vol.185, No.1, (July 2005), pp:247-252, ISSN 0361-803X

Maleux, G.; Pirenne, J.; Aerts, R. & Nevens, F. Case report: hepatic artery pseudoaneurysm after liver transplantation: definitive treatment with a stent-graft after failed coil embolisation. *Br J Radiol,* Vol.78, No.929, (May 2005), pp:453-456, ISSN 0007-1285

Margreiter, C.; Aigner, F.; Orozco, H.; Wechselberger, G.; Ollinger, R.; Bosmuller, C.; Sucher, R.; Mark, W. & Margreiter, R. Hepatic artery reconstruction with inferior mesenteric vein graft in pediatric living donor liver transplantation. *Pediatr Transplant,* Vol.12, No.3, (May 2008), pp:324-328, ISSN ISSN 1399-3046

Matsuda, H.; Yagi, T.; Sadamori, H.; Matsukawa, H.; Shinoura, S.; Murata, H; Umeda, Y. & Tanaka N. Complications of arterial reconstruction in living donor liver transplantation: a single-center experience. *Surg Today,* Vol.36, No.3, (2006), pp:245-251, ISSN 0941-1291

Miyagi, S.; Enomoto, Y.; Sekiguchi, S.; Kawagishi, N.; Sato, A.; Fujimori, K. & Satomi, S. Microsurgical back wall support suture technique with double needle sutures on hepatic artery reconstruction in living donor liver transplantation. *Transplant Proc,* Vol.40, No.8, (October 2008), pp:2521-2522, ISSN 0041-1345

Mun, H.S.; Kim, K.W.; Song, G.W.; Ahn, C.S.; Kim, S.Y; Hwang, S. & Lee, S.G. Evaluation of the hepatic artery anastomosis by intraoperative sonography with high-frequency transducer in right-lobe graft living donor liver transplantation. *Journal Clinical Ultrasound,* Vol.38, No.1, (January 2010), pp:10-16, ISSN 1097-0096

Muradali, D. & Wilson, S. (2005). Organ transplantation, In *Diagnostic ultrasound,* Rumack, C.; Wilson, S.; Charboneau, J., (Eds), 657-701, Elsevier Mosby, ISBN 0323020232

Okochi, M; Ueda, K.; Hirose, T.; Okochi, H.; Watanabe, H.; Suzuki, Y. & Kajikawa A. A modified technique for hepatic artery reconstruction in living donor liver transplantation. *Microsurgery,* Vol.30, No.7, (October 2010), pp:541-544, ISSN 0738-1085

Renz, J.F. & Busuttil, R.W. Adult-to-adult living-donor liver transplantation: a critical analysis. *Semin Liver Dis,* Vol.20, No.4, (2000), pp:411-424, ISSN 0272-8087

Saad, W.E.; Davies, M.G.; Sahler, L.; Lee, D.E.; Patel, N.C.; Kitanosono, T.; Sasson, T. & Waldman, D.L. Hepatic artery stenosis in liver transplant recipients: primary treatment with percutaneous transluminal angioplasty. *J Vasc Interv Radiol,* Vol.16, No.6, (June 2005), pp:795-805, ISSN 1051-0443

Sahani, D.; D'souza, R.; Kadavigere, R.; Hertl, M.; McGowan, J.; Saini, S. & Mueller, P.R. Evaluation of living liver transplant donors: method for precise anatomic definition by using a dedicated contrast-enhanced MR Imaging Protocol. *RadioGraphics*, Vol.24, No.4, (July0August 2004), pp: 957-967 ISSN 02171-5333

Sakamoto, Y.; Harihara, Y.; Nakatsuka, T.; Kawarasaki, H.; Takayama, T.; Kubota, K.; Kimura, W.; Kita, Y.; Tanaka, H.; Ito, M.; Hashizume, K. & Makuuchi M. Rescue of liver grafts from hepatic artery occlusion in living-related liver transplantation. *Br J Surg*, Vol.86, No.7, (July 1999), pp:886-889, ISSN 0007-1323

Stell, D.; Downey, D.; Marotta, P.; Solano, E.; Khakhar, A.; Quan, D.; Ghent, C.; McAlister, V. & Wall W. Prospective evaluation of the role of quantitative Doppler ultrasound surveillance in liver transplantation. *Liver Transpl*, Vol.10, No.9, (September 2004), pp:1183-1188, ISSN 1527-6465

Stemmler, B.J.; Paulson, E.K.; Thornton, F.J.; Winters, S.R.; Nelson, R.C. & Clary, B.M. Dual-phase 3D MDCT angiography for evaluation of the liver before hepatic resection. *AJR Am J Roentgenol*, Vol.183, No.6, (December 2004), pp:1551-1557, ISSN 0361-803X

Tanaka, K.; Uemoto, S.; Tokunaga, Y.; Fujita, S.; Sano, K.; Nishizawa, T.; Sawada, H.; Shirahase, I.; Kim, H.J. & Yamaoka, Y. Surgical techniques and innovations in living related liver transplantation. *Ann Surg*, Vol.217, No.1, (January 1993), pp:82-91, ISSN 0003-4932

Tannuri, U.; Maksoud-Filho, J.G.; Silva, M.M.; Suzuki, L.; Santos, M.M.; Gibelli, N.E.; Ayoub, A.A.; Velhote, M.C.; Pinho-Apezzato, M.L. & Maksoud, J.G. An alternative method of arterial reconstruction in pediatric living donor liver transplantation with the recipient right gastroepiploic artery. *Pediatr Transplant*, Vol.10, No.1, (February 2006), pp:101-104, ISSN 1399-3046

Tobben, P.J.; Zajko, A.B.; Sumkin, J.H.; Bowen, A.; Fuhrman, C.R.; Skolnick, M.L.; Bron, K.M.; Esquivel, C.O. & Starzl T.E. Pseudoaneurysms complicating organ transplantation: roles of CT, duplex sonography, and angiography. *Radiology*, Vol.169, No.1, (October 1988), pp:65-70, ISSN 0033-8419

Uchiyama, H.; Harada, N.; Sanefuji, K.; Kayashima, H.; Taketomi, A.; Soejima, Y.; Ikegami, T.; Shimada, M. & Maehara, Y. Dual hepatic artery reconstruction in living donor liver transplantation using a left hepatic graft with 2 hepatic arterial stumps. *Surgery*, Vol.147, No.6, (June 2010), pp:878-886, ISSN 0039-6060

Uchiyama, H.; Hashimoto, K.; Hiroshige, S.; Harada, N.; Soejima, Y.; Nishizaki, T.; Shimada, M. & Suehiro, T. Hepatic artery reconstruction in living-donor liver transplantation: a review of its techniques and complications. *Surgery*, Vol.131, No.1 Suppl, (January 2002), pp:S200-S204, ISSN 0039-6060

Uchiyama, H.; Ikegami, T.; Soejima, Y.; Ninomiya, M.; Kayashima, H.; Taketomi, A.; Shirabe, K. & Maehara, Y. Use of recipient's left hepatic artery for artery reconstruction in right lobe living donor liver transplantation with duct-to-duct anastomosis. *Transplantation*, Vol.89, No.8, (April 2010), pp:1016-1021, ISSN 1534-0608

Uchiyama, H.; Shirabe, K.; Taketomi, A.; Soejima, Y.; Ninomiya, M.; Kayashima, H.; Ikegami, T. & Maehara, Y. Extra-anatomical hepatic artery reconstruction in living donor liver transplantation: can this procedure save hepatic grafts? *Liver Transpl*, Vol.16, No.9, (September 2010), pp:1054-1061, ISSN 1527-6465

Ulusal, B.G.; Cheng, M.H.; Ulusal, A.E.; Lee, W.C. & Wei, F.C. Collaboration with microsurgery prevents arterial complications and provides superior success in partial liver transplantation. *Microsurgery*, Vol.26, No.7, (2006), pp:490-497, ISSN 0738-1085

3

Microvascular Hepatic Artery Reconstruction in Living Donor Liver Transplantation

Hideaki Uchiyama et al.*
Department of Surgery and Science, Graduate School of Medical Sciences, Kyushu University
Japan

1. Introduction

Even with the recent technical advances in the surgical procedures used for living donor liver transplantation (LDLT), hepatic artery reconstruction is still one of the most difficult procedures in LDLT (Matsuda et al., 2006; Eguchi et al., 2008). Because hepatic artery complications in liver transplantation, such as hepatic artery thrombosis (HAT) or hepatic artery dissection (HAD), often lead to devastating consequences, such as graft loss or patient death (Yanaga et al., 1990a; Settmacher et al., 2000; Stange et al., 2003), hepatic artery reconstruction should be performed using the most reliable procedure. A graft hepatic artery to be reconstructed in LDLT usually has a narrower caliber and a shorter stump compared to the arteries used during cadaveric liver transplantation. We introduced microvascular surgery for hepatic artery reconstruction in LDLT at the beginning of our LDLT program (Uchiyama et al., 2002). The use of microvascular surgery in LDLT was first reported in 1992 (Mori et al., 1992). Thereafter, many transplant centers introduced this technique for hepatic artery reconstruction in LDLT and confirmed that its application to hepatic artery reconstruction in LDLT decreased the number of hepatic artery complications (Inomoto, et al., 1996; Millis et al., 2000; Wei et al., 2004; Takatsuki et al., 2006; Panossian et al., 2009). We performed 401 cases of LDLT between October 1996 and June 2011 and almost all hepatic artery reconstructions were performed by microvascular surgery under a microscope. Microvascular surgery for hepatic artery reconstruction has been performed by general surgeons in our department. In this chapter, we present our microvascular surgical techniques used for hepatic artery reconstructions in LDLT and the outcomes of these reconstructions in 401 LDLT cases.

2. Preoperative anatomical evaluation of graft hepatic arteries

In our early experience, the donors underwent invasive conventional angiography to assess the anatomy of the hepatic arteries. Now, we use only CT angiography for the assessment of the donor's hepatic artery anatomy. Current CT angiography methods can be used to assess the donor's hepatic artery anatomy preoperatively with almost 100% accuracy (Saylisoy et

* Ken Shirabe, Akinobu Taketomi, Yuji Soejima, Tomoharu Yoshizumi, Toru Ikegami, Noboru Harada, Hiroto Kayashima and Yoshihiko Maehara

al., 2005; Apisarnthanarak et al., 2011). Graft hepatic arteries are usually reconstructed using the recipient hepatic arterial branches (Fig. 1).

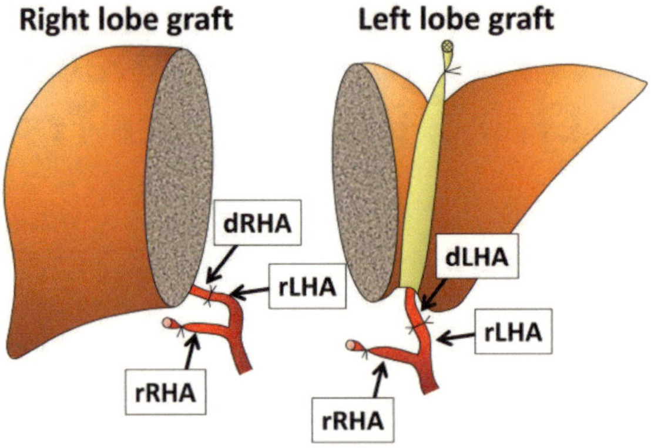

Fig. 1. A schematic diagram of hepatic artery reconstruction. dLHA, left hepatic artery of the donor; dRHA, right hepatic artery of the donor; rLHA, left hepatic artery of the recipient; rRHA, right hepatic artery of the recipient

When assessing the donor's hepatic artery anatomy, the most important consideration is to precisely predict how many hepatic arterial stumps there will be on a graft (Fig. 2). Sometimes, a hepatic graft has multiple hepatic arterial stumps, which usually have a very narrow caliber (Uchiyama et al., 2010a). Thus, LDLT using such graft makes hepatic artery reconstruction difficult. Some transplant surgeons regard such a graft as a contraindication for LDLT (Broelsch et al., 1991; Kostelic et al., 1996), and others have reported various arterial manipulations in donors that can be used to make the hepatic artery reconstruction easier (Takatsuki et al., 2006; Douard et al., 2002). On rare occasions, a hepatic graft is expected to have three or more hepatic arterial stumps by CT angiography, in which hepatic artery reconstructions are extremely difficult. In such cases, the other side graft (i.e., right lobe) or a graft from another donor may be selected.

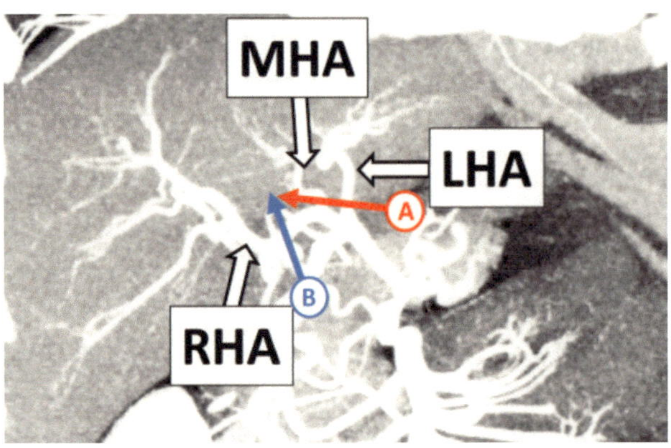

Fig. 2. The results of a CT angiographic examination of a donor. The arrow (A) indicates the dividing point of the middle and left hepatic arteries when the left lobe graft is selected, while the arrow (B) indicates the dividing point of the right hepatic artery. LHA, left hepatic artery; MHA, middle hepatic artery; RHA, right hepatic artery

3. Preparation of graft hepatic arteries for hepatic artery reconstruction

The arterial flows into the donor's remnant liver should never be compromised. In procuring a graft liver, special care should be paid not to make wall dissections of graft arteries by ligating the proximal site of the hepatic artery with excessive force, because wall dissection of the arterial stump is usually irreparable. On the backtable, it is not necessary to flush the graft artery with preservation solution because the preservation time is very short in LDLT. In fact, cannulating a flushing tube into the narrow graft artery increases the risk of making a wall dissection. Furthermore, there is no need to trim the graft artery on the backtable.

After the portal vein is reperfused and hemostasis is obtained to a certain degree, microvascular hepatic artery reconstruction is started. The micro-instruments and the microscope we usually use are shown in Figs. 3 and 4, respectively. Microvascular hepatic artery reconstruction is performed by 3 surgeons (Fig. 5). The primary surgeon and the first assistant face each other looking into the lens of the microscope. The second assistant exposes the surgical field.

First, the hepatic graft is brought up or rotated in a proper position to fully visualize the graft hepatic arteries (Fig. 6). The graft hepatic arteries in a right lobe graft usually exist deep in the right subdiaphragmatic space. By putting several piles of folded gauze under the graft liver, the graft artery is brought up, which makes the hepatic artery reconstruction easier. The graft hepatic arteries in a left lobe graft are usually covered by the graft itself. By pulling the round ligament upward or using a brain retractor, the graft hepatic artery can be exposed. It is very difficult to expose the graft hepatic arteries on a lateral graft used for small infants because of the very small abdominal cavity relative to the hepatic graft. However, by rotating the graft liver clockwise and pushing it into the left subdiaphragmatic space made by pulling down the spleen, the graft hepatic artery can be exposed.

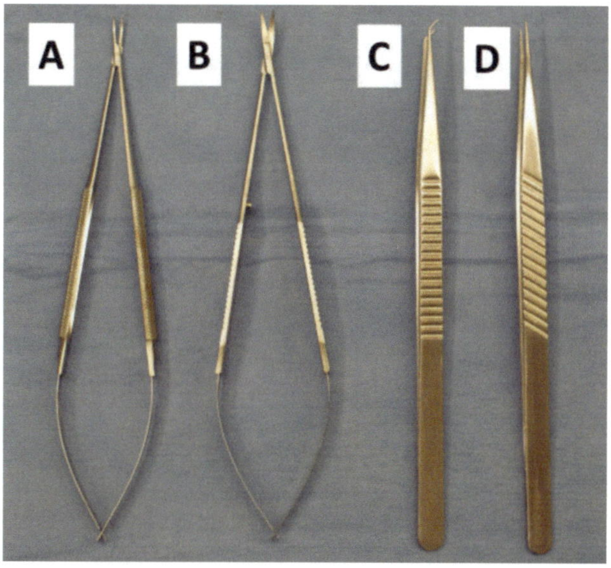

Fig. 3. Instruments used for microvascular hepatic artery reconstruction (A) Needle holder (Aesculap, FD245R). (B) Micro scissors (Aesculap, FD023R). (C) Angulated micro forceps (S & T, JFAL-3-18). (D) Straight micro forceps (S & T, JF-3-18)

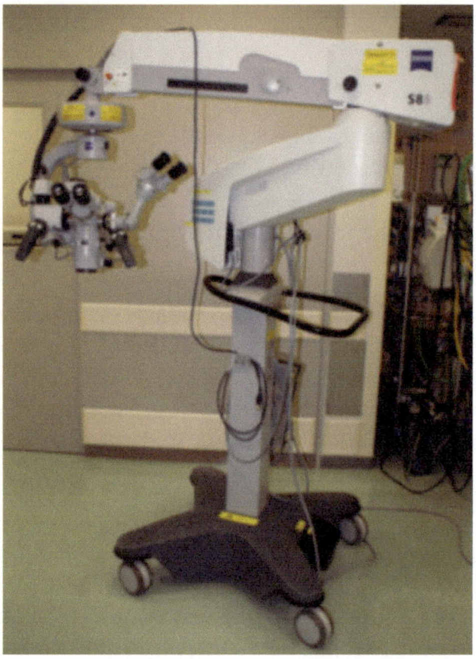

Fig. 4. The surgical microscope used for microvascular hepatic artery reconstruction (Carl Zeiss, OPMI VARIO S88). This microscope has a foot pedal. The surgeon can adjust the microscope using this foot pedal without interrupting the procedure

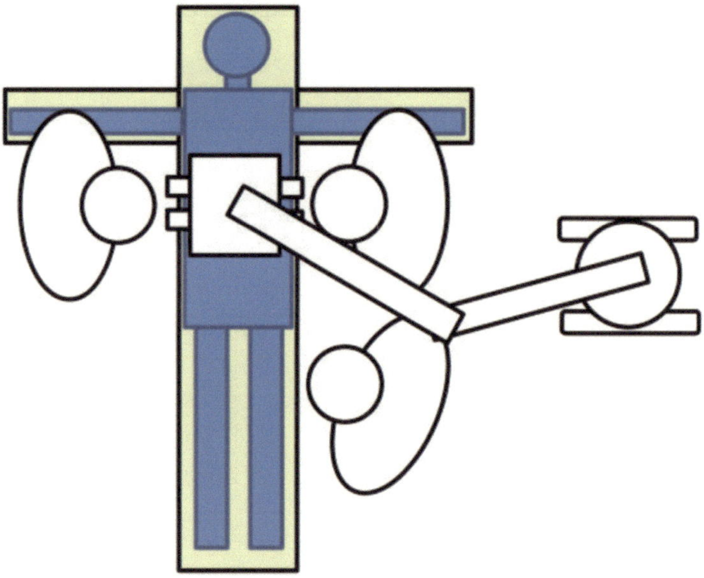

Fig. 5. The positioning of the microvascular surgeons. The primary surgeon stands on the right side of the recipient. The first assistant stands on the left side of a recipient, looking into the other lens of a microscope. The second assistant stands next to the first assistant and exposes the surgical field

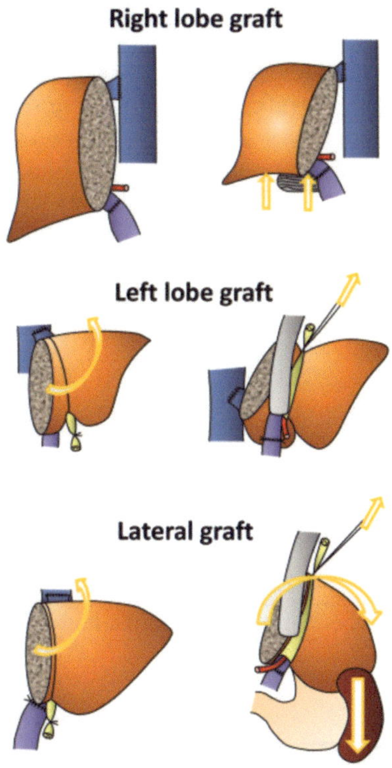

Fig. 6. The positioning of the hepatic grafts required to visualize the graft hepatic artery. Hepatic grafts are positioned in order to fully expose the graft arteries

In preparing the graft hepatic arteries for anastomosis, they should be gently manipulated so as not to injure the arterial wall (Fig. 7). When a surgeon wants to move the arterial stump, only the surrounding connective tissue should be grasped.

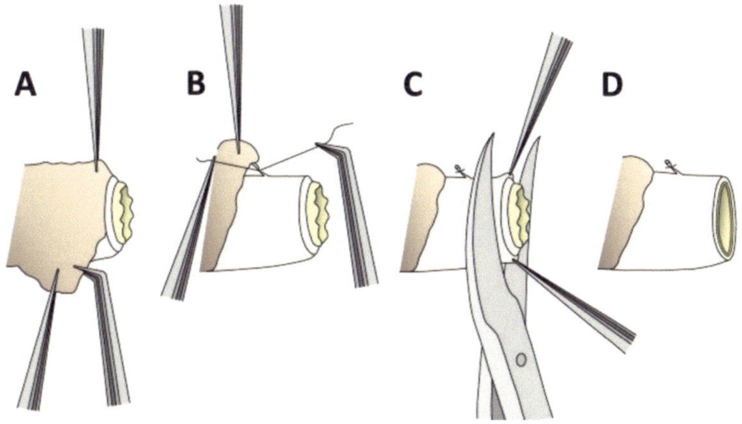

Fig. 7. Preparation of the graft hepatic artery. (A) The outer surrounding connective tissue is removed from the artery. (B) Sometimes, small branches are encountered. These are ligated with 8-0 Prolene™ string and cut. (C) The edge of the arterial stump is trimmed off. (D) Then, the graft hepatic artery is ready to be anastomosed

4. Preparation of recipient hepatic arteries for hepatic artery reconstruction

The recipient arteries to be used for hepatic artery reconstruction are usually hepatic arterial branches, such as the left hepatic artery, the middle hepatic artery, and the right hepatic artery. First, we determine how many graft hepatic arteries should be reconstructed. In our experience, 28% of hepatic grafts have two or more graft hepatic arteries (Table 1).

Most of them are left hepatic grafts. Despite the greater difficulty of hepatic artery reconstruction when selecting left hepatic grafts with multiple hepatic arteries, we prefer to use a left hepatic graft because it increases donor's safety (Nishizaki et al., 2001; Soejima et al., 2006; Taketomi et al., 2009).

Graft type No. of arterial stumps	N	No. of reconstructed arteries	N (total number of reconstructed arteries)
Left lateral	**33**		
One stump	27	One reconstruction	27 (27)
Two stumps	6	One reconstruction	3 (3)
		Two reconstructions	3 (6)
Left	**240**		
One stump	146	No reconstruction	1 (0)
		One reconstruction	145 (145)
Two stumps	88	One reconstruction	30 (30)
		Two reconstructions	58 (116)
Three strumps	6	One reconstruction	1 (1)
		Two reconstructions	2 (4)
		Three reconstructions	3 (9)
Right	**124**		
One stump	117	One reconstruction	117 (117)
Two stumps	7	One reconstruction	0 (0)
		Two reconstructions	7 (14)
Posterior	**5**		
One stump	5	One reconstruction	5 (5)
Total	402		(477)

Table 1. A summary of hepatic artery reconstruction. Note: Because one recipient received dual grafts, the total number of hepatic grafts is 402 in 401 LDLTs

Most of the reported donor deaths are the result of right hepatic lobe donation (Miller et al., 2004; Akabayashi et al., 2004; Trotter et al., 2006; Ghobrial et al., 2008). Although some surgeons have stated that it is not always necessary for all graft hepatic arteries to be reconstructed when backflows are observed from the second graft hepatic artery after reconstruction of the first artery (Ikegami et al., 1996; Kubota et al., 2000) because of the collateral arterial blood supply of the liver (Plengvanit et al., 1972), our policy for a graft with two or more graft hepatic arteries is that all graft hepatic arteries should be reconstructed if it is technically feasible (Uchiyama, 2010a). Incomplete hepatic artery reconstruction may result in relative arterial ischemia in a hepatic graft, which leads to biliary stricture, abscess formation, and so on (Yanaga, et al. 1990b; Suehiro, et al. 2002).

To increase the number of candidate recipient hepatic arteries and in cases of very short graft hepatic arteries, the recipient hepatic arterial branches must be divided as peripherally as possible. When dividing hepatic arterial branches, a surgeon should pay special attention not to make a wall dissection. Patients with end-stage liver disease have enlarged hepatic arteries to compensate for their decreased portal venous flow, and as a result, they tend to have fragile hepatic arterial walls. Once an arterial wall dissection occurs, it often extends to the proximal celiac trunk and none of the tributary arteries of the celiac trunk can then be used for hepatic artery reconstruction. To avoid this devastating complication, we first gently tie a hepatic artery, then we place the second knot with a relatively secure force just above the first knot. The artery is then divided just above the second knot.

In selecting which hepatic arterial branch to use as an inflow artery, we prefer to use the left hepatic artery (Uchiyama et al., 2010b). Patients with end-stage liver disease usually have a relatively large left hepatic arteries, of the proper size for hepatic artery reconstruction, because of the compensation for the decreased portal venous flow. Furthermore, our first choice for biliary reconstruction is currently duct-to-duct biliary reconstruction, which makes hepatic artery reconstructions using the recipient right hepatic artery relatively difficult. The recipient bile duct is partly nourished by small branches of the right hepatic artery. To make the right hepatic artery easy to use for reconstruction, the connective tissues between the common hepatic duct and the right hepatic artery are somewhat divided, which may disrupt those small nourishing arteries flowing into the common hepatic duct (Chen et al., 1999; Gunji et al., 2006). The ischemia of the bile duct is considered to be one of the leading causes of anastomotic biliary stricture (Fan et al., 2002). On the other hand, if the connective tissue is untouched for fear of disrupting the nourishing arteries, not only is it more difficult to reconstruct the hepatic artery using the right hepatic artery because the right hepatic artery does not have good flexibility, but also there will be a kink at the anastomosis site after performing duct-to-duct anastomosis.

When the recipient hepatic arterial branches cannot be used for an inflow artery, as in the case of a stiff arterial wall caused by repeated transarterial chemoembolization for hepatocellular carcinoma (Lin et al., 2009), or intraoperative arterial injury, a surgeon should use any recipient arteries other than hepatic arterial branches, such as the gastric arteries (Wang et al., 2008; Ikegami et al., 2000), as an inflow artery because a hepatic graft without any arterial flow may often succumb to graft failure or sepsis. We call this mode of hepatic artery reconstruction *extra-anatomical hepatic artery reconstruction* (Uchiyama et al., 2010c). In reconstructing graft hepatic arteries extra-anatomically, we use the right gastroepiploic artery, the right gastric artery, the gastroduodenal artery, and so on (Table 2).

Inflow artery	N
Anatomical inflow	**445**
Left hepatic artery	245
Right hepatic artery	107
Middle hepatic artery	53
Anterior branch of the right hepatic artery	11
Posterior branch of the right hepatic artery	9
Replaced left hepatic artery	8
Proper hepatic artery	6
Common hepatic artery	3
Replaced right hepatic artery	1
A2 artery	1
A3 artery	1
Extra-anatomical inflow	**32**
Right gastroepiploic artery	12
Right gastric artery	7
Gastroduodenal artery	7
Cystic artery	3
Splenic artery	2
Left gastric artery	1
Total	477

Table 2. A summary of the recipient inflow arteries used in hepatic artery reconstructions

So far, we have used only 3 interposition vessel grafts for hepatic artery reconstruction, namely one right gastric vein graft (Uchiyama et al., 2007), one splenic artery graft and one superior rectal artery graft. The right gastric vein graft was used to fill a gap between the graft artery and the recipient inflow artery. The Y-shaped splenic artery graft was used to reconstruct two graft arteries from one inflow artery. The superior rectal artery graft was used to taper the caliber of a large recipient inflow artery. Because the use of an interposition graft necessitates at least two anastomoses, which may increase the rate of hepatic artery complications, it should be considered a last resort for hepatic artery reconstruction.

In preparing the recipient arteries, the outer surrounding tissue around the recipient candidate hepatic arteries has to be meticulously removed (Fig. 8).

Recipients with end-stage liver disease often have dense nerve fibers and lymphatic vessels around the hepatic arteries. These fibers and vessels are obstacles for hepatic artery reconstruction and should be removed. Adequate blood flow is confirmed by releasing the proximal forceps.

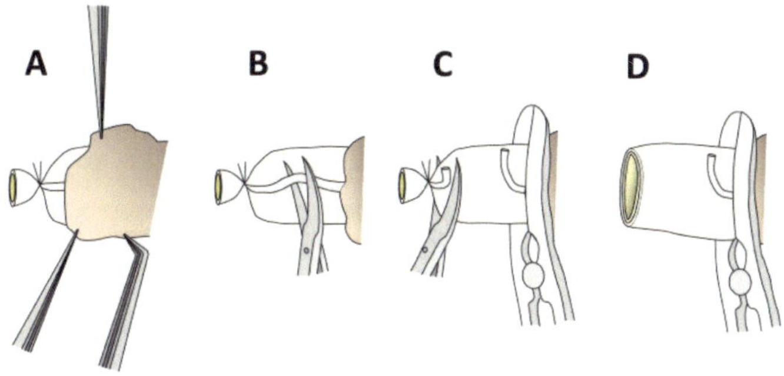

Fig. 8. Preparation of the recipient hepatic artery. (A) The outer surrounding tissue is removed from the recipient hepatic artery. (B) Sometimes, nerve fibers are firmly attached to the artery. These are dissected from the artery and divided. (C) After the proximal portion of the artery is clamped, the distal end of the artery is cut open. (D) The intact arterial flow is confirmed by temporary declamping of the artery, and the recipient artery is ready to be anastomosed

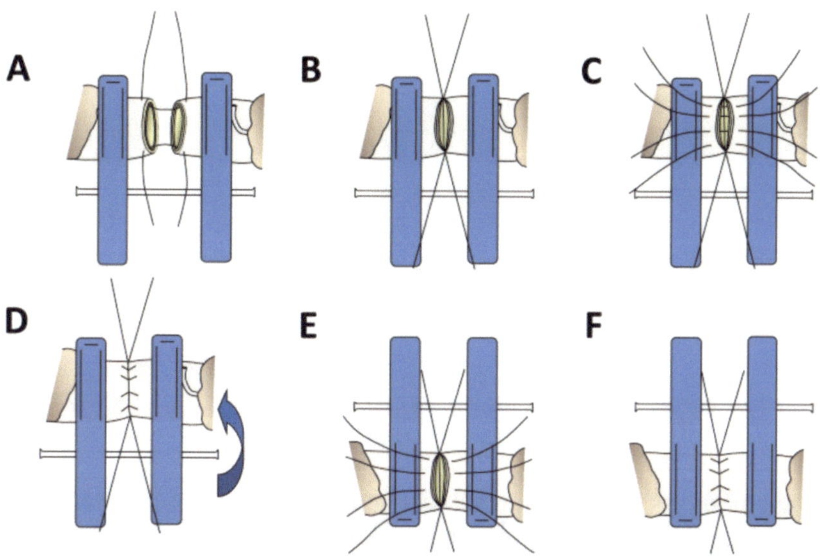

Fig. 9. Hepatic artery reconstruction using a double-clip. (A) After removal of the outer connective tissue surrounding both the donor and recipient arteries, these are secured by a double-clip. Angle stitches (8-0 or 9-0 non-absorbable sutures) are placed on both edges of the arteries. (B) After the clips are moved inward so that both arteries are attached to each other, the angle stitches are tied. (C) Several stitches (usually 4 or 5 stitches) are placed between the angle stitches. The number of stitches is determined according to the diameter of the arteries. These stitches are left untied until all stitches are placed, because it is easier to place each stitch correctly before they are tied, which is called the untied suture technique (Harashina, 1977). (D) These stitches are tied one-by-one. Then, the double-clip is turned over. (E, F) Several stitches are placed on the other side of the arteries in the same manner

5. Hepatic artery anastomosis

After the preparation of both the donor and recipient hepatic arteries is complete, then the final step is to actually reconstruct the graft hepatic arteries. When considering the hemodynamics of the arterial flow, a direct end-to-end anastomosis is the preferred mode of reconstruction. All hepatic artery reconstructions we experienced were done by a direct end-to-end anastomosis. A size-discrepancy up to 2 times is usually acceptable. However, anastomosing so large a recipient artery to a thin graft artery may lead to a rupture of the anastomosis. In such cases, another recipient artery should be selected. So far, we have never experienced a case that required end-to-side anastomosis.

5.1 Hepatic artery anastomosis using a double-clip

We prefer to use a disposable double-clip for performing anastomosis (Fig. 9). The desired grasp force is 45 to 60 grams. By fixing both the graft and recipient arteries, excessive forces at the anastomosis can be avoided.

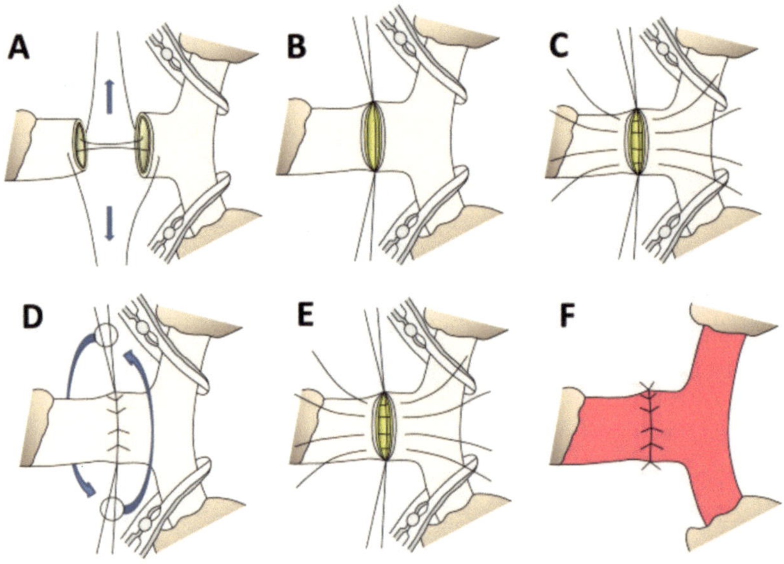

Fig. 10. Hepatic artery reconstruction without a double-clip. (A) After removal of the outer connective tissue surrounding both the donor and recipient arteries, angle stitches are placed on the 6 o'clock and the 12 o'clock positions. (B) After the angle stitches are tied, these stitches are pulled in opposite directions using light clamps so that the arterial walls between the angle stitches are held horizontal with appropriate tension. (C) Several stitches (usually 4 or 5 stitches) are placed between the angle stitches. The number of stitches is determined according to the diameter of the arteries. These stitches are left untied until all stitches are placed, because it is easier to place each stitch correctly before they are tied, which is called the untied suture technique (Harashina, 1977). (D) These stitches are tied one-by-one. The arteries being anastomosed are turned over by pulling each angle stitch in the opposite direction. (E, F) Several stitches are placed on the other side of the arteries in the same manner

5.2 Hepatic artery anastomosis without a double-clip

Sometimes, surgeons encounter a situation where a double-clip cannot grasp the arteries to be anastomosed because of the stiffness of the arteries or because the stump is too short. In such situations, hepatic arteries are reconstructed using two tension stitches placed at the 6 o'clock and 12 o'clock positions (Fig. 10).

6. Posttransplant management

Daily Doppler ultrasound should be performed to check for intact hepatic arterial flows for 7 days after transplantation (Fig. 11). We use neither anti-coagulant nor anti-platelet agents for the purpose of preventing hepatic artery thrombosis. Current Doppler ultrasound machines are so accurate (Kaneko et al., 2004) that they rarely give false positive results (good pulsatile hepatic arterial flows in the graft are detected even when there is a hepatic arterial problem). Whenever there is no pulsatile hepatic arterial flow on Doppler ultrasonography, the patient should immediately undergo contrast-enhanced CT. If there is a suspicion of hepatic artery complications, invasive angiography should be performed, and any attempts to restore the hepatic arterial flow into the graft need to be made within several hours, or devastating consequences (graft failure, sepsis, etc.) will occur.

With regard to repairing hepatic artery complications, our first choice is surgical revision of the HA anastomosis, although there have been some reports regarding non-surgical interventional therapy or retransplantation (Maleux et al., 2005; Kodama et al., 2006; Fistouris et al., 2006).

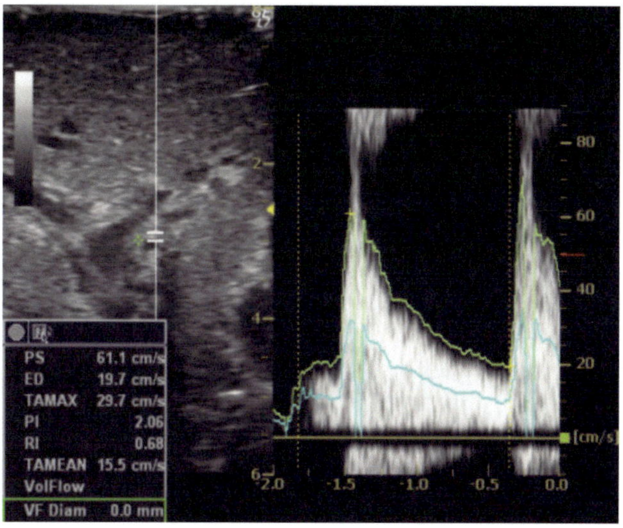

Fig. 11. Doppler ultrasonography is used to detect the intact hepatic arterial flow in the graft liver

7. Hepatic artery complications after living donor liver transplantation

So far, we have experienced 6 hepatic artery complications (Table 3, Fig. 12). Most of them occurred in our early experience.

Patient #17 underwent an auxiliary partial orthotopic LDLT. The case was previously reported as a case report (Uchiyama et al., 2007). The left hepatic graft had a single left hepatic artery, which was reconstructed using the right gastric artery interposed by the right gastric vein graft. There was a restriction on the use of recipient inflow arteries because the native residual liver also had to receive arterial inflows. The patient underwent a follow-up CT examination at 4 years after the LDLT without any symptoms, and an aneurysm at the vein graft was found incidentally. Six months later, the patient underwent a follow-up CT examination again, and the aneurysm was found to be growing. We performed an aneurysm resection and hepatic artery re-reconstruction using the right gastroepiploic artery. The patient is now alive and still doing well at 12 years and 3 months post-transplant.

Patient #18 suffered refractory anastomotic bile leakage after the first LDLT and had to undergo repeated drainage tube insertions to drain infected biloma. On posttransplant day 28, the serous transaminases were steeply elevated and the pulsatile hepatic arterial flows disappeared on Doppler ultrasonography. Emergency angiography was performed which revealed that there was no hepatic artery inflow into the hepatic graft. Although we tried to re-reconstruct the hepatic artery, the tissues around the hepatic hilum had become very fragile because of the infected biloma and we could not perform hepatic artery re-reconstruction. The patient underwent re-LDLT and is still alive at 12 years and 2 months posttransplant.

Patient #39 experienced an unstable clinical course after LDLT, in which hypotension, atrial fibrillation, and oliguria persisted. On posttransplant day 7, the serum transaminases were steeply elevated and no pulsatile arterial flows in the hepatic graft could be detected. Emergency angiography revealed that there was a hepatic artery thrombosis at the anastomosis. An emergency operation was performed to restore the hepatic arterial flows into the graft. The thrombus partially extended into the graft from the origin at the anastomosis. After the thrombus was removed from the graft hepatic artery as much as possible, the arterial re-reconstruction was accomplished using the recipient gastroduodenal artery. Nevertheless, the patient died of multiple organ failure with intact hepatic arterial flows on postransplant day 10.

Patient #73 received a right hepatic graft and the right hepatic artery was anastomosed to the right hepatic artery of the recipient. On posttransplant day 7, the pulsatile flows on Doppler ultrasonography were shown to be weakened, and emergency angiography revealed there was an arterial wall dissection which extended 3 cm proximally from the anastomosis. The dissected wall was resected, and the graft hepatic artery was re-reconstructed using the left gastric artery.

Patient #203 received a right hepatic graft with two hepatic arterial stumps. The main right hepatic artery and the accessory A6 artery were each reconstructed using the anterior branch of the right hepatic artery and the posterior branch of the posterior branch of the right hepatic artery, respectively. This was an ABO-incompatible case, and a cannulation tube was inserted into the hepatic artery for local graft infusion therapy (Egawa et al., 2008), which was considered to have caused the later hepatic artery complication. On the posttransplant day 10, the pulsatile flows on Doppler ultrasonography were shown to be weakened, and emergency angiography revealed there was an arterial wall dissection which extended proximally from the anastomosis with intact A6 arterial flow. We considered that

LDLT No.	Complication	Presentation	Treatment	Outcome
#17	Hepatic artery aneurysm	Incidental finding on a follow-up CT	Aneurysmal resection and hepatic artery re-reconstruction	12 y and 3 m posttransplant, alive
#18	Hepatic artery thrombosis	Elevation of transaminases	Unable to re-reconstruct the hepatic artery. Living donor re-transplantation was performed.	12 y and 2 m posttransplant, alive
#39	Hepatic artery thrombosis	Elevation of transaminases	Hepatic artery re-reconstruction	10 days posttransplant, died of multiple organ failure
#73	Hepatic artery dissection	Dullness of hepaic arterial flow on Doppler ultrasonography	Hepatic artery re-reconstruction	11 y and 5 m posttransplant, alive
#203	Hepatic artery dissection	Dullness of hepaic arterial flow on Doppler ultrasonography	Hepatic artery re-reconstruction	5 y and 8 m posttransplant, alive
#292	Hepatic artery aneurysm	Incidental finding on a follow-up CT	Hepatic artery re-reconstruction	2 y and 10 m posttransplant, alive

Table 3. The hepatic artery complications in our series

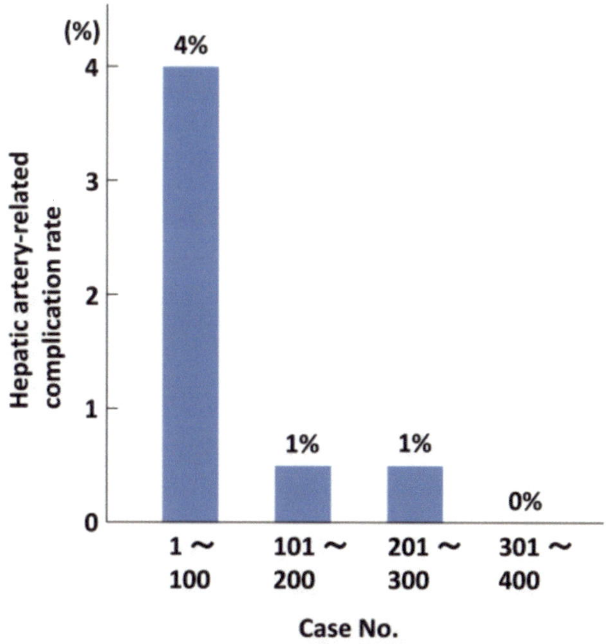

Fig. 12. The hepatic artery-related complication rate in our series

this tiny A6 artery could not sustain the right hepatic graft, and a reoperation was performed. The dissected wall was resected, and the graft main right hepatic artery was re-reconstructed using the recipient right gastroepiploic artery.

Patient #292 received a left lobe graft with two graft hepatic arteries. The graft replaced left hepatic artery and the graft middle hepatic artery were anastomosed to the recipient left hepatic artery and the recipient middle hepatic artery, respectively. The patient was incidentally found to have an aneurysm at the anastomosis between the graft replaced left hepatic artery and the recipient left hepatic artery. The aneurysm was resected and the graft replaced left hepatic artery was re-reconstructed.

8. Conclusion

With the technical advances made in hepatic artery reconstruction, plus our experience with the procedures, we have not recently encountered any hepatic artery-related complications. Although mastering microvascular surgical techniques is time-consuming, we think that this is the most reliable procedure for hepatic artery reconstruction, especially in LDLT for small recipients. The next issue that must be addressed is how to securely pass these techniques to the next generation.

9. References

Akabayashi, A., Slingsby, B.T. & Fujita, M. (2004) The first donor death after living-related liver transplantation in Japan. Transplantation Vol. 77(No. 4): 634.

Apisarnthanarak, P., Raman, S.S., Ghobrial, R.M., Busuttil, R.W., Saab, S. & Lu, D.S. (2011) Efficacy of CT angiography for preoperative vascular mapping in adult to adult living related liver transplant donors. J Med Assoc Thai Vol. 94(No. 1): 98-105.

Broelsch, C.E., Whitington, P.F., Emond, J.C., Heffron, T.G., Thistlethwaite, J.R., Stevens, L., Piper, J., Whitington, S.H. & Lichtor, J.L. (1991) Liver transplantation in children from living related donors. Surgical techniques and results. Ann Surg Vol. 214(No. 4): 428-437.

Chen, W.J., Ying, D.J., Liu, Z.J. & He, Z.P. (1999) Analysis of the arterial supply of the extrahepatic bile ducts and its clinical significance. Clin Anat Vol. 12(No. 4): 245-249.

Douard, R., Ettorre, G.M., Sommacale, D., Jan, D., Révillon, Y., Farges, O. & Belghiti, J. (2002) A two-step strategy for enlargement of left arterial branch in a living related liver graft with dual arterial supply. Transplantation Vol. 73(No. 6): 993-994.

Egawa, H., Teramukai, S., Haga, H., Tanabe, M., Fukushima, M. & Shimazu, M. (2008) Present status of ABO-incompatible living donor liver transplantation in Japan. Hepatology Vol. 47(No. 1): 143-152.

Eguchi, S., Takatsuki, M., Hidaka, M., Tajima, Y. & Kanematsu, T. (2008) Evolution of living donor liver transplantation over 10 years: experience of a single center. Surg Today Vol. 38(No. 9): 795-800.

Fan, S.T., Lo, C.M., Liu, C.L., Tso, W.K. & Wong, J. (2002) Biliary reconstruction and complications of right lobe live donor liver transplantation. Ann Surg Vol. 236(No. 5): 676-683.

Fistouris, J., Herlenius, G., Bäckman, L., Olausson, M., Rizell, M., Mjörnstedt, L. & Friman, S. (2006) Pseudoaneurysm of the hepatic artery following liver transplantation. Transplant Proc Vol. 38(No. 8): 2679-2682.

Ghobrial, R.M., Freise, C.E., Trotter, J.F., Tong, L., Ojo, A.O., Fair, J.H., Fisher, R.A., Emond, J.C., Koffron, A.J., Pruett, T.L., Olthoff, K.M. & A2ALL Study Group. (2008) Donor morbidity after living donation for liver transplantation. Gastroenterology Vol. 135(No.2): 468-476.

Gunji, H., Cho, A., Tohma, T., Okazumi, S., Makino, H., Shuto, K., Mochizuki, R., Matsubara, K., Hayano, K., Mori, C., Murakami, G. & Ochiai, T. (2006) The blood supply of the hilar bile duct and its relationship to the communicating arcade located between the right and left hepatic arteries. Am J Surg Vol. 192(No. 3): 276-280.

Harashina, T. (1977) Use of the untied suture in microvascular anastomoses. Plast Reconstr Surg Vol. 59(No. 1): 134-135.

Ikegami, T., Kawasaki, S., Hashikura, Y., Miwa, S., Kubota, T., Mita, A., Iijima, S., Terada, M., Miyagawa, S. & Furuta, S. (2000) An alternative method of arterial reconstruction after hepatic arterial thrombosis following living-related liver transplantation. Transplantation Vol. 69(No. 9): 1953-1955.

Ikegami, T., Kawasaki, S., Matsunami, H., Hashikura, Y., Nakazawa, Y., Miyagawa, S., Furuta, S., Iwanaka, T. & Makuuchi, M. (1996) Should all hepatic arterial branches be reconstructed in living-related liver transplantation? Surgery Vol. 119(No. 4): 431-436.

Inomoto, T., Nishizawa, F., Sasaki, H., Terajima, H., Shirakata, Y., Miyamoto, S., Nagata, I., Fujimoto, M., Moriyasu, F., Tanaka, K. & Yamaoka, Y. (1996) Experience of 120 microsurgical reconstructions of hepatic artery in living related liver transplantation. Surgery Vol. 119(No. 1): 20-26.

Kaneko, J., Sugawara, Y., Akamatsu, N., Kishi, Y., Niiya, T., Kokudo, N., Makuuchi, M. & Mizuta, K. (2004) Prediction of hepatic artery thrombosis by protocol Doppler ultrasonography in pediatric living donor liver transplantation. Abdom Imaging Vol. 29 (No. 5): 603-605.

Kodama, Y., Sakuhara, Y., Abo, D., Shimamura, T., Furukawa, H., Todo, S. & Miyasaka, K. (2006) Percutaneous transluminal angioplasty for hepatic artery stenosis after living donor liver transplantation. Liver Transpl Vol. 12 (No. 3): 465-469.

Kostelic, J.K., Piper, J.B., Leef, J.A., Lu, C.T., Rosenblum, J.D., Hackworth, C., Kahn, J., Thistlethwaite, J.R. & Whitington, P.F. (1996) Angiographic selection criteria for living related liver transplant donors. AJR Am J Roentgenol Vol. 166(No. 5): 1103-1108.

Kubota, K., Makuuchi, M., Takayama, T., Harihara, Y., Hasegawa, K., Aoki, T., Asato, H. & Kawarasaki, H. (2000) Simple test on the back table for justifying single hepatic-arterial reconstruction in living related liver transplantation. Transplantation Vol. 70(No. 4): 696-697.

Lin, T.S., Chiang, Y.C., Chen, C.L., Concejero, A.M., Cheng, Y.F., Wang, C.C., Wang, S.H., Liu, Y.W., Yang, C.H. & Yong, C.C. (2009) Intimal dissection of the hepatic artery following transarterial embolization for hepatocellular carcinoma: an intraoperative problem in adult living donor liver transplantation. Liver Transpl Vol. 15(No. 11): 1553-1556.

Maleux, G., Pirenne, J., Aerts, R. & Nevens, F. (2005) Case report: hepatic artery pseudoaneurysm after liver transplantation: definitive treatment with a stent-graft after failed coil embolisation. Br J Radiol Vol. 78(No. 929): 453-456.

Matsuda, H., Yagi, T., Sadamori, H., Matsukawa, H., Shinoura, S., Murata, H., Umeda, Y. & Tanaka, N. (2006) Complications of arterial reconstruction in living donor liver transplantation: a single center experience. Surg Today Vol. 36(No. 3): 245-251.

Miller, C., Florman, S., Kim-Schluger, L., Lento, P., De La Garza, J., Wu, J., Xie, B., Zhang, W., Bottone, E., Zhang, D. & Schwartz, M. (2004) Fulminant and fatal gas gangrene of the stomach in a healthy live liver donor. Liver Transpl Vol. 10(No. 10): 1315-1319.

Millis, J.M., Cronin, D.C., Brady, L.M., Newell, K.A., Woodle, E.S., Bruce, D.S., Thistlethwaite, J.R. & Broelsch, C.E. (2000) Primary living-donor liver transplantation at the University of Chicago: technical aspects of the first 104 recipients. Ann Surg Vol. 232(No. 1): 104-111.

Mori, K., Nagata, I., Yamagata, S., Sasaki, H., Nishizawa, F., Takada, Y., Moriyasu, F., Tanaka, K., Yamaoka, Y., Kumada, K., et al. (1992) The introduction of microvascular surgery to hepatic artery reconstruction in living-donor liver transplantation - its surgical advantages compared with conventional procedures. Transplantation Vol. 54(No. 2): 263-268.

Nishizaki, T., Ikegami, T., Hiroshige, S., Hashimoto, K., Uchiyama, H., Yoshizumi, T., Kishikawa, K., Shimada, M. & Sugimachi, K. (2001) Small graft for living donor liver transplantation. Ann Surg Vol. 233(No. 4): 575-580.

Panossian, A., Diamond, I., Fecteau, A., Grant, D. & Zuker, R. (2009) Hepatic artery microvascular anastomosis in pediatric living donor liver transplantation: a review of 35 consecutive cases by a single microvascular surgeon. J Reconstr Microsurg Vol. 25(No. 7): 439-443.

Plengvanit, U., Chearanai, O., Sindhvananda, K., Dambrongsak, D., Tuchinda, S. & Viranuvatti, V. (1972) Collateral arterial blood supply of the liver after hepatic artery ligation, angiographic study of twenty patients. Ann Surg Vol. 175(No. 1): 105-110.

Saylisoy, S., Atasoy, C., Ersöz, S., Karayalçin, K. & Akyar, S. (2005) Multislice CT angiography in the evaluation of hepatic vascular anatomy in potential right lobe donors. Diagn Interv Radiol Vol. 11(No. 1): 51-59.

Settmacher, U., Stange, B., Haase, R., Heise, M., Steinmüller, T., Bechstein, W.O. & Neuhaus P. (2000) Arterial complications after liver transplantation. Transpl Int Vol. 13(No. 5): 372-378.

Soejima, Y., Taketomi, A., Yoshizumi, T., Uchiyama, H., Harada, N., Ijichi, H., Yonemura, Y., Shimada, M. & Maehara, Y. (2006) Feasibility of left lobe living donor liver transplantation between adults: an 8-year, single-center experience of 107 cases. Am J Transplant Vol. 6(No. 5): 1004-1011.

Stange, B.J., Glanemann, M., Nuessler, N.C., Settmacher, U., Steinmüller, T. & Neuhaus P. (2003) Hepatic artery thrombosis after adult liver transplantation. Liver Transpl Vol. 9(No. 6): 612-620.

Suehiro, T., Ninomiya, M., Shiotani, S., Hiroshige, S., Harada, N., Minagawa, R., Soejima, Y., Shimada, M. & Sugimachi, K. (2002) Hepatic artery reconstruction and biliary stricture formation after living donor adult liver transplantation using the left lobe. Liver Transpl Vol. 8(No. 5): 495-499.

Takatsuki, M., Chiang, Y.C., Lin, T.S., Wang, C.C., Concejero, A., Lin, C.C., Huang, T.L., Cheng, Y.F. & Chen, C.L. (2006) Anatomical and technical aspects of hepatic artery reconstruction in living donor liver transplantation. Vol. 140(No. 5): 824-828.

Taketomi, A., Kayashima, H., Soejima, Y., Yoshizumi, T., Uchiyama, H., Ikegami, T., Yamashita, Y., Harada, N., Shimada, M. & Maehara, Y. (2009) Donor risk in adult-to-adult living donor liver transplantation: impact of left lobe graft. Transplantation Vol. 87(No. 3): 445-450.

Trotter, J.F., Adam, R., Lo, C.M. & Kenison, J. (2006) Documented deaths of hepatic lobe donors for living donor liver transplantation. Liver Transpl Vol. 12(No. 10): 1485-1488.

Uchiyama, H., Harada, N., Sanefuji, K., Kayashima, H., Taketomi, A., Soejima, Y., Ikegami, T., Shimada, M. & Maehara, Y. (2010a) Dual hepatic artery reconstruction in living donor liver transplantation using a left hepatic graft with 2 hepatic arterial stumps. Surgery Vol. 147(No. 6): 878-886.

Uchiyama, H., Hashimoto, K., Hiroshige, S., Harada, N., Soejima, Y., Nishizaki, T., Shimada, M. & Suehiro, T. (2002) Hepatic artery reconstruction in living-donor liver transplantation: a review of its techniques and complications. Surgery Vol. 131 (1 Suppl): S200-204.

Uchiyama, H., Ikegami, T., Soejima, Y., Ninomiya, M., Kayashima, H., Taketomi, A., Shirabe, K. & Maehara, Y. (2010b) Use of recipient's left hepatic artery for artery reconstruction in right lobe living donor liver transplantation with duct-to-duct anastomosis. Transplantation Vol. 89(No. 8): 1016-1021.

Uchiyama, H., Shirabe, K., Taketomi, A., Soejima, Y., Ninomiya, M., Kayashima, H., Ikegami, T. & Maehara, Y. (2010c) Extra-anatomical hepatic artery reconstruction in living donor liver transplantation: can this procedure save hepatic grafts? Liver Transpl Vol. 16(No. 9): 1054-1061.

Uchiyama, H., Soejima, Y., Taketomi, A., Yoshizumi, T., Harada, N., Ijichi, H., Yonemura, Y. & Maehara, Y. (2007) Hepatic artery aneurysm arising from an interposition vein graft four years after auxiliary partial orthotopic liver transplantation. Transpl Int Vol. 20(No. 2): 197-200.

Yanaga, K., Lebeau, G., Marsh, J.W., Gordon, R.D., Makowka, L., Tzakis, A.G., Todo, S., Stieber, A.C., Iwatsuki, S. & Starzl, T.E. (1990a) Hepatic artery reconstruction for hepatic artery thrombosis after orthotopic liver transplantation. Arch Surg Vol. 125(No. 5): 628-631.

Yanaga, K., Tzakis, A.G. & Starzl, T.E. (1990b) Partial dearterialization of the liver allograft. Transpl Int Vol. 3(No. 4): 185-188.

Wang, C.C., Lin, T.S., Chen, C.L., Concejero, A.M., Iyer, S.G. & Chiang, Y.C. (2008) Arterial reconstruction in hepatic artery occlusions in adult living donor liver transplantation using gastric vessels. Surgery Vol. 143(No. 5): 686-690.

Wei, W.I., Lam, L.K., Ng, R.W., Liu, C.L., Lo, C.M., Fan, S.T. & Wong, J. (2004) Microvascular reconstruction of the hepatic artery in live donor liver transplantation: experience across a decade. Arch Surg Vol. 139(No. 3): 304-307.

4

Small-for-Size Syndrome After Living Donor Liver Transplantation

Yuzo Umeda, Takahito Yagi, Hiroshi Sadamori and Toshiyoshi Fujiwara
Department of Gastroenterological Surgery,
Okayama University Graduate School of Medicine,
Dentistry and Pharmaceutical Sciences
Japan

1. Introduction

Patients scheduled for liver transplantation frequently have portal hypertension and consequently they are likely to have a high portal blood flow in the transplanted graft. When the graft volume is small in adult living donor liver transplantation with partial liver transplantation, various problems that may affect the prognosis often occur because the partial graft cannot sustain excessive portal blood perfusion. It is widely known that liver transplant recipients can potentially develop a specific syndrome known as "small-for-size syndrome", when a small for size graft causes size mismatch in the presence of portal hypertension. The small-for-size syndrome can result in large-volume ascites, hyperbilirubinemia, and coagulopathy. The pathologic mechanism of small-for-size syndrome includes graft failure caused by excessive and destructive portal inflow into the small for size graft. The small-for-size syndrome is widely recognized by transplant surgeon as one of the important post-transplant events. Thus, sufficient graft volume is one of the important determinants of successful transplant and clinically satisfactory outcome. Particularly in the case of living donor liver transplantation, there is the added problem of insufficient donor pool and donor safety, but it is essential to maintain graft function under the given circumstances. The decision on the type of liver graft depends on various factors, such as recipients' status and donor safety: a small for size graft tends to be selected due to problems related to donor selection and to ensure the safety of the donor. In this regard, many centers stipulate the absolute lack of various pre-transplant risk factors and a minimal graft size in order to prevent the development of this syndrome and good outcome.

2. Pathophysiological mechanisms of small-for-size syndrome

Small-for-size syndrome can occur in the special situation of partial liver graft transplantation, especially in adult living donor liver transplantation, with resultant size mismatching between graft size and recipient hepato-portal circulation. Once the partial liver volume graft is subjected to excessive portal inflow, portal hyperperfusion results in the development of the small-for-size syndrome. The basic pathophysiology in this syndrome relates to graft injury after transplantation, which is caused by graft size mismatch and portal hypertension, followed by the appearance of various clinical abnormalities such as excessive ascites, hyperbilirubinemia, coagulopathy, encephalopathy, and renal dysfunction. Transplant recipients develop symptoms related to the above abnormalities after transplantation and post-transplant prognosis is reported to be less than ideal.

To understand the pathophysiological mechanism of the small-for-size syndrome, several studies examined post-transplant biopsies. These studies reported histopathological evidence of mechanical injury and graft failure caused by destructive portal hyperperfusion. The main histopathological findings are: (1) Portal vein and periportal sinusoidal endothelial denudation and focal hemorrhage into the portal tract connective tissue; and (2) poor arterial flow and vasospasm, resulting in ischemic cholangitis and parenchymal infarct. Furthermore, electron microscopic examination showed sinusoidal congestion, excessive swelling of the mitochondria in hepatocytes, irregular large gaps of sinusoidal lining cells, and collapse of the space of Disse. These findings are considered to represent progressive damage of the graft resulting from microcirculatory failure due to irreversible endothelial injury after reperfusion. On the other hand, other studies examined the molecular basis of graft damage by analyzing intragraft gene expression. The results of these studies provided evidence for sinusoidal damage. Cases of small-for-size syndrome and associated graft dysfunction due to portal hyperperfusion, showed intragraft upregulation of endothelin-1 and down regulation of heme-oxigenase-1 and heat shock protein-70. Others showed low portal venous plasma nitric oxide levels. In addition, experimental studies using animal models of the small-for-size syndrome showed intragraft over-expression of endothelin-1, early growth response -1 (Egr-1) and endotherin-1A receptor and significant changes in intragraft mRNA levels as well as plasma levels of inflammatory cytokines (interleukin [IL]-6, IL-15, tumor necrosis factor [TNF]-alpha). Furthermore, the small for size isografts and allografts, with volumes measuring 50% or 30% of the liver graft volume, demonstrated higher expression levels of vascular endothelial growth factor (VEGF) and fetal liver kinase (Flk)-1 than the whole isograft and allograft. In addition, Flk-1-positive activated macrophages were also detected in small for size isografts and allografts, which were probably induced by VEGF. In this regard, the expression of VEGF and its interaction with Flk-1 could mediate the inflammatory response, early activation of macrophages. Thus, the above changes in the small for size graft injury likely play important roles in the accelerated acute rejection process of the small for size allograft.

Previous studies indicated that liver regeneration begins in the early period after partial liver transplantation. Although the detailed mechanism remains unknown at present, the high portal flow rate and high portal pressure are considered important triggers of liver regeneration. In partial liver transplantation, a high level of liver regeneration is observed when the graft size is small, or when portal pressure is high in cirrhotic patients. On the other hand, liver tissue damage and ischemic reperfusion injury caused by high portal pressure in small-for-size syndrome result in serious interference with the process of liver regeneration. Interestingly, IL-6 and TNF-alpha play key roles in liver regeneration, though they are also considered to represent markers of acute-phase tissue damage. Local activation and excessive production of these cytokines is associated with poor liver regeneration, since they can act as negative regulators of cell proliferation. In fact, TNF-alpha could trigger the cell death pathway after binding to the TNF-receptor. Thus, although the role of these cytokines remains controversial, they are considered to function as inflammatory cytokines, rather than as liver regenerative factors, in patients with small-for-size syndrome.

Furthermore, accumulation of oxygen free radicals in the graft could possibly contribute to graft dysfunction.

3. Treatment strategy for small-for-size syndrome

The most important step is prevention of small-for-size syndrome through perioperative treatment strategies that include approaches aimed at reducing excessive portal inflow as the major cause of small-for-size syndrome, and lowering the graft perfusion pressure. Furthermore, efforts should be made to prevent hepatic venous congestion due to insufficient vascular orifices or mechanical stenosis and kinking.

An important factor in determining portal inflow volume and pressure is the blood perfusion level in the spleen, thus highlighting the benefits of splenectomy and ligation of the splenic artery. However, patients with end-stage hepatic failure exhibit a hyperdynamic state of splanchnic blood flow, compared with normal state, and are at increased risk of hemorrhage associated with seriously invasive surgical procedures. Thus, careful attention should be paid to the expansion of the dissection area during surgery, especially in patients with collateral circulation around the splenic artery, such as gastric coronary vein and spleno-renal shunt. However, the development of new surgical technique and advances in medical devices have allowed a reduction in blood loss during surgical dissection procedures and splenectomy. Although the invasiveness of surgical procedure such as splenectomy and splenic artery ligation could be diminished further, adverse events such as increased susceptibility to infection caused by low immunity and portal vein thrombosis, may occur after splenectomy. Thus, patients should be carefully selected for splenectomy and splenic artery ligation.

Portosystemic shunt is currently considered an efficacious procedure in the treatment of portal hypertension. Especially adequate portosystemic shunt, which achieves favorable portal decompression to below 15 mmHg, could dramatically improve the post-transplant prognosis of patients with small for size graft. The procedure has allowed lowering the cut-off value for graft weight-to-recipient body weight ratio from 0.8% to 0.6%. This procedure is anticipated to become the main strategy in the future to prevent the development of the small-for-size syndrome. However, the separation of the graft portal route, as seen in portosystemic shunt, may result in portal steal to the extrahepatic route, which sometimes leads to fatal events especially in cases with decreased graft portal vascular compliance, such as the case of steatotic liver graft or accute cellular rejection. Based on this potential complication, some centers have adopted certain precautionary measures against such complications using modifications of the shunt closing technique.

The recently introduced approach of splenic artery embolization could be an effective procedure for portal decompression instead of the conventional treatment. Splenic artery embolization is described by some investigators as a rescue treatment for post-transplant small-for-size syndrome. In this regard, we previously reported that preoperative portal decompression by splenic artery embolization efficaciously reduced blood loss during operation and shortened the operating time, and that it contributed to favorable prognosis without serious complications related to the procedure itself. In our institution, preoperative embolization is selected for patients considered at risk of development of shunt in the peri-celiac trunk. The risk assessment is based on preoperative radiography showing possible problems with safety of splenic artery ligation. In each patient scheduled for preoperative splenic artery embolization, abdominal angiography was performed 12 to 18 hours before transplantation. As a rule, a metallic coil was placed in the area adjacent to the root of the splenic artery and proximal to the bifurcation of the major pancreatic artery, to produce total embolization of the splenic artery trunk (Figure 1). Evaluation of post-transplantation graft hemodynamics by Doppler ultrasonography showed a significant reduction in the level of graft portal perfusion following splenic artery ligation and splenic artery embolization in the portal modulation group, compared with the non-portal modulation group (Figure 2). In the portal modulation group, the efficacy of portal decompression following splenic artery embolization was equivalent to that after splenic artery ligation. Furthermore, hepatic arterial flow was significantly higher during the postoperative phase in the portal modulation group, reflecting arterial flow shift from the spleen to the hepatic artery or hepatic arterial buffer response (Figure. 1).

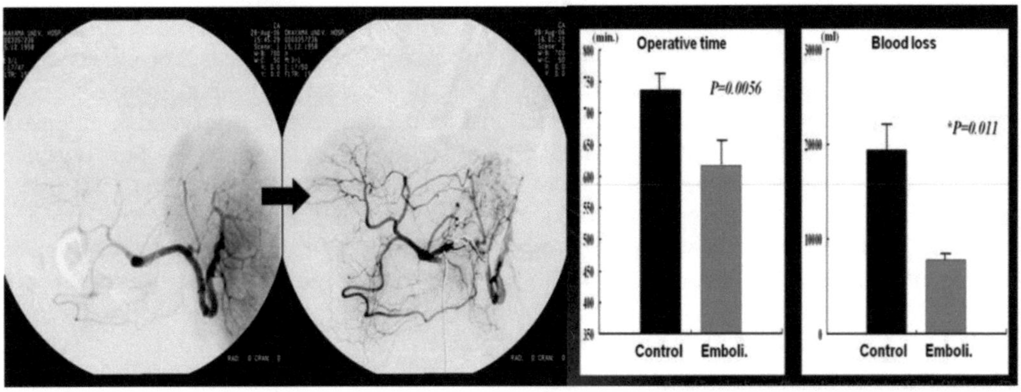

Fig. 1. Preoperative splenic artery embolization as a prophylactic procedure for the prevention of small-for-size syndrome. Splenic artery was totally embolized adjacent to the root of celiac artery, 12-18 hours before liver transplantation. Splenic artery embolization reduced portal flow and increased hepatic arterial flow. Preoperative portal decompression also decreased blood loss and shortened operative time

As a result, such change in arterial blood flow could also contribute to the prevention of splenic artery steal syndrome, which causes poor arterial blood supply. Based on this procedure, none of the patients developed portal vein thrombosis or septicemia, which are sometimes observed after splenectomy.

Another issue related to liver transplantation is the post-transplant course. In this regard, high level liver regeneration is observed when the graft size is small, or when portal pressure is high in cirrhotic patients. Importantly, high serum IL-6 concentrations are considered to reflect high hemodynamic shear stress, which could lead to regenerative signaling pathway. However, in patients with extra small for size graft, regeneration of the graft liver does not occur sometimes, and liver tissue damage and ischemic reperfusion injury could result in increased release of inflammatory cytokines, such as IL-6 and TNF-alpha, which lead to poor liver regeneration, i.e., these cytokines act as negative regulators of cell proliferation. Thus, although the role of these cytokines remains controversial, they are considered to function as inflammatory cytokines, rather than as liver regenerative factors, in patients with small-for-size syndrome, and thus, are considered as markers of graft injury. The postoperative outcome depends on the extent of graft injury immediately after the transplantation and portal decompression can protect the liver graft from destructive portal hyperperfusion and reduce the levels of these inflammatory cytokines. Our previous study reported that prophylactic splenic artery embolization and ligation decreased serum IL-6 and TNF-alpha after graft reperfusion and resulted in certain graft liver regeneration and favorable outcome. Based on these new findings, in terms of treatment strategy in small-for-size syndrome, prophylactic treatment would be favorable compared with rescue therapy.

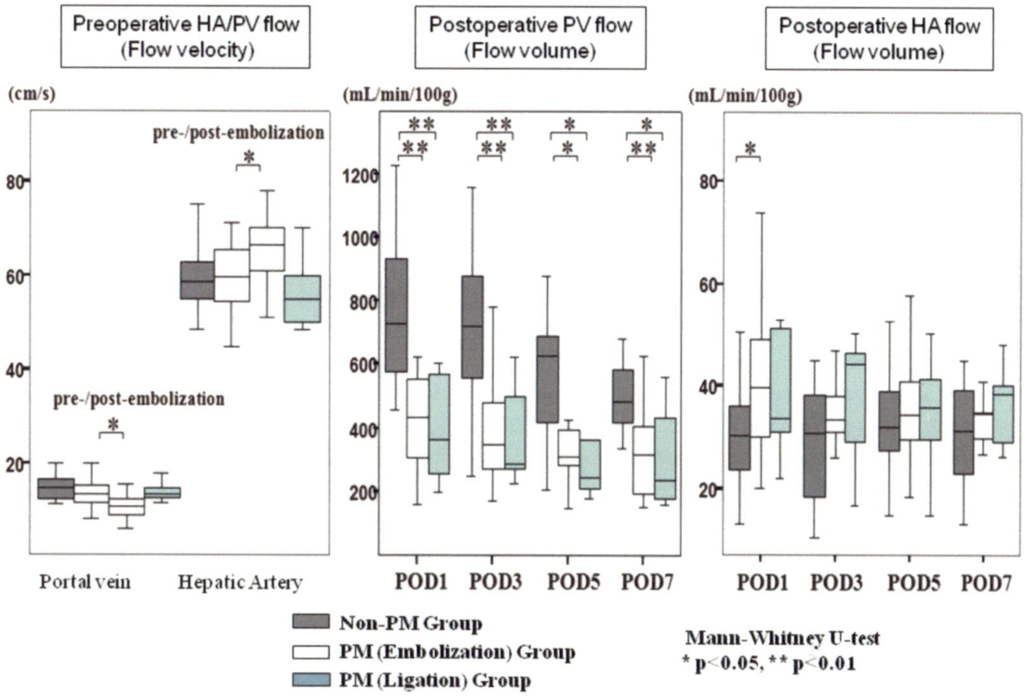

Fig. 2. Box-and-whisker plots of portal vein flow and hepatic artery flow in patients of the non-portal modulation (PM) and PM groups during postoperative days (POD) 1, 3, 5 and 7

Any decision regarding the treatment strategy for small-for-size syndrome, flexible stance is often needed. Among the various approaches, either decision could be suitable depending on the individual patient. For example, the patient characteristics and institutional operative policies could influence the final decision. While portosystemic shunt is widely used for the prevention of small-for-size syndrome, there is no doubt that splenectomy and splenic artery ligation are also suitable and effective techniques to produce portal decompression. Furthermore, splenic artery embolization prior to transplantation could be an alternative effective treatment modality especially in patients with severe portal hypertension, and with established collateral circulation in the peri-celiac trunk, which makes it difficult to perform splenic artery ligation or splenectomy. In this regard, when sufficient portal decompression cannot be achieved through a single technique, a combination of two or more procedures should be applied. In essence, a proper portal decompression therapy can inhibit portal overperfusion injury and prevent small-for-size syndrome and also have beneficial effects on liver generation as well as improvement of post-transplantation prognosis. In addition to the reduction in the mortality rate after the development of the technique of living donor liver transplantation, from medical and economic standpoints, the cost benefits of liver transplantation can be fully expected based on the reduced use of blood products, and shorter hospitalization through improvement of perioperative clinical condition.

4. Prediction of small-for-size syndrome and hospital mortality

Theoretically, small-for-size syndrome is expected in cases of small for size graft with high portal inflow. However, several studies have demonstrated that small-for-size syndrome does not necessarily occur even in such situations. In other words, the development of small for size syndrome and post-transplant graft function could not be predicted from the graft size only. We hypothesized that early graft function does not only depend on graft size, but also on portal hypertension, donor age and recipient status. To test our hypothesis, we determined the perioperative risk factors in small-for-size syndrome and post-transplant hospital death. In this regard, there are only a few studies that have dealt with the prediction of small-for-size syndrome in living donor liver transplantation.

We analyzed retrospectively 200 consecutive adult patients who underwent living donor liver transplantation in our hospital during the period from August 1998 to January 2010. We used multivariate analysis of hospital deaths for this purpose and various clinical, pathological and surgical parameters, after employment of cut-off values for these parameters using ROC analysis. Patients were divided into two groups according to the treatment protocol for the prevention of small-for-size syndrome. The first 50 patients had not received any prophylactic portal decompression. There were significant differences in the clinical parameters based on the time trend between the groups with and without prophylactic portal decompression. Interestingly, an aggressive operative stance was identified in the late time group and this correlated with the recipient age, donor age, MELD, and graft volume. Meanwhile, there was a significant learning curve, which seemed to reflect the development of the operative procedure, including the cold ischemic time, blood loss, and operative time (Figure 3). In the first 50 cases, the in-hospital mortality rate and 1-year survival rates of patients with a graft weight (GW)/recipient body weight (RBW) rate less than 0.8% were 27.3% and 63.6%, respectively (Figure 4). Multivariate analysis identified a single factor, which was a graft weight (GW)/recipient body weight (RBW) rate less than 0.8%, as a significant determinant of post-transplant hospital death (Table 1). From the 51th patients onward, prophylactic portal decompression was used in 70 of the 150 patients in order to prevent small-for-size syndrome. The prophylactic portal decompression consisted of splenic artery embolization in 50 patients, splenic arterial ligation in 14, splenectomy in 5, and portocaval shunt in 1 patient. After the introduction of the prophylactic portal decompression in the later 150 cases, the hospital mortality rate and 1-year survival rate of patients with GW/RBW less than 0.8% were 7.2% and 86%, respectively. After the introduction of prophylactic portal decompression, post-transplant prognosis did not correlate with a cut-off value of 0.8% for the GW/RBW ratio (Figure 4). Multivariate analysis of post-transplant hospital mortality rate in the later 150 cases identified donor age more than 54 years and MELD score more than 23, but not the GW/RBW, as significant perioperative risk factors (Table 2). In other words, the minimum GW/RBW ratio could be safely lowered to 0.68% with adequate portal modulation.

Variables	n	Odds ratio	P-Value
Recipient factors			
Age ≥ 50 (vs < 50 years)	22 / 28	23.4	0.99
MELD ≥ 20 (vs < 20)	2 / 48	6.29	0.23
Disease			
Cholestatic disease vs PLC	22 / 19	0.34	0.21
Acute liver failure vs PLC	9 / 19	1.39	-
Donor factors			
Age ≥ 53 (vs < 53 years)	10 / 40	1.15	0.92
Graft type (right lobe vs left lobe graft)	38 / 12	0.29	0.46
GW/RBW < 0.8% (vs ≥ 0.8%)	12 / 38	8.44	0.02
Treatment and Operative factors			
Blood loss ≥ 50 (vs < 50ml/kg)	39 / 11	3.59	0.99
CIT ≥ 80 (vs < 80min)	16 / 34	1.16	0.91
WIT ≥ 50 (vs < 50min)	14 / 36	1.92	0.40
Operating time ≥10 (vs <10 hrs)	38 / 12	4.56	0.74

Table 1. Logistic regression analysis of post-transplant hospital mortality (the first 50 cases). PLC, Post-necrotic Liver cirrhosis; MELD, Model for End-stage Liver Disease; GW/RBW, Graft weight to recipient body weight ratio; CIT, Cold ischemic time; WIT, Warm ischemic time

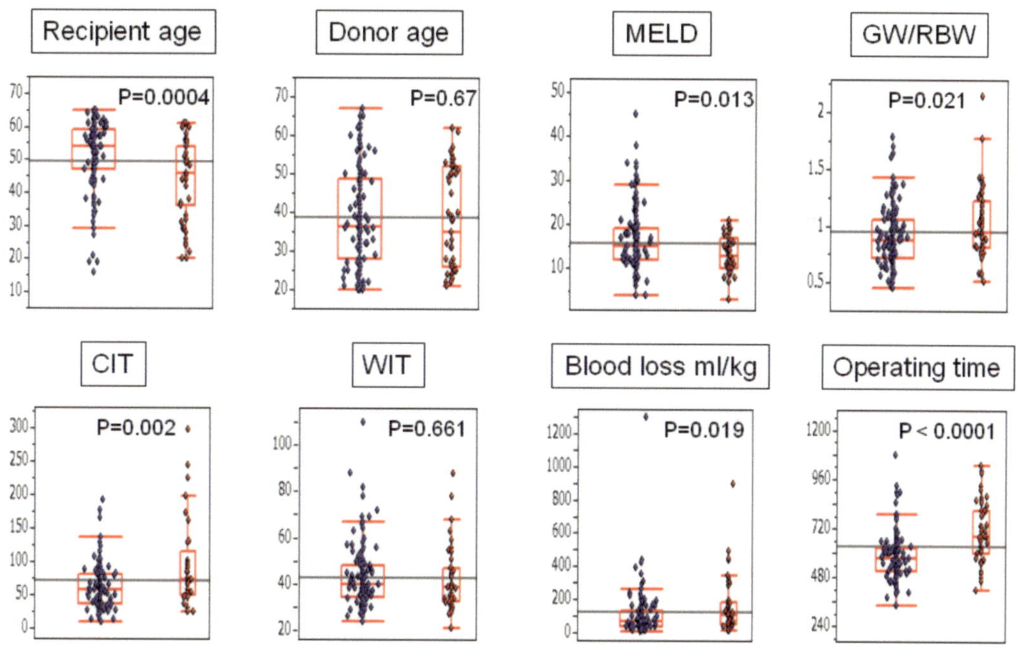

Abbreviations: MELD, Model for End-stage Liver Disease; GW/RBW, Graft weight to recipient body weight ratio; CIT, Cold ischemic time; WIT, Warm ischemic time.

Fig. 3. Box-and-whisker plots of clinical factors in the first 50 cases (right side) and the later 150 cases (left side)

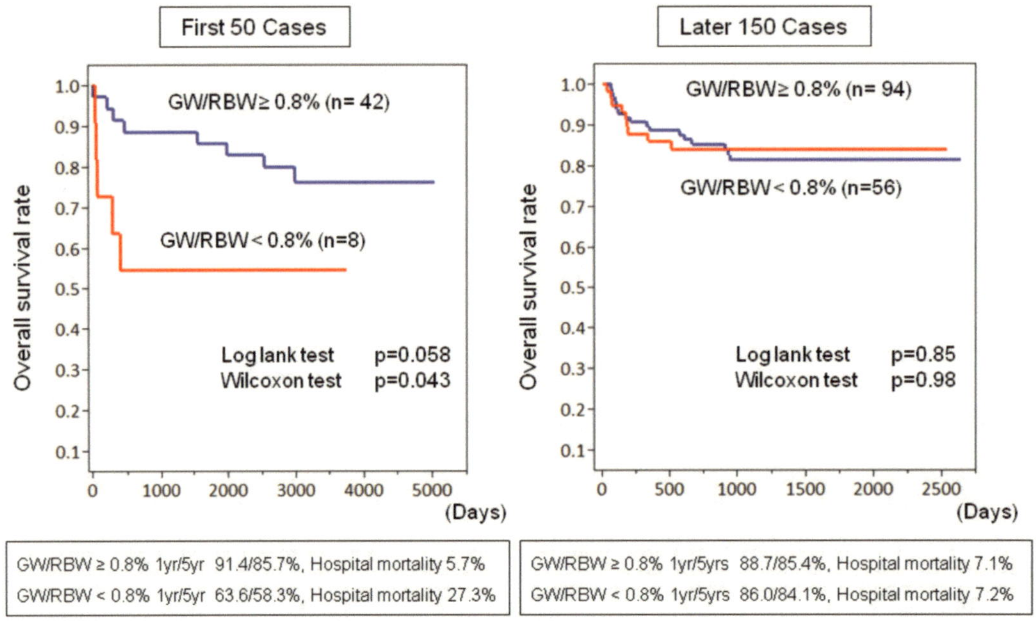

Fig. 4. Overall survival curves and hospital mortality before and after the introduction of portal modulation

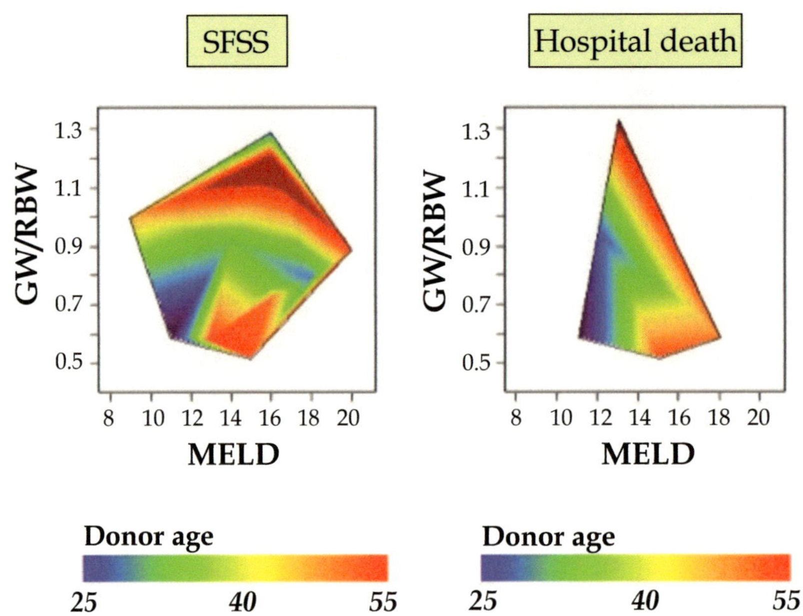

Fig. 5. Correlation between graft size, MELD, and donor age in cases of small-for-size syndrome and hospital death

To evaluate the impact of small for size graft on the outcome, we defined small-for-size syndrome as both prolonged functional cholestasis and intractable ascites. Prolonged functional cholestasis was defined as total bilirubin >10 mg/dL at postoperative day 14, without any other cause of cholestasis. Intractable ascites was defined as daily production of ascites of more than one liter at postoperative day 14 or >500 mL at postoperative day 28. Production of ascites represented the daily volume of ascites estimated by discharge from the abdominal drain. According to this diagnostic criterion, small-for-size syndrome occurred in 21 of 200 cases (10.5%) and 5 cases had fatal outcome. Patients with the small-for-size syndrome consisted of 11 cases (22%) in the first 50 cases and 10 cases (6.7%) in the later 150 cases, respectively. Furthermore, early hospital death was noted in 16 of 200 cases (8%).

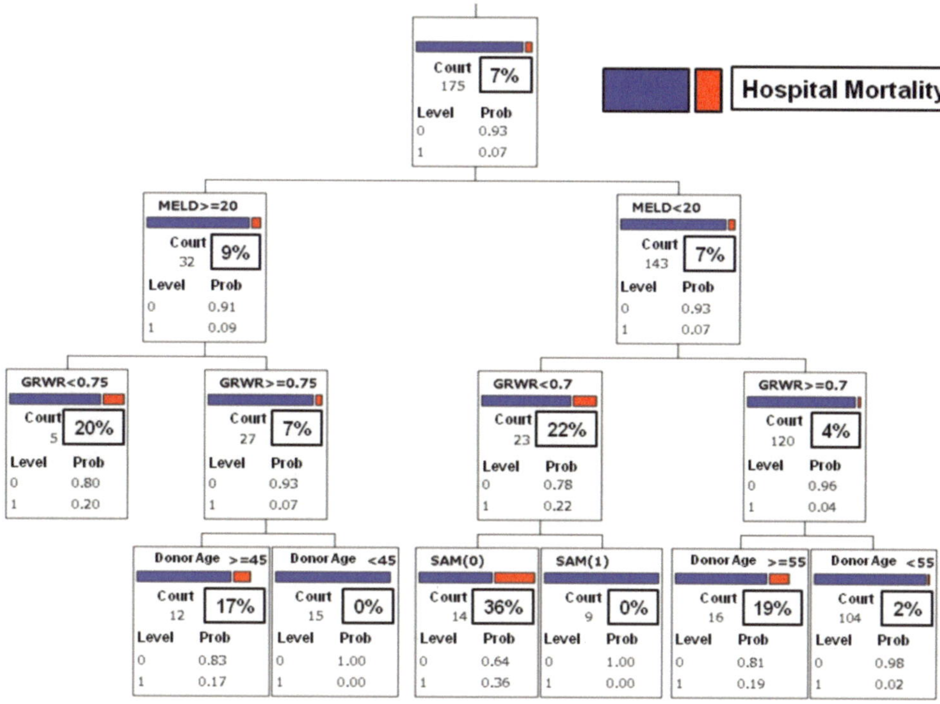

Fig. 6. Decision tree analysis of post-transplant hospital mortality (175 cases). MELD, model for end-stage liver disease; GRWR, graft weight to recipient body weight ratio; SAM, splenic artery embolization as portal modulation

The occurrence of small-for-size syndrome and hospital death depends on the specific combination of graft size, donor age, and MELD. Even using large-size graft, the use of grafts with high MELD and from old-age donors tended to result in the development of small-for-size syndrome and hospital mortality (Figure 5). These results indicated that the use if sufficient graft volume does not prevent the development of small-for-size syndrome graft, and that the incidence of this syndrome depends on other risk factors, which affect the post-transplant prognosis. Concerning the prediction of small-for-size syndrome or post-transplant prognosis, none of the analyses used could find significant risk factors. The decision tree analysis for hospital mortality indicated that the value of any one risk factor should affect the cut-off values of other risk factors (Figure 6). Thus, early graft function and hospital mortality are determined not only by graft size, but also by donor age and recipient status. Donor age and graft size should be matched to the recipient status when possible, and when not possible, portal modulation should be considered. Splenic artery embolization could help reduce the morbidity and mortality rates, as well as increase the survival rates, and should be considered along with the other perioperative risk factors.

Variable	n	Odds ratio	P-Value
Recipient factors			
Age ≥ 54 (vs < 54 years)	78 / 72	1.54	0.59
MELD ≥ 23 (vs < 23)	24 / 126	3.66	0.001
Disease			
Cholestatic disease vs PLC	21 / 115	0.61	0.73
Acute liver failure vs PLC	14 / 115	1.39	
Donor factors			
Age ≥ 53 (vs < 53 years)	33 / 117	6.84	0.03
Graft type (Right lobe vs Left lobe graft)	80 / 70	0.47	0.44
GW/RBW < 0.68% (vs ≥ 0.68%)	26 / 124	1.41	0.72
Treatment and Operative factor			
Portal modulation	70 / 80	0.61	0.54
Blood loss ≥ 50 (vs < 50ml/kg)	101 / 49	1.90	0.61
CIT ≥ 80 (vs < 80min)	35 / 115	1.91	0.40
WIT ≥ 50 (vs < 50min)	42 / 108	1.87	0.74
Operating time ≥ 10 (vs < 10hrs)	59 / 91	3.98	0.39

Table 2. Logistic regression analysis of post-transplant hospital mortality (the later 150 cases). LC, post-necrotic liver cirrhosis; MELD, model for end-stage liver disease; GW/RBW, graft weight to recipient body weight ratio; CIT, cold ischemic time; WIT, warm ischemic time

5. Conclusion

Recently published clinical trials and basic research conducted by several groups have uncovered the mechanism of small-for-size syndrome, allowing the design and implementation of new treatment strategies. These advances have resulted in significant improvement in prognosis after living donor transplantation. Further improvement of liver transplantation and liver surgery techniques should result in better outcome of patients with small for size syndrome.

6. Acknowledgement

This work was supported by a Grant-in-Aid for scientific research from the Ministry of Education, Culture, Sports, Science and Technology of Japan

7. References

Botha, JF; Campos, BD & Johanning J, et al. (2009). Endovascular closure of a hemiportocaval shunt after small for size adult-to-adult left lobe living donor liver transplantation. *Liver Transplantation*; 15:1671-1675.

Broering, DC; Walter, J & Bassas AF. (2005) Overcoming the portal steal phenomenon in auxiliary partial orthotopic liver transplantation by modulation of the venous outflow of the native liver. *Liver Transplantation;* 11: 1140-1143.

Dahm, F; Georgiev, P & Clavien, PA, et al. (2005). Small for size syndrome after partial liver transplantation: Definition, mechanisms of disease and clinical implications. *American Journal of Transplantation;* 5: 2605-2610.

Eguchi, S; Yanaga, K & Sugiyama, N, et al. (2003). Relationship between portal venous flow and liver regeneration in patients after living donor right-lobe liver transplantation. *Liver Transplantation;* 9: 547-551.

Eipel, C; Glanemann, M & Nuessler, AK, et al. (2005). Ischemic preconditioning impairs liver regeneration in extended reduced-size livers. *Annals of Surgery;* 241: 477-484.

Hessheimer, AJ; Fondevila, C & Taurá, P, et al. (2011).Decompression of the portal bed and twice-baseline portal inflow are necessary for the functional recovery of a "small for size" graft. *Annals of Surgery;* 253:1201-1210.

Hill, MJ; Hughes, M & Jie T, et al. (2009). Graft weight/recipient weight ratio: how well does it predict outcome after partial liver transplants? *Liver Transplantation;* 15:1056-1062.

Ikegami, T; Masuda, Y & Ohno Y, et al. (2009). Prognosis of adult patients transplanted with liver grafts < 35% of their standard liver volume. *Liver Transplantation;* 15:1622-1630.

Ikegami, T; Toshima, T & Takeishi, K, et al. (2009).Bloodless splenectomy during liver transplantation for terminal liver diseases with portal hypertension. *Journal of the American College of Surgeons;* 208:e1-4.

Kiuchi , T; Kasahara, M & Uryuhara K, et al. (1999). Impact of graft size mismatching on graft prognosis in liver transplantation from living donors. *Transplantation;* 67: 321-327.

Marcos, A; Fisher, RA & Ham, JM, et al. (2000). Liver regeneration and function in donor and recipient after right lobe adult to adult living donor liver transplantation. *Transplantation;* 69: 1375-1379.

Navasa, M; Feu, F & Garcia-Pagan, JC, et al. (1993). Hemodynamic and humoral changes after liver transplantation in patients with cirrhosis. *Hepatology* 1993; 17: 355-360.

Ogura, Y; Hori, T & El, Moghazy WM, et al. (2010). Portal pressure <15 mm Hg is a key for successful adult living donor liver transplantation utilizing smaller grafts than before. *Liver Transplantation;* 16:718-728.

Park, A & Baichwal, VR (1996). Systematic mutational analysis of the death domain of the tumor necrosis factor receptor 1-associated protein TRADD. *Journal of Biological Chemistry;* 271: 9858-9862.

Piscaglia, F; Zironi, G & Gaiani S, et al. (1999). Systemic and splanchnic hemodynamic changes after liver transplantation for cirrhosis: A long-term prospective study. *Hepatology* 1999; 30: 58-64.

Sterpetti, AV; Cucina, A & Morena, AR, et al. (1993). Shear stress increases the release of interleukin-1 and interleukin-6 by aortic endothelial cells. *Surgery;* 114: 911-914.

Tian, Y; Graf, R & Jochum, W, et al. (2003). Arterialized partial orthotopic liver transplantation in the mouse: A new model and evaluation of the critical liver mass. *Liver Transplantation;* 9: 789-795.

Tian, Y; Jochum, W & Georgiev, P, et al. (2006). Kupffer cell-dependent TNF-alpha signaling mediates injury in the arterialized small for size liver transplantation in the mouse. *Proceedings of the National Academy of Sciences USA* 2006; 103: 4598-4603.

Tian, Y; Jochum, W & Georgiev P, et al. (2006). Kupffer cell-dependent TNF-alpha signaling mediates injury in the arterialized small for size liver transplantation in the mouse. *Proceedings of the National Academy of Sciences USA* 2006; 103: 4598-4603.

Troisi, R & de Hemptinne, B. (2003). Clinical relevance of adapting portal vein flow in living donor liver transplantation in adult patients. *Liver Transplantation;* 9: 36-41.

Umeda, Y; Yagi, T & Sadamori, H, et al. (2007). Preoperative proximal splenic artery embolization: A safe and efficacious portal decompression technique that improves the outcome of live donor liver transplantation. *Transplantation International;* 20: 947-955.

Umeda, Y; Yagi, T & Sadamori, H, et al. (2008). Effects of prophylactic splenic artery modulation on portal overperfusion and liver regeneration in small for size graft. *Transplantation* 15; 86: 673-80.

Yagi, S; Iida, T & Taniguchi, K, et al. (2005). Impact of portal venous pressure on regeneration and graft damage after living-donor liver transplantation. *Liver Transplantation;* 11: 68-75.

Zhong, Z; Schwabe, RF & Kai, Y, et al. (2006). Liver regeneration is suppressed in small for size liver grafts after transplantation: Involvement of c-Jun N-terminal kinase, cyclin D1, and defective energy supply. *Transplantation;* 82: 241-250.

Part 2

Deceased Donor Liver Transplantation: Surgical Techniques

5

Vascular and Biliary Anastomoses in Deceased Donor Orthotopic Liver Transplantation

Steven Cohn, Julie Stein, Alan Koffron and Vandad Raofi
Oakland University William Beaumont School of Medicine / Beaumont Health System
USA

1. Introduction

The purpose of this chapter is to review the various techniques of implantation for deceased donor liver transplants (DDLT). Given the overall broad nature of the topic, the focus will be exclusively on adult DDLT, without including split liver and living donor liver transplants.

There are a total of five structures that have to be reconstructed in DDLT. These include the suprahepatic and infrahepatic vena cava, the portal vein, the hepatic artery and the bile duct. Prior to describing the various methods of implantation of the donor liver, we will briefly review the different options available for the recipient hepatectomy, as the surgeon's choice of reconstruction of the vena cava will dictate the type of hepatectomy performed. For a bicaval anastomosis, the hepatectomy involves completely dissecting out the supra- and infrahepatic vena cava, mobilizing the inferior vena cava (IVC) off of the retroperitoneum, achieving full vascular isolation and subsequently removing the intrahepatic portion of the IVC with the native liver. In this scenario, the use of venovenous bypass may be required for hemodynamic stability of the patient. The traditional method involves reconstruction of the suprahepatic and infrahepatic donor cava to the corresponding structures in the recipient.

A second option is to preserve the vena cava by dissecting the native liver off of the IVC completely. Subsequently, we describe several ways in which the cava is reanastomosed in the setting of caval preservation. One method is commonly known as the "piggyback" technique where two or all three recipient hepatic veins are joined together into a common orifice which is used as the site of anastomosis. Other configurations of caval anastomosis are also used, including side-to-side and end-to-side techniques. Finally, we discuss a modification of the lateral cavo-cavostomy.

The remainder of the implantation is similar regardless of the method chosen for caval reconstruction. The next anastomosis is usually the portal vein (PV). For the most part, portal vein reconstruction is straightforward unless there is partial or complete thrombosis of the recipient portal vein. If thrombectomy fails, then a venous conduit may be necessary. Other salvage maneuvers are used if even a conduit is not possible.

At this point, the liver is usually reperfused. In some situations, hepatic arterial reperfusion is performed simultaneously with portal, or even precedes portal reconstruction. Close cooperation between the surgical and anesthesia team is necessary at this critical time as reperfusion instability may result.

Hepatic arterial reconstruction probably has the most options, as anatomic variations are common, and depending on surgeon preference, different techniques of reconstruction are available. If there is inadequate inflow from the recipient's hepatic artery or its branches, an arterial conduit between the recipient aorta and donor artery may be necessary.

The last anastomosis is the biliary, which has been dubbed the "Achilles heel" of DDLT. Options for reconstructing the bile duct include common duct to common duct anastomosis for the donor and recipient. The second method is a Roux-en-Y hepaticojejunostomy. We will discuss the indications for a Roux reconstruction, and mention some controversies regarding biliary reconstruction.

While an attempt is made to mention many variations in technique, the reader should bear in mind the fact that there are numerous small modifications that are done on a case by case basis based upon the surgeon's preference and personal experience.

2. Recipient hepatectomy

Deceased donor liver transplantation (DDLT) can be divided into several distinct steps. The first is the recipient hepatectomy, followed by the anhepatic phase, and finally reperfusion of the donor graft and completion of the arterial and biliary reconstruction. It would be difficult to simply focus on the implantation of the donor graft without mentioning the recipient hepatectomy, as the choice of vascular reconstruction during the implantation essentially dictates the type of hepatectomy performed.

A key factor to improving outcomes in DDLT is minimizing the cold ischemic time especially in marginal donors or in donation after cardiac death. Therefore, we prefer to have two surgical teams. Once the procurement team has visualized the donor liver and reviewed any biopsies if indicated, the decision is made to proceed or abort the recipient case. If the donor liver is deemed suitable, the recipient is brought to the operating room in preparation for the procedure. Our preference is to have both a pulmonary artery catheter placed for close hemodynamic monitoring, as well as a large bore bypass line placed in the right internal jugular vein in case of need for venovenous bypass.

The hepatectomy can be quite challenging depending on factors such as the degree of portal hypertension, presence of adhesions, and clinical stability of the recipient. Typically, it is started by a bilateral subcostal incision with a vertical midline incision (Figure 1). Previous incisions or anatomy (e.g. presence of ostomy) may dictate where the incision is made. Also, if a combined liver and kidney transplant is planned, the subcostal portion can be made lower on the abdominal wall to facilitate placement of the kidney. With the standard incision, the right side is extended laterally to at least to the mid-axillary line to allow for adequate exposure for both dissection and placement of clamps on the IVC. The upper midline extension is carried to the xiphoid process, and, if necessary, the xiphoid is removed for better exposure of the suprahepatic IVC. The falciform ligament is then taken down and the coronary ligament is dissected until the anterior border of the suprahepatic IVC is identified. Next the left triangular ligament is divided and the left lateral lobe is mobilized. The next step is to mobilize the gastro-hepatic ligament, which would expose the left side of the IVC and the caudate lobe. If there is a replaced left hepatic artery it is ligated at this time.

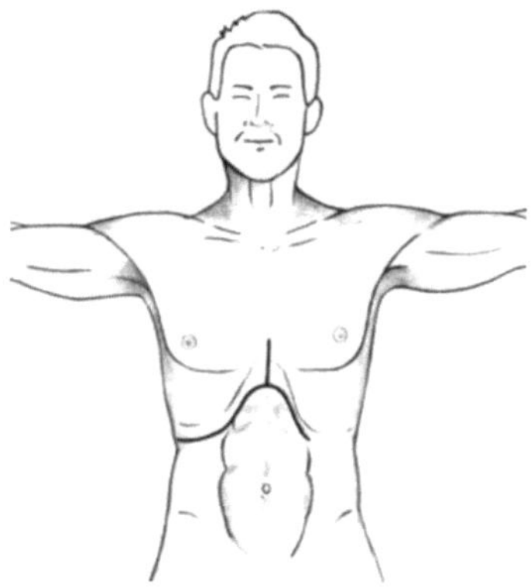

Fig. 1. Typical bilateral subcostal incision with upper midline extension

Dissection of the portal structures proceeds from the left or right side depending on the surgeon's preference. From the left, the gastro-hepatic ligament is divided anterior to the caudate lobe, and the lateral aspect of the portal vein is identified. Staying anterior to the PV, the proper hepatic artery is dissected out and transected. We do not routinely dissect out and divide the right and left hepatic artery individually high up in the hilum. However, some teams prefer to maintain length on the native artery if their preference is to use the bifurcation of the proper hepatic artery for reconstruction. Once the hepatic artery is divided, the only structure anterior to the PV is the common bile duct. This structure is taken down immediately distal to the insertion of the cystic duct. Finally, the only remaining structure in the hilum is the portal vein. At this time the PV is completely skeletonized from its bifurcation distally to near the first pancreatic branch proximally. One needs to ensure that the PV is completely mobilized circumferentially from the surrounding lymphatic and loose areolar tissue.

The next step is mobilization of the IVC. The initial step is to dissect out and obtain control of the infrahepatic IVC. Once the plane of the IVC is established, we continue to the left and mobilize the lateral aspect of the caudate lobe off of the IVC. This is carried in a cephalad direction until the lateral aspect of the suprahepatic IVC is identified immediately above the insertion of the left hepatic vein. When the left side of the IVC is exposed, attention is then directed toward mobilizing the right lobe of the liver. The right triangular and hepatorenal ligaments are taken down and the right lobe is mobilized fully until the suprahepatic IVC is exposed immediately superior to the insertion of right hepatic vein.

At this point, the dissection differs between the standard and caval sparing technique.

2.1 Bicaval hepatectomy

For the standard bicaval technique, both the suprahepatic and infrahepatic IVC are circumferentially dissected out. Generally, the right adrenal vein has to be taken down to provide for adequate infrahepatic exposure. Care is taken near the right renal vein, adrenal gland, and right hepatic vein. Gently, the surgeon's index finger is passed behind the suprahepatic IVC and the soft tissue posterior to the IVC is ensnared and retracted forward (Figure 2). This tissue is taken down either with electrocautery or tied off with silk tie if there is any concern for bleeding or retroperitoneal varices.

Once the intrahepatic cava is fully mobilized a test clamp is performed. For this, the surgeon manually compresses both the infrahepatic IVC and the PV, then checks with the anesthesia team to ensure patient stability. If the patient remains hemodynamically stable, then we proceed with the hepatectomy. Initially a clamp is placed on the PV proximally and the distal aspect of the PV is tied off with a silk tie at the level of its bifurcation and transected. Subsequently a vascular clamp is place on the infrahepatic IVC. This clamp can be either placed in a horizontal or vertical position. Finally, a clamp is placed on the suprahepatic IVC. The recipient's IVC is transected between the clamps and the liver is passed off the field.

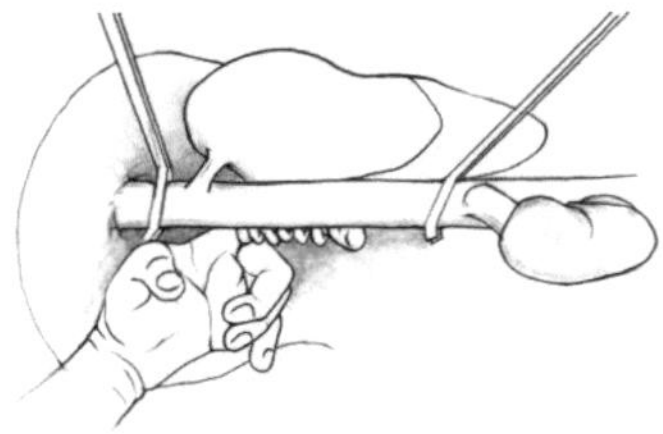

Fig. 2. Hepatectomy with mobilization of retrohepatic vena cava

While this technique avoids the extra time for going on venovenous bypass, two concerns arise. First, is that the recipient may initially be hemodynamically stable, but may become unstable during the anhepatic phase. Second, if there is concern for lack of exposure, such as edematous viscera, small recipient, or a large donor liver, proceeding in the anhepatic phase without bypass can lead to significantly worsening bowel edema and a more technically challenging implantation. For these reasons, we have a very low threshold for going on bypass. In general, however, venovenous bypass is used selectively nowadays depending on the recipient status and the bias of the surgical team (Reddy, 2005).

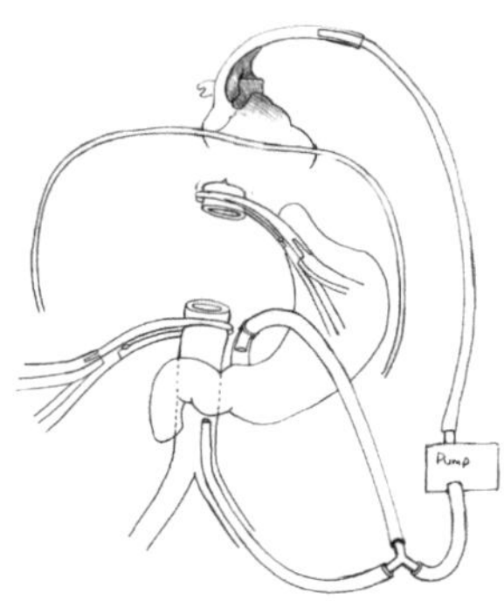

Fig. 3. Venovenous Scheme: Systemic and mesenteric flow travels out of patient through centrifugal pump, and is reintroduced into systemic circulation through either the axillary or jugular vein

To start systemic bypass, a femoral cannula is placed by cut-down or percutaneous technique in either groin, and the infrarenal cava is cannulated. Systemic return is through a cannula placed through cutdown in the axillary vein, or (as we prefer) through a percutaneously placed jugular cannula. Systemic bypass is then initiated while leaving the portal cannula of the circuit still clamped. Subsequently, the PV is clamped and taken down, and the PV cannula is then inserted and full venovenous bypass initiated (Figure 3). In certain situations,only the systemic and/or portal bypass portion of the venovenous circuit is utilized. Once on venovenous bypass, the infrahepatic and suprahepatic IVC are clamped and the liver is explanted. Rarely, as with a very large liver (e.g. polycystic liver), the hepatectomy is facilitated by removing the left lateral segment of the liver first.

2.2 Caval sparing hepatectomy

For the caval sparing technique, the caudate and right lobes are mobilized as before. However, the right adrenal vein is left alone, and no dissection is carried out behind the cava. Instead, starting from the region of the infrahepatic cava, the liver is mobilized off the anterior surface of the IVC. Dissection proceeds either from left to right (or visa versa) depending on the anatomy. All short hepatic veins are dissected out and either tied with silk ties or oversewn with 5-0 prolene for larger branches. Larger retrohepatic veins may also be stapled.

While the PV can be left intact during most of the piggyback dissection, many surgeons prefer to create a temporary end-to-side portacaval shunt to minimize mesenteric congestion and improve hemodynamic stability (Cherqui et al., 1994; Llado´ & Figueras, 2004). Other reasons to use a shunt include decreased bleeding, improved renal function, reduced liver congestion,and improved exposure and mobility of the liver.. Shunting is more important when the patient has not developed chronic mesenteric collateralization (e.g. fulminant hepatitis). When partial clamping of the cava is used in conjunction with a shunt, both systemic and mesenteric flow are preserved without the need for venovenous bypass. If no portal decompression is used, the portal vein is left intact as long as possible prior to removing the liver in order to prevent splanchnic congestion (Lerut, 2003).

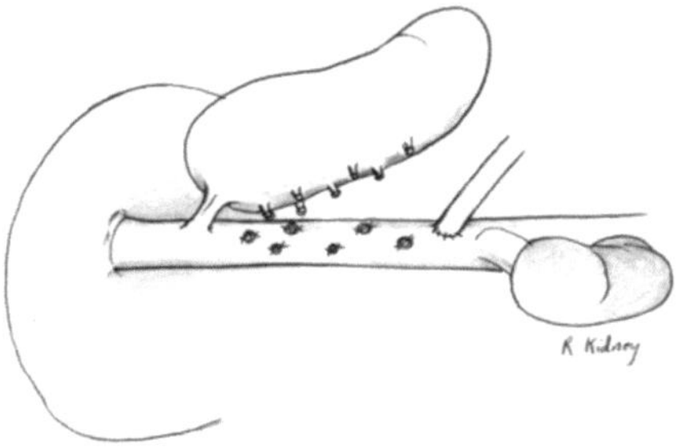

Fig. 4. Caval preservation: Liver is mobilized off retrohepatic cava in a caudal to cephalad direction. Shown above right renal vein is a temporary end-to-side portal caval shunt

The dissection is carried cephalad anterior to the IVC until the IVC ligament is identified, dissected out, and transected. We prefer to use an endovascular stapler on "thick" caval ligaments however one can clamp and cut the IVC ligament, and subsequently suture the remnant stump (large caudate lobes may increase the difficulty). Finally, the hepatic veins are isolated and completely dissected out. Many times, it helps to divide the right hepatic vein which facilitates exposure of the common middle and left trunk.

If a portacaval shunt has not been created, at this time the PV is taken down, and depending on the reconstruction technique, the hepatic veins are either taken with a stapler or a Satinsky clamp is placed on the caval side of the hepatic veins, and the liver is removed. If the hepatic vein cuffs are to be used as part of the recipient anastomosis, the veins are transected intrahepatically to preserve length. The liver is now removed.

Caval sparing techniques are used in large part to maintain systemic (and portal flow, if a temporary portal caval shunt is used) without requiring venovenous bypass. Thus, the dissection is carried out without disturbing systemic flow of the cava. Sometimes, however, either a partially occluding clamp, or complete caval clamping is necessary if troublesome bleeding ensues. (Belghiti et al., 2001). Also, if necessary, venovenous bypass can be used, although proponents of caval preservation usually are striving to avoid systemic bypass.

During the anhepatic phase, once the liver is explanted, the operative field is meticulously examined to ensure adequate hemostasis. This is the best opportunity to visualize the retrohepatic space before the new liver is implanted.

3. Anhepatic phase

The anhepatic phase consists of the IVC and PV reconstruction.

The initial anastomosis in the implantation of the donor liver is the IVC reconstruction. There are several different techniques which we will discuss here. These include the standard bicaval method, the piggyback technique, the lateral cavocavostomy and a modification of the cavocavostomy technique.

3.1 Bicaval technique

For the standard bicaval reconstruction, both the suprahepatic and infrahepatic IVC of the recipient are already fully clamped. Depending on the patient's clinical status and the surgeon's preference, the patient may already be on venovenous bypass. The donor liver is brought onto the operative field. Some teams prefer to maintain a slow, continuous antegrade flush through the portal vein to keep the liver cold. For the suprahepatic IVC, 3-0 prolene suture is used. Initially the corner stitches are placed on both the donor and recipient suprahepatic IVC and the liver is gently lowered into the surgical field. Both ends are tied and the posterior wall o f the IVC is anastomosed first from inside the lumen of both veins. An imbrication technique is used to prevent posterior leaks, and to exclude potentially thrombogenic adventitial surfaces. Subsequently the anterior wall is sutured.

After the suprahepatic IVC anastomosis is complete, attention is turned to the infrahepatic IVC. The anastomosis is created with 4-0 prolene in similar fashion to the suprahepatic IVC. Prior to completing the lower caval anastomoses, the liver needs to be flushed with approximately 1 liter of cold crystalloid solution to remove by products of metabolism, air, and preservation solution. This is especially true if using University of Wisconsin solution which is high in potassium and can cause arrhythmias post-reperfusion. The crystalloid is flushed through the donor's PV and the effluent is drained via the infrahepatic IVC.

When the drainage is complete, the lower IVC anastomosis is completed. Sometimes the lower caval anastomosis is left untied to allow egress of blood if the surgical team prefers to also vent the liver with blood prior to final reperfusion. (Figure 5).

3.2 Classic piggyback technique

In the case of the piggyback technique, there is no infrahepatic IVC reconstruction. In this case the orifice of the right hepatic vein can be tied or stapled off, and the common opening of the middle and left hepatic veins of the recipient are sewn to the donor's suprahepatic IVC. However, joining all three hepatic veins and using a common orifice may be associated with less incidence of venous outflow obstruction (Parrilla et al., 1999; Tayar et al, 2011). Usually, it is technically difficult to place a clamp that will include all three veins during the hepatectomy phase. Therefore, in most instances, the orifice of the right hepatic vein and the common orifice of the left and middle hepatic veins are initially clamped separately. Once the liver is removed, a second clamp is placed to include all three veins The initial clamps are removed and the opening of all three veins are joined together. (Figure 6). Another technique described involves making a horizontal enlargement of the middle/left trunk to decrease outflow obstruction (Lerut et al, 1997).

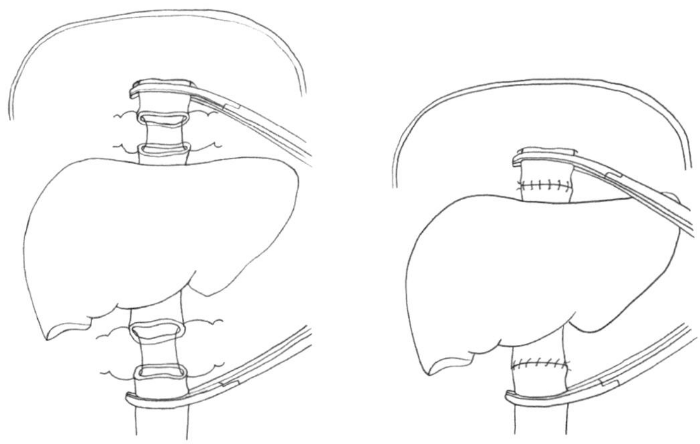

Fig. 5. Bicaval reconstruction: Suprahepatic anastomosis preceedes infrahepatic anastomosis

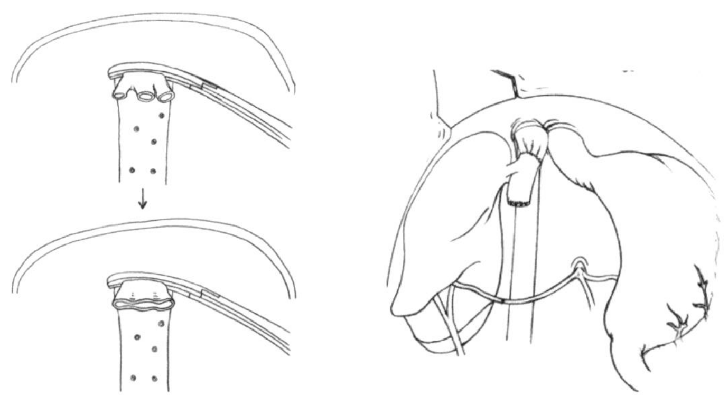

Fig. 6. Classic piggyback reconstruction: Recipient hepatic veins are joined together (all three in this picture), and anastomosed to donor cava

The donor liver is brought onto the operative field. Using 3-0 prolene, the donor's suprahepatic cava is anastomosed to the common orifice of all three hepatic veins of the recipient. Similar to the bicaval technique the posterior wall is created first. Once the suprahepatic anastomoses is complete, one liter of cold crystalloid solution is flushed through the donor's PV and the effluent is drained through the donor infrahepatic cava. Once the flush is complete, the orifice of the donor infrahepatic IVC is stapled off with a TA stapler, or double tied off with 0 silk ties. Once again, some teams leave the infrahepatic side open for further blood venting prior to reperfusion.

3.3 Piggyback modifications

As surgeons gained more experience with the original piggyback concept, other variations of the caval reconstruction evolved ((Belghiti et al., 1992; Bismuth et al., 1992; Cherqui et al., 1994,Lerut et al, 1997). These were developed to allow preservation of caval flow, and to decrease venous outflow complications. Configurations include lateral side-to-side cavocavostomy and end-to-side cavocavostomy (Figure 7).

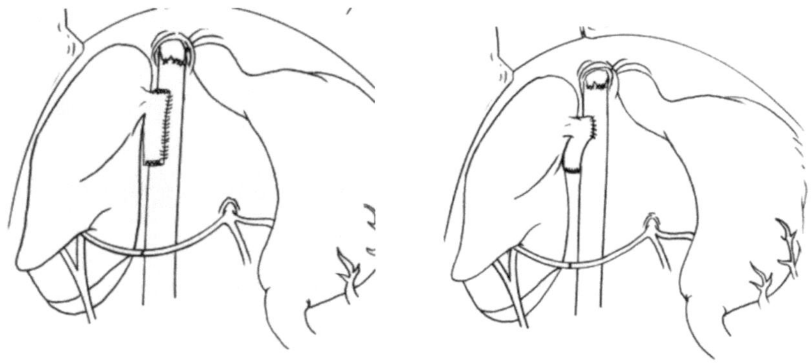

(a) (b)

Fig. 7. Piggyback modifications: (a) side-to-side and (b) end-to-side. The recipient hepatic veins have been stapled closed

The hepatectomy for these techniques is similar to that described above for the classic piggyback technique. A portacaval shunt can be created depending on the operating team's preference and the patient's clinical status. To perform the side-to-side anastomosis, the recipient hepatic veins are transected and the donor cava's suprahepatic and infrahepatic openings are eventually closed. A partially occluding clamp is placed on the recipient's cava, and a longitudinal cavotomy is created (approximately 6 cm). A corresponding cavotomy is made on the donor cava, and a side-to-side anastomosis is carried out between the recipient and donor (Figure 8). This anastomosis is usually done from the left side of the table using an intraluminal technique. Depending on the placement of the stay sutures, a triangulated anastomosis can also be fashioned (Dasgupta, 2006).

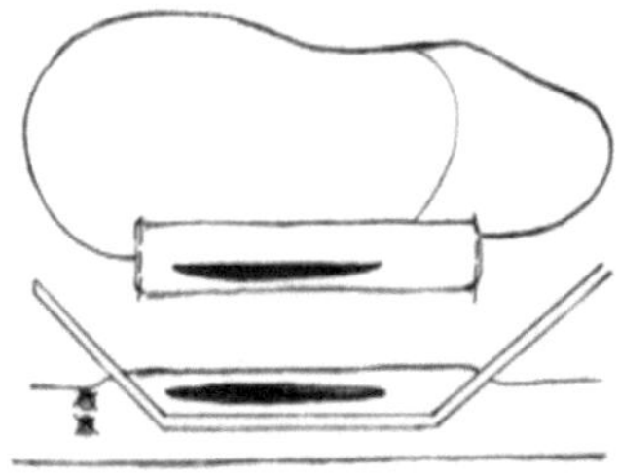

Fig. 8. Lateral-to-lateral cavocavostomy. The recipient hepatic vein orifices have been closed. A partially occluding clamp is placed on recipient side to preserve caval flow

The liver can be flushed with either cold crystalloid solution through the PV prior to completing the PV anastomosis, or blood can be introduced though the completed PV anastomosis and allowed to vent through the open end of the donor cava, which is subsequently stapled closed.

One issue to keep in mind with this technique, is that even though the recipient IVC is not fully clamped, in order to create a longitudinal cavotomy, one needs to partially clamp the IVC and the patient's hemodynamic status needs to be carefully monitored. Advantages of the cavostomy technique include a widely patent anastomoses which minimizes outflow obstruction. Furthermore, this technique allows for better exposure and easier anastomoses in cases with difficult exposure, such as a large donor liver. The mobility and positioning of the liver may even facilitate the biliary anastomosis (Sonnenday et al., 2008).

Other variations of the piggyback technique include the end-to-side configuration (Figure 7a) which may involve enlarging the donor opening with a longitudinal cavotomy through the suprahepatic portion of the donor cava. Also, the recipient hepatic vein orifices may be included, for example, by creating a longitudinal cavotomy through the common trunk of the middle/left veins (Figure 9) (Klintmalm & Busuttil, 2005).

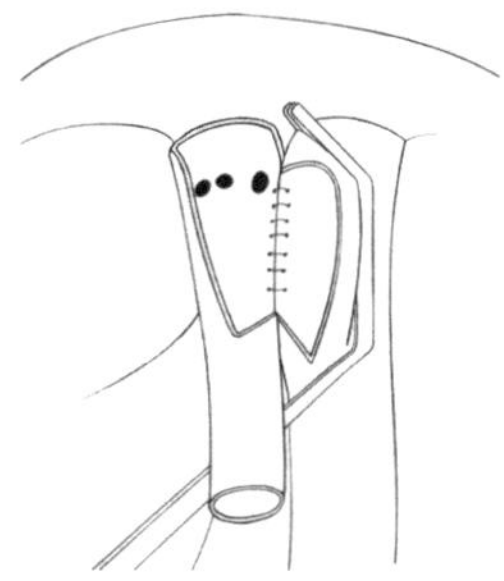

Fig. 9. Another variation utilizing partial caval clamping

3.4 Modification of the cavocavostomy

A final variant of the caval anastomoses is to combine the cavocavostomy incision with the orifice of the hepatic veins on both the donor and recipient. This has been referred to as a suprahepatic cavoplasty (Wu et al., 2001) or a triangulating cavocavostomy (Dasgupta et al., 2006). It is similar to the variant of the piggyback technique described above (Figure 9) but creates a much larger cavotomy. Also, this method requires full clamping of the IVC and, therefore, the hemodynamic changes are similar to the standard bicaval technique and the recipient may require the use of complete venovenous bypass.

However, unlike the bicaval technique there is no need for retroperitoneal dissection of the IVC, nor is there a need for piggyback dissection.

For this method, the recipient suprahepatic and infrahepatic IVC are fully dissected out. If the patient tolerates a test clamp, we will proceed with the hepatectomy, otherwise venovenous bypass is initiated. The PV is clamped and transected at its bifurcation. The suprahepatic and infrahepatic IVC are also clamped. Using Metzenbaum scissors, the short hepatics are sharply divided until the level of the hepatic veins. A small patch of the anterior IVC can also be resected along with short hepatics. Subsequently the hepatic veins are also transected intrahepatically, creating a large "triangular" opening along the length of the intrahepatic IVC which also includes the orifice of the hepatic veins. The orifice of the short hepatic veins are either included in the segment of the anterior IVC that was removed, or for the most part can be excluded by the suture line.

Transected veins that will not become part of the anastomosis are suture repaired, and the three hepatic vein orifices are converted into one opening continuous with the cavotomy. Extraneous tissue on the remnant hepatic veins is trimmed in preparation for the anastomosis (Figure 10).

For the donor liver, a slit is created in the posterior aspect of the IVC starting from and incorporating the suprahepatic caval opening. This cavotomy is created to match the opening of the recipient IVC, but does not extend fully to the infrahepatic IVC of the donor (Figure 10). Using 3-0 prolene, the three corner sutures are placed. Care is taken to avoid compromising the hepatic vein orifices on the donor liver. Initially the right lateral wall is created, followed by the left side, and finally the superior aspect. Sometimes, it may be easier to perform the entire anastomosis from the left side by doing the right suture line intraluminally. Again, one liter of cold crystalloid solution is perfused through the donor PV and effluent is drained through the infrahepatic IVC. The infrahepatic donor cava is stapled closed (or left open for blood venting).

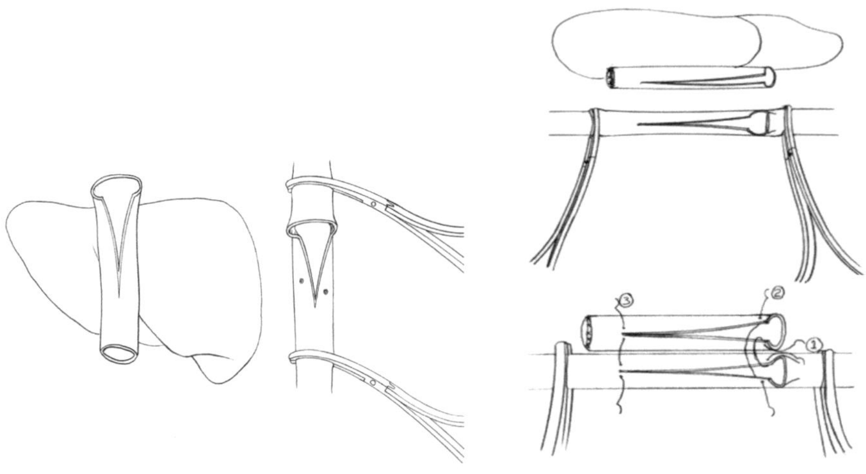

Fig. 10. "Modified" cavocavostomy (triangulated anastomosis). The recipient hepatic vein orifices are incorporated into the anastomosis. The cava is totally occluded. Three corner stitches are shown

Though this modification requires full IVC clamping with potential need for venovenous bypass, it is our preferred method for several reasons. First, it does create the largest possible outflow. Second, in cases with poor exposure, there is no posterior suprahepatic caval anastomosis, and there is better exposure during both the caval reconstruction and after reperfusion to allow examination of the suture line. Finally, since the short hepatic veins will be either removed with the patch of IVC or incorporated into the anastomoses, the hepatectomy phase is considerably shortened since one can simply "cut off" the anterior wall of the cava once the clamps are placed. There is no need to meticulously dissect the liver off the IVC. Furthermore, bleeding during this phase of the hepatectomy is minimized since there is full isolation of the IVC during mobilization of the liver off of the IVC.

The technique can be done expeditiously, and, thus, as experience is gained with the technique, it may be possible to forego systemic and/or portal bypass. In addition, size mismatch problems between donor and recipient are decreased (Wu et al., 2001).

A variant of this technique has been called the "infrahepatic" cavocavostomy. (Khanmoradi, et al., 2009) In this case, the donor cava is opened from the infrahepatic side and the suprahepatic side is closed. A side-to-side anastomosis is created. This technique has been touted as an alternative when either recipient or donor characteristics make using the suprahepatic cava hazardous. For example, if a transjugular shunt is present or if there is a significant size mismatch between donor and recipient. It has also been used as a rescue technique if there is outflow obstruction following a piggyback anastomosis. (Quintini et al., 2008).

To summarize, each of the relative pros/cons of the above techniques have been debated. Advocates for the classic bicaval technique state that most cases can still be done without the need for cava preservation unless, for example, the donor graft is relatively small, or if retroperitoneal inflammation precludes dissection (Klintmalm and Busuttil,2005). Also, venous outflow complications may be lower with end-to-end anastomosis vs piggyback technique (Glanemann et al., 2002). Some teams have found that, in their hands, venovenous bypass may not even be necessary a majority of the time, even with the classic technique (Vieira de Melo et al., 2011). In cases of unfavorable anatomy, as with a large liver or caudate lobe, classic caval resection may be easier (Navarro et al., 1997).

Advocates for caval preservation state that greater hemodynamic stability, less bleeding, decreased warm ischemic time, improved renal flow, better visualization are advantages of caval preservation. Technical modifications have reduced venous outflow complications (Mehrabi et al., 2009).Also,venovenous bypass with its inherent problems (e.g. air embolism, nerve injury, wound infections) can often be avoided, and splanchnic congestion can be handled with temporary portal caval shunting (Belghiti et al., 1995; Llado' & Figueras, 2004). In many cases,portal shunting can also be avoided if the portal vein is maintained until the hepatectomy is finished (Lerut et al., 2003). With experience, cases originally thought too difficult can be performed with caval preservation (e.g. large polycystic livers, Budd-Chiari, retransplantation) (Belghiti et al., 2001).

Many comparisons have been studied, but it is difficult to achieve large numbers with prospective studies (Perkins, 2007; Kahn et al., 2006; Lai et al., 2011). Ideally, a surgeon can become familiar with all the techniques in order to adapt to different situations (Eghtesad et al., 2005).

3.5 Portal vein anastomosis

Generally speaking, the PV reconstruction is usually the most straightforward of all the anastomoses. This is due to a lack of extra-hepatic PV anatomic variability (unlike the hepatic artery), and the fact that an end to end anastomoses is essentially the only feasible way of reconstructing the donor and recipient portal veins.

There are however two key points that need to be addressed. One is to ensure that there is no redundancy in the PV anastomoses as this can lead to kinking, poor flow, and increased risk of post-transplant PV thrombosis. The second point is the management of chronic PV thrombus in the recipient.

If the patient has been on venovenous bypass, at this time the PV cannula is removed and the PV clamp is replaced back on. Systemic venovenous bypass is continued. In cases where a portacaval shunt has been created, a vascular clamp is placed on the pancreas side, the caval aspect of the shunt stapled off, and subsequently the shunt is transected.

In order to avoid redundancy in the PV anastomoses, one must keep in mind that the distance between the donor and recipient PV is greatly exaggerated during the anhepatic phase. The rib cage is significantly retracted in a cephalad direction and the visceral contents of the abdomen, including the stomach and duodenum, are retracted down during the caval anastomoses.

Though this provides optimal exposure to the IVC and retroperitoneum, one must keep in mind that this does increase the space between the recipient and donor PV stumps. If this is not accounted for, once the retractors are removed, there could be a noticeable kinking and redundancy in the PV anastomoses. To avoid this complication, an attempt must be made to bring the two PV stumps as close to their natural position as possible. Loosening the rib cage retractors or placing folded laparotomy pads behind the dome of the liver are two ways of bringing the donor liver closer to its natural position. On the recipient side, relaxing the bowel retractors allows the foregut, including the duodenum to return to its normal position. We prefer to put a spoon clamp on the donor PV approximately one to one and a half inches proximal to its bifurcation. This helps us gauge both the length of the donor PV needed and also maintains its orientation. The vascular clamps on the donor and recipient PV are lined up to avoid twisting of the two veins. Any excess length on both the recipient and donor PV are trimmed off. The anastomoses is created with either 5-0 or 6-0 prolene. Again, similar to the IVC anastomoses, the back wall is anastomosed initially followed by the front wall (Figure 11). Near the completion of the PV anastomoses, the donor PV clamp is kept on, the recipient clamp is removed, and about 300-500ml of blood is flushed out to remove any potential clots that may have formed and also to flush out the stagnant blood from the viscera. The PV anastomoses is completed while leaving a "growth factor". Essentially, the running prolene is not tied fully down, and an air knot which would be around one half the diameter of the PV is left to allow for the expansion of the anastomoses once blood flow is restored. This step is done to avoid narrowing at the suture line.

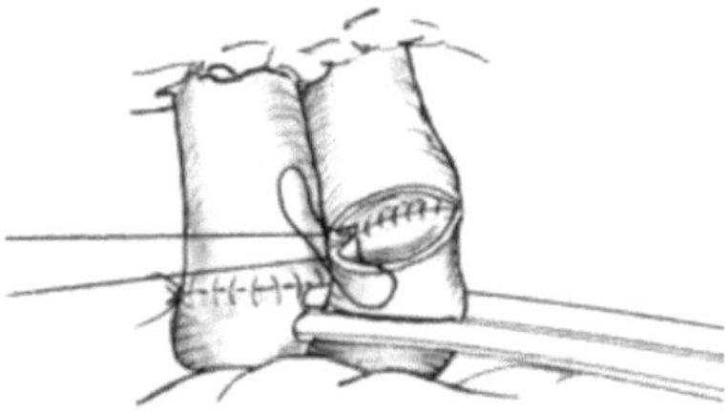

Fig. 11. Portal vein anastomosis. The posterior wall is completed intraluminally. The completed infrahepatic anastomosis is shown

The second potential problem with the PV anastomoses is the chronic PV thrombus that can be encountered in about 15-10% of liver transplant recipients (Yerdel et al., 2000). In the vast majority of cases, this clot is non-occlusive and a simple eversion thrombectomy re-establishes flow. (Dumortiera et al., 2002). This is performed by grasping the edges of the recipient PV with non-crushing clamps, elevating the thrombus away from the wall of the PV using a dissector, and continuing circumferentially. Once a substantial portion of the clot is mobilized, a grasping instrument- such as ring forceps, can be used to forcefully extract the thrombus (Figure 12). The vascular clamp on the recipient PV will have to be periodically released to allow for full extraction of the thrombus as well as to check inflow. Once adequate thrombectomy has been performed the anastomoses can be completed as described above.

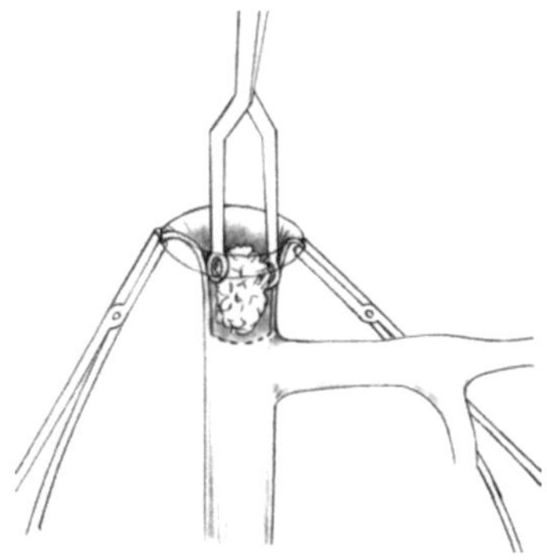

Fig. 12. Eversion thrombectomy of portal vein

If one fails to re-establish flow through the main recipient PV, several options exist. A venous jump graft to the proximal portal vein or the superior mesenteric vein may be constructed using donor iliac vein. This graft is passed behind the stomach and anterior to the pancreas. To perform this, the recipient SMV has to be patent. This structure is dissected out below the level of the transverse colon and proximal to the insertion of the middle colic vein into the SMV. (Nikitin et al., 2009) (Figure 13).

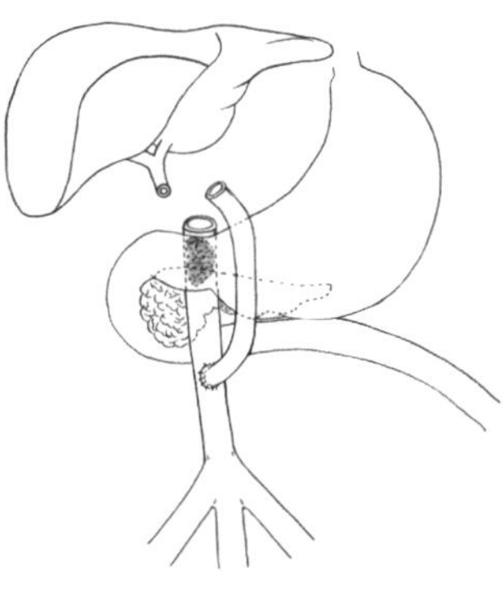

Fig. 13. Venous conduit: Donor iliac vein connects superior mesenteric vein to donor portal vein

In case there is no good target SMV, the inferior mesenteric vein can be used as a potential inflow. Other potential inflow sources include the splenic vein or a large collateral. Finally, if a conduit is not an option, a caval hemi-transposition can be performed. In this technique, the donor PV is anastomosed to the recipient infrahepatic IVC and subsequently the recipient IVC is stapled above the level of the PV anastomoses to divert all flow through the transplanted liver. Unfortunately, outcomes with this method are inferior as may be expected (Yan et al., 2008; Selvaggi et al., 2007). Even more rarely, a conduit may be constructed using donor vessels to supply arterial blood to the portal vein (arterialization).

4. Reperfusion phase

After the IVC and PV anastomoses are complete, the next step is reperfusion of the donor liver. Prior to re-establishing flow, one must closely communicate with the anesthesia team to ensure that the patient is ready for reperfusion. During the initial portion of the reperfusion phase, the right heart is exposed to a large volume of cold preservation solution, which may also be high in potassium, and also contains elevated levels of cytokines secondary to the ischemia of the donor organ. This can potentially lead to right heart failure of arrhythmias. Therefore, ensuring that the anesthesia team is ready for reperfusion is of paramount importance.

The sequence of unclamping and reperfusing the liver depends on the method of IVC reconstruction. In the standard bicaval method or the "triangulation" technique where both the suprahepatic and infrahepatic portions are clamped, initially the suprahepatic IVC clamp is removed and the caval suture lines are closely examined for hemostasis. Second the infrahepatic caval clamp is removed. Finally the PV clamp is removed slowly. If the surgeon's preference is to vent the first several hundred cc's of blood, this is done through the untied infrahepatic caval anastomosis, which is subsequently tied. Once reperfusion is complete, all suture lines and the operative field is examined for full hemostasis prior to proceeding. If the patient had been on venovenous bypass, at this time the femoral vein is decannulated.

In the piggyback and cavocavostomy techniques, there is only one caval clamp. Once this clamp is removed and hemostasis is achieved, the PV clamp is removed. If blood is to be vented, this is achieved through an opening in the donor cava which is subsequently closed. As above, reperfusion syndrome is diminished by slowly reestablishing portal flow.

After reperfusion, the liver is assessed. The liver should attain a normal appearance. flow is poor if the liver is soft and dusky; outflow is poor if the liver is abnormally tense and swollen. Some surgeons use a flow meter to assess the portal and arterial flow.

5. Hepatic artery reconstruction

Usually, hepatic arterial reconstruction follows reperfusion. The order of portal vs arterial reperfusion does not seem to matter; however, sometimes it may be necessary to complete the artery first and reestablish flow to the liver to decrease warm ischemic time (e.g. unexpected difficulty dealing with a portal vein thrombosis) (Busuttil & Klintmalm, 2005).

Unlike the PV, the hepatic artery (HA) anastomoses can be performed in a variety of different ways. This is due in part to variations in the donor and recipient anatomy, the need to optimize inflow and the surgeon's preference.

For a donor HA with standard anatomy and no replaced or accessory branches, several options exist for reconstruction. The celiac axis with or without a patch of aorta can be used. Alternatively, the celiac axis can be shortened near the take-off of the splenic artery.

Subsequently, the celiac axis and splenic artery orifice are joined to create a fishmouth patch. The stump of the left gastric artery is tied off.

On the recipient side, if the HA had been dissected out above the bifurcation of the left and right hepatic arteries, a small vascular clamp or bulldog can be placed on the proper hepatic artery distal to the gastroduodenal artery (GDA) and the right and left branches of the HA are be joined to form a common orifice. A second option is to dissect the proper HA, identify and dissect out the GDA and continue by mobilizing the common HA proximal to the GDA. A vascular clamp is then placed on the common HA, the distal aspect of the GDA is tied off, and a patch is created between the orifice of the GDA and proper HA at this time.

While any combination of the above mentioned options can be used, the main concern with the HA reconstruction is that any excessive length can lead to twisting and looping once the retractors are removed and the liver returns to its native position. This can lead to an increased incidence of HA thrombosis. Therefore, in order to avoid redundancy, our preference is to resect the excess celiac trunk and use the celiac-splenic patch on the donor, which is then anastomosed to the recipient proper HA - GDA patch (Figure 14).

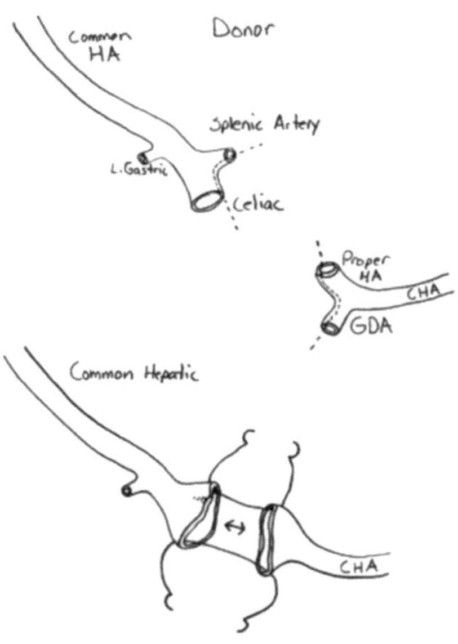

Fig. 14. Typical arterial reconstruction with "common" anatomy. Branch patches are created on both the donor and recipient ends

The two most common variations encountered in the HA anastomoses are replaced (or accessory) right and left hepatic arteries. In case of a replaced or accessory left HA, the reconstruction is simple. The left HA is kept in continuity with the left gastric artery. On the backtable, the main trunk of the left gastric artery is ligated distal to the take-off of the replaced left HA. There are several small branches coming off the left HA which are also dissected out and tied off. If the splenic-celiac axis patch can be created on the donor without compromising the take-off of the left gastric artery, a standard reconstruction is performed similar to previously described. The second option would be to use the celiac trunk on the donor side and tie off the stump of the splenic artery (Figure 15a).

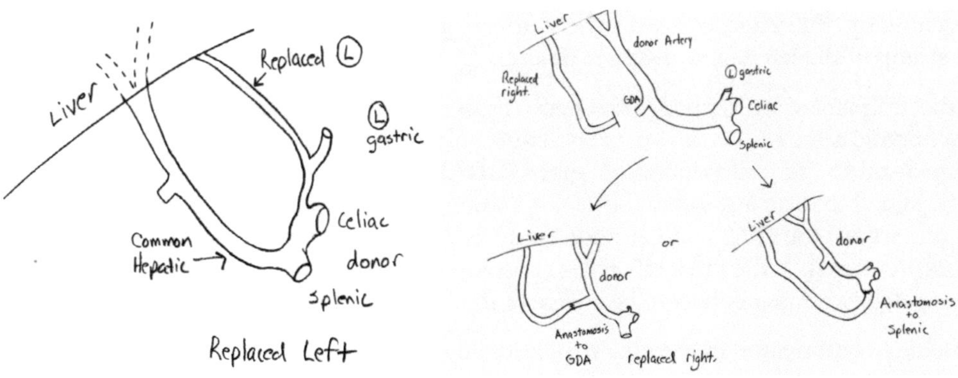

(a) (b)

Fig. 15. Hepatic reconstruction examples with (a) replaced left on donor, and (b) replaced right on donor

For a replaced right HA, the reconstruction is technically more challenging. This structure is usually procured with a segment of the superior mesenteric artery (SMA). While several methods have been described, a common technique used is to resect the excess right HA and SMA trunk and subsequently anastomose the lumen directly to the orifice of the donor splenic artery or GDA. Our preference is to use the GDA to minimize the chance of a kink or twist during the reconstruction on the backtable. The replaced right HA orifice is spatulated and the orifice of the GDA is extended onto the common hepatic artery to create for a wider anastomoses and better outflow (Figure 15b).

If variations in recipient anatomy result in inadequate inflow from the common hepatic artery, another inflow source can be used. For example, if the celiac is inadequate (as in arcuate ligament syndrome), the gastroduodenal artery may be dominant. Likewise, if a replaced right is dominant, it may be more appropriate as the recipient vessel. If no vessel is adequate, an aorta to donor artery conduit is created using donor iliac artery. Usually, the infrarenal aorta is chosen as the recipient side, although sometimes the supraceliac aorta is chosen as the proximal side. Similar to a portal venous conduit, it is tunneled retrocolic between the stomach and the pancreas. The tunnel location may vary depending on the anatomy. The aortic side is created with 5-0 prolene and the donor side with 6-0 prolene (Figure 16).

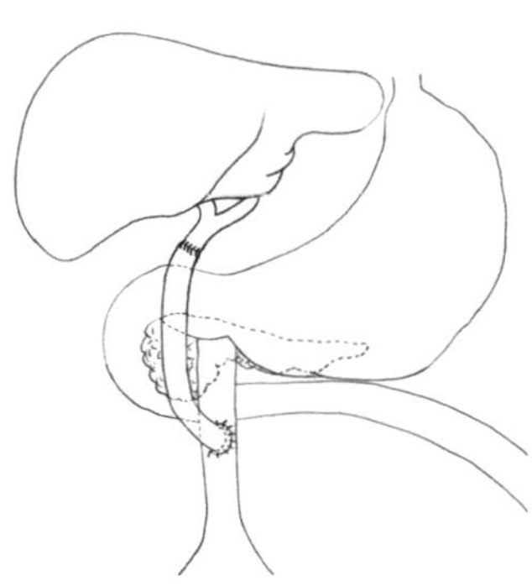

Fig. 16. Arterial conduit: Donor iliac artery connects infrarenal aorta to donor hepatic artery

While the incidence of HA thrombosis is low, both arterial reconstruction of multiple vessels and increased time to arterial reperfusion are risk factors for this complication. (Warner et al., 2011; Oh et al., 2001; Pastacaldi et al., 2001). Therefore, both technique and time are of essence.

6. Biliary anastomosis

Once the liver is reperfused, biliary reconstruction is initiated. An end-to-end anastomosis (choledochocholedochostomy) is the most commonly used configuration. Otherwise, a Roux-en-Y is usually chosen as the second choice. Indications for a Roux include technical difficulty apposing the two duct ends (e.g. after removing a large polycystic recipient liver),size discrepancy, and poor condition or blood supply of recipient duct (e.g. during retransplantation).

Another indication for a Roux is a diseased recipient duct. This can be related to choledocholithiasis, biliary atresia, secondary biliary cirrhosis, or primary sclerosing cholangitis. Recently, the tradition of using a Roux for a disease such as primary sclerosing cholangitis has been readdressed, and some authors have reported the use of duct-to-duct anastomosis when there is no evidence of extra-hepatic stricturing involving the distal duct and/or the duct appears visually healthy (Distante et al., 1996; Heffron et al., 2003). The use of choledochoduodenostomy has also been reported. Also, duct to duct anastomosis has been used during retransplantation (Sibulesky et al., 2011)

Whatever technique is chosen, the goal is to achieve a tension-free anastomosis between two well vascularized structures. To start the end-to-end anastomosis, it is helpful to elevate the liver with several packs placed behind the right lobe. The donor and recipient ends are trimmed to achieve healthy, bleeding surfaces. Bleeders are controlled with suture ligation. Cautery is avoided. If the donor side contains the lumen of the cystic duct, a small septotomy is made between the cystic and common hepatic duct to create a common orifice. If the cystic duct opening is not in continuity with the common duct, it is marsupialized to avoid creating a fluid-filled "sac" that may eventually contort the main duct. The anastomosis is accomplished with 5-0 or 6-0 absorbable, monofilament (PDS) creating the posterior wall first. Although many surgeons interrupt the anastomosis, we run the suture line. If size discrepancies exist, one end may need to be spatulated or partially closed to allow anastomosis. Most of the time, this does not seem necessary.

Traditionally, a T-tube is used. It's purpose is to provide access to the biliary system, to allow monitoring of the quantity and quality of bile, and to "splint" the anastomosis. The current trend, however, is to avoid the use of T-tubes. This is due to the recognition that T-tubes may be associated with biliary leaks as well as other technical problems (Riediger et al., 2010; Sotropoulos et al., 2009).

A Roux-en-Y is constructed in a standard fashion, usually dividing the small bowel 15-20 cm distal to the ligament of Treitz, and making a 40cm defunctionalized limb. The bowel anastomosis can be sewn or stapled. The end of the limb is reinforced with a seromuscular imbricating stitch. The limb is brought to the porta through a retro- or antecolic approach. If the colon is present, and the patient has inflammatory bowel disease, a retrocolic position will make subsequent colectomy easier. The donor duct is anastomosed to the

Roux limb with absorbable monofilament. Some surgeons use an internal or external stent (Figure 17).

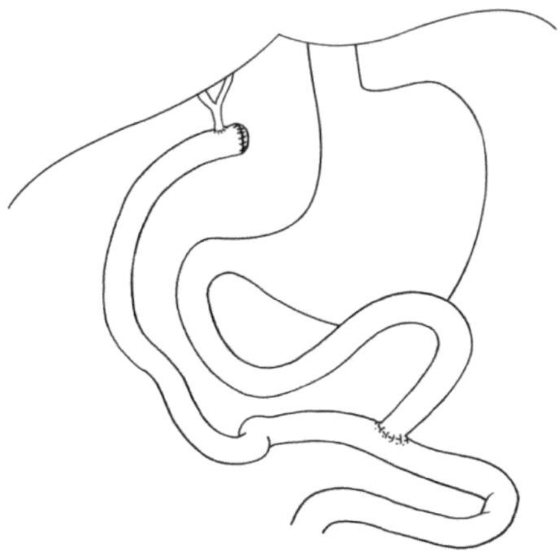

Fig. 17. Roux-en-y biliary anastomosis

7. Closure

Once the biliary reconstruction is complete, systematic inspection of the field is carried out. Mechanical hemostasis is achieved. Non-mechanical bleeding is addressed by the anesthesia team. Generally, two drains are left, one behind the right lobe towards the supahepatic cava, and one near the biliary anastomosis in an infrahepatic position. The midline incision is closed in a single layer, the bilateral subcostal incisions in two layers.

8. References

Belghiti, J, Fekete F, Gayet B, Panis Y, & Sauvanet A,. (1992) A New technique of Side to Side Caval Anastomoses During Orthotopic HepaticTransplantation Without Caval Occlusion. Surg Gynecol Obstet, Vol 75, No.3 (Sep 1992) pp. 75:270-2.

Belghiti J, Noun R, & Sauvanet A. (1995) Temporary Portocaval Anastomosis with Preservation of Caval Flow During Orthotopic Liver Transplantation. Am J Surg, Vol 169, No 2 (1995), pp. 277-279, ISSN 0002-9610

Belghiti J, Durand F, Ettore G.M., Farges O, Jerius J, Sauvanet A, & Sommacale D,. (2001)Feasibility and Limits of Caval-Flow Preservation During Liver Transplantation, Liver Transplantation, Vol 7, No. 11, (November 2001), pp. 983-987, Online ISSN 1527-6473

Bismuth H, Castaing D, Shellock DJ. (1992) Liver Transplantation by "Face to Face" Venacavaplasty, Surgery, Vol 111, (1992) pp.151-5, ISSN 0039-6060

Busuttil, R., & Klintmalm, G, (2005) *The Recipient Hepatectomy and Grafting, In: Transplantation of the Liver,* Busuttil and Klintmalm, (Editors), pp. 575-588, Elsevier Saunders, ISBN 0-7216-01118-9, Philadelphia, PA, USA

Cherqui, D, Dhumeaux, N, Duvoux, D, Fagniez, PL, Julien, M, Lauzet, JV, & Rotman, C,.(1994) Orthotopic Liver Transplantation with Preservation of the Caval and

Portal Flows:Technique and Results in 2 Cases. *Transplantation,* Vol 58, No. 7 (Oct 1994), pp.793-796, ISSN:0041-133

Dasgupta, D, Sharpe, J, Prasad KR, Asthana S, Toogood GJ, Pollard, SG, & Lodge, JP. (2006). Triangular and Self-triangulating Cavocavostomy for Orthotopic Liver Transplantation Without Posterior Suture Lines: a Modified Surgical Technique. *Transpl Int.,* Vol 19, No. 2 (Feb 2006), pp. 117-21, ISSN 0934-0874

Distante V, Farouk M, Kurzawinski TR, Ahmed SW, Burroughs AK, Davidson BR,& Rolles K. (1996) Duct-to-Duct Biliary Reconstruction Following Liver Transplantation for Primary Sclerosing Cholangitis. *Transpl Int,* Vol 9, No. 2 (1996), pp. 126-30, ISSN 0934-0874

Dumortiera, J, Czyglika, B, Poncet, G, Blanchet M-C, Boucaud, C, Henry, L, & Boillot. Eversion Thrombectomy for Portal Vein Thrombosis During Liver Transplantation. (2002). *American Journal of Transplantation,* Vol 2, No. 10(Nov 2002), pp. 934–938, ISSN 1600-6135

Eghtesad, B, Fung, J & Kadry, Z. (2005) Technical Considerations in Liver Transplantation: What a Hepatologist Needs to Know (and Every Surgeon Should Practice), *Liver Transplantation,* Vol 11, No 8 (August 2005),pp. 861-871, online ISSN 1572-6473

Glanemann, M, Settmeacher, U, Langrehr, JM, Stange, B, Haase, R, Nuessler, NC, Lopez-Hanninen,E, Podrabsky, P, Bechstein, WO, & Neuhaus, P. (2002). Results of end-to-end Cavocavostomy During Adult Liver Transplantation. *World J Surg,* Vol 26, No. 3 (Mar 2002), pp.342-7, ISSN 0364-2313

Heffron, T, Smallwood, G, Ramcharan, T, Davis, L, Connor, K, Martinez, E, & Stiebeer, (2003).Duct-to-Duct Biliary Anastomosis for Patients with Sclerosing Cholangitis Undergoing Liver Transplantation. *Transplantation Proceedings,* Vol 35, No.8 (Dec 2003), pp. 3006-7, ISSN 0041-1345

Khan S, Silva MA, Tan YM, John A, Gunson B, Buckels JA, Mayer D, Bramhall SR, & Mirza DF (2006). Conventional versus piggyback technique ofcaval implantation: without extra-corporealvenovenous bypass. A comparative study. *Transpl Int,* Vol, 19, No. 10 (2006), pp.795-801, ISSN 0934-0874, online ISSN 1432-2277

Khanmoradi K, Defaria W, Nishida S, Levi, D, Kato, T, Moon J, Selvaggi, G & Tzakis, A. (2009). Infrahepatic Vena Cavocavostomy, a Modification of the Piggyback Technique for Liver Transplantation. *Am Surgeon,* Vol 75, No. 5 (2009), pp. 421-425, ISSN 0003-1348, online ISSN 1555-9823

Lai, Q, Nudo, F, Molinaro, A, Mennini, G, Spoletini, G, Melandro, F, Guglielmo, N, Parlati, L, Mordenti, M, Corradini, S, Berloco, P, & Rossi, M. (2011). Does Caval Reconstruction Technique Affect Early Graft Function after Liver Transplantation? A Preliminary Analysis. *Transplantation Proceedings,* Vol 43,,No. 4 (2011), pp.1103-1106, ISSN 0041-1345

Lerut, J, Molle, G, Donataccio, M,De Kock, M, Ciccarelli, O, Laterre, PF, Van Leeuw, V, Bourlier, P, Ville de Goyet, J, Reding, R, Gibbs, P, & Otte, JB. (1997) Cavocaval Liver Transplantation Without Venovenous Bypass and Without Temporary Portocaval Shunting: The Ideal Technique for Adult Liver Grafting? Transpl Int, Vol 10, No. 3 (1997), pp.171-179 ISSN 0934-0874

Lerut, J, Ciccarelli, O, Roggen, F, Laterre P.F.,Danse, E, Goffette, P, Aunac, S, Carlier, M, De Kock M,Van Obbergh, L, Veyckemans, F, Guerrieri, C, Reding, R, & Otte, J.B. (2003). Cavocaval Adult Liver Transplantation and Retransplantation Without Venovenous Bypass and Without Portocaval Shunting: a Prospective Feasibility Study in Adult Liver transplantation. *Transplantation*, Vol 25, No. 10 (May 2003), pp.1740-5 ISSN 0041-1337

Llado', L., & Figueras, J. (2004) Techniques of Orthotopic Liver Ttransplantation. *HPB*,Vol. 6, Number 2 (2004) pp. 69-75, ISSN 1477-2574

Mehrabi, A, Zhoobin, A.M., Hamidreza, F, Kashfi, A, Hillebrand, N, Mëller, S.A., Encke, J, Bëchler, M.W., & Schmidt, J. (2009). A Single-Center Experience of 500 LiverTransplants Using the Modified Piggyback Technique by Belghiti. *Liver Transplantation*, Vol 15, No. 5 (2009), pp.466-474, online ISSN 1527-6473

Navarro,F., Moine, Marie-Christine Le, Fabre, Jean-Michel, Belghiti, J, Cherqui D., Adam R., Pruvot, F, Letoublon, C, & Domergue J Specific Vascular Complications of Orthotopic Liver Transplantation with Preservation of the Retrohepatic Vena Cava: Review of 1361 Cases. *Transplantation*, Vol 68 No.5 (Sept 15 1999), pp.646-650 ISSN 0041-1337

Nikitin, D, Jennings, L, Khan, T, Vasani, S, Ruiz, R, Sanchez, E, Chinnakotla, S, Levy, M, Goldstein, R.M., & Klintmalm. (2009). Twenty Years' Follow-Up of Portal Vein Conduits in Liver Transplantation. *Liver Transplantation*, Vol. 15, No. 4 (2009), pp.400-406, online ISSN 1527-6473

Oh CK, Pelletier SJ, Sawyer RG, Dacus AR, McCullough CS, Pruett TL, & Sanfey HA. Uni- and Multivariate Analysis of Risk Factors for Early and Late Hepatic Artery Thrombosis After Liver Transplantation. (2001) *Transplantation*, Vol 71, No. 6 (Mar 2001), pp.767-772, ISSN 0041-1337

Parrilla,P, Sanchez-Bueno, F, Figueras, J, Jaurrieta, E, Mir, J, Margarit, C, Lazaro, J, Herrera, L, Gomez-Fleitas, M, Varo, E,Vicente, E,Robles, R,& Ramirez, P. Analysis of the Complications of the Piggy Back Technique in 1,112 Liver Transplants. *Transplantation*, Vol 67, No. 9 (May 1999), pp. 1214-1217, ISSN 0041-1337

Pastacaldi S, Teixeira R, Montalto P, Rolles K,& Burroughs AK. Hepatic Artery Thrombosis After Orthotopic Liver Tansplantation: A Review of Nonsurgical Causes. *Liver Transpl*, Vol 7, No. 2(2001) pp.75-81, online ISSN 1527-6473

Perkins, J. D. (2007). The Evolution of Caval Implantation in Liver Transplantation. *Liver Transplantation* Vol 13, No. 3(Mar 2007),pp.463-467, online ISSN 1527-6473

Qunintini, C, Miller, C.M., Hashimoto, K, Philip, D, Diago Uso, T., Aucejo, F., Kelly, D., Winans, C., Eghtesad, B., Vogt, D., & Fung J. (2008). Side-to-Side Cavocavostomy with an Endovascular Stapler: Rescue Technique for Severe Hepatic Vein and/or Inferior Vena Cava Outflow Obstruction After Liver Transplantation Using the Piggyback Technique. *Liver Transplantation*, Vol 15, No.1 (2008), pp.49-53, online ISSN 1527-6473

Reddy, K, Mallett, S, Peachey, T (2005). Venovenous Bypass in Orthotopic Liver Transplantation: Time For a Rethink. *Liver Transplantation*, Vol 11, No.7 (July 2005),pp.741-749, online ISSN 1527-6473

Riediger, C, Muller, M, Michalski, C, Huser, N, Schuster, T, Kleeff, J, & Friess, H. (2010). T-Tube or No T-Tube in the Reconstruction of the Biliary Tract During Orthotopic Liver Transplantation: Systematic Review and Meta-Analysis. *Liver Transplantation*, Vol 16, No. 6 (2010), pp. 705-717, online ISSN 1527-6473

Selvaggi, G., Weppler, D., Nishida, S., Moon, J., Levi, D., Kato, T., and Tzakis A.G. (2007). Ten-Year Experience in Porto-Caval Hemitransposition for Liver Transplantation in the Presence of Portal Vein Thrombosis. *American Journal of Transplantation*, Vol. 7, No. 2 (2007), pp.454-460, ISSN 1600-6135

Sibulesky, L, Heckman, M, Perry, D, Taner, C, Willingham, D, & Nguyen. (2011). A Single-Center Experience With Biliary Reconstruction in Retransplantation: Duct-to- Duct or Roux-en-Y Choledochojejunostomy. *Liver Transplantation*, Vol 17, No. 6 (2011), pp. 710-716, online ISSN 1527-6473

Sonnenday, C, Englesbe, M, Mathur, A, Heidt, D, Magee, J, Punch, J, Sung, R, Welling, T, Woodside, K, & Pelletier, S. (2008). Side-to-Side Cavocavostomy Technique. (video) Accessed Aug 2011, available at http:/www.med.umich.edu/trans/public/liver/cavoplasty.htm

Sotiropoulos, G, Sgourakis, G, Radtke, A, Molmenti, E, Goumas, K, Mylona, S, Fouzas, I, Karaliotas, C, & Lang, H. (2009). Orthotopic Liver Transplantation: T-tube or not T-tube? Systematic Review and Meta-analysis of Results. *Transplantation*, Vol 87, No. 11 (June 2009), pp. 1672-80, ISSN 0041-1337

Tayar, C., Kluger, M.D., Laurent, A., & Cherqui, D. (2011). Optimizing Outflow in Piggyback Liver Transplantation Without Caval Occlusion: The Three-Vein Technique. *Liver Transplantation*, Vol 17, No 1 (Jan 2011), pp.88-92., online ISSN 1527-6473

Vieira de Melo, P, Miranda, L., Batista, L., Neto, O, Amorim, B, Sabat, B, Candido, H, Adeodato, L, Lemos, R, Carvalho, G, & Lacerda, C (2011). Orthotopic Liver Transplantation Without Venovenous Bypass Using the Conventional and Piggyback Techniques.*Transplantation Proceedings*, Vol 43, No. 4 (May 2011), pp.1327-1333, ISSN 0041-1345

Warner, P, Fusai, G, Glantzouniz, GK, Sabin, CA, Rolando, N, Patch, D, Sharma D, Davidson BR, Rolles, K, & Burroughs, AK. (2011). Risk Factors Associated With Early Hepatic Artery Thrombosis After Orthotopic Liver Transplantation - Univariable and Multivariable Analysis. *Transplant Int*, Vol 24, No.4 (April 2011), pp. 401-408, ISSN 0934-0874

Wu, Y, Voigt, M, Rayhill, S, Katz, D, Rou-Yee, C, Schmidt, W, Miller, R, Mitros, F & Labrecque (2001). Suprahepatic Venacavplasty (Cavaplasty) With Retrohepatic Cava Extension in Liver Transplantation: Experience With First 115 Cases. *Transplantation* 2001; vol 72, No. 8 (Oct 2001), pp.1389-1394, ISSN 0041-1337

Yan, Mao-Lin,Zeng, Y, Li, B, Xu, Ming-Qing, Wen,Tian-Fu, &Wang, Wen-Tao. (2008). Postoperative Complications After Liver Transplantation with Cavoportal Hemitransposition. *Hepatobiliary Pancreat Dis Int*, Vol. 7, No. 3 (Jun 2008), pp.322-324, ISSN 1499-3872

Yerdel, M, Gunson, B, Mirza, D, Karayalcin, K, Olliff, S, Buckels, J, Mayer, D, McMaster, P & Pirenne, J (2000). Portal Vein Thrombosis in Liver Transplantation: Risk Factors, Screening, Management, and Outome. *Transplantation*, Vol 69, No.9 (2000), pp.1873-1881, ISSN 0041-1337

6

The Routinely Use of "Piggyback" Technique in Adult Orthotopic Liver Transplantation

Luis Herrera et al.*
Hospital Universitario "Marqués de Valdecilla"
Spain

1. Introduction

1.1 Liver transplantation relevance

Liver transplantation is a surgical technique designed for the treatment of patients suffering from end stage liver disease and who would not otherwise have a chance to survive. After the first liver transplantation, performed by Thomas Earl Starzl on the first of March, 1963 in Denver, Colorado, thousands of procedures have been performed all around the world. 5300 liver transplantations were performed in the USA during 2002 and 5142 in Europe. The European liver transplantation registry has 93634 transplantations registered until December 2009 (www.eltr.org).

The evolution of liver transplantation was not easy initially, and survival was inferior to one year until 1967. Liver transplantation was not considered as the gold standard treatment for end stage liver diseases by National Institutes of Health until 1984 (National Institutes of Health Consensus Development Conference on Liver Transplantation, 1984). Two years later, this procedure was included by the Public Health department of the USA as a treatment modality (U.S. Department of Health and Human Services, Public Health Service, Health Resources and Services, 1986).

2. Principles and techniques for liver transplantation

Orthotopic liver transplantation requires total hepatectomy and substitution of the native liver by another one in the right hypochondrium. Vascular reconstruction is needed for the inferior vena cava, portal vein, and the hepatic artery. Biliary reconstruction is also needed, by either an end to end biliary anastomosis or a biliodigestive anastomosis.

Classic technique for orthotopic liver transplantation requires resection of the intrahepatic part of the inferior vena cava, and the use of a veno-venous bypass to keep venous return to the heart. This technique has a considerable morbidity and mortality in some cases, and can

---

* Federico Castillo, Marcos Gómez, Gonzalo Gutiérrez, Roberto Fernández, Elena García, Antonio López, Mónica González, Juan Carlos Rodríguez, Francisco González, Fernando Casafont and Manuel G. Fleitas
Hospital Universitario "Marqués de Valdecilla" Spain

be avoided if resection of the inferior vena cava is not done, preserving it during the procedure.

3. Anatomy of hepatic veins

Couinaud described eight segments of the liver in which each segment has an independent vascular inflow and outflow and biliary drainage. Based on the location of the hepatic veins, the right liver is divided into the anterior section (segments V and VIII) and the posterior section (segments VI and VII). On the left, the falciform ligament demarcates the left lateral section (segments II and III) from the left medial section (segment IV). The caudate lobe (segment I) lies anterior to the IVC.

The venous drainage of the liver is through the hepatic veins that ultimately coalesce into three hepatic veins that drain into the IVC superiorly. The left and middle hepatic veins may drain directly into the IVC but more commonly form a short common trunk before draining into the IVC. The right hepatic vein is typically larger, with a short extra hepatic course and drains directly into the IVC. Additional drainage occurs directly into the IVC via short retro hepatic veins and, on occasion, an inferior right accessory hepatic vein. The hepatic veins within the parenchyma are unique in that, unlike the portal venous system, they lack the fibrous, protective, encasing the Glisson capsule (Ger, 1989)

The liver has a rather constant anatomic pattern, the knowledge of which allows for a safe surgical approach. There are some anatomic irregularities, in these cases a computed three-dimensional reconstruction of anatomic detail is possible following computed tomographic or magnetic resonance imaging contrast scan. Software packages are currently available that allow for the mapping of the individual anatomy as well as for the calculation of volumes corresponding to the whole liver, liver sectors, and segments (Molmenti, 2007)

Ultrasonography facilitates intraoperative mapping of the internal anatomy of the liver. The portal venous anatomy can readily be identified by the hyperechogenic Glisson capsule surrounding the portal veins, whereas the hepatic veins lack this.

The IVC maintains an important and intimate association with the liver as it courses in a cranial-caudal direction to the right of the aorta. As the IVC travels cranially, it courses posterior to the duodenum, pancreas, porta hepatis, caudate lobe, and posterior surface of the liver as it approaches the bare area where it receives the hepatic venous outflow from the hepatic veins. Multiple small retro hepatic veins enter the IVC along its course, mostly from the right hepatic lobe. Hence, in mobilizing the liver or during major hepatic resections, it is imperative to maintain awareness of the IVC and its vascular tributaries at all times (Abdel-Misih, 2010)

4. Recipient implantation

In the Classic technique of orthotopic liver transplantation (OLT) the retrohepatic inferior vena cava (IVC) is included in the hepatectomy of the native liver (Starzl, 1968). To limit the hemodynamic complications associated with complete caval clamping, the routine use of the veno-venous bypass (VVB) was accepted particularly in noncirrhotic patients. (Shaw, 1984). Although VVB has been proposed in order to reduce these hemodynamic disorders it is associated with high morbidity and increased operation time (Veroli, 1992 & Khoury, 1987, 1990)

Preservation of the inferior vena cava (IVC) during orthotopic liver transplantation (OLT), described by Calne and Williams in 1968, was popularized in 1989 by Tzakis as the piggyback procedure (PB). The main advantages of this procedure were to avoid retrocaval dissection, to reduce the risk for bleeding and facilitate caval anastomosis in patients receiving large-for-size grafts (Tzakis, 1989 & Parrilla, 1999).

5. Caval anastomosis

Several methods of graft-to-inferior vena cava (IVC) implantation during orthotopic liver transplantation with preservation of the caval flow have been described. Large studies have shown that optimal outflow is essential to a successful piggyback procedure (Navarro & Parrilla, 1999). In the series by Tzakis (Tzakis, 1989) the caval anastomosis was performed between the supra hepatic part of donor IVC and the common orifice of all three hepatic veins or the common orifice of two hepatic veins (left and middle or right and middle). This is the so-called PB technique.

In 1992, Belghiti developed a technique of caval anastomosis in a side-to-side fashion (Belghiti, 1992). In this technique, both ends of the donor IVC are closed. Anastomosis is made between two newly created openings: one on the anterior wall of the recipient IVC and one on the posterior wall of the donor IVC , but because of insufficient exposure during implantation of large grafts and to facilitate postoperative trans-jugular biopsy, they used an end-to-side fashion after 1993. (Belghiti, 1995)

The third type of caval anastomosis is the end-to-side (ES) technique and can be found in the literature some modifications of this technique. Cherqui et al. described in their series, the distal end of the donor infra hepatic IVC was closed and the anastomosis was made between the end of the donor supra hepatic IVC and a longitudinal incision on the anterior wall of the recipient IVC. Additionally, a temporary portocaval shunt was routinely used (Cherqui, 1994). Other authors report several variations of the technique, the middle and left hepatic veins are exposed and a Satinsky side clamp is applied to the caval side with partial IVC occlusion. The middle and left hepatic veins are divided, and the recipient liver is removed. A single hepatic venous outflow orifice is created from the middle and left hepatic venous trunks, and this orifice can be extended caudally (Fleitas, 1994 & Belghiti, 1995).

Some authors suggest that the technique the 3-vein appears to be the most physiological way of achieving this goal. Although it has often been mentioned, the approach to creating a large 3-vein stoma without complete occlusion of the IVC is difficult. As Tayar reported (Tayar, 2011), anastomosis of the graft IVC to the joined orifice of the 3 main hepatic veins with partial caval occlusion was first mentioned by Lazaro (Lazaro, 1997).

PB technique can be associated with some disadvantages and complications, including hepatic venous outflow obstruction (Cescon, 2005) and thrombosis in up to 10%, because of the inappropriate size of the hepatic vein outlet, which results in venous congestion of the liver allograft. This congestion increases the chance of post-transplant ascites and Budd-Chiari syndrome (BCS) (Bilbao & Cirera, 2000; Mehrabi, 2009)

6. History of the "piggyback" technique

During the 5th and the 6th decade of 20th century, two pioneers in liver transplantation, Francis Daniels Moore and Thomas Earl Starzl, in Boston and Chicago respectively, were trying to perform with success an experimental transplantation. Unfortunately, their model in dogs, did not tolerate blood flow interruption neither at the IVC, nor at the portal vein because they supposed half of the venous return of the animal. Bypass dispositive had to be developed to avoid the hemodynamic compromise that the total hepatectomy supposed in the animal (Moore, 1959) and, in the end, they were included as routine tools for transplantation surgery in the first era. Nevertheless, Calne and Starzl noticed that in human adults, it was not always necessary to bypass neither portal nor inferior cava vein blood flow during the anhepatic phase of the transplantation (Calne, 2008).

Liver transplantation with IVC preservation was first performed by Sir Roy Calne in February 1968, at the Addenbrooke´s Hospital in Cambridge (UK) (Calne, 1968). Patient was a 46 year old female suffering from cholangiocarcinoma and donor was a 5 year old child that had virus related encephalitis. Because of the anatomical difference, Calne had to drain liver graft to the supra hepatic veins of the patient, completely preserving inferior cava vein during the procedure. The patient survived for 11 weeks, and it was the 3rd liver transplantation in Europe, and the 19th all around the world.

Later, Tzakis and cols. (Tzakis, 1989) described this technique in 24 cases, in the early 1988 with an indication index of 19%. They reported a greater technical difficulty of the procedure, the possibility of affected margins in the oncological indications at that moment, and a case with transitory thrombosis of the infra hepatic remnant cava vein, not recommending the routine use of inferior cava vein preservation.

7. Our technique for venous outflow drainage in orthotropic liver transplantation

In order to avoid the use of veno-venous bypass and to routinely preserve the IVC in our liver transplantation program, we adjusted our technique to the anatomical differences in the venous drainage of the liver. We designed our own model as follows (G. Fleitas, 1994):

7.1 Total hepatectomy with complete preservation of the IVC

Once identified and isolated, the liver pedicle elements are dissected adequately. With the vascular exclusion performed, we practice complete section of the falciform and triangular ligament in order to expose the confluence of the right hepatic vein and the left set (medial and left hepatic veins that usually drain together). After that, through the cavo-hepatic space, we perform a caudo-cranial dissection of the caudate lobe, with selective ligation of the hepatic veins. Their number varies, but the lesser the caliber, the greater the number is. The presence of a greater "inferior hepatic vein" that drains segment VI is very frequent. Usually, dissection extends by the left side of the IVC; dividing IVC and the caudate lobe until the arcuate ligament of the cavodiaphragmatic hiatus, very close to the mouth of the left phrenic vein, which usually has no venous drainage.

Once this space has been dissected, and the anterior hepatic veins have been tied and cut (usually sagittal to the IVC) and inferior and medial part of caudate lobe is dissected (usually hypertrophied because of cirrhosis) it is possible to easily pass in between both hepatic veins, at their mouth in the IVC. We isolate and clamp the left venous set and cut it, leaving enough margins for a safe cavo-caval anastomosis. After this, usually the right hepatic vein mouth in to the liver is exposed at a coronal level of the IVC, approximately

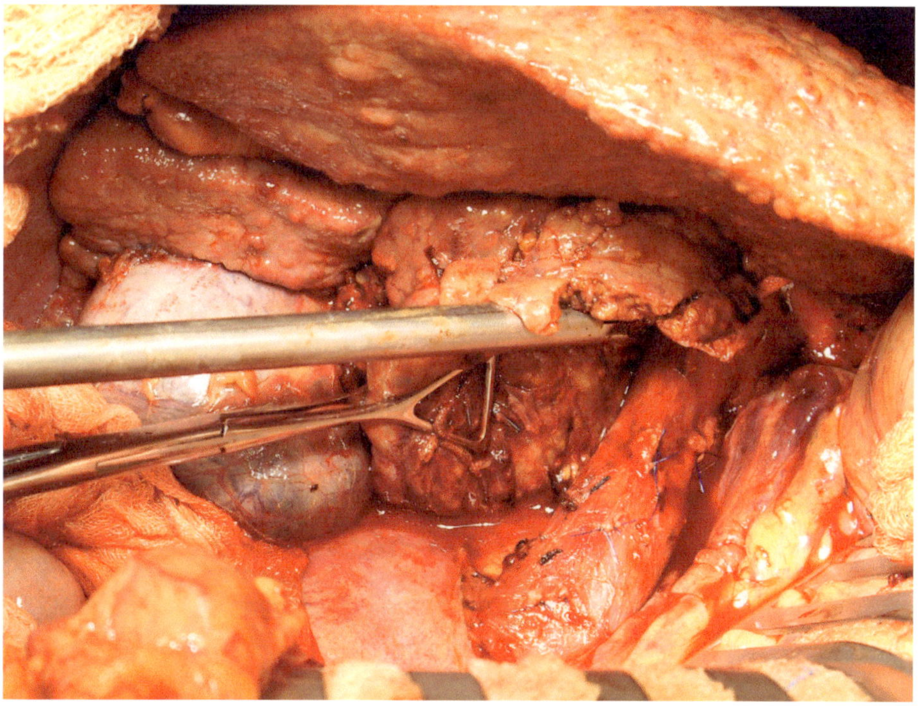

Fig. 1. Dissection of the infrahepatic IVC and left caudate lobule

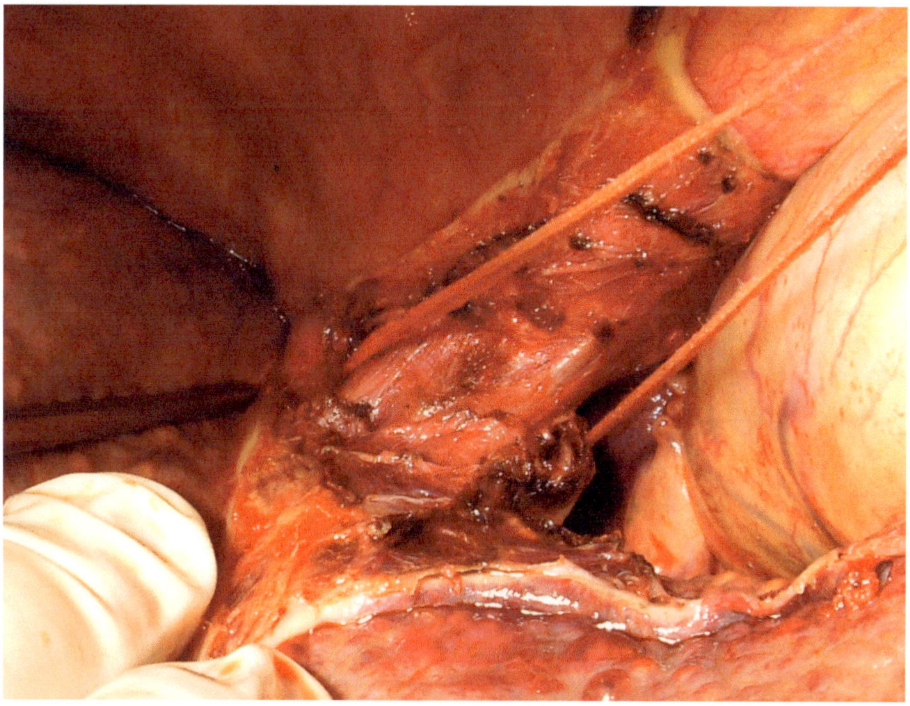

Fig. 2. Suprahepatic left and middle hepatic veins dissection

3 cm. far from the left venous set, suturing it with a continuous 3/0 polypropylene. After that, the right triangular ligament is cut, and right side of the IVC is dissected, cutting the corresponding veins, until caudate lobe is completely free from the IVC. This is the way how total hepatectomy is completed.

7.2 Carving liver graft drain mouth

This is an essential part of our technique. During this part, we clean the IVC of the graft, removing the tissues that are around its supra hepatic portion, cutting it at a level next to the supra hepatic veins mouth, at the level of the phrenic veins mouth, leaving a vascular sleeve to avoid the supra hepatic veins mouth being involved in the anastomosis.

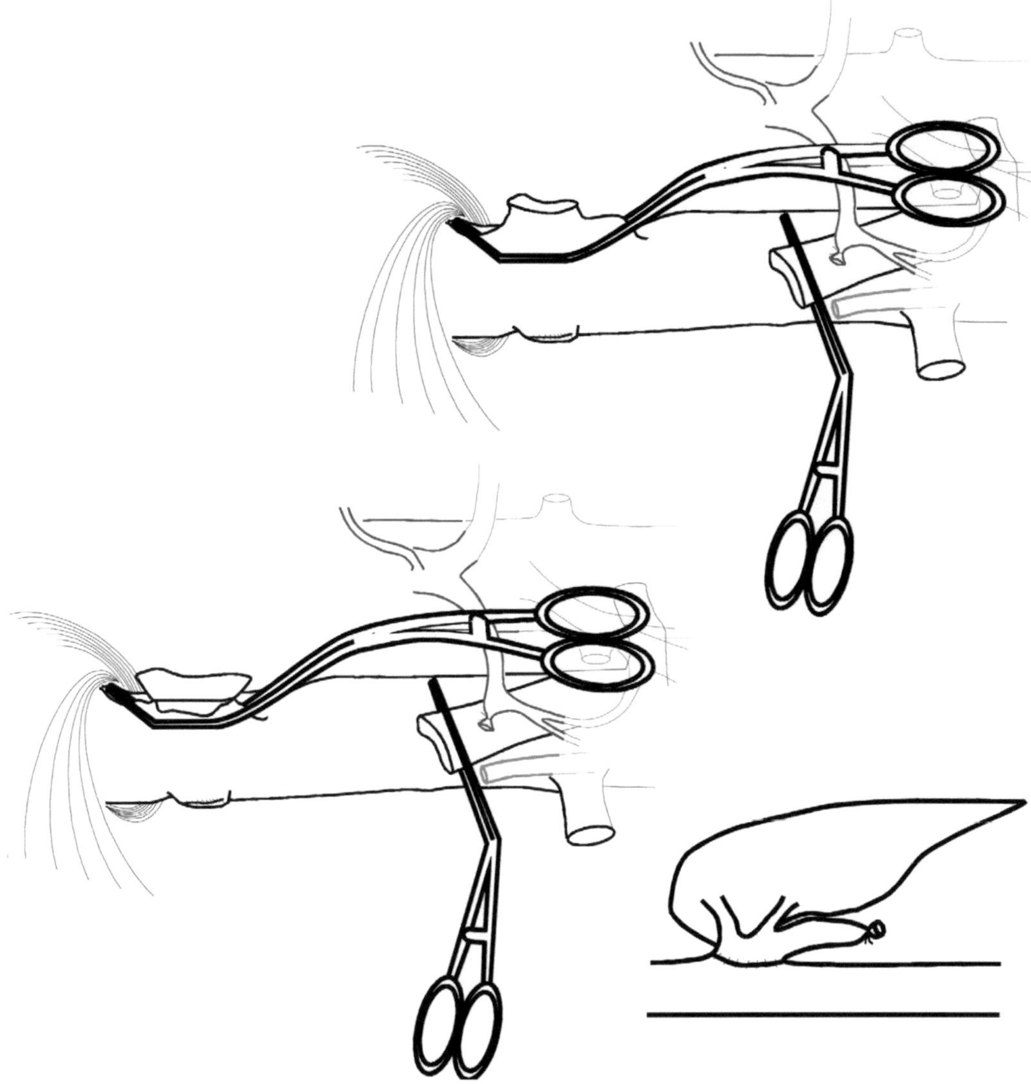

Fig. 3. Schematic lateral caval vein clamping and final result

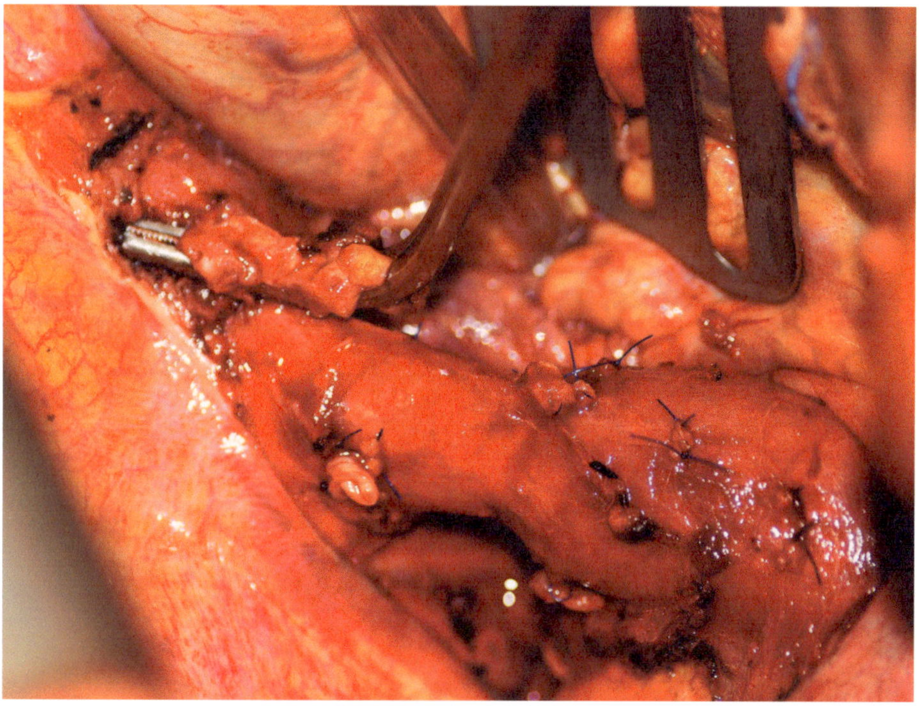

Fig. 4. Total Hepatectomy completed. Clamping of the left and middle hepatic veins

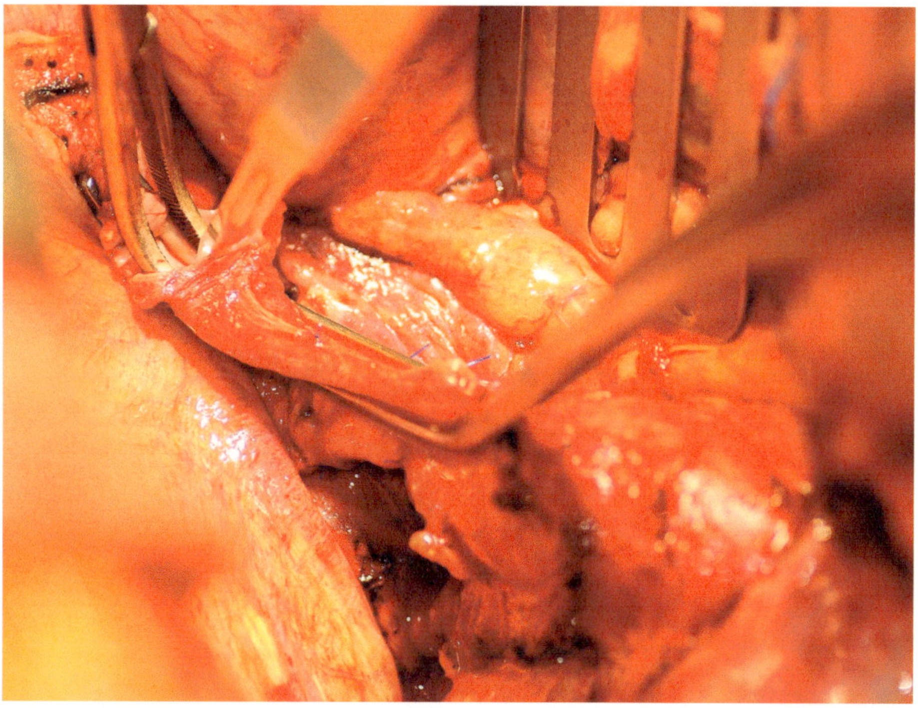

Fig. 5. Inferior caval vein cavotomy

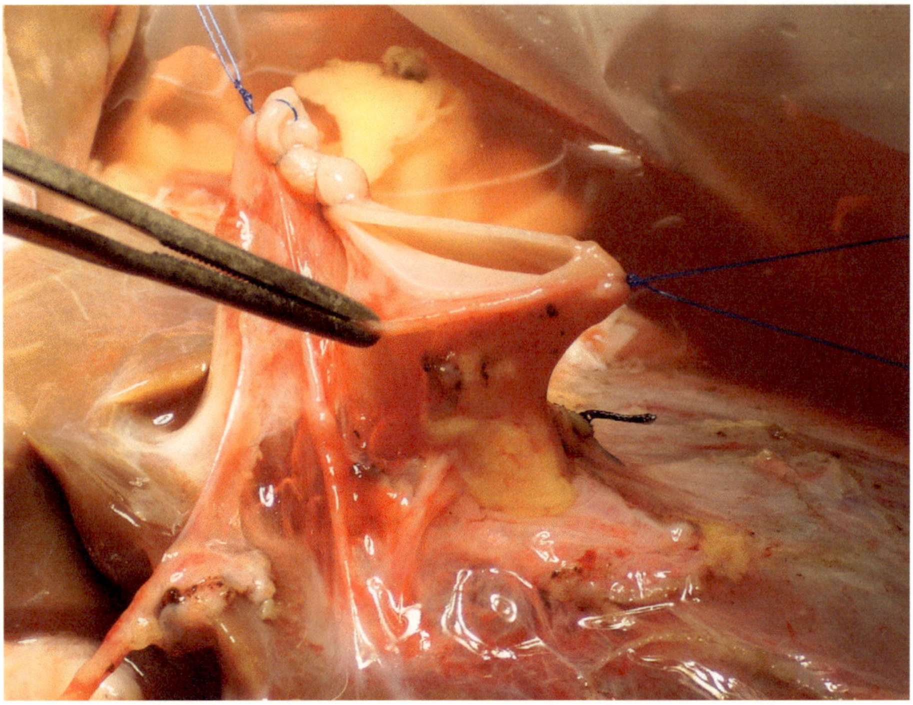

Fig. 6. Preparing liver graft. Infra hepatic caval vein stump partial closure

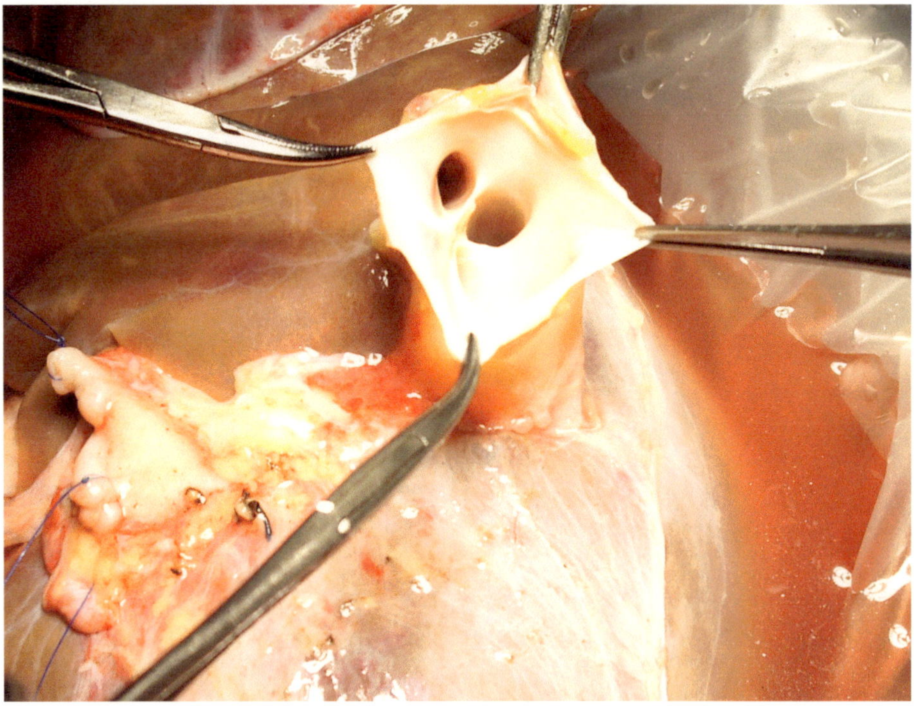

Fig. 7. The outlet and the entire graft IVC prepared for implantation

7.3 Left supra hepatic veins set cavoplasty

While monitoring hemodynamic parameters (Cardiac output and pressure at the inferior cava vein), we perform a lateral partial clamp of the cava vein, enough to carve a good venous sleeve made at the confluence of the left and medial supra hepatic veins, concordant in size to the graft venous sleeve made before. This clamping also allows temporal porto-cava anastomosis in case it is required without hemodynamic damage.

7.4 Inferior vena cavotomy

In some cases, when a left venous set can not be well defined or does not exist, and replace by a group of tiny veins interfering with safe anastomosis with a good drainage, we perform a craneocaudal cavotomy "de novo" in the IVC, as close to the right atrium as possible to achieve a negative pressure that allows better venous drainage of the liver graft, particularly in cases of Budd-Chiari Syndrome.

7.5 Enlargement of the venous outflow orifice of the graft

In order to achieve wider drainage of the supra hepatic veins, caudal cavotomy can be performed in the medial posterior side of the graft IVC, until supra hepatic veins orifices can be easily seen.

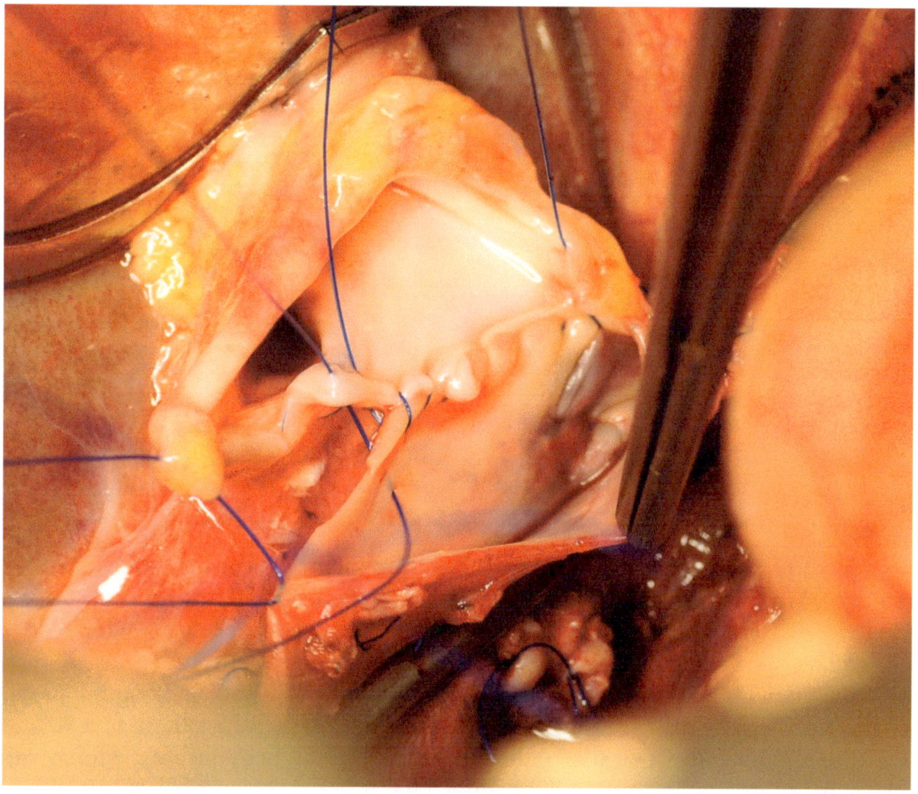

Fig. 8. Piggyback posterior side anastomosis close to right hepatic vein outlet

7.6 Graft implantation

Once adequate corresponding anastomotic orifices are achieved, and while keeping the vascular clamp on the recipient side of the IVC, we perform end to side, cavo-caval anastomosis using continuous 3/0 polypropylene. The aim is to provide wide anastomosis trying to achieve good outflow drainage of the graft. The distal end of the graft IVC is left open to allow "washing" of the graft after reperfusion, once the porto-portal anastomosis is done.

8. Advantages of the piggyback technique

Although initial attempts at preservation of the inferior vena cava in orthotopic liver transplantation by Sir Roy Calne, the so-called piggyback (PB) technique, was not initially worldwide accepted, it has become the most commonly used procedure in liver transplantation. Twenty years were necessary for Tzakis to describe the technique and its advantages over the classical caval reconstruction technique. Progressively in the 90's more transplant groups reported the utility and feasibility of the piggyback.

In addition, some modifications of the initial technique has been described, as the latero-lateral cavoplasty which added some benefits as well as the use of different types veno-venous bypass or portocaval shunts. These two options are controversial, with some benefits and drawbacks, and are not widely used. (G. Fleitas, 1994; Ducerf, 1996; Lai & Vieira, 2011).

The advantages of the piggyback come from the disadvantages of the classical technique, due to clamping of the IVC next to the diaphragm and above the renal veins, during the anhepatic phase. This results in decreased venous return to the heart and reduction in cardiac output by as much as 50% and in blood pressure (Vieira, 2011). On the contrary, PB technique preserves caval flow, reduces hemodynamic instability, the needs of transfusions with less hemorrhage and allows shorter ischemia and operative times as will be explained.

During the anhepatic phase, the PB technique allows adequate venous return to the heart, which maintains the patient hemodynamics and renal venous outflow (Lázaro, 1997). Partial clamping of the cava at the level of the hepatic veins does not usually cause significant changes in the mean arterial pressure, IVC pressure, systemic vascular resistance index and cardiac index. The urine output before, during and after revascularization do not change significatly (G. Fleitas, 1994). Acute renal failure is less frequent (Sakai, 2010), and, cyclosporine or tacrolimus therapy can be started early. (Busque, 1998)

The PB procedure shortens the time of the liver transplant procedure, specially the warm ischemia time. Most groups report that with PB, and its modifications, no porto-caval shunt is needed. Even though there may be some exceptions, (situations in which no porto-systemic collaterals exist as fulminant hepatitis). The significant reduction in the time improves the patient and graft survival (Lai, 2011; Nishida, 2006; Busque, 1998). This permits early extubation and shorter intensive care unit stay. In fact there is a 30% shorter intensive care unit stay and a similar reduction in the overall hospital stay. Moreover, these advantages have an impact on total hospital charges for about 85% of the transplants procedures, with a significant mean reduction of $23500 (Hossein, 2000).

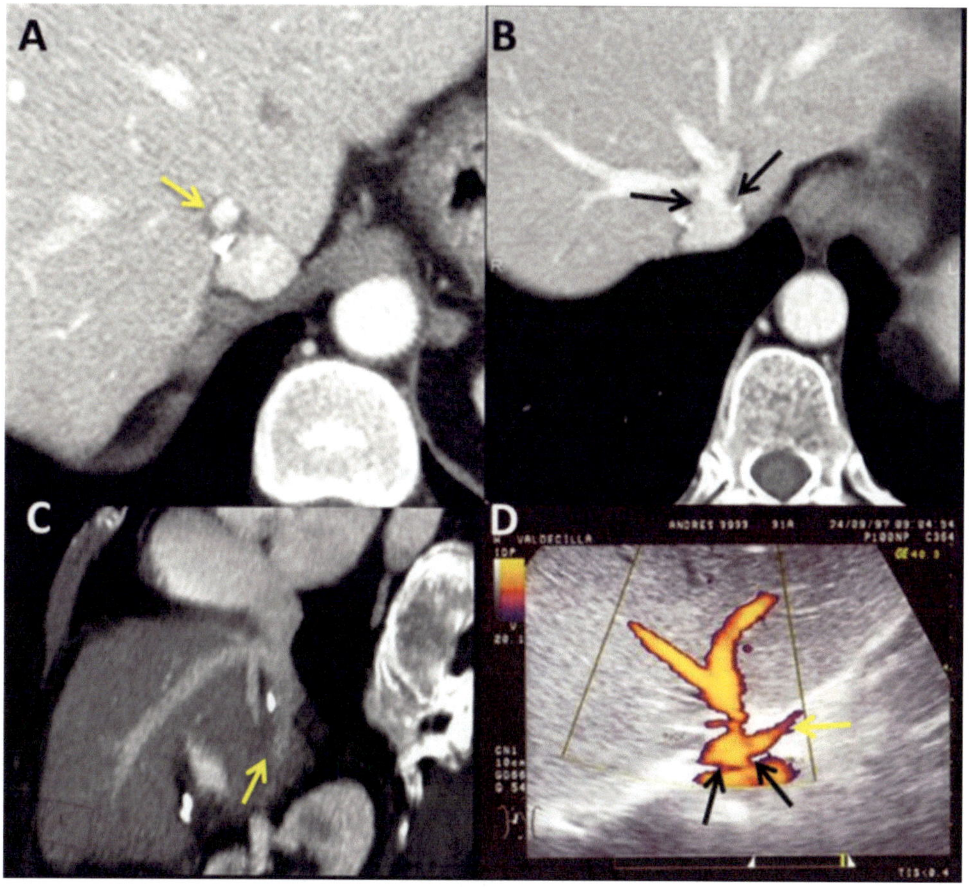

Fig. 9. Duplex-Doppler and CT Image showing the appearance of the normal caval stump. Yelow arrows pointing normal appearance of the graft caval stump and the black ones show the caval anastomotic outlet with adequate graft venous outflow drainage

Comparing the classical and the PB techniques, the more extensive dissection involving the cava and suprarenal veins from the liver causes more profuse bleeding with the former technique. The latter is associated with less extentive dissection which shortens the procedure and reduces the blood loss (Vieira, 2011). According to this, several papers confirmed that PB technique decreases blood requirements (Busque, 1998; Hossein, 2000; Nishida, 2006), and therefore the incidence post-transfusion problems are much less. Other advantages of PB technique include, better maintenance of core body temperature, avoidance of external venous bypass which is usually required in the classical technique with its associated intraoperative coagulopathy and third-spacing of fluid are significantly reduced, and in turn, the needs for transfusion is reduced (Hossein, 2000)

In addition, retransplantation may be easier if PB technique has been performed. Lateral clamping of the cava is again possible, and usually sufficient part of the wall of the IVC will be available for the anastomosis (Busque, 1998). This technique also makes easier to solve problems posed by mismatched recipient and donor IVC size, particularly in pediatrics, reduced-size, split, or living donor liver transplantation (Figueras, 2001; Calne, 1968).

In summary, adoptions of surgical techniques that minimize ischemia time, blood loss and shortens surgical times represent a surgical goal. PB technique seems to achieve the target. However some controversial points exist. General agreement is that PB technique can be used in almost any case of liver transplant. However, the exact procedure whether latero-lateral cavoplasty or bypass porto-caval shunt, remains unclear or at least, lacks of definitive evidence. As pointed out by (Gurusamy, 2011) in a Cochrane review, there are very few prospective randomized papers comparing the classical with the PB technique and the existing ones present important bias. According to this paper no important differences exist between both procedures.

9. Complications of piggyback technique

Complications of PB technique are well described in the literature although some distinction should be done according to the type of modification within the PB technique.

The reported morbidity is as low as 4% and the overall mortality is 0.7% (Navarro, 1999).

The main concern about PB technique is venous outflow obstruction. However, some other adverse effects related to PB technique and its modifications must be taken into consideration.

Intraoperative complications are basically related to bleeding or malposition of the graft and account for 2.5 %. Tears in the cava and release of the anastomosis running suture, were described as well as congestion of the graft after portal revascularization due to graft rotation. All of these complications can be satisfactorily resolved during the operation (Parrilla, 1999).

The most significant complication of the PB technique in the postoperative period is the occlusion of the venous outflow. This can be a dramatic situation and may occur in the perioperative, immediate postoperative period, after the first postoperative week (25%) (Horton, 2008) or years after the transplant (Brosstoff, 2008). The incidence is rather low, 0.54-7%, but the mortality rate in such cases may be as high as 24% (Navarro, 1999; Nishida, 2006). The causes of outflow obstruction include inappropriate size of the hepatic anastomosis, malrotation or twisting of the anastomosis, direct compression of the graft, excessively tight sutures, and caval thrombosis. Late causes are likely secondary to intimal hyperplasia and fibrotic changes resulting in anastomotic stricture formation.

Hepatic venous outflow obstruction results in Budd-Chiari syndrome. The patient presents with, abdominal pain, weight gain, ascites, lower extremity edema, pleural effusion, hepato-splenomegaly, worsening hepatic function and eventually loss of the graft (Wang, 2005). A recurrent Budd-Chiari syndrome has been also described with an incidence as high as 27% (Horton, 2008). In these cases lifelong anticoagulation is recommended. A chronic outflow obstruction may occur after several weeks with massive ascites as main symptom (Parrilla, 1999).

In order to prevent this adverse event some modifications of the piggyback technique have been described in the last decades. One modification consists on a side-to-side anastomosis at the anterior face of the recipient cava (Belghiti, 1992). The incidence of Budd-Chiari syndrome is reported to be lower, 0.7% compared to 2.4% in the classic PB technique (Navarro, 1999) and 7 out of 500 cases in Meherabi series (Meherabi, 2009). Parrilla also reported a decrease in the incidence from 1.6 to 0.28% when using a patch obtained by joining three instead of two hepatic veins when doing the anastomosis (Parrilla, 1999). The anastomosis performed, as previously described by the authors, is wide enough to allow a good flow and the liver is anchored securely.

After graft reperfusion the restoration of the venous return results in a sudden central volume overload that can cause pulmonary edema. A decrease greater of 50% in median arterial pressure for more than one minute is described as "reperfusion syndrome" and has been reported in 30% of cases (Figueras, 2001) and two cases out of 1361 transplants presented with hemodynamic shock on reperfusion (Navarro, 1999). The PB technique has been found to be associated with more pulmonary infiltrates (Isern, 2004), but this was not clinically relevant or statistically significant when compared with the classic technique (Gurusamy, 2011).

10. Treatment of complications of piggyback technique

Hemorrhagic complications during the anastomosis performance or in the early postoperative are usually well controlled. Tears, anastomotic bleeding, loose running sutures are repaired. However in some cases, new anastomosis or modifications must be done, as a new side-to-side cavo-caval reanastomosis. Special care must be taken in these situations since gaseous embolism and graft ischemia due to vascular clamping have been reported with negative consequences. (Navarro, 1999)

Intraoperative liver simple congestion due to outflow problems because of malrotation or excessive tension of the anastomosis for discrepancies in size of the graft might be resolved by accommodating the liver to recipient bed, suturing the falciform ligament to the diaphragm or even using breast prosthesis as the authors have used in a case with poor positional drainage (Fig. 10.).

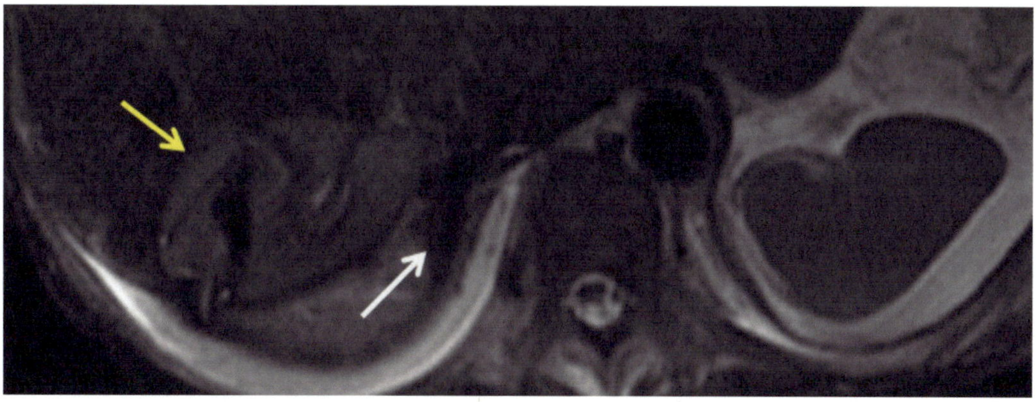

Fig. 10. Picture showing the breast prosthesis (yellow arrow) and the partially compromised caval flow (white arrow)

Treatment of Budd-Chiari syndrome varies from simple rotation of the graft to re-transplantation. Nevertheless, depending on the mode of onset of the syndrome the therapeutic procedure will vary. Acute presentation, in the first hours-days, will be more suitable for open surgery. This may involve re-anastomosis (with thrombectomy if necessary), conversion to standard liver transplant technique or emergency retransplantation, if the graft is seriously injured. Also a "bridge" end-to-side anastomosis with infrahepatic caval stump (Stieberg, 1997) could be performed, as we had performed twice before this technical solution was reported (Fig. 11.).

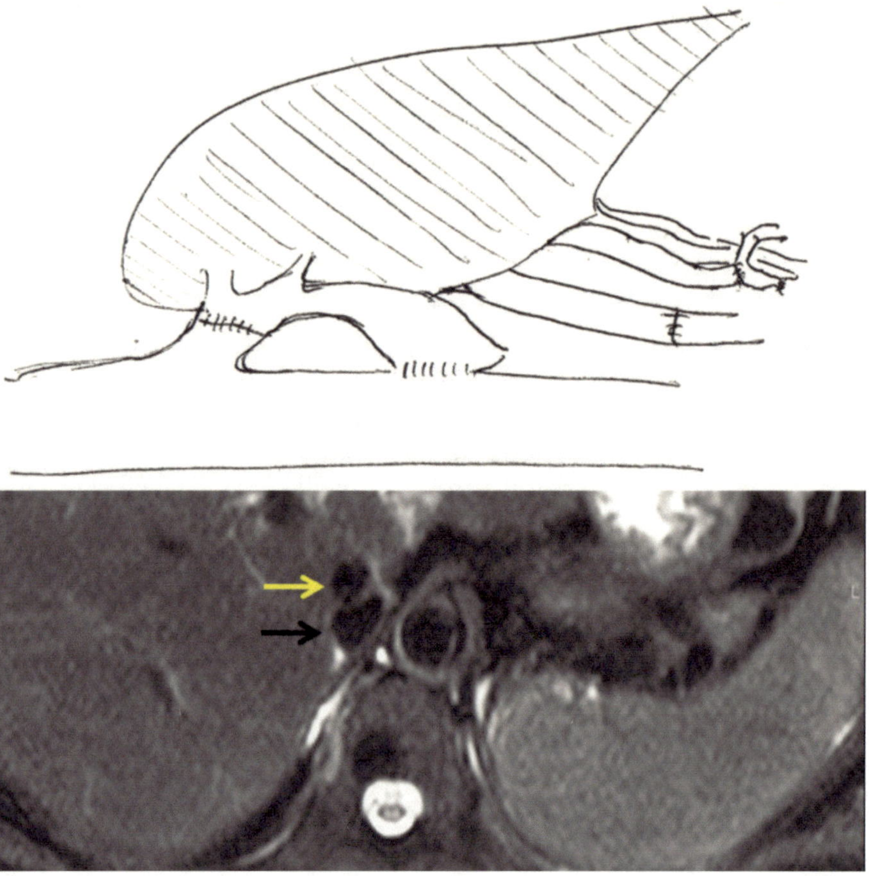

Fig. 11. Above: Drawing from operation report form of our first "bridge" case on November, 23th 1993. Below: Cholangio-NMR, 173 monts after the transplant showing adecuate flow through graft's caval stump. Black arrow: Recipient's cava. Yelow arrow: Graft's caval stump, functioning as bridge flow (compare with Fig. 9. Image A)

In a later onset of the obstruction, or even in an acute phase, non-surgical approaches have been described. A variety of treatment options have been proved useful. Thrombolysis with streptokinase was successfully used in a caval thrombosis. Diuretics can be used to control late and chronic BCS that manifests as massive ascites (Parrilla, 1999). However, the most commonly reported non-surgical approach is endovascular stent placement and endoluminal anastomotic dilatation (venoplasty). In the setting of a scarring and fibrotic stenosis, the endovascular route represents a less invasive and less risky option (Sze, 1999) and 100% success rate has been reported. The only reported complication is stent migration. Balloon dilatation can be repeated, if single dilatation does not resolve the stenosis permanently.

Late diagnosis is the most important single factor that affects the outcome. Delayed diagnosis can lead to a hepatic failure that will in turn make the treatment ineffective. In fact the best way to treat outflow problems is to prevent its occurrence. The length of the upper IVC of the graft should be kept short to prevent kinking; the length of the anastomosis is also important to allow good venous outflow. In addition, when the anastomosis is constructed using two hepatic veins (middle and left) instead of the three hepatic veins, the incidence of intraoperative congestion and acute and chronic BCS are significantly higher 2.4% vs. 0.7% (Parrilla, 1999).

In summary, outflow obstructions related to PB technique must be rapidly addressed and resolved since the risks of liver failure and mortality are high. Surgical approach may be inevitable but less aggressive non-surgical measures can be also effective, even in the first postoperative days, with a fresh anastomosis (Wang, 2005)

11. Evolution of IVC preservation as the technique of choice for venous outflow drainage in the OLT

Since the first case of our transplantation program on November 1990, we have performed 503 orthotropic liver transplantations. Piggyback technique was performed in 502. The "classic" technique was performed in only one case with a huge liver due to polycystic disease.

Since 1994, there were no series in the literature supporting the routine use of the piggyback technique although it seemed to us that it could be routinely used in a safe way (G. Fleitas, 1994). Subsequently, larger series have demonstrated its utility (Parrilla, 1999), although the variability of the technique, mainly regarding to the venous outflow handling is very big.

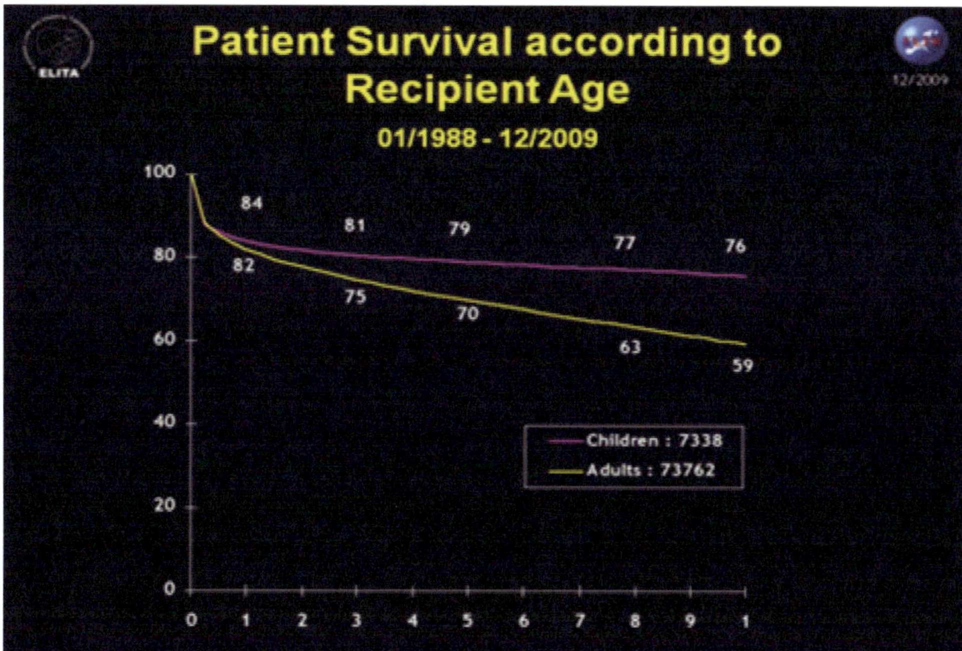

Fig. 12. European group patient survival (Source: European Liver Transplant Registry)

12. Valdecilla liver transplantation program

Our liver transplantation series started in November 1990, having already performed until 24 August 2011, 503 liver transplantations in adult patients (460 transplants, 41 retransplantations and 2 third transplantations). Their main characteristics are summarized in the following table, being similar to the other Spanish and European groups.

DONOR AGE n = 503	media (SD)	46.5 (18.8)
	median (Range)	47 (30-62)
RECEPTOR AGE n = 460	media (SD)	59 (11)
	median (Range)	65 (27-84)
INDICATIONS n = 503	OH related Cirrhosis	35.5%
	Virus Related Cirrhosis	22.25% (Ratio CVRC/BVRC = 8:1)
	Hepatocellular carcinoma	29.75%
	Fulminant Hepatitis	4.75%
	Others	7.75%
RE-TRANSPLANTATION	Normal Re-Transplantation	43 (8.54%)
	Urgent Re-Transplantation	5 (0.99%)
SD=Standard deviation; CVRC=C Virus Related Cirrhosis; BVRC=B Virus Related Cirrhosis		

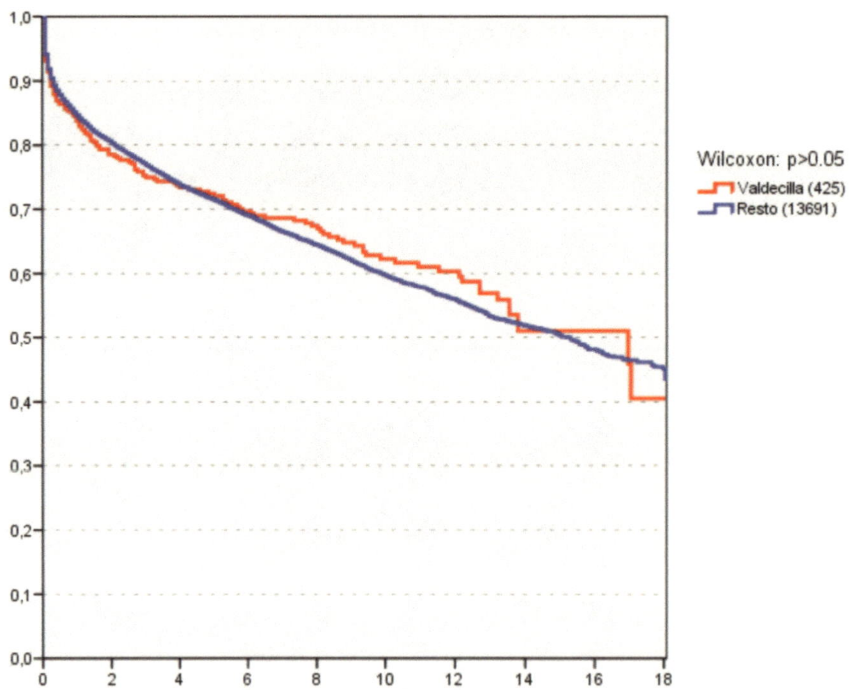

Table 1. Year survival rate comparing our series with the rest of the spanish liver transplant team (Source: Spanish Liver Transplant Registry; Dec. 2009). Resto=Others

In all cases of our series, the piggyback technique has been used, with the exception of one case of policystosis and inflammatory adhesions at the retrohepatic IVC. There was a case of the "situs inversus"; the donor, graft implantation was made to the right hepatic vein of the recipient by making necessary the caudal cavotomy enlargement (Herrera, 1996). In five cases, "de novo" cavotomy was performed, because of hypoplasia or "malposition" of the hepatic veins.

CASE	PROBLEM	SOLUTION	RESULT	SURVIVAL
1º	Huge graft	Re Tx 48 h.	Alive	241 months
2º	Technical	Hanging liver and Re Tx	Dead	8 days
3º	Technical	Bridge	Alive	226 months
4º	Unknown	Bridge	Alive	221 months
5º	Huge graft	Re Tx	Alive	74 months
6º	Poor drain	Breast Prosthesis	Dead (HCC recurrence)	73 months
7º	Budd-Chiari	Endo-prosthesis cava	Dead	1 month

(Re Tx=Retransplantation; HCC=Hepatocellular carcinoma)

Table 2. Complications and mortality related to a bad drain of the graft in our series

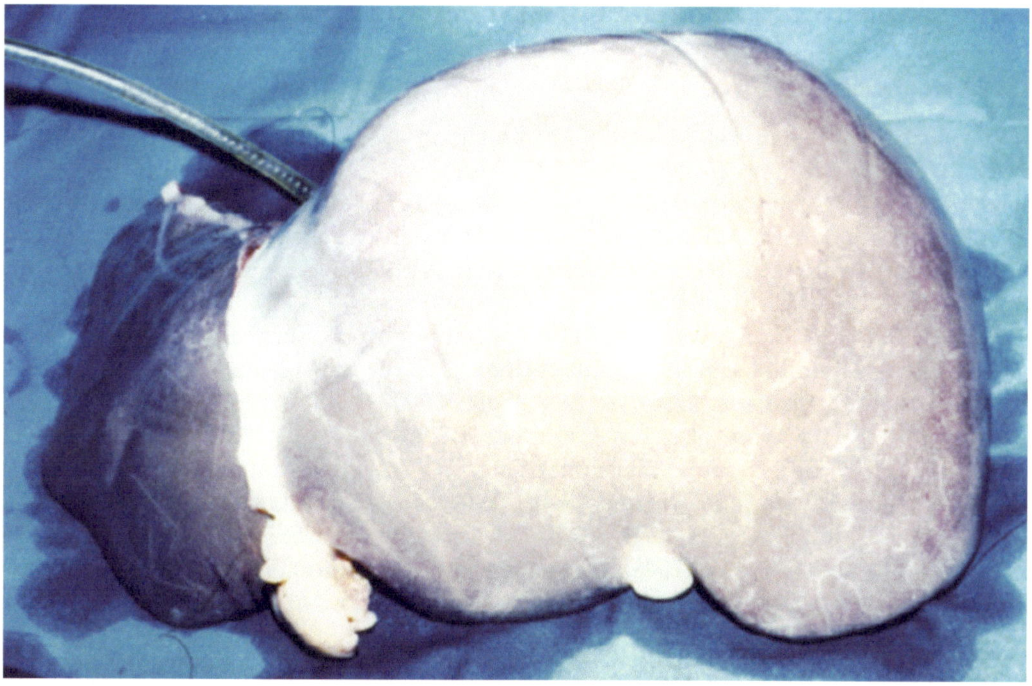

Fig. 13. Liver graft from a "*situs inversus*" donor

13. Conclusion

The main advantage of liver transplantation with caval preservation are of hemodynamic nature including, maintenance of the venous return to the heart during the procedure, thus providing, considerable hemodynamic stability, and avoiding the use of the veno-venous bypass to keep a good infrarenal venous pressure that provides an adequate renal filtration (Casanova, 2002). The extended use of piggyback technique in liver transplantation is mainly due to its hemodynamic advantages (Moreno, 2003). It has allowed to the performance of liver transplantation without the need for temporary veno-venous bypass. Although controversial issues have been raised, the use of veno-venous bypass is related to the preferences in each institution (Fonouni, 2008) rather than to its advantages, for which there is no supporting evidence nowadays (Gurusamy, 2011). In addition, avoiding the use of veno-venous bypass, minimizes the coagulation problems that happen on the surface of the bypass tubings. Another important advantage of the Piggyback technique is the better exploitation of grafts that allows using smaller grafts, with the accompanying disparity in the size or with unfavorable anatomy, as the case in "situs inversus" donors (Herrera, 1996) (Fig. 13.).

14. Acknowledgment

The authors would like to thank the transplantation nursing team at our institution for their support and dedicated profession: Carmen García, Mª Eugenia Bustillo, Mª Antonia Barros, Laura Briones, Sagrario Espinosa, Concepción Fernández, Mª Jóse Gómez, Mª Jesús Larrañaga, Guiomar Ortiz, Claribel Ortiz, Mª José Velasco and Isabel Villaverde.

15. References

Abdel-Misih, R. & Bloomston, M. (2010). Liver anatomy. *Surg Clin North Am.*, Vol. 90, No. 4, (August 2010), pp. (643-53), ISSN 0039-6109

Belghiti, J; Panis, Y; Sauvanet, A; Gayet, B. & Fékété, F. (1992). A new technique of side to side caval anastomosis during orthotopic hepatic transplantation without inferior vena caval occlusion. *Surg Gynecol Obstet*, Vol.175 No.3, (Sep 1992), pp. (270-2), ISSN 0039-6087

Belghiti, J; Noun, R. & Sauvanet, A. (1995). Temporary portocaval anastomosis with preservation of caval flow during orthotopic liver transplantation. *Am J Surg.* Vol. 169, No. 2, (February 1995), pp. (277-9), ISSN 0002-9610

Bilbao, J; Herrero, J; Martinez-Cuesta, A; Quiroga, J; Pueyo, J; Vivas, I; Delgado, C. & Pardo, F. (2000) Ascites due to anastomotic stenosis after liver transplantation using the piggyback technique: treatment with endovascular prosthesis. *Cardiovasc Intervent Radiol,* Vol. 23, No. 2, (March-April 2000), pp. (149-151), ISSN 0174-1551

Brostoff , J; Bhati, C & Syn, W. (2008). Late venous outflow obstruction after liver transplant: The 'piggy-back' syndrome. *Eur J Intern Med,* Vol. 19, No. 5, (Jul 2008), pp. (374-6), ISSN 0953-6205

Busque, S; Esquivel, C; Concepcion, W & So, S. (1998). Experience with the piggyback technique without caval occlusion in adult orthotopic liver transplantation. *Transplantation,* Vol. 65, No. 1, (Jan 1998), pp. (77-82), ISSN 0041-1337

Calne, R. & Williams, R. (1968). Liver transplantation in man. I. Observations on technique and organization in five cases. British Medical Journal, Vol. 4, 1968, pp. (535-540), ISSN 0959 8138

Calne, R. (2008) Early Days of Liver Transplantation. American Journal of Transplantation, Vol.8, No. 9, (September 2008), pp. (1775–1778), ISSN 1600-6135.

Casanova, D; Rabanal, J; Solares, D; G.Fleitas, M; Martino, E; Herrera, L; Hernanz, F; Castillo, J; Rodriguez, J; Casanueva, J & Izquierdo, M. (2002) Inferior Vena Cava Preservation Technique in Orthotopic Liver Transplantation: Haemodynamic Advantages. Transplantation Proceedings, Vol. 34, No. 1 (February 2002), p. (259), ISSN 0041-1345

Cecchis, L; Hribrnik, M; Ravnik, D & Gadzijev, EM. (2000). Anatomical variations in the pattern of the right hepatic veins: possibilities for type classification. J. Anat, Vol.197, 2000, pp. (487-493), ISSN 0021-8782

Cherqui, D; Lauzet, J; Rotman, N; Duvoux, C; Dhumeaux, D; Julien, M. & Fagniez, P. (1994). Orthotopic liver transplantation with preservation of the caval and portal flows. Technique and results in 62 cases. Transplantation, Vol. 58, No. 7, (October 1994), pp. (793-796), ISSN 0041-1337

Cirera, I; Navasa, M; Rimola, A; Garcia-Pagan, JC; Grande, L; Garcia-Valdecasas, J; Fuster, J; Bosch, J. & Rodes, J. (2000). Ascites after liver transplantation. *Liver Transpl.*, Vol. 6 No. 2 (March 2000), pp. (157-162), ISSN 1525-6465

Ducerf, C; Rode, A; Adham, M; De la Roch,e E; Bizollon, T; Baulieux, J & Pouyet, M. (1996). Hepatic outflow study after piggyback liver transplantation. *Surgery*. Vol.120, No.3, (Sep 1996), pp. (484-7), ISSN 0039-6060

Figueras, J; Llado, L; Ramos, E; Jaurrieta, E; Rafecas, A; Fabrega,t J; Torras, J; Sabate, A. & Dalmau, A. (2001). Temporary portocaval shunt during liver transplantation with vena cava preservation. Results of a prospective randomized study. *Liver Transp*, Vol.7, No.10, (October 2001), pp. (904-11), ISSN 1527-6465

Fonouni, H; Mehrabi, A; Soleimani, M; Mu¨ Ller, S; Bu¨ Chler, M & Schmidt, J. (2008). The need for venovenous bypass in liver transplantation. *HPB (Oxford)*, Vol.10, 2008, pp. (196-203), ISSN 1365-182X

Ger R. (1989). Surgical anatomy of the liver. *Surg Clin North Am*, Vol.69, No.2 (April 1989), pp. 179-92, ISSN 0039-6109

G.Fleitas, M; Casanova, D; Martino, E; Maestre, J; Herrera, L;Hernanz, F; Rabanal, J; Pulgar, S & Solares, G. (1994). Could the Piggyback Operation in Liver Transplantation Be Routinely Used? *Arch. Surg*, Vol.129, No. 1, (July 1994), pp. (842-845), ISSN 0004-0010

Gurusamy, K; Pamecha, V. & Davidson B. (2011). Piggy-back graft for liver transplantation. *Cochrane Database Syst Rev.* Vol.19, No.1 (Jan 2011), ISSN 1469-493X (Electronic)

Gurusamy, KS; Koti, R; Pamecha, V. & Davidson, BR. (2011) Veno-venous bypass versus none for liver transplantation. *Cochrane Database of Systematic Reviews* 2011, Issue 3. Art. No.: CD007712. DOI: 10.1002/14651858.CD007712.pub2. ISSN 1469-493X (Electronic)

Herrera, L; Castillo, J; Martino, E; Rabanal, J & G.Fleitas, M (1996) Orthotopic liver transplantation from a donor with abdominal situs inversus. *Transplantation*, Vol.62, 1996 pp. (133-135), ISSN 0041-1337

Horton, J; San Miguel, F; Membreno, F; Wright, F; Paima, J; Foster, P. & Ortiz, J. (2008). Budd-Chiari syndrome: illustrated review of current management. *Liver Int*, Vol.28, No.4, (Apr 2008), pp. (455-66), ISSN 1478-3223

Hossein, M; Osama, A; Bagous, W; Grewal, H; Hathaway, D; Vera, S; Stratta, R; Bagous, T. & Kizilisik T. (2000). Choice of surgical technique influences perioperative outcomes in liver transplantation. *Ann Surg, Vol.* 231, No.6, (Jun 2000), pp. (814-23), ISSN 0003-4932

Isern, MR; Massarollo, PC; de Carvalho, EM; Vaía, C; Kavakama, J; de Andrade, P. & Mies, S. (2004). Randomized trial comparing pulmonary alterations after convencional with venovenous bypass versus piggyback liver transplantation. *Liver Transpl,* Vol.10, No.3, (Mar 2004), pp. (425-33), ISSN 1527-6465

Khoury, G; Mann, M; Porot, M; Abdul-Rasool, I. & Busuttil, R. (1987). Air embolism associated with venovenous bypass during orthotopic liver transplantation. *Anesthesiology,* Vol. 67 No. 5, (November 1987), pp. (848-851), ISSN 0003-3022

Khoury, G; Kaufman, R. & Musich, J. (1990). Hypothermia related to the use of veno-venous bypass during liver transplantation in man. *Eur J Anaesthesiol.* Vol. 7 No. 6 (November 1990) pp. (50 l-503), ISSN 0265-0215

Lai, Q; Nudo, F; Molinaro, A; Mennini, G; Spoletini, G; Melandro, F; Guglielmo, N; Parlati, L; Mordenti, M; Ginanni, S; Berloco, PB & Rossi, M. (2011) Does caval reconstruction technique affect early graft function after liver transplantation? A preliminary analysis. *Transplantation Proceedings,* Vol.43, No.4, (May 2011), pp. (1103-6), ISSN 0041-1345

Lázaro, J; Charco, R; Revhaug, A; Murio, E; Balsells, J; Hidalgo, E; Mora, A; Cortés, C & Margarit, C. (1997). Hemodynamics in human liver transplantation with inferior vena cava preservation. techniques *Transplantation Proceedings,* Vol.29, No. 7, (Nov 1997), pp. (2851-2), ISSN 0041-1345

Mehrabi, A; Mood, ZA; Fonouni, H; Kashfi, A; Hillebrand, N; Müller, S; Encke, J; Büchler, M. & Schmidt J. (2009). A single-center experience of 500 liver transplants using the modified piggyback technique by Belghiti. *Liver Transpl,* Vol.15, No.5, (May 2009), pp. (466-74), ISSN 1527-6465

Molmenti, P; Radtke, A; Sotiropoulos, C. & Malago, M. (2007). Anatomy and physiology of the liver. In: Shackelford's Surgery of the Alimentary Tract, 6th Ed., Yeo, C; Dempsey, D; Klein, A; Pemberton, J. & Peters, J. (Ed), pp. (1597-1610), Saunders Elsevier, ISSN 9781416023579, Philadelphia.

Moore, F, Smith, L, Burnap, T, Dallenbach, F, Dammin, G, Gruber, U, Shoemaker, W, Steenburg, R, Ball, M. & Belko, J. (1959). One-stage homotransplantation of the liver following total hepatectomy in dogs. *Transpl Bull,* Vol.6, No.1, (Jan 1959), pp. (103-7), ISSN 0564-1217

Moreno-Gonzalez, M; Meneu-Diaz, J; Fundora, Y; Ortega, P; Moreno, A; García I; Jimenez C, Loinaz, C.; Gomez, R. &, Abradelo, M. (2003). Advantages of the Piggy Back Technique on Intraoperative Transfusion, Fluid Compsumption, and Vasoactive Drugs Requirements in Liver Transplantation: A Comparative Study. *Transplantation Proceedings,* Vol.35, No.5, (August 2003) pp. (1918-9), ISSN 0041-1345

National Institutes of Health Consensus Development Conference Statement: Liver transplantation—June 20-23, 1983. (1984) *Hepatology,* Vol.4, (1Suppl) pp. (107-110), ISSN 0270-9139

Navarro, F; Le Moine, M; Fabre, J; Belghiti, J; Cherqui D; Adam, R; Pruvot, F; Letoublon, C. & Domergue J. (1999). Specific vascular complications of orthotopic liver transplantation with preservation of the retro hepatic vena cava: review of 1361 cases. *Transplantation,* Vol.68, No.5, (Sep 1999), pp. (646-50), ISSN 0041-1337

Nishida, S; Nakamura, N; Vaidya, A; Levi, D; Kato, T; Nery, J; Madariaga, J; Molina, E; Ruiz, P; Gyamfi, A. & Tzakis A. (2006). Piggyback technique in adult liver transplantation: an analysis of 1067 liver transplants at a single center. *HPB (Oxford),* Vol.8, No.3, 2006 pp. (182-8), ISSN 1365-182X

Parrilla, P; Sánchez-Bueno, F; Figueras, J; Jaurrieta, E; Mir, J; Margarit, C; Lázaro, J; Herrera, L; G.Fleitas, M; Varo, E; Vicente, E; Robles, R & Ramirez, P. (1999). Analysis of the complications of the piggy-back technique in 1112 liver transplants. *Transplantation,* Vol.67, No.9, (May 1999), pp. (1214-7), ISSN 0041-133

Sakai, T; Matsusaki, T; Marsh, J; Hilmi, I. & Planinsic, R. (2010). Comparison of surgical methods in liver transplantation: retro hepatic caval resection with venovenous bypass (VVB) versus piggyback (PB) with VVB versus PB without VVB. *Transpl Int,* Vol.23, No.12, (December 2010), pp. (1247-58), ISSN 0934-0874

Stieberg, C; Gordon D. & Bassi, N. (1997). A simple solution to a technical complication in "piggyback" liver transplantation. *Transplantation,* Vol.64, No.4, (August 1997), pp. (653-654), ISSN 0041-1337

Shaw, B; Martin, D; Marquez, J; Kang, Y; Bugbee, A; Iwatsuki, S; Griffith, BP; Hardesty, R; Bahnson, H. & Starzl T. (1984), Venous bypass in clinical liver transplantation. *Ann Surg,* Vol. 200 No. 4, (October 1984) pp. (524-34), ISSN 0003-4932

Starzl, T; Groth, C; Brettschneider, L; Penn, I; Fulginiti, V; Moon, J; Blanchard, H; Martin, A. & Porter, K. (1968). Orthotopic homotransplantation of the human liver. *Ann Surg,* Vol. 168 No. 3, (September 1968), pp. (392-415), ISSN 0003-4932

Sze, DY; Semba, CP; Razavi, MK; Kee, ST; Dake, MD. (1999). Endovascular treatment of hepatic venous outflow obstruction after piggyback technique liver transplantation. *Transplantation,* Vol.68, No.3, (August 1999), pp. (446-9), ISSN 0041-1337

Tayar, C; Kluger, M; Laurent, A. & Cherqui D. (2011). Optimizing Outflow in Piggyback Liver Transplantation Without Caval Occlusion: The Three-Vein Technique. *Liver Transpl.,* Vol. 17, No. 1, (January 2011), pp. (88-92), ISSN 1525-6465

Tzakis A, Todo S & Starzl TE. (1989). Orthotopic liver transplantation with preservation of the inferior vena cava. *Ann Surg,* Vol.210, No. 5, (November 1989), pp. (649-652), ISSN 0003-4932

United States, Task Force on Organ Transplantation. (1986). Organ transplantation: issues and recommendations: report of the Task Force on Organ Transplantation U.S. Dept. of Health & Human Services, Public Health Service, Health Resources and Services, Administration, Office of Organ Transplantation, April 1986, pp. 141-152.

Veroli, P; El Hage, C. & Ecoffrey, C. (1992). Does adult liver transplantation without venovenous bypass result in renal failure? *Anesth Anal.,* Vol. 75, No. 4, (October 1992), pp. (489-494), ISSN 003-2999

Vieira, P; Miranda, L; Batista, L; Neto, O; Amorim, A; Sabat, B; Candido, H; Adeodato, L; Lemos, R; Carvalho, G. & Lacerda, C. (2011). Orthotopic liver transplantation without venovenous bypass using the conventional and piggyback techniques

Transplantation Proceedings, Vol.43, No.4, (May 2011), pp. (1327-33), ISSN 0041-1345

Wang, SL; Sze, D; Busque, S; Razavi, M; Kee, S; Frisoli, J. & Dake, D.(2005). Treatment of hepatic venous outflow obstruction after piggyback liver transplantation. *Radiology,* Vol.236, No.1, (July 2005), pp. (352-9), ISSN 0033-8419

Part 3

Cell and Experimental Liver Transplantation

7

Cell Transplantation – A Possible Alternative to Orthotopic Liver Transplant (OLT)

Kristen J. Skvorak et al.*
University of Pittsburgh
USA

1. Introduction

The progress made in the field of liver organ transplantation has revolutionized the treatment of a wide spectrum of liver diseases. Orthotopic liver transplantation (OLT), which requires removal of the entire native liver and transplantation of a high quality graft, has become an almost routine procedure with 1-year survival rates higher than 80%. However, with the ensuing interminable increase in the waiting list, the current major limitation is the considerable shortage in organ donors and the need of timely availability of suitable livers. As a result, although death rate after surgery is slowly decreasing, the number of total deaths in waiting list patients is steadily rising. Several solutions have been proposed to overcome this problem, such as legislative measures, mass media campaigns, optimization of available organ allocation, or innovative surgical techniques such as split-liver, living donor, non-heart beating donor, and domino transplantation. However, these measures have been met with only limited success in providing enough liver grafts (Neuberger, 2000; Thalheimer & Capra, 2002). Hence, the research community endeavoured to establish clinical alternatives to liver transplantation. Cell-based therapies are emerging as an alternative to whole-organ transplantation, which has shown initial promise in both animal models and clinical cases. This novel technique may provide functional liver support while the native liver regenerates in patients of acute liver failure, may provide a short-term "bridge" to sustain critical patients until OLT, or may aid in replacing a missing enzyme function in metabolic conditions with the aim of avoiding OLT. Some of the most promising cells types that could be used in this emerging field are hepatocytes, embryonic stem cells (ESC), mesenchymal stromal cells (MSC), amnion epithelial (AE) cells, and induced pluripotent stem cells (iPSC).

2. Cell transplant versus OLT

Although still in the experimental stages, cell transplant (CTx) has a variety of potential advantages over whole liver transplant. OLT requires major invasive surgery associated with long recovery times and a high prevalence of post-surgical complications such as infections, renal failure, and acute rejection, which could all contribute to patient mortality. The financial cost of OLT and subsequent lifelong immunosuppression therapy is substantial,

---

* Roberto Gramignoli, Marc C. Hansel, Suleyman Uraz, Veysel Tahan, Kenneth Dorko, Fabio Marongiu and Stephen C. Strom

and long term immunosuppression has also been linked to an increased incidence in cancers. Finally, the number of livers needed for transplant greatly outnumbers available livers, and timing is critical. In contrast, CTx is less invasive, less expensive, and is associated with less severe and fewer complications as well as shorter recovery times. Theoretically, stable patients, such as those with a metabolic disease, could potentially be given an infusion of cells as an outpatient procedure. Cells for transplant can be banked and cryopreserved for almost instant availability; therefore, procedural timing would no longer be a major concern. One significant benefit of CTx is that patients would retain their native liver. This is of particular relevance for patients with metabolic liver diseases. For example, a patient with Maple Syrup Urine Disease (MSUD) has a mutation in the enzyme complex that catalyzes the permanent degradation of branched-chain amino acids (BCAA), but can perform all other necessary liver functions. Therefore, transplanted cells would not need to provide complete liver support. In addition, since a metabolic disease patient is not reliant on the donor cells for other liver functions, loss of a graft or failure of the cells to perform would only return the recipient to pretransplant conditions. Cells can also be infused into patients multiple times, and OLT remains an option if CTx proves insufficient. Less immunosuppression may also be required, though this would likely depend on the type of cells used, the number of cells infused, and each patient's individual needs.

3. Cell types, utility for transplant, and major benefits / concerns

Cell transplant may be clinically useful for cell support for acute liver failure, as a "bridge" therapy to whole liver transplantation, or for the treatment of metabolic liver disease (Strom & Ellis, 2011). Hepatocytes, as well as many stem or stem-like cells (ESC, MSC, AE, and iPSC), are all being investigated for use in this novel yet promising branch of regenerative medicine. Each cell type has its own associated risks and benefits, which will be discussed separately.

3.1 Hepatocytes

The adult human liver consists of approximately 250 billion hepatocytes organized in about one million hepatic lobules. Each capillary leads to a lobule. Hepatocytes, the basic metabolic cell of the liver, constitute approximately 65–80% of the cell population of the liver. These cells are involved in protein synthesis, storage and transformation of carbohydrates, synthesis of cholesterol, bile salts and phospholipids, detoxification, and modification and excretion of exogenous and endogenous substances (Kaplowitz, 1992). The hepatocyte also initiates the formation and secretion of bile. Other important cells of the liver include Kupffer cells, stellate cells, and endothelial cells. Kupffer cells are specialized macrophages located in the liver that form part of the reticuloendothelial system. Their development begins in the bone marrow with the genesis of peripheral blood monocytes, and completing their differentiation into Kupffer cells in the liver. The primary functions of Kupffer cells are to recycle old and non-functional red blood cells, phagocytosis, and clearance of pathogens. Stellate cells, also known as Ito cells, are pericytes found in the perisinusoidal space (space of Disse) and represent ~5-8% of the total liver cell number. In normal liver, stellate cells are largely quiescent, store vitamin A, and have cell body protrusions that wrap around sinusoids. The stellate cell is the major cell type involved in liver fibrosis, which is the formation of scar tissue in response to liver damage. When liver is damaged, stellate cells can change into an activated state, and are responsible for secreting collagen and other extra-cellular molecules which can lead to cirrhosis. Endothelial cells constitute the wall of the liver sinusoids. They lie on a discontinuous extracellular matrix, creating a narrow extravascular fluid compartment into which hepatocytes project microvilli. This arrangement maximizes the surface area of hepatocytes with the extravascular fluid space and permits free movement of solutes into contact with the hepatocyte plasma membrane.

In healthy individuals, regeneration is slow; it is commonly accepted that liver is replaced by normal tissue renewal approximately once a year. The liver is largely quiescent with only 1:1000 hepatocytes in mitosis at any given time. This number decreases with increasing age, making regeneration slower and less complete in older animals (Steer, 1995). However, this slow cellular turnover is quickly altered when a chemical or physical trauma occurs to cause a significant loss to the liver. Sudden and massive hepatocyte proliferation then occurs due to a rapid increase in mitotic division resulting in restoration of functional liver mass (Bucher, 1963).

3.1.2 Hepatocyte transplantation and route of administration

Hepatocytes are capable of rapid proliferation as well as complete and functional regeneration of the liver following injury. Thus, this capacity for self-renewal has led some to regard the hepatocyte as essentially a "unipotent" stem cell. As early as 1977, hepatocyte transplantation (HTx) has been recognized as an attractive option for the management of metabolic liver disease (Groth et al., 1977). Groth and colleagues demonstrated that intraportal HTx in glucuronosyltransferase-deficient rats improved hyperbilirubinemia. Since then, continuing preclinical research determined that HTx can support liver function and improve survival in animal models of acute liver failure suggesting it had potential clinical application (Gupta & Chowdhury, 2002). There have also been a large number of studies with various animal models that show the efficacy of hepatocyte transplantation to correct metabolic liver disease (as reviewed in Malhi & Gupta, 2001; Strom et al, 2006). Importantly, Harding's group showed the correction of murine phenylketonuria (PKU) despite low engraftment of cells (Hamman et al., 2005); Harding & Gibson (2010) later suggest only 10-20% repopulation may be sufficient to correct PKU clinically. Our group also recently reported a significant partial correction of murine intermediate MSUD despite very low (~3%) repopulation of the liver (Skvorak et al., 2009a; 2009b). As a result, HTx has gained attention as a potential therapeutic intervention for a number of liver diseases, and transplantation of hepatocytes corresponding to 1-5% of total liver mass (1.5-9.0 billion hepatocytes) can be expected to have a positive impact. It has been determined that approximately 3.5-7.5% of liver mass can safely be transplanted in one transplant event (Fox et al., 1998), whereby the transplant may be divided in up to 6 separate infusions over a number of hours. CTx is generally associated with an increase in portal pressures as blood flow is restricted by plugs of donor hepatocytes (Gupta et al., 1999). However, if transplanted cells are in the range of 5% of the total liver mass, this increased portal pressure usually resolves within minutes or hours. When portal pressures return to normal, or at least decrease to acceptable levels, it is then safe to infuse more cells. At present, the majority of hepatocyte transplant procedures have been performed in adults with acute or chronic liver failure, though HTx as a therapeutic alternative to treat metabolic hepatic disease is becoming more accepted. Thus far, there have been four reported clinical cases of recovery from acute liver failure following HTx (Table 1), though the use of cell transplant as a "bridging" therapy to OLT is more common in both acute and chronic liver failure. Most published articles report a positive impact of HTx in clinical studies, and results are in general agreement with preclinical data using animal models. Table 1 summarizes clinical hepatocyte transplant studies to date, as well as significant results of those studies.

HTx as an alternative treatment for metabolic liver disease is an appealing proposal. The progression of inherited metabolic liver disease usually varies less than cases of liver failure. In addition, objective parameters such as laboratory data (i.e. bile acid, clotting factors, etc.) can be determined to unequivocally assess the efficacy of the treatment. On the other hand, the situation is rarely immediately life threatening and often acceptable conventional therapies are available, such as a special diet. Therefore, the potential benefit must be carefully weighed against any possible complications, such as immunosuppression, embolisation of the pulmonary vascular system, sepsis, or hemodynamic instability. HTx is more often done as therapy for inborn errors of hepatic metabolism in which a specific absent protein can be measured from transplanted unmodified donor hepatocytes expressing the gene. The use of hepatocyte infusions to correct inborn errors of metabolism is logical when a specific metabolic deficiency, with well-studied animal modelling, can be measured. Then, after infusion of donor liver cells natively expressing the required gene, objective measures of required hepatocyte mass, engraftment percent, and survival advantage can be obtained. Thus far, therapeutic benefit has been seen clinically in the treatment of disorders of the urea cycle (citrullinemia, OTC, argininosuccinase lyase deficiency), familial cholesterolemia, Crigler-Najjar, biliary atresia, infantile refsum disease, Factor VII, and Glycogen storage disease type 1a & 1b (summarized in Table 1). To avoid the need for immunosuppression or the risk of rejection, transplantation of genetically modified autologous hepatocytes may also be an option, such as in a clinical study to treat familial cholesterolemia (Grossman et al., 1991). In this study, retrovirus was used to transduce and correct a patient's deficient hepatocytes, which were then infused back into the patient to yield a partial correction of the disease. HTx to treat progressive familiar intrahepatic cholestasis and A1AT were also attempted, but no clinical benefit was determined likely due to the presence of fibrosis in the native liver (Strom et al., 1997a; Strom et al., 1999; Hughes et al., 2005). With respect to long-term engraftment, it will be important whether the transplanted hepatocytes will gain a selection advantage over the recipient's cells. Damage or injury to the native liver triggers rapid proliferation of healthy hepatocytes; theoretically this would provide transplanted hepatocytes a selected growth advantage over native cells in patients with acute or chronic liver failure. Importantly, the livers of metabolic disease patients are not injured or damaged in most cases; transplanted cells would likely not receive selection advantage over the recipient's cells. Therefore, higher numbers of transplanted hepatocytes, a need for better cell engraftment, and repeated transplantations may be necessary for the successful treatment of metabolic liver diseases.

Cell therapy of end-stage liver disease (i.e. cirrhotic livers) is more problematic. Infusion into the liver via the portal vein is the preferred method of transplant in cases where liver architecture is intact (i.e., metabolic diseases, or in the case of acute liver failure). It is known from animal studies that hepatocytes infused via the portal vein disperse with the portal blood flow and finally translocate to the hepatic sinusoids in the periportal region of the liver lobules (Sokal et al., 2003). Single cells succeed in traversing the endothelial barrier and integrate into the parenchyma. After re-establishing intercellular contacts with neighbouring

Liver Disease	Outcome	References
α1-antitrypsin (A1AT)	No clinical benefit likely due to the presence of fibrosis	(Strom et al., 1997a; Strom et al., 1999)
Acute liver failure	Reversal of disease	(Fisher et al., 2000; Soriano, 2002; Fisher & Strom, 2006; Ott et al., 2006)
Argininosuccinate lyase deficiency	Complete correction	(Stephenne et al., 2006)
Biliary atresia	Partial correction - slow and continuous decrease in bilirubin levels	(Khan et al., 2008)
Chronic liver failure	Bridge to OLT	(Bilir et al. 200; Strom et al. 1997b; Fisher & Strom, 2006; Strom et al., 1999)
Citrullinemia	Partial correction – decreased citrulline and circulating ammonia at 6 months post- cell infusion	(Meyburg et al., 2009a)
Crigler-Najjar type 1	Partial correction - slow and continuous decrease in bilirubin levels; evidence of long term correction by hepatocyte graft (one patient was followed for > 1.5 years)	(Fox et al., 1998; Dhawan et al., 2004; Ambrosino et al., 2005)
Familial cholesterolemia	Partial correction – cholesterol decrease and transgenic expression >4 months	(Grossman et al., 1991) *
Glycogen storage disease type 1a & 1b	Partial correction – patients could maintain blood glucose between meals as well as higher and sustained glucose levels at meals	(Muraca et al., 2002; Lee et al., 2007)
Infantile refsum disease	Partial correction – improved fatty acid metabolism, reduced pipecolic acid and bile salt levels, improved strength and weight gain	(Sokal et al., 2003)
Inherited Factor VII deficiency	Partial correction – reduced FVII requirement 80%	(Dhawan et al., 2004)
Ornithine transcarbamylase deficiency (OTC)	Partial correction – ammonia and glutamine levels were normalized following transplant. Most required OLT at a later date.	(Strom et al., 1997a; Horslen et al., 2003; Mitry et al., 2004; Stephenne et al., 2005; Puppi et al., 2008; Meyburg et al., 2009a; 2009b)
Progressive familiar intrahepatic cholestasis	No clinical benefit likely due to the presence of fibrosis	(Hughes et al., 2005)

* use of genetically modified autologous hepatocytes

Table 1. Summary of clinical HTx to treat chronic liver failure, acute liver failure, and inherited metabolic diseases host cells, transplanted hepatocytes may start to proliferate when sufficient space is made for the infused cells. Donor cells and their descendents form gradually increasing clusters, thus finally repopulating the recipient liver. However, cirrhotic livers contain abnormalities of the hepatic architecture, as well as loss of functional hepatocytes, which contributes to the decrease in liver function. In addition, intrahepatic portal venous shunts may prevent an efficient exchange between hepatocytes and blood plasma, and cell infusions may cause prolonged portal hypertension and embolization in the lung (Strom et al., 1999). Preclinical HTx studies conducted on rat cirrhosis models discovered significantly increased intrapulmonary translocation of donor cells due to portal shunting (Gupta et al., 1993). Due to cirrhotic changes in the liver and associated portal hypertension, the infusion of donor hepatocytes into the liver via the portal vein without first restoring the normal liver architecture would likely cause serious complications in patients with portal hypertension. For safety purposes, transplantation into the spleen is preferable (Strom et al., 1997b; Fisher & Strom, 2006). Direct intrasplenic injection produced engraftment that was far superior to that obtained using splenic artery infusion and resulted in fewer serious complications (Nagata et al.; 2003). However, it is still unknown whether the human spleen is capable of accommodating a sufficient number of functional hepatocytes to compensate for the cirrhotic liver. For example, alcoholic cirrhotic patients showed only transient clinical improvement after treatment by splenic HTx (Strom et al., 1999; Sterling & Fisher, 2001). Another strategy that has been getting recent attention is the use of a bioartificial liver (BAL) to support metabolic function and regeneration (Koenig et al., 2005; Carpentier et al., 2009). Several devices are being tested clinically (as reviewed in Carpentier et al., 2009). However, current limitations of BAL devices are cost and, due to the shortage of allogenic hepatocytes, their prevalent use of porcine hepatocytes, which carry the risk of infection with porcine endogenous retrovirus and anaphylaxis (Chamuleau et al., 2005). Treatment of cirrhotic livers by CTx requires extra consideration regarding transplant site, cell number, and overall safety of the procedure. The continuing development of BAL is promising, but there are more challenges to overcome in this area before these devices can be considered a cost-effective and safe option for the treatment of liver disease.

3.1.3 Hepatocyte isolation, culture, and cryopreservation

The major source of hepatocytes for HTx are livers that were rejected for OLT. Some of the most common reasons that procured livers are not used for transplantation are as follows: unavailability of a matched recipient, physical damage to the liver, pre-existing liver diseases, breach of sterility during the procurement process, high liver fat content (steatosis), inappropriate age (too old), or inappropriate warm ischemic time or cold storage time (cold ischemia). Though these organs may not be therapeutically useful for OLT, viable cells for CTx may still be acquired.

Hepatocyte isolation was first employed in the late-1960s for rat livers (Howard et al., 1967; Berry & Friend, 1969). In 1976, the traditional two-step collagenase perfusion technique was developed for rat tissue (Seglan, 1976), which was later adapted for use with human tissue (Bojar et al., 1976). Another widely used method, which yields a high number of viable cells per gram of whole liver tissue, is the three-step collagenase perfusion technique (Dorko et al., 1994; Nakazawa et al., 2002; Mitry et al., 2004; Alexandrova et al.; 2005). More recently, the increasing application of these approaches in clinical grade cell therapies require the standardization of cell isolation procedures in accordance with GMP conditions (Gramignoli et al., 2011). In general, after collagenase has disassociated the hepatocytes from the connective tissue, cells are separated by low speed centrifugation, and the hepatocyte pellets are washed with ice-cold buffer solution to purify the cells. The number and quality of the isolated hepatocytes vary depending on the composition of perfusion buffer solutions, the type and concentration of enzyme, and the type and quality of the tissue source used. Further purification of viable cells can be obtained through the use of the Percoll centrifugation technique (Olinga et al., 2000), though extensive loss in cell number (20-40% cell recovery) is a major disadvantage of this method (Dorko et al., 1994). Cell viability is determined using trypan blue exclusion. However, *in vitro* viability may not reflect good cell function *in vivo*.

The primary requirement for both short-term and long-term culture of hepatocytes is their ability to efficiently attach to the culture plate. The culture dish should be pre-coated with a suitable attachment factor such as collagen (type I or IV) or Matrigel, which contains a mixture of extracellular matrices (Blaauboer & Paine, 1979; Chen et al., 1998). However, even under currently optimal *in vitro* cell culture conditions, mature human hepatocytes typically do not survive or maintain mature functionality for periods longer than 1-2 weeks, proliferation is extremely poor, and they appear to de-differentiate and lose hepatic potential (Tanaka et al., 2006, Nahmias et al., 2007).

A shortage of donor liver tissue for the isolation of human hepatocytes necessitates the development of improved cryopreservation techniques for long-term storage. There are several reports describing various cryopreservation techniques and some of the associated complexities of the procedure (Diener et al., 1993; Terry et al., 2005; 2007). Hepatocytes are typically cryopreserved in suspension, which can occur immediately following isolation. No culture step is needed. The ultimate goal of any improved cryopreservation protocol is to minimize sudden intracellular formation of ice crystals that could result in ultrastructural damage, and thus maintain cell viability, attachment, and metabolic activity upon thawing. Storage time of cryopreserved hepatocytes at temperatures well below −100°C (e.g. liquid nitrogen or -140°C freezers) may play an important role in the quality of thawed cells. Cells are resuspended in ice-cold media (usually Belzer solution, also known as UW) containing cryoprotective agents. UW has been well established in the literature to have the best results in terms of viability and recovery. The cryoprotectants used can be permeating (e.g., DiMethylSulfoxide (DMSO), glycerol) or non-permeating molecules (e.g., polymers, sugars). DMSO is the cryoprotectant of choice because it is permeating and highly soluble. It is able to enter cells and reduce injury through reduction of ice crystal formation during freezing. DMSO, being a polar solvent, may also stabilize the plasma membrane by electrostatic interactions. The concentration of these cryoprotectants, as well as the rate at which they are added, final cell density, and freezing rate may also be crucial factors contributing to viability upon thawing. The standard optimum thawing protocol for hepatocytes is rapid thawing at 37°C with slow dilution of the cryoprotectant (to reduce osmotic imbalances) at 4°C (to reduce possible toxicity of the cryoprotectant) (Karlsson et al., 1993; 1996; Pegg, 2002). Upon thawing, cells are then washed to remove cryoprotectant to avoid potential adverse affects in patients.

3.1.4 Benefits / concerns

Due to the undeniable success of OLT, it is reasonable to use all suitable donor livers for organ transplantation. Therefore, an advantage of HTx is that it would not require obtaining livers that could be used for OLT, which would only further stress an already stressed system. HTx would be using liver tissue that would otherwise be discarded. In addition, multiple patients could be treated with hepatocytes from a single tissue donor, and potentially, in cases of metabolic disease, a patient's autologous hepatocytes could be collected, genetically manipulated to correct the deficiency, and infused back into the patient. Nonetheless, there are still many problems associated with the use of hepatocytes. Despite the use of discarded tissue, the current major limitation is the availability of human hepatocytes. Although hepatocytes *in vivo* have remarkable proliferation potential, primary hepatocytes proliferate very poorly *in vitro*, appear to de-differentiate and lose their hepatic potential, and display very limited survival (Tanaka et al., 2006, Nahmias et al., 2007). Therefore, the collection of hepatocytes for HTx is still limited by the availability of fresh liver tissue as cells cannot be expanded in culture. The numbers and/or quality of hepatocytes isolated from non-transplantable livers will not allow a widespread application of HTx. A second major limitation is the need for timely availability of hepatocytes. If hepatocytes cannot be successfully cryopreserved and thawed, some advantages of CTx over OLT are lost. Successful cryopreservation is needed for establishment of cell banks, which would allow cryopreserved hepatocytes to be available for emergency use in acute and chronic liver diseases, or for planned or repeated use in patients with liver-based metabolic disorders. A third major limitation is the consistently poor quality of cells after cryopreservation. Hepatocytes are very sensitive to freezing damage, and three distinct modes of cell death have been identified: cell rupture by the formation of ice crystals, necrosis, and apoptosis (Baust, 2002). Loss of membrane integrity, and thus leakage of important enzymes and cofactors which affect liver function, low attachment efficiency, and a loss in viability of 50% or greater is typical. This situation will remain unaltered until alternatives to primary hepatocytes becomes available, which are discussed in the next sections of this chapter, or more efficient methods of cryopreservation and storage of hepatocytes, as well as cell recovery from cryopreservation are determined.

3.2 Embryonic stem cells

Embryonic stem cells (ESC) are derived from totipotent cells of the inner cell mass of the blastocyst, an early stage of the developing embryo (Thomson et al., 1998). ESCs are pluripotent, meaning they can differentiate into all three germ layers (ectoderm, mesoderm, and endoderm), and express many specific gene factors that have come to be known as cell markers of pluripotency. Common markers of "stemness" include stage specific embryonic antigens (SSEA) 3 & 4, and the tumor rejection antigens (TRA) 1-60 & 1-81 (Thomson et al., 1998), while some common molecular markers include OCT-4, SOX-2, and Nanog, as well as high expression of telomerase reverse transcriptase (TERT) (Thomson et al., 1998; Chambers et al., 2003). Telomerase maintains telomere length and adds telomere repeats to chromosome ends, which is important in a cell's replicative lifespan (Vaziri & Benchimol, 1998). However, high levels of telomerase activity are also found in 80-90% of human tumor samples (Chen & Chen, 2011). ESCs will readily become tumorigenic *in vivo* when injected into severe combined immunodeficient (SCID) mice forming either teratomas, tumors comprised of cells from all three germ layers, or teratocarcinomas, which are more aggressive, malignant teratomas (Ben-David & Benvenisty, 2011). In fact, teratoma formation is so characteristic of ESCs, it has become one of the most informative tests of pluripotency for ESC-like cells, such as induced pluripotent stem cells (iPSC). ESCs also display genetic instability (i.e. aneuplody) *in vitro*, another unfortunate characteristic they share with cancer cells (Spits et al., 2008). Furthermore, ESCs express very low human leukocyte antigen (HLA) class I antigens (Baroja et al., 2004), and almost undetectable levels of HLA class II antigens and co-stimulatory factors (Drukker et al., 2006). ESCs are still subject to immune system targeting, however. Low expression of HLA class I molecules is sufficient to induce acute rejection through the action of cytotoxic T-cells and affect treatment tolerance (Robertson et al., 2007; Drukker et al., 2006), which suggests that immunosuppression would still be required if patients recieved stem cell-derived CTx.

Sustaining pluripotency *in vitro* requires continued expression of Nanog and OCT-4 (Chambers et al., 2003). The expression of these factors are maintained through co-culture with a feeder cell layer, most commonly mouse embryonic fibroblasts (MEFs), and either the addition of basic fibroblast growth factor (bFGF) for human ESC, or leukemia inhibitory factor (LIF) for mouse ESC. Without optimal culture conditions, ESC will rapidly and spontaneously differentiate into cells from all three germ layers (Chambers et al., 2003). Finally, ESCs are indefinitely self-renewing theoretically providing an unlimited therapeutic source of cells for regenerative medicine (Thomson et al., 1998).

3.2.1 Inducing hepatic differentiation in ESC and laboratory / clinical data

ESCs will spontaneously differentiate simply by removing factors and/or allowing the formation of spheroid clumps known as embryoid bodies (EB) in culture. ESCs can also be made to differentiate along a defined lineage through exposure to specific growth factors. In a developing embryo, signals from the cardiac mesoderm and septum transversum mesenchyme specify endoderm to accept a hepatic fate. It was eventually determined that FGFs and bone morphogenic proteins (BMPs) can mimic the appropriate signals and thus induce endoderm towards a hepatic fate (Jung et al., 1999). From there, targets of BMPs and FGFs, as well as other *in vivo* hepatic regulatory genes, such as FoxA genes and the GATA and hepatocyte nuclear factor (HNF) transcription factors, defined additional molecules tested in differentiation studies to produce hepatocyte-like cells from ESC. Currently there are many published protocols to differentiate ESC into various cell types from all three germ layers, which have been reviewed elsewhere (Trounson, 2006; Zaret & Grompe, 2008; Soto-Gutierrez et al., 2008; Sancho-Bru et al., 2009). Hepatocyte-like cells that express α-fetoprotein (AFP), albumin, cytochrome P450 (CYP450), cytokeratin (CK) 18, and display epithelial-like morphology have all been extensively described. However, expression of these few factors does not guarantee the differentiated stem cell is a "hepatocyte"; hepatocyte-like stem cells may express a few hepatic genes, but they could also be negative for many others important to hepatic function (Soto-Gutierrez et al., 2008). In addition, some of these hepatic markers are not limited to hepatocyte expression, such as CYP450. Therefore, there must be a more stringent check list to determine when a stem cell is considered to be completely differentiated.

There have been many articles describing ESC derived hepatocyte-like cells transplanted into liver-damaged mice (e.g. review by Banas et al. 2007) but few have determined the cells significantly contribute to improved liver function and regeneration. Induction rates remain low regardless of the method used, and general hepatic function of the cells, even once transplanted, were very limited when compared to mature hepatocytes (Sharma et al., 2008). However, a successful report described ESCs demonstrating liver function able to overcome liver damage in mice (Heo et al., 2006). This is encouraging for the field of liver disease, but more efficient differentiation and transplantation techniques must be established. Clinical ESC therapy for liver disease is not currently realistic, but at present there are four ongoing ESC clinical trials targeting other organs in the United States (Trounson et al., 2011). Two trials are in Phase I and are targeting spinal cord injuries or spinal muscular atrophy, while the remaining two are in Phase I/II and are targeting Macular Degeneration. All trials involve ESCs that were first differentiated in culture prior to transplantation.

3.3 Mesenchymal stromal cells

Mesenchymal stromal cells (MSC), formerly known as mesenchymal stem cells, are multipotent non-hematopoietic adult stem cells that have been isolated from a variety of tissues, including bone marrow, adipose tissue, Wharton's jelly, umbilical cord blood, and different compartments of the placenta (Parolini et al., 2008). Since they originate from mesoderm, MSCs show *in vitro* differentiation potential into three cell lineages (adipogenic, chondrogenic, and osteogenic). These cells are highly proliferative fibroblast-like cells that display plastic adherence in culture and express specific surface markers (i.e. positive for CD105/CD90/CD73, and negative for CD34/CD45/CD11b, or CD14/CD19, or CD79α/HLA-DR1) (Dominici et al., 2006). Importantly, MSCs are TERT-negative (Zimmerman et al., 2003). Although tumorigenicity is lower than ESC, MSCs have been shown to assist tumor growth by transformation and suppression of the antitumor immune response (Ren et al., 2009).

Similar to ESCs, MSCs display reduced immunogenicity, but MSCs also demonstrate a powerful immunomodulatory response *in vivo* (Hematti, 2008; Bifari et al., 2010). MSCs interfere with antigen-presenting cells and suppress B-cell differentiation causing inhibition of Natural Killer (NK) cells and cytotoxic T cells. They also express a broad number of anti-inflammatory factors, such as a variety of cytokines and chemokines (Banas et al.; 2008). MSCs also inhibit local and systemic proinflammatory responses through inhibition of TNF-α and interleukin (IL)-1, which functions to prevent tissue damage (Lin et al., 2011), and can nonspecifically inhibit allogeneic lymphocyte proliferation. In addition, MSCs express low levels of HLA class I antigens and lymphocyte function-associating antigen (LFA)-3, and do not express HLA class II antigens or many co-stimulatory molecules which could function to upregulate HLA class II antigens *in vivo* (Bifari et al., 2010). By far, the most exciting and potentially useful characteristics of these cells are their immunomodulatory behaviors. MSCs significantly lower the incidence of graft-versus-host disease, autoimmune diseases, and can induce tolerance upon transplantation (Le Blanc et al, 2004; 2005; 2007). Nonetheless, it should be noted that MSC therapy may also increase the vulnerability to viral infections such as herpes (Sundin et al., 2006).

3.3.1 Differentiation of MSCs and laboratory / clinical data

Similar to ESC, MSCs are able to differentiate into various cell types by stimulation with specific growth factors, and there are many published protocols for differentiating MSCs along various cell lineages. For example, a recent review describes a number of protocols for differentiating along a hepatic lineage (Puglisi et al., 2011). The ability of MSCs to differentiate into hepatocyte-like cells was first reported in 2002 (Schwartz et al., 2002). The resulting hepatocyte-like cells performed hepatic functions such as albumin production, urea synthesis, glycogen storage, and low-density lipoprotein uptake (Jiang et al., 2002).

MSCs are able to differentiate into hepatocyte-like cells by stimulation with hepatocyte growth factor (HGF), epidermal growth factor (EGF), and FGF (Lange et al., 2005). MSC-derived hepatocytes were able to engraft in the liver upon transplantation and have been shown to contribute towards improved hepatic function and regeneration (Kuo et al., 2008). Conversely, another report using bone marrow MSCs significantly increased the number of hepatic stellate cells and myofibroblasts, which could contribute to the fibrotic cascade (Russo et al., 2006). Despite the availability of many hepatic differentiation protocols, it is currently unclear whether MSCs are able to become hepatic cells through differentiation or by cell fusion, as evidenced by Sharma, et al. (2005). In addition, the homing mechanism by which intravenously injected MSCs can preferentially recruit to the injured liver is interesting (Sakaida et al., 2004), but also not well understood. MSCs preferentially target tissues undergoing remodeling; it has been suggested that inflammation might provide key regulatory factors in the targeted migration of MSCs into the diseased location (Kuo et al., 2008).

Due to their impressive immunomodulatory features, MSCs have been used to treat acute graft-versus-host disease and osteogenesis imperfecta in children (Le Blanc et al., 2005). MSCs also secrete several factors able to suppress hepatocyte apoptosis, inflammatory responses, and liver fibrosis, as well as stimulate hepatocyte proliferation and function (Lin et al., 2011; Zhou et al., 2009). Many such factors, for example HGF, can also aid in liver regeneration. Preclinical and clinical studies have suggested that MSC transplantation can moderately restore liver function and enhance survival rates in fulminant hepatic failure and end-stage liver disease (Yagi et al., 2009; Kuo et al., 2008; Banas et al., 2009), though it has been suggested that the benefits MSCs provide to damaged livers have more to do with the expression of immunomodulatory factors than engraftment and subsequent hepatic function of the transplanted cells (Banas et al., 2008). There is little evidence to date that verifies whether MSCs are able to form mature hepatocytes, either in culture or once transplanted. However, growing evidence does suggest that MSCs may improve cirrhotic liver function once infused into patients. For example, bone marrow MSCs transplantation reduced liver fibrosis, and improved liver function and survival in mice (Sakaida et al., 2004) and rats (Abdel Aziz et al., 2007). This provided rationale for the use of autologous bone marrow MCSs for cell therapy to treat cirrhosis, which spurred several clinical trials investigating cell safety and feasibility (Kharaziha et al., 2009; Mohamadnejad et al., 2007; Salama et al., 2010). At present, there are 123 ongoing clinical trials involving MSCs investigating a variety of applications including bone, cartilage, and heart repair, immune rejection and autoimmune diseases, as well as treatment for cancer, gastrointestinal, and neurodegenerative diseases (Trounson et al., 2011).

3.4 Benefits / concerns of ESCs and MSCs

Since ESCs possess the ability of unlimited self-renewal, this relieves some pressure to identify new cell sources for regenerative medicine. However, although self-renewal is generally viewed as a powerful benefit, it is also a double-edged sword. Self-renewal, genetic instability, and tumorigenicity are characteristics shared by ESCs and cancer cells. In both differentiated and undifferentiated ESCs, there is a risk of malignancy due to their associated tumorigenicity and genetic instability (Stutchfield et al., 2010). The generation of spontaneous tumors is of particular concern for clinical applications, and much of the current research is dedicated to reducing and eventually overcoming this risk. Perhaps with more complete differentiation protocols, this will become a concern of the past. In addition to safety issues, ESCs also carry religious, political, and ethical concerns, and there is legislation restricting or banning their use in certain countries, such as the United States and United Kingdom. In contrast to ESCs, MSCs have fewer ethical concerns, as these cells are easily accessible from a variety of postnatal tissues. They exhibit a lower risk of spontaneous tumors, and their impressive ability to hide from and modulate the immune response is of considerable interest. However, MSCs have been shown to contribute to tumor growth *in vivo* and increased risk of viral infections. Therefore, high-risk patients may not be feasible candidates for MSC transplantation.

Despite many promising therapeutic reports in the literature stating stem cells are able to contribute to liver regeneration, particularly with MSCs, there are still many problems associated with their use. Even with the considerable number of differentiation protocols available to produce various cell types, differentiation methods have not been optimized. Though stem cells are abundantly proliferative, high induction rates of hepatic cells are currently not possible to provide the required number of cells for transplantation to treat disorders of the liver, an organ which contains several billion cells. Furthermore, differentiated cells display minimal hepatocyte function both *in vitro* and *in vivo*. Once transplanted, engraftment is very low with low contributions towards tissue regeneration. For these reasons, it is relatively unknown whether stem cell-derived hepatocyte-like cells will be useful to treat and correct liver disease. More research is required to determine more efficient ways to induce hepatocyte-like cells, and a standardized list of requirements should be established to verify complete differentiation. In brief, stem cell derived hepatocyte-like cells should demonstrate characteristic hepatic gene expression and function, express appropriate transport proteins and transcription factors, metabolize ammonia and billirubin, produce albumin and/or bile acids, and no longer express genes characteristic of ESC or other cell types. Therapeutically useful hepatocyte-like cells must be safe (i.e. nontumorigenic), contribute to liver function *in vivo*, and importantly, must express hepatic genes at a level comparable to mature hepatocytes. Currently there are no definitive reports of any stem cell-derived hepatocytes with these ideal characteristics.

3.5 Human placenta as a source for stem cells

The human full term placenta is comprised of three distinct layers: amnion, chorion, and decidua (Figure 1). The amnion and chorion are fetal-derived while the decidua originates from maternal tissue. The trophoblast layer gives rise to the chorion; the amnion is derived from the pluripotent epiblast, which also gives rise to all three germ layers of the embryo. The amnion layer is established as early as day 8 following fertilization, well before gastrulation when cell fate is specified (day 15-17). The amnion is derived at a time when the epiblast remains pluripotent, and amnion epithelial (AE) cells retain some of these characteristics. AE cells are easily isolated from full term placenta following live birth, which would normally be discarded after delivery. Placenta is readily available and easily procured without invasive procedures or causing harm to either mother or baby. In 2007, there were 1.4 million cesarean births in the United States, which equates to ~32% of all U.S. births (Hamilton et al., 2009). Placentas for cell isolation are typically obtained from cesarean deliveries due to sterility concerns; however, all placentas should be considered a useful source for stem cells. Theoretically, placental stem cells could be isolated from all term births and cryopreserved in a cell bank for future use. Since it has been estimated that as little as 30 stem cell lines would be needed to match HLA haplotypes in >80% of the Japanese population (Nakatsuji et al., 2008), global banking of placental stem cells containing all HLA haplotypes worldwide may be considered a realistic and attainable goal. Therefore, placental amnion may provide a useful source of pluripotent stem cells that are plentiful and free from most ethical, religious, or political concerns.

3.5.1 Amnion epithelial (AE) cells

The amniotic layer is composed of a single-celled epithelial layer of cuboidal and columnar cells and a deeper mesodermal layer composed of an upper compact acellular layer and a lower fibroblast-containing layer (Figure 1). The epithelial layer of the amnion is in contact with the amniotic fluid, which serves to protect and cushion the fetus through gestation. The chorionic layer is comprised of a mesodermal layer and an extravillious trophoblast layer. The maternally derived decidua, which interacts with the fetal derived trophoblast, serves to support the fetus through gas, nutrition, and waste exchange, and protect the fetus from the maternal immune system.

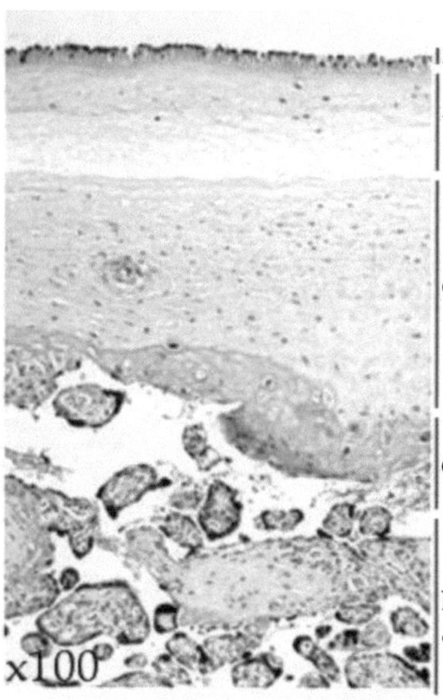

Fig. 1. Cross-sectional representation of the human placenta. The amnion and chorion are fetal-derived membranes while the decidual membrane is maternally-derived. The amniotic layer is composed of a single-celled epithelial layer and a deeper mesodermal layer. The chorionic layer is comprised of a mesodermal layer and a trophoblast layer. The maternal decidua is intermingled with the fetal chorionic trophoblast. (AE: amniotic epithelium; AM: amniotic mesoderm; CM: chorionic mesoderm; CT: chorionic trophoblast.)

AE cells in culture express stem cell surface markers (e.g. SSEA-3 & 4, TRA 1-60 & 1-81) as well as molecular markers of stem cells (e.g. OCT-4, Nanog, SOX-2, FGF-4, and Rex-1), and unlike ESC, do not require feeder cell layers to maintain OCT-4 and Nanog expression (Miki et al., 2005; Miki & Strom, 2006). Interestingly, AE cells do not express the stem cell marker TERT (Miki et al., 2005). Telomerase activity is found in human ESC, multipotent adult progenitor stem cells, human germ cells, and 80-90% of human tumor samples (Chen & Chen, 2011). Telomerase-positive stem cells display an unstable karyotype and can become tumorigenic, most commonly forming teratomas, when transplanted into SCID mice. Conversely, AE cells consistently display a normal karyotype and are nontumorigenic when transplanted into SCID mice (Miki & Strom, 2006; Marongiu et al., 2011). In addition, AE cells are derived from neonatal tissue and should therefore naturally possess less environmental and age-acquired DNA damage (Miki, 2011). It is commonly known in the field that amnion does not express HLA class II antigens and only expresses class I antigens at low levels, which later led to the premise that AE would be able to bypass the immune system. AE cells were also found to secrete anti-inflammatory and immunosuppressive factors, which inhibited inflammation and reduced the proliferation of T- and B-cells *in vitro* (Li et al., 2005). Volunteers transplanted with AE cells did not experience any immunological reaction, and to date no tumors have ever formed as a result (Akle et al., 1981; Yeager et al, 1985; Scaggiante et al, 1987; Sakurgawa et al., 1992). Many of these characteristics identify AE cells as similar to ESC, but not identical.

3.5.2 AE cell isolation and differentiation methods

Placental tissues are obtained with local Institutional Review Board (IRB) approval in the U.S., or under appropriate Ethical Committee approval, as well as patient approval. The amnion membrane is easily stripped from the underlying layers of the placenta by carefully peeling it away from the chorion (Figure 2). The amnion membrane contains AE cells and amniotic mesenchymal (AM) fibroblasts. AE and AM cells can be isolated from the amnion membrane following simple protocols (Miki et al., 2010; Marongiu, 2010). In brief, for collection of AE, the amnion membrane is first washed several times to remove blood contamination. The membrane is then subjected to several trypsinization steps, which releases the AE cells from the amnion mesenchymal fibroblasts and the connective tissue. The trypsin digests are then centrifuged to pellet the AE cells and resuspended in standard

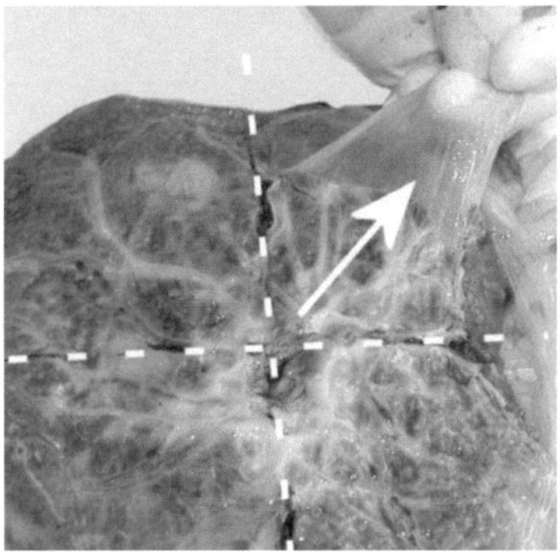

Fig. 2. Isolation of the amnion membrane from the chorion of the placenta. The maternal side of the placenta is placed face down and a shallow X-shaped incision (dashed lines) is made through the center of the placenta. The thin, nearly transparent amnion membrane is then peeled from the chorion starting at the center of the cut and progressing outward (direction of the arrow)

culture medium. A density separation step is done to enrich the population of SSEA-4 positive AE cells similar to the process used for hepatocytes. Cell viability is determined by trypan blue exclusion and counted with a hemocytometer. An estimated AE cell yield from one term placenta is 80-300 million cells (Miki et al.; 2010). When AE cells are cultured in the presence of epidermal growth factor (EGF), they readily proliferate with numerous mitotic events (Terada et al., 2000), though senescence routinely occurs after 6-10 passages (Miki & Strom, 2006).

AE cells have previously shown the potential to differentiate into all three germ layers *in vitro* (Miki et al., 2005). Similar to ESC, differentiation of AE cells to other cell types is dependent upon the culture substrate, as well as which growth factors are added and at what concentration (Parolini et al., 2007; Miki, 2011). Our group previously published efficient methods to differentiate AE cells along a hepatic lineage (Miki, et al., 2009; Marongiu, et al., 2011); after differentiation, AE cells expressed many endodermal/hepatic marker genes such as A1AT, hepatocyte nuclear factor-4 (HNF4-α), albumin, CAAT enhancer binding protein-alpha (C/EBP-α), many CYP450 genes, CK 8, 18, and 19, CYP7A1, plus several others at the level of fetal hepatocytes. Interestingly, cultured AE hepatocyte-like cells express both CYP3A7 and CYP3A4, which indicates that AE differentiates along a pathway similar to human fetal liver. Furthermore, the ratio of CYP3A4 to CYP3A7 implies that cells are progressing towards mature hepatocytes (Miki et al., 2009). Early studies demonstrated proof of principle for AE cell transplantation through the production of dopamine-expressing cells from AE, which could survive and function in a rat model of Parkinson's disease (Kakishita et al, 2000; 2003). Importantly, it was found that when undifferentiated AE cells were transplanted into the livers of immunodeficient mice, cells displaying hepatic morphology were observed that expressed mature liver genes such as transporters, cytochromes, and albumin or A1AT; circulating A1AT was also detected in transplanted mice confirming functional engraftment (Miki & Strom, 2006; Marongiu et al.; 2011).

3.5.3 AE cell transplantation

Amnion epithelial cells, due to their stem cell-like pluripotent characteristics, low immunogenicity, and anti-inflammatory properties, show exciting promise in the field of regenerative medicine. Recently, studies have shown lung protection following human AE cell transplantation in a SCID mouse model of bleomycin-induced lung injury (Moodley et al., 2010; Murphy et al., 2010). Studies have also shown the efficacy of AE cells on corneal resurfacing in horses (Plummer, 2009), rabbits (Wan et al., 2011), and humans patients (Nubile et al., 2011), in which amniotic membranes were transplanted as a graft over the injury site. These studies were done without immunosuppression and without evidence of acute rejection. Differentiated AE have also been used to treat a rat model of Parkinson's disease (Kakishita et al, 2000; 2003). Important for the treatment of liver diseases by CTx, AE cells demonstrate hepatic gene expression and functions at a level of mature hepatocytes following implantation into the livers of SCID mice, which suggest they differentiate into hepatocyte-like cells once engrafted in the liver parenchyma (Miki & Strom, 2006; Marongiu et al., 2011). Undifferentiated AE cells were able to functionally engraft into the livers of immunocompromised mouse models of liver damage resulting in a reduction of hepatic fibrosis, inflammation, and hepatocyte apoptosis (Manuelpillai et al., 2010; Marongiu et al., 2011). In addition, AE cells have also been used in clinics to correct lysosomal storage diseases with no adverse effects (Yeager et al, 1985; Scaggiante et al, 1987; Sakurgawa et al., 1992). Finally, our group recently determined that AE cells could partially rescue a mouse model of intermediate MSUD (Skvorak et al., 2010), an inborn error of metabolism characterized by deficiency of the branched-chain keto-acid dehhydrogenase (BCKDH) enzyme complex and high levels of BCAA (Homanics et al., 2006). iMSUD mice were given multiple infusions of undifferentiated AE cells, either freshly isolated or cryopreserved, directly into the liver parenchyma. AE cell transplantation partially corrected iMSUD mice similarly to the partial correction previously obtained with hepatocyte transplantation (Skvorak et al, 2009a; 2009b). While untreated iMSUD mice grew sickly and all died prior to 27 days of age, iMSUD-treated mice displayed improved BCKDH enzyme activity, reduced BCAA and other relevant metabolites in the brain and blood, their body weight mimicked that of healthy wildtype littermates, and >70% of animals survived to day of life 100 (Skvorak et al., 2010). Immunosuppression was not used and there was no evidence of rejection.

3.5.4 Benefits / concerns of AE cells

Current research suggests that stem cells isolated from discarded placenta may be an abundant, noncontroversial, and safe source of cells for regenerative medicine. There are a multitude of reports in the literature, some going as far back as 1947, which describe the successful use of AE and amniotic membranes to treat a variety of disorders both preclinically and clinically. Furthermore, isolation is relatively easy, and does not require a special laboratory set up (Miki et al., 2007). An average of 100 million cells can be isolated from a single term placenta, and AE is able to proliferate robustly in culture; Miki, et al. (2005) estimates that 100 million AE cells could be expanded to 10-60 billion cells within six passages. Unlike hepatocytes, AE cell viability and morphology are also very stable when cryopreserved long term at -80°C. Taken together, these benefits greatly encourage the establishment of a placental cell bank. Current umbilical cord blood stem cell guidelines could be used as a template to set up similar procurement and banking procedures for placental-derived stem cells (Serrano-Delgado et al., 2009).

AE cells meet many important criteria for clinically relevant cells: expression of anti-inflammatory factors, nonimmunogenic, maintains a stable karyotype, and consistently nontumorigenic *in vivo* in both SCID mice and humans. Undifferentiated AE cells are proposed to become hepatocyte-like once engrafted in the liver parenchyma and have contributed to liver function in animal models of disease. There are also many published differentiation protocols describing induction along many cell lineages, including hepatic. However, though these cells exhibit many advantages, particularly over other stem cell types, the ability to produce therapeutically useful cells to treat liver diseases has still not been developed from AE cells. Though it is unknown whether differentiation prior to transplantation will be necessary, one should assume that differentiation into the required cell type will be the most clinically efficient and effective method of treatment. Therefore, hepatocyte-like cells derived from AE should be held to the same standardized list of requirements, outlined in Section 3.4, as cells differentiated from other classifications of stem cells. As with other types of stem cells, more research is required to establish better induction of therapeutically useful cells. However, the safety of these cells has been exhaustively established and they already have a long history of clinical use. Clinical application of AE for liver and other diseases may be in our near future.

3.6 Discovery and characterization of induced pluripotent stem cells (iPSC)

Once an embryo reaches the blastocyst stage, highly specific (i.e. spatially and temporally controlled) molecular signaling events coordinate directed differentiation of cells to their appropriate cell fate. Therefore, a cell becomes specified not by changing its DNA sequence, but by controlling the expression of certain genes through specific signals. The first attempt to manipulate a cell's developmental potential was known as somatic cell nuclear transfer, which led to the birth of live lambs (Wilmut et al., 1997). "Dolly" the sheep provided evidence that differentiation of a cell towards a somatic state is not accomplished by irreversible genetic manipulation.

Almost a decade later, Yamanaka's group successfully derived pluripotent ESC-like cells from murine somatic cells through forced expression of the reprogramming factors OCT-3/4, SOX-2, c-MYC, and KLF-4 by lentiviral induction (Takahashi & Yamanaka, 2006). These "induced pluripotent stem cells" (iPSC) were similar to ESCs in morphology, growth properties, expression of ESC marker genes, display of an unstable karyotype, tumorigenicity and teratoma formation in SCID mice, and injection into a blastocyst yielded cells that contributed to mouse development. Human iPSC from adult skin fibroblasts were also generated using the same four factors as mice (Takahashi et al., 2007), and also by forced expression of a new set of four factors: OCT-4, SOX-2, Nanog, and Lin-28 (Yu et al., 2007). Pluripotent iPSC should express the stem cell markers SSEA3, SSEA-4, TRA-1-60, TRA-1-81, OCT-4, alkaline phosphatase, TERT, SOX-2 and Nanog, and form teratomas *in vivo*. It has also been reported that a specific expression profile of stem cell markers corresponds to either a completely or partially reprogrammed cell (Chan et al., 2009). Recently, iPSCs have been derived from a variety of human tissues, such as umbilical cord matrix (Cai et al., 2010), fetal and juvenile tissues (Park et al., 2008a; Li et al., 2010; Aasen et al., 2008), placental tissue (Nagata et al., 2009; Cai et al., 2010; Zhao et al., 2010), and primary human hepatocytes. However, evidence that iPSC retain epigenetic memory of their cells of origin exist for both mouse (Kim et al., 2010; Polo et al., 2010) and human (Hu et al., 2010), which can affect their differentiation potential. This is a concern, but it also suggests that the best cell source to generate iPSC for the treatment of liver disease would be hepatocytes; hepatic-like cells differentiated from hepatocyte-derived iPSC would most closely resemble their primary cell counterparts.

Currently, iPSC research is largely dedicated to reducing the tumorigenicity of the cells. The use of retroviruses and lentiviruses is a concern, which integrates into the target cell genome in a random fashion potentially causing cancer. The generation of mouse iPSC through the use of non-integrating adenoviruses (Stadtfeld et al., 2008) determined reprogramming could be achieved through transient expression. Vector integration-free human iPSCs have since been derived using Epstein-Barr virus-derived episomes (Yu et al., 2009), mRNA transfection (Yakubov et al., 2010), bacterial DNA-free episomal vectors (Jia et al., 2010), and proteins (Kim et al., 2009). However, viral integration is only one problem contributing to the tumorigenicity of iPSC. c-MYC is a well established oncogene, and the remaining factors (OCT-4, SOX-2, KLF-4) are also known to be highly expressed in cancers (Schoenhals et al., 2009). Recent studies have shown that reprogramming could be successful without using c-MYC and KLF-4 (Li et al., 2010; Huangfu et al., 2008). However, the use of viral-free vectors or the omission of c-MYC and KLF-4 drastically reduces reprogramming efficiency, and one study found no difference in tumorigenicity between viral and viral-free methods

(Moriguchi et al., 2010). More recently described epigenetic factors such as cell memory and genetic imprinting may also contribute to the tumorigenicity of iPSC, which is not yet understood (Ben-David & Benvenisty, 2011).

3.6.1 iPSC for disease modeling, hepatic differentiation, and transplantation

Now that iPSC technology has been well established, disease-specific iPSC to model diseases *in vitro* and *in vivo* may help researchers better understand diseases in order to develop new treatments. Park et al. (2008b) described the generation of iPSC from a variety of inherited diseases, such as Huntington's, Duchene's and Beckers's muscular dystrophy, diabetes mellitus type 1, Down's syndrome, and Parkinson's. iPSC have also been generated from inherited metabolic disease patients with A1AT, Crigler-Najjar, tyrosinemia type 1, familial hypercholesterolemia, and glycogen storage disease type 1a (Rashid et al., 2010), which were then differentiated into hepatocytes to more accurately model the disease *in vitro*. More recently, iPSC-derived hepatocyte-like cells generated from the dermal fibroblasts of a Wilson's disease patient was shown to mimic the disease phenotype *in vitro* (Zhang et al., 2011). Importantly, iPSCs of metabolic disease could be genetically corrected in culture, differentiated into hepatocytes possessing the ability to make normal protein, and potentially infused back into patients to cure their disease. The use of autologous cells would also reduce the risk of immune issues and rejection theoretically avoiding the need for immunosuppression. Human artificial chromosome technology was used to deliver the entire dystrophin gene to genetically correct patient fibroblasts with Duchenne muscular dystrophy *in vitro*, and iPSC were generated from the corrected cells (Kazuki et al., 2010). In addition, iPSC-derived hepatocyte-like cells modeling Wilson's disease were corrected *in vitro* using either lentiviral gene therapy or treatment of the drug curcumin (Zhang et al., 2011).

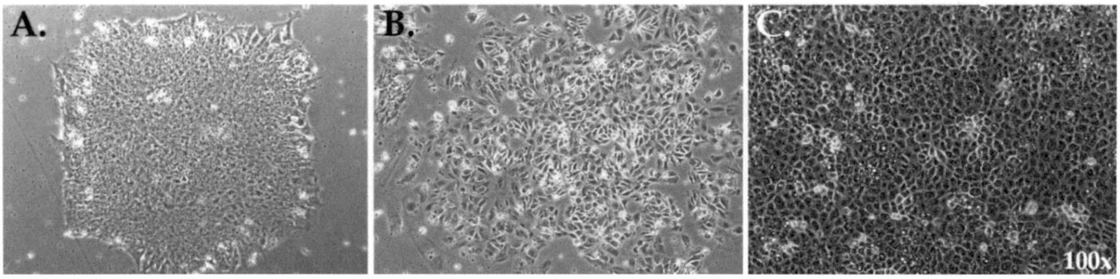

Fig. 3. Examples of iPSC *in vitro*. A. undifferentiated iPS cell colony; B. a spontaneously differentiating iPS cell colony; C. iPS cell-derived hepatocytes formed after following an *in vitro* protocol adapted from Si-Tayeb et al. 2010. All cells were cultured on matrigel in mTeSR1 media

Using established differentiation protocols for ESCs, researchers have been able to differentiate iPSCs into all three germ layers in culture, further proving these cells are truly pluripotent. Figure 3 shows examples of cultured iPSC in either an undifferentiated state (Figure 3A) or spontaneous differentiation (Figure 3B). Furthermore, there are several reports of differentiation of iPSC along a hepatic lineage (Figure 3C) using ESC protocols (Si-Tayeb et al., 2010; Song et al., 2009; Liu et al., 2011). However, in most reported cases iPSC-derived hepatocytes displayed very low hepatic function and gene expression *in vitro* when compared to primary hepatocytes. However, blastocysts from tyrosinema type 1 mouse models deficient in the FAH gene were injected with MEF-derived iPSC, and resulting pups with high chimerism could survive without NTBC drug (Espejel et al., 2010). FAH-negative pups with low levels of chimerism were dependent on NTBC to survive. These data demonstrate the potential for iPSC to form "mature" hepatocytes which can express sufficient levels of protein to correct a metabolic defect. However, Espejel et al. differentiated iPSC through injection into a blastocyst. As with other stem cells, improved *in vitro* differentiation protocols are needed to yield high amounts of therapeutically useful cells.

3.6.2 Benefits / concerns of iPS cells

Similar to ESC, the major benefits of iPSC are their self-renewal abilities and differentiation potential. iPSC could theoretically provide an unlimited pluripotent source of cells that could be banked and differentiated into hepatocytes for transplant when needed. Nakatsuji et al. (2008) estimated that an iPSC bank with only 30 stem cell lines could match the HLA haplotypes in >80% of the Japanese population. Unlike ESC, patient specific iPSC could be generated, corrected, and infused back into a patient avoiding immune problems and the need for immunosuppression. Importantly, there are no religious, ethical, or political controversies associated with the use of iPSCs. However, the field of iPSC research is very new and there are still a lot of unknowns. The major concern with iPSC use is a question of safety; iPSC have a high risk of tumorigenicity. Just like ESC, iPSC exhibit genetic instability, express TERT, and can produce teratomas *in vivo*. Furthermore, rapidly accumulating evidence suggests these two cell types have important genetic and epigenetic differences that influence their tumorigenicity, and that iPSC are likely more tumorigenic than ESC (reviewed by Ben-David & Benvenisty, 2011). Furthermore, the most reliable, reproducible, and efficient method to currently generate iPSC is through an integrating viral vector process that could induce cancers, and both integrating and non-integrating methods use reprogramming factors that are highly expressed in many tumor samples. Aside from the issue of safety, cell differentiation protocols and methods to enhance engraftment have not yet been optimized, and it is currently unknown whether long term survival of iPSCs *in vivo* is possible. Further research is needed to generate iPSC that are safe, effective, and therapeutically useful before these cells can be used for clinical cell therapies.

4. Conclusions

Alternatives to OLT must be found in order to circumvent the increasing amount of patient deaths due to long organ wait times and insufficient numbers of available livers. CTx has shown a great deal of promise, and the progress made over the past several decades of preclinical and clinical studies provides a growing amount of rationale for its use to treat a variety of liver disorders. Cells isolated from donor livers have been proven to provide safe and effective liver support for both short- and long-term function. There have been several reported clinical cases of disease reversal in acute liver failure, and HTx has provided partial correction for a variety of inherited metabolic diseases (Table 1). *In vitro* gene modification to correct allogenic hepatocytes is also possible to avoid immunogenicity of transplanted cells and a lifelong immunosuppression regimen. However, complete correction of a metabolic disorder by HTx has not yet been achieved, and more than one treatment would likely be required to sustain a patient through his/her lifetime. There are still several challenges to overcome. For HTx, the first major challenge is the availability of donor livers for the isolation of hepatocytes. There are not enough donor livers rejected for OLT, thus making them available for HTx, to provide for everyone requiring treatment. The second is regarding reliable storage of isolated hepatocytes. Current cryopreservation and thawing protocols result in massive cell loss and decreased viability; this reduces the number of cells available for transplant, and cell quality influences cell engraftment, cell function, and thus patient outcome. These drawbacks emphasize our need for alternative cell sources. Research to use stem cells and stem-like cells (e.g. ESC, MSC, AE, iPSC) for CTx are currently in preclinical and, for some, early clinical stages. Though there have been some advances made in animal models, the safety and efficacy of these cells must be unequivocally determined. All the aforementioned alternative cell types display varying levels of immunomodulatory properties making them potentially less immunogenic than hepatocytes. However, ESC, MSC, and iPSC all have tumorigenicity risks associated with their use *in vivo*. It has been suggested that more complete differentiation of cells into hepatocyte-like cells may reduce tumor formation, though it is not known whether this strategy will completely ablate the risk. In addition, the recently discovered epigenetic factors in iPSC must be more thoroughly investigated. These epigenetic differences may influence differentiation efficiencies, and it has been suggested that they may make iPSC more tumorigenic than ESC (Ben-David & Benvenisty, 2011). AE cells are nontumorigenic in both an undifferentiated and differentiated state, are nonimmunogenic, and have been used in clinical studies for more than sixty years without immunosuppression and without evidence of acute rejection. AE cells are clearly the safest alternative to hepatocytes from the stem cells discussed in this chapter, but their effectiveness to correct liver disease is currently unknown.

In summary, considerable progress has been gained in cell transplantation thus far, though future work is required to enhance utility of this novel branch of regenerative medicine. Improvement of cell engraftment remains the single biggest challenge to overcome. New methods to modulate the immune reaction and relieve changes in vascular pressures after cell transplant are currently being investigated to enhance engraftment and improve patient outcome. Preconditioning protocols of the recipient liver, such as hepatic irradiation, portal vein embolization, and surgical resection, may also help to improve engraftment by giving donor cells selected growth advantage (Soltys et al., 2010; Puppi et al., 2011), which will be of particular importance in patients of metabolic disease. Though hepatocytes remain the most preferred cell for cell transplantation, stem cells may provide a useful cell alternative to hepatocytes once the question of safety has been resolved and the ability to provide therapeutically useful cells at a scale suitable for transplantation is achieved.

5. Acknowledgements

Stephen Strom was supported in part by N01-DK-7-0004/HHSN267200700004C, the Liver Tissue and Cell Distribution System. Kristen Skvorak and Roberto Gramignoli were supported by fellowships from the National Phenylketonuria Alliance.

6. References

Aasen, T.; Raya, A.; Barrero, M.J.; et al. (2008). Efficient and rapid generation of induced pluripotent stem cells from human keratinocytes. *Nat Biotechnol.* Vol. 26, pp. 1276-1284.

Abdel Aziz, M.T.; Atta, H.M.; Mahfouz, S.; et al. Therapeutic potential of bone marrow-derived mesenchymal stem cells on experimental liver fibrosis. *Clin Biochem*. Vol. 40, No. 12, pp. 893-899

Akle, C.A.; Adinolfi, M.; Welsh, K.I.; et al. (1981) Immunogenicity of human amniotic epithelial cells after transplantation into volunteers. *Lancet*. Vol. 2, No. 8254, pp. 1003-1005

Alexandrova, K.; Griesel, C.; Barthold, M.; et al. (2005) Large-scale isolation of human hepatocytes for therapeutic application. *Cell Transplant*. Vol. 14, pp. 845

Ambrosino, et al., 2005; Ambrosino, G.; Varotto, S.; Strom, S.C.; et al. (2005) Isolated hepatocyte transplantation for Crigler–Najjar syndrome type 1. *Cell Transplant*. Vol. 14, pp. 151–157

Banas, A.; Yamamoto, Y.; Teratani, T. & Ochiya, T. (2007) Stem cell plasticity: learning from hepatogenic differentiation strategies. *Developmental Dyn*. Vol. 236, pp. 3228-3241

Banas, A.; Teratani, T.; Yamamoto, Y.; et al. (2008) *In vivo* therapeutic potential of human adipose tissue mesenchymal stem cells (AT-MSCs) after transplantation into mice with liver injury. *Stem Cells*. Vol. 26, pp. 2705-2712

Banas, A.; Teratani, T.; Yamamoto, Y.; et al. (2009) Rapid hepatic fate specification of adipose-derived stem cells and their therapeutic potential for liver failure. *J Gastroenterol Hepatol*. Vol. 24, No. 1, pp. 70-77

Baust, J.M. (2002) Molecular mechanisms of cellular demise associated with cryopreservation failure. *Cell Preservation Technol*. Vol. 1, pp. 17–31

Ben-David, U. & Benvenisty, N. (2011) The tumorigenicity of human embryonic and induced pluripotent stem cells. *Nature Rev. Cancer*. Vol. 11, pp. 268-277

Berry, M.N. & Friend, D.S. (1969) High-yield preparation of isolated rat liver parenchymal cells: a biochemical and fine structural study. *J Cell Biol*. Vol. 43, pp. 506–520

Bifari, F., Pacelli, L. & Krampera, M. (2010) Immunological properties of embryonic and adult stem cells. *World J. Stem Cells*. Vol. 2, No. 3, pp. 50-60

Bilir, B.M.; Guinette, D.; Karrer, F.; et al. (2000) Hepatocyte transplantation in acute liver failure. *Liver Transplant*. Vol. 6, pp. 32–40

Blaauboer, B.J. & Paine, A.J. (1979) Attachment of rat hepatocytes to plastic substrata in the absence of serum requires protein synthesis. *Biochem. Biophys. Res. Commun*. Vol. 90, pp. 368–74

Bojar, H.; Basler, M.; Fuchs, F.; et al. (1976) Preparation of parenchymal and non-parenchymal cells from adult human liver—morphological and biochemical characteristics. *J. Clin. Chem. Clin. Biochem*. Vol. 14, pp. 527–532

Bucher, N.L.R. (1963) Regeneration of the mammalian liver. *Int. Rev. Cytol.*,Vol. 15, pp. 245-300

Cai, J.; Li, W.; Su, H.; et al. (2010). Generation of human induced pluripotent stem cells from umbilical cord matrix and amniotic membrane mesenchymal cells. *J Biol Chem*. Vol. 285, pp. 11227-11234.

Cai, J.; Zhao, Y.; Liu, Y.; et al. (2007). Directed differentiation of human embryonic stem cells into functional hepatic cells. *Hepatology*.Vol. *45*, pp. 1229-1239.

Chan, E.M.; Ratanasirintrawoot, S.; Park, I.H.; et al. (2009). Live cell imaging distinguishes bona fide human iPSC from partially reprogrammed cells. *Nat Biotechnol*. Vol. 27, pp. 1033-1037.

Carpentier, B.; Gautier, A. & Legallais, C. (2009) Artificial and bioartificial liver devices: present and future. *Gut*. Vol. 58, pp. 1690-1702.

Chambers, I.; Colby, D.; Robertson, M; et al. (2003) Functional expression cloning of Nanog, a pluripotency sustaining factor in embryonic stem cells. *Cell.* Vol. 113, pp. 643-655

Chamulearu, R.A.; Beurhold, T. & Hoekstra, R. (2005) What are the right cells to be used in the bioartificial liver? *Metab. Brain. Disease.* Vol. 20, pp. 327-335

Chen, H.L.; Wu, H.L. ; Fon, C.C. ; et al. (1998) Long-term culture of hepatocytes from human adults. *J Biomed Sci.* Vol. 5, pp. 435–40

Chen, C.H. & Chen, R.J. (2011) Prevalence of telomerase activity in human cancer. *J. Formos. Med. Association.* Vol. 110, No. 5, pp. 175-189

Diener, B.; Utesch, D.; Beer, N.; et al. (1993) A method for the cryopreservation of liver parenchymal cells for studies of xenobiotics. *Cryobiology.* Vol. 30, pp. 116-117

Dhawan, A.; Mitry, R.R.; Hughes, R.D.; et al. (2004) Hepatocyte transplantation for inherited factor VII deficiency. *Transplantation.* Vol. 78, pp. 1812-1814

Dominici, M.; Le Blanc, K.; Mueller, I.; et al. (2006) Minimal criteria for defining multipotent mesenchymal stromal cells. The International Society for Cellular Therapy Position Statement. Cytotherapy. Vol. 8, No. 4, pp. 315-317

Dorko, K.; Freeswick, P.D.; Bartoli, F.; et al. (1994) A new technique for isolating and culturing human hepatocytes from whole or split livers not used for transplantation. *Cell Transplant.* Vol. 3, pp. 387–395

Drukker, M.; Katchman, H.; Katz, G.; et al. (2006) Human embryonic stem cells and their differentiated derivatives are less susceptible to immune rejection than adult cells. *Stem Cells.* Vol. 24, pp. 221–229

Espejel, S.; Roll, G.R.; McLaughlin, K.J.; et al. (2010). Induced pluripotent stem cell-derived hepatocytes have the functional and proliferative capabilities needed for liver regeneration in mice. *J Clin Invest.* Vol. 120, pp. 3120-3126.

Fisher, R.A.; Bu, D.; Thompson, M.; et al. (2000) Defining hepatocellular chimerism in a liver failure patient bridged with hepatocyte infusion. *Transplantation.* Vol. 69, pp. 303-307

Fisher, R.A. & Strom, S.C. (2006) Human hepatocyte transplantation: worldwide results. *Transplantation.* Vol. 82, pp. 441-449

Fox, I.J.; Chowdhury, J.R.; Kaufman, S.S.; et al. (1998) Treatment of the Crigler-Najjar syndrome type 1 with hepatocyte transplantation. *New England J. Medicine.* Vol. 228, pp. 1422-1426

Gramignoli, R.; Green, M.L.; Tahan, V.; et al. (2011) Development and application of purified tissue dissociation enzyme mixtures for human hepatocyte isolation. *Cell Transplant*, in press.

Grossman, M.; Raper, S.E. & Wilson, J.M. (1991) Towards liver-directed gene therapy: retrovirus-mediated gene transfer into human hepatocytes. Somat. Cell Mol. Gen. Vol. 17, No. 6, pp. 601-607

Groth, C.G.; Arborgh, B.; Björkén, C.; et al. (1977) Correction of hyperbilirubinemia in the glucuronyltransferase-deficient rat by intraportal hepatocyte transplantation. *Transplant Proc.* Vol. 9, No. 1, pp. 313-316

Gupta, S.; Yerneni, P.R.; Vemura, R.P.; et al. (1993) Studies on the safety of intrasplenic hepatocyte transplantation: relevance to ex vivo gene therapy and liver repopulation in acute hepatic failure. *Human Gene Ther.* Vol. 4, pp. 249-257

Gupta, S.; Rajvanshi, P.; Sokhi, R.; et al. (1999) Entry and integration of transplanted hepatocytes in rat liver plates occur by disruption of hepatic sinusoidal endothelium. *Heptatology.* Vol. 29, pp. 509-519

Gupta, S. & Chowdhury, J.R. (2002) Therapeutic potential of hepatocyte transplantation. *Semin Cell Dev Biol.* Vol. 13, No. 6, pp.439-46

Hamilton, B.E.; Martin, J.A. &Ventura, S.J. (2009) Births: Preliminary data for 2007. National vital statistics reports. *National Center for Health Statistics.* Hyattsville, MD., Vol. 57, No. 12. (March 18, 2009). Available from: http://www.cdc.gov/nchs/data/nvsr/nvsr57/nvsr57_12.pdf

Harding, C.O. & Gibson, K.M. (2010) Therapeutic liver repopulation for phenylketonuria. *J. Inherited. Metabolic Dis.* Vol. 33, No. 6, pp. 681-7

Hamman, K., Clark, H., Montini, E.; et al. (2005) Low therapeutic threshold for hepatocyte replacement in murine phenylketonuria. *Molecular Therapy.* Vol. 12, No. 2, pp. 337-344

Hematti, P. (2008) Role of mesenchymal stromal cells in solid organ transplantation. *Transplant Rev (Orlando).* Vol. 22, No. 4, pp. 262-73

Heo, J.; Factor, V.M.; Uren, T.; et al. (2006) Hepatic precursors derived from murine embryonic stem cells contribute to regeneration of injured liver. Hepatology. Vol. 44, pp. 1478-1486

Homanics, G.E.; Skvorak, K.; Ferguson, C.; et al. (2006) Production and characterization of murine models of classic and intermediate maple syrup urine disease. *BMC Medical Genetics.* Vol. 7, No. 1, pp. 33

Horslen, S.P.; McCowan, T.C.; Goertzen, T.C.; et al. (2003) Isolated hepatocyte transplantation in an infant with a severe urea cycle disorder. *Pediatrics* Vol. 111, pp. 1262–1267

Howard, R.B.; Christensen, A.K.; Gibbs, F.A. & Pesch, L.A. (1967) The enzymatic preparation of isolated intact parenchymal cells from rat liver. *J Cell Biol.* Vol. 35, pp. 675–684

Hu, Q.; Friedrich, A.M.; Johnson, L.V.; et al. (2010) Memory in induced pluripotent stem cells: reprogrammed human retinal pigmented epithelial cells show tendency for spontaneous redifferentiation. Stem Cells. Vol. 28, pp. 1981-1991

Huangfu, D.; Osafune, K.; Maehr, R.; et al. (2008). Induction of pluripotent stem cells from primary human fibroblasts with only Oct4 and Sox2. *Nat Biotechnol.* Vol. 26, pp.1269-1275.

Hughes, R.D.; Mitry, R.R. & Dhawan, A. (2005) Hepatocyte transplantation for metabolic liver disease: UK experience. *J R Soc Med.* Vol. 98, pp. 341–345

Jia, F.; Wilson, K.D.; Sun, N.; et al. (2010). A nonviral minicircle vector for deriving human iPSC. *Nat Methods.* Vol. 7, pp. 197-199.

Jiang, Y.; Jahagirdar, B.N.; Reinhardt, R.L.; et al. (2002) Pluripotency of mesenchymal stem cells derived from adult marrow. *Nature.* Vol. 41, No. 6893, pp. 41-9.

Jung, J.; Zheng, M.; Goldfarb, M. & Zaret, K.S. (1999) Initiation of mammalian liver development from endoderm by fibroblast growth factors. Science. Vol. 284, pp. 1998-2003

Kakishita, K.; Elwan, M.A.; Nakano, N.; Itakura, T. & Sakuragawa, N. (2000) Human amnionic epithelial cells produce dopamine and survive after implantation into the struatum of a rat model of Parkinson's disease: a potential source of donor for transplantation therapy. *Experimental Neurology.* Vol. 165, No. 1, pp. 27-34

Kakishita, K.; Nakao, N.; Sakuragawa, N. & Itakura, T. (2003) Implantation of human amniotic epithelial cells prevents the degeneration of nigral dopamine neurons in rats with 6-hydroxydopamine lesions. *Brain Research.* Vol. 980, Vol. 1, pp. 48-56

Kaplowitz, N. (1992) Structure and function of the liver. In: *Liver and Biliary Diseases*, Kaplowitz, N., ed, pp. 5, Williams &Wilkins, ISBN 0683045458, Baltimore, Maryland

Karlsson, J.O.M.; Cravalho, E.G.; Borel Rinkes, I.H.M.; et al. (1993) Nucleation and growth of ice crystals inside cultured hepatocytes during freezing in the presence of dimethylsulphoxide, *Biophys. J.* Vol. 65, pp. 2524–2536

Karlsson, J.O.M. & Toner, M. (1996) Long-term storage of tissues by cryopreservation: critical issues. *Biomaterials.* Vol. 17 pp. 243–256

Kazuki, Y.; Hiratsuka, M.; Takiguchi, M.; et al. (2010). Complete genetic correction of iPSC from Duchenne muscular dystrophy. *Mol Ther.* Vol. 18, pp. 386-393

Khan, et al. (2008) Management of hyperbilirubinemia in biliary atresia by hepatic progenitor cell transplantation through hepatic artery: a case report. Transplant Proc. Vol. 40, pp. 1153-1155

Kharaziha, P.; Hellström, P.M.; Noorinayer, B.; et al. (2009) Improvement of liver function in liver cirrhosis patients after autologous mesenchymal stem cell injection: a phase I-II clinical trial. *Eur J Gastroenterol Hepatol.* Vol. 21, No. 10, pp. 1199-1205

Kim, D.; Kim, C.H.; Moon, J.I.; et al. (2009). Generation of human induced pluripotent stem cells by direct delivery of reprogramming proteins. *Cell Stem Cell.* Vol. 4, pp. 472-476.

Kim, K.; Doi, A.; Wen, B.; et al. (2010). Epigenetic memory in induced pluripotent stem cells. *Nature.* Vol. 467, pp. 285-292.

Koenig, S.; Stoesser, C.; Krause, P.; et al. (2005) Liver repopulation after hepatocellular transplantation: integration and interaction of transplanted hepatocytes in the host. *Cell Transplant.* Vol. 14, pp. 31–40

Kuo, T.K.; Hung, S.P.; Chuang, C.H.; et al. (2008) Stem cell therapy for liver disease: parameters governing the success of using bone marrow mesenchymal stem cells. *Gastroenterology.* Vol. 134, No. 7, pp. 2111-2121

Lange, C.; Bassler, P.; Lioznov, M.V.; et al. (2005) Liver-specific gene expression in mesenchymal stem cells is induced by liver cells. *World J Gastroenterol.* Vol. 11, No. 29, pp. 4497-504

Le Blanc, K.; Rasmusson, I.; Sundburg, B.; et al. (2004) Treatment of severe acute graft-versus-host disease with third party haploidentical mesenchymal stem cells. *Lancet.* Vol. 363, pp. 1439-1441

Le Blanc, K.; Gotherstrom, C.; Ringden, O., et al. (2005) Fetal Mesenchymal Stem-Cell Engraftment in Bone after In Utero Transplantation in a Patient with Severe Osteogenesis Imperfecta. *Transplantation.* Vol. 79, pp. 1607-1614

Le Blanc, K. & Ringden, O. (2007) Immunomodulationby mesenchymal stem cells and clinical experience. *J Intern Med.* Vol. 262, pp.509–525.

Lee, K.W.; Lee, J.H.; Shin, S.W.; et al. (2007) Hepatocyte transplantation for glycogen storage disease type 1b. *Cell Transplant.* Vol. 16, pp. 629-637

Li, H.; Niederkorn, J.Y.; Neelam, S.; et al. (2005) Immunosuppressive factors secreted by human amniotic epithelial cells. *Invest. Ophtalmol. Visual Science.* Vol. 46, No. 3, pp. 900-907

Li, L.; Baroja, M.L.; Majumdar, A.; et al. (2004) Human embryonic stem cells possess immune-privileged properties. *Stem Cells.* Vol. 22, pp. 448–456

Li, Y.; Zhao, H.; Lan, F.; et al. (2010). Generation of human-induced pluripotent stem cells from gut mesentery-derived cells by ectopic expression of OCT4/SOX2/NANOG. *Cell Reprogram.* Vol. 12, pp. 237-247.

Lin, H.; Xu, R.;Zhang, Z.; et al. (2011) Implications of the immunoregulatory functions of mesenchymal stem cells in the treatment of human liver diseases. *Cell Mol Immunol.* Vol. 8, No. 1, pp. 19-22.

Liu, H.; Kim, Y.; Sharkis, S.; et al. (2011). In vivo liver regeneration potential of human induced pluripotent stem cells from diverse origins. *Sci Transl Med.* Vol. 3, pp. 82ra39.

Mali, H. & Gupta, S. (2001) Hepatocyte transplantation: new horizons and challenges. J. *Hepatobiliary Pancreat. Surg.* Vol. 8, pp. 40-50

Marongiu, F.; Gramignoli, R.; Sun, Q.; et al. (2010) Isolation of amniotic mesenchymal stem cells. *Current Protocols Stem Cell Biol.* Chapter 1, Unit 1E.5

Marongiu, F.; Gramignoli, R.; Dorko, K.; et al. (2011) Hepatic differentiation of amnion epithelial cells. *Hepatology.* Vol. 53, No. 5, pp. 1719-29

Manuelpillai, U.; Tchongue, J.; Lourensz, D.; et al. (2010) Transplantation of human amnion epithelial cells reduces hepatic fibrosis in immunocompetant CCl_4-treated mice. *Cell Transplant.* Vol. 19, No. 9, pp. 1157-1168

Meyburg, J.; Das, A.M.; Hoerster, F.; et al. (2009a) One liver for four children: first clinical series of liver cell transplantation for severe neonatal urea cycle defects. *Transplantation.* Vol. 87, No. 5, pp. 636-641

Meyburg, J.; Das, A.M.; Hoerster, F.; et al. (2009b) Liver cell transplantation: basic investigations for safe application in infants and small children. *Cell Transplant.* Vol. 18, pp. 777-786

Miki, T.; Lehmann, T.; Cai, H.; Stoltz, D. & Strom, S.C. (2005) Stem cell characteristics of amnion epithelial cells. *Stem Cells.* Vol. 23, pp. 1549-1559

Miki, T. & Strom, S.C. (2006) Amnion-derived pluripotent/multipotent stem cells. *Stem Cell Reviews.* Vol. 2, pp.133-142

Miki, T.; Marongiu, F.; Dorko, K.; et al. (2010) Isolation of amnion epithelial stem cells. *Curr. Protocols in Stem Cell Biol.* Chapter 1, Unit 1E.3

Miki, T.; Marongiu, F.; Ellis, E.C.S.; et al. (2009) Production of hepatocyte-like cells from human amnion. *Methods Molecular Biology.* Vol. 481, pp. 155-168

Miki, T. (2011) Amnion-derived stem cells: in quest of clinical applications. *Stem Cell Research & Therapy.* Vol. 2, No. 25.

Mitry, R.R.; Dhawan, A.; Hughes, R.D.; et al. (2004) One liver, three recipients: segment IV from split-liver procedures as a source of hepatocytes for cell transplantation. *Transplantation.* Vol. 77, pp. 1614–1616

Mitry, R.R.; Hughes, R.D.; Aw, M.M.; et al. (2003) Human hepatocyte isolation and relationship of cell viability to early graft function. *Cell Transplantation.* Vol. 12, pp. 69-74

Mohamadnejad, M.; Namiri, M.; Bagheri, M.; et al. (2007) Phase 1 human trial of autologous bone marrow-hematopoietic stem cell transplantation in patients with decompensated cirrhosis. *World J Gastroenterol.* Vol. 13, No. 24, pp. 3359-3563

Moodley, Y.; Ilancheran, S.; Samuel, C.; et al. (2010) Human amnion epithelial cell transplantation abrogates lung fibrosis and augments repair. *American Journal of Respiratory and Critical Care Medicine.* Vol. 182, No. 5, (September 2010), pp.643-651

Moriguchi, H.; Chung, R.T. & Sato, C. (2010) Tumorigenicity of human induced pluripotent stem cells depends on the balance of gene expression between p21 and p53. Hepatology. Vol. 51, pp. 1088-1089

Muraca, M.; Gerunda, G.; Neri , D.; et al. (2002) Hepatocyte transplantation as a treatment for glycogen storage disease type 1a. *Lancet.* Vol. 359, pp. 317–318

Murphy, S.; Lim, R.; Dickinson, H.; et al. (2010). Amnion epithelial cells prevent bleomycin-induced lung injury and preserve lung function. *Cell Transplant*. November 2010, ePub ahead of print, PMID: 21092408

Nagata, S.; Toyoda, M.; Yamaguchi, S.; et al. (2009). Efficient reprogramming of human and mouse primary extra-embryonic cells to pluripotent stem cells. *Genes Cells*. Vol. 14, pp. 1395-1404.

Nahmias, Y.; Berthiaume, F. & Yarmush, M.L. (2007) Integration of technologies for hepatic tissue engineering. *Adv. Biochem. Eng. Biotechnol*. Vol. 103, pp. 309-329

Nakatsuji, N.; Nakajima, F. & Tokunaga, K. (2008) HLA-haplotype banking and iPS cells. *Nature Biotechnology*. Vol. 26, pp. 739-740

Nakazawa, F.; Cai, H.; Miki, K.; et al. (2002) Human hepatocyte isolation from cadaver donor liver, In: *Proceedings of Falk Symposium, Hepatocyte Transplantation*. Vol. 126, pp. 147-158, Lancaster, UK, Kluwer Academic Publishers

Neuberger, J. (2000) Liver Transplantation. J, *Hepatology*, Vol. 32, pp.198-207

Nubile, M.; Dua, H.S.; Lanzini, M.; et al. (2011) In vivo analysis of stromal integration of multilayer amniotic membrane transplantation in corneal ulcers. *American Journal of Ophthalmology*. Vol. 151, No. 5, pp.809-822.e1.

Olinga, P.; Maring, J.K.; Merema, M.; et al. (2000) The capability of isolated hepatocytes and liver slices of donor livers to predict graft function after liver transplantation. *Liver*. Vol. 20, pp. 374–380

Ott, M.; Schneider, A.; Attaran, M & Manns, M.P. (2006) Transplantation of hepatocytes in liver failure. *Deutsch Med. Wochenschr*. Vol. 131, pp. 888-891

Park, I.H.; Zhao, R.; West, J.A.; et al. (2008a). Reprogramming of human somatic cells to pluripotency with defined factors. *Nature*. Vol. 451, pp. 141-146.

Park, I.H.; Arora, N.; Huo, H; et al. (2008b). Disease-specific induced pluripotent stem cells. *Cell*. Vol. 134, pp. 877-886.

Parolini, O.; Alviano, F.; Bagnara, G.P.; et al. (2008) Concise review: Isolation and characterization of cells from human term placenta: Outcome of the first International Workshop on Placenta Derived Cells. *Stem Cells*. Vol. 26, pp. 300-311

Pegg, D.E. (2002) The history and principles of cryopreservation., *Semin. Reproduct. Med*. Vol. 20, pp. 5-13

Plummer, C.E.; Ollivier, F.; Kallberg, M.; et al. (2009) The use of amniotic membrane transplantation for ocular surface reconstruction: a review and series of 58 equine clinical cases (2002-2008). *Vet Ophtamology*. Suppl. 1, pp.17-24

Polo, J.M.; Liu, S.; Figueroa, M.E.; et al. (2010). Cell type of origin influences the molecular and functional properties of mouse induced pluripotent stem cells. *Nat Biotechnol*. Vol. 28, pp.848-855.

Puglisis, M.A.; Saulnier, N.; Piscaglia, A.C.; et al. (2011) Adipose tissue-derived mesenchymal stem cells and hepatic differentiation: old concepts and future perspectives. *Eur. Rev. Med. Pharmacol. Sci*. Vol. 15, No. 4, pp. 355-64

Puppi, J.; et al. (2008) Hepatocyte transplantation followed by auxillary liver transplantation - a novel treatment for ornithine transcarbamylase deficiency. *Am J Transplant*. Vol 8, pp. 452-457

Puppi, J.; Strom, S.C.; Hughes, R.D.; et al. (2011) Improving the techniques for human hepatocyte transplantation: report from a consensus meeting in London. *Cell Transplant*. April 1, ePub ahead of print, PMID: 21457616

Rashid, S.T.; Corbineau, S.; Hannan, N.; et al. (2010). Modeling inherited metabolic disorders of the liver using human induced pluripotent stem cells. *J Clin Invest*. Vol. 120, pp. 3127-3136.

Ren, G.; Su, J.; Zhang, L.; et al. (2009) Species variation in the mechanisms of mesenchymal stem cell-mediated immunosuppression. *Stem Cells*. Vol. 27, No. 8, pp. 1954-62.

Robertson, N.J.; Brook, F.A.; Gardner, R.L.; et al. (2007) Embryonic stem cell-derived tissues are immunogenic but their inherent immune privilege promotes the induction of tolerance. *Proc Natl Acad Sci USA*. Vol. 104, pp. 20920–20925

Russo, F.P.; Alison, M.R.; Bigger B.W.; et al. (2006) The bone marrow functionally contributes to liver fibrosis. *Gastroenterology*. Vol. 130, No. 6, pp. 1807-1821

Sakaida, I.; Terai, S.; Yamamoto, N.; et al. (2004) Transplantation of bone marrow cells reduces CCl4-induced liver fibrosis in mice. *Hepatology*. Vol. 40, No. 6, pp. 1304-1311

Sakuragawa, N.; Yoshikawa, H. & Sasaki, M. (1992) Amniotic tissue transplantation: clinical and biochemical evaluations for some lysosomal storage diseases. *Brain Development*. Vol. 14, pp. 7-11

Salama, H.; Zekri, A.N., Bahnassy, A.A.; et al. (2010) Autologous CD34+ and CD133+ stem cells transplantation in patients with end stage liver disease. *World J. Gastroenterology*. Vol. 16, No. 42, pp. 5297-5305

Sancho-Bru, P.; Najimi, M.; Caruso, M.; et al. (2009) Stem and progenitor cells for liver repopulation: can we standardize the process from bench to bedside? *Gut*. Vol. 58, No. 4, pp. 594-603

Scaggiante, B.; Pineschi, A.; Sustersich, M.; et al. (1987) Successful therapy of Niemann-Pick disease by implantation of human amniotic membrane. *Transplantation*. Vol. 44, pp. 59-61

Schoenhals, M.; et al. (2009) Embryonic stem cell markers expression in cancers. *Biochem. Biophys Res. Commun*. Vol. 383, pp. 171-162

Schwartz, R.E.; Reyes, M.; Koodie, L.; et al. (2002) Multipotent adult progenitor cells from bone marrow differentiate into functional hepatocyte-like cells. *J Clin Invest*. Vol, 109, No. 10, pp. 1291-302.

Seglen, P.O.(1976) Preparation of isolated rat liver cells. *Methods Cell Biol*. Vol. 13, pp. 29–83

Serrano-Delgado, V.M.; Novello-Garza, B. &Valdez-Martinez, E. (2009) Ethical issues relating to the banking of umbilical cord blood in Mexico. *BMC Medical Ethics*. Vol. 10, pp. 12

Sharma, A.D.; Cantz, T.; Richter, R.; et al. (2005) Human cord blood stem cells generate human cytokeratin 18-negative hepatocyte-like cells in injured mouse liver. *Am. J. Pathology*. Vol. 167, pp. 555-564

Sharma, A.D.; Cantz, T.; Vogel, A.; et al. (2008) Murine embryonic stem cell-derived hepatocyte progenitor cells engraft in recipient livers with limited capacity of liver tissue formation. *Cell Transplant*. Vol. 17, No. 3, pp. 313-323

Si-Tayeb, K.; Noto, F.K.; Nagaoka, M.; et al. (2010). Highly efficient generation of human hepatocyte-like cells from induced pluripotent stem cells. *Hepatology*. Vol. 51, pp. 297-305.

Skvorak, K.J.; Paul, H.S.; Dorko, K.; et al. (2009a) Hepatocyte transplantation improves phenotype and extends survival in a murine model of intermediate maple syrup urine disease. *Molecular Therapy*. Vol. 17, No. 7, pp. 1266-1273

Skvorak, K.J.; Hager, E.J.; Arning, E.; et al. (2009b) Hepatocyte transplantation (HTx) corrects selected neurometabolic abnormalities in murine intermediate maple syrup urine disease (iMSUD). *Biochim. Biophys. Acta.* Vol. 1792, No. 10, pp. 1004-10

Skvorak, K.J.; Dorko, K.; Hansel, M.C.; et al. (2010) Human amnion epithelial (hAE) stem cell transplant significantly improves disease phenotype and survival in the Intermediate Maple Syrup Urine Disease (iMSUD) mouse model. *Hepatology.* Vol. 52, No. 4 Supplimental, pp. 413A, abstract #181, *Proceedings of AASLD Annual Meeting, Boston, MA, Oct. 29-Nov. 2, 2010*

Sokal, E.M.; Smets, F.; Bourgois, A.; et al. (2003) Hepatocyte transplantation in a 4-year-old girl with peroxisomal biogenesis disease: technique, safety, and metabolic follow-up. *Transplantation.* Vol. 76, pp. 735–738

Soltys, K.; Soto-Gutierrez, A.; Nagaya, M.; et al. (2010) Barriers to the successful treatment of liver disease by hepatocyte transplantation. Hepatology. Vol. 53, pp. 769-774

Song, Z.; Cai, J.; Liu, Y.; et al. (2009). Efficient generation of hepatocyte-like cells from human induced pluripotent stem cells. *Cell Res.* Vol. 19, pp. 1233-1242.

Soriano, H.E. (2002) Liver cell transplantation: human applications in adults and children. In: *Proceedings of Falk Symposium, Hepatocyte Tranplantation.* Kluwer Academic Publishers, Vol. 126, pp. 99-115. Lancaster, UK

Soto-Gutierrez, A.; Basma, H.; Navarro-Alvarez, N.; et al. (2008) Differentiating stem cells into liver. *Biotech. Genetic Enginering Rev.* Vol. 25, pp. 149-164

Spitz, C.; Mateizel, I.; Geens, M.; et al. (2008) Recurrent chromosomal abnormalities in human embryonic stem cells. *Nature Biotech.* Vol. 26, pp. 1361-1363

Steer, C.J. (1995) Liver regeneration, *FASEB Journal,* Vol. 9, pp.1396-400Stephenne, X.; Najimi, M.; Smets, F. ; et al. (2005) Cryopreserved liver cell transplantation controls ornithine transcarbamylase deficient patient while awaiting liver transplantation. *Am J Transplant.* Vol. 5, pp. 2058–2061

Stephenne, X.; Najimi, M.; Sibille, C.; et al. (2006) Sustained engraftment and tissue enzyme activity after liver cell transplantation for argininosuccinate lyase deficiency. *Gastroenterology.* Vol. 130, pp. 1317-1323

Sterling, R.K. & Fisher, R.A. (2001) Liver Transplantation: Living Donor, Hepatocyte, and Xenotransplantation. In: *Current Future Treatment Therapies for Liver Disease. Clinics in Liver Disease,* Gish, R. (ed.) Philadelphia: WB Saunders

Strom, S.C.; et al. (1997a) Transplantation of human hepatocytes. *Transplant Proc.* Vol. 29, pp. 2103-2106

Strom, S.C.; Fisher, R.A.; Thompson, M.T.; et al. (1997b) Hepatocyte transplantation as a bridge to orthotopic liver transplantation in terminal liver failure. *Transplantation.* Vol. 63, pp, 559–569

Strom, S.C.; Choudhury, J.R. & Fox, I.J. (1999) Hepatocyte transplantation for the treatment of human disease. *Semin Liver Dis.* Vol. 19, pp. 39-48

Strom, S.C. & Ellis, E.C.S. (2011) Cell therapy of liver disease: From hepatocytes to stem cells, In: *Principles of Regenerative Medicine, 2nd Edition,* Atala, A.; Lanza, R.; Thomson, R.A. & Nerem, R. (eds.), Elsevier, pp. 305-326, ISBN 9780123814227

Stadtfeld, M.; Nagaya, M.; Utikal, J.; et al. (2008). Induced pluripotent stem cells generated without viral integration. *Science.* Vol. 322, pp. 945-949.

Stutchfield, B.M.; Forbes, S.J. & Wigmore, S.J. (2010) Prospects for stem cell transplantation in the treatment of hepatic disease. *Liver Transplantation.* Vol. 16, pp. 827-836

Sundin, M.; Orvell, C.; Rasmusson, I.; et al. (2006) Mesenchymal stem cells are susceptible to human herpes viruses, but viral DNA cannot be detected in the healthy seropositive individual. *Bone Marrow Transplant*. Vol. 37, No. 11, pp. 1051-9

Takahashi, K.; Tanabe, K.; Ohnuki, M.; et al. (2007). Induction of pluripotent stem cells from adult human fibroblasts by defined factors. *Cell*. Vol. 131, pp. 861-872.

Takahashi, K. & Yamanaka, S. (2006). Induction of pluripotent stem cells from mouse embryonic and adult fibroblast cultures by defined factors. *Cell*. Vol. *126*, pp. 663-676.

Tanaka, K.; Soto-Gutierrez, A.; Navarro-Alvarez, N.; et al. (2006) Functional hepatocyte culture and its application to cell therapies. *Cell Transplant*. Vol. 15, pp. 855-864

Terada, S.; Matsuura, K.; Enosawa, S.; et al. (2000) Inducing proliferation of human amniotic epithelial (HAE) cells for cell therapy. *Cell Transplant*. Vol. 9, No. 5, pp.701-704

Terry, C.; et al. (2005) The effects of cryopreservation on human hepatocytes obtained from different sources of liver tissue. *Cell Transplant*. Vol. 14, pp. 585-594

Terry, C.; Hughes, R.D.; Mitry, R.R.; et al. (2007) Cryopreservation-induced non-attachment of human hepatocytes: role of adhesion molecules. *Cell Transplant*. Vol. 16, pp. 639-647

Thalheimer, U. and Capra, F. (2002), Liver transplantation: making the best of what we have. *Dig Dis Sci*. Vol. 5, pp.945-53.

Thomson, J.A.; Itskovitz-Eldor, J.; Shapiro, S.S.; et al. (1998) Embryonic stem cell lines derived from human blastocysts. *Science*. Vol. 282, pp. 1145-1147

Trounson, A. (2006) The production and directed differentiation of human embryonic stem cells. *Endocr Rev*. Vol. 2, No. 2, pp. 208-19

Trounson, A.; Thakar, R.G.; Lomax, G. & Gibbons, D. (2011) Clinical trials for stem cell therapies. *BMC Medicine*. Vol 9, pp. 52-58

Wan, P.; Wang, X.; Ma, P.; et al. (2011) Cell delivery with fixed amniotic membrane reconstructs corneal epithelium in rabbits with limbal stem cell deficiency. *Investigative Ophthalmology & Visual Science*. Vol.52, No.2, pp.724-30.

Wilmut, I.; Schnieke, A.E.; McWhir, J.; et al. (1997). Viable offspring derived from fetal and adult mammalian cells. *Nature*. Vol. 385, pp. 810-813.

Vaziri, H. & Benchimol, S. (1998) Reconstitution of telomerase activity in normal human cells leads to elongation of telomeres and extended replicative life span. *Current Biol*. Vol. 8, No. 5, pp. 279-282

Yagi, H.; Parekkadan, B.; Suganuma, K.; et al. (2009) Long-term superior performance of a stem cell/hepatocyte device for the treatment of acute liver failure. *Tissue Eng Part A*. Vol. 1, No. 11, pp. 3377-88

Yakubov, E.; Rechavi, G.; Rozenblatt, S. & Givol, D. (2010). Reprogramming of human fibroblasts to pluripotent stem cells using mRNA of four transcription factors. *Biochem Biophys Res Commun*. Vol. 394, pp. 189-193.

Yeager, A.M.; Singer, H.S.; Buck, J.R.; et al. (1985) A therapeutic trial of amniotic epithelial cell implantation in patients with lysosomal storage diseases. *Am. J. Medical Genetics*. Vol. 22, pp. 347-355

Yu, J.; Hu, K.; Smuga-Otto, K.; et al. (2009). Human Induced Pluripotent Stem Cells Free of Vector and Transgene Sequences. *Science*. Vol. 324, pp. 797-801.

Yu, J.; Vodyanik, M.A.; Smuga-Otto, K.; et al. (2007). Induced pluripotent stem cell lines derived from human somatic cells. *Science*. Vol. 318, pp. 1917-1920.

Zaret, K.S. & Grompe, M. (2008) Generation and regeneration of cells of the liver and pancreas. Science. Vol. 322, No. 5907, pp. 1490-1494

Zhang, S.; Chen, S.; Li, W.; et al. (2011) Rescue of ATP7B function in hepatocyte-like cells from Wilson's disease induced pluripotent stem cells using gene therapy or the chaperon drug curcumin. *Human Mol. Genetics*. Vol. 20, No. 16, pp. 3176-3187

Zhao, H.X.; Li, Y.; Jin, H.F.; et al. (2010). Rapid and efficient reprogramming of human amnion-derived cells into pluripotency by three factors OCT4/SOX2/NANOG. *Differentiation*. Vol. 80, pp. 123-129.

Zhou, P.; Hohm, S.; Olusanya, Y.; et al. (2009) Human progenitor cells with high aldehyde dehydrogenase activity efficiently engraft into damaged liver in a novel model. *Hepatology*. Vol. 49, No. 6, pp. 1992-2000

Zimmermann, S.; Voss, M.; Kaiser, S.; et al. (2003) Lack of telomerase activity in human mesenchymal stem cells. *Leukemia*. Vol. 17, pp. 1146-1149

8

Experimental Liver Transplantation

Mirela Patricia Sîrbu Boeți, Sadiq Shoaib,
Alaa Elshorbagy, Cătălin Iulian Efrimescu and Irinel Popescu
Fundeni Clinical Institute, Department of General Surgery and Liver Transplantation
Romania

1. Introduction

The development and implementation of different surgical techniques and immunosuppressive regimens in liver transplantation have been based upon animal experimental studies. The first experimental attempt for liver transplantation was reported on dogs, in 1955, by Welch (Welch, 1955), who described the insertion of a heterotopic auxiliary liver, engrafted in either the pelvis or right paravertebral gutter. The portal vein was anastomosed to the inferior vena cava and the hepatic artery to the aorta or iliac artery, and no immunosuppression was used. The first experimental liver replacement with orthotopic liver transplantation (OLT) was reported by Cannon at the University of California at Los Angeles in 1956, but none of those dogs survived. (Cannon, 1956)

Surgical techniques for experimental orthotopic liver transplantation on pigs were started by Garnier and colleagues in 1965 (Garnier et al., 1965), and continued by Cordier and colleagues in 1966 (Cordier et al., 1966), Mieny and colleagues in 1967 (Mieny et al., 1967), Calne and colleagues in 1968 (Calne et al., 1968). Surgical techniques and vascular bypass methods used on pigs were transposed from dogs. Methods of passive venous bypass used by Moore (external portal and systemic bypass) (Moore et al., 1959) and Starzl (external side-to-side portacaval bypass) (Kaupp & Starzl 1960) on dog models facilitated the development and use by Calne of portal-jugular and portal-caval-jugular passive venous bypass methods and later the active venous bypass method on pigs (Calne et al., 1968).

Pig orthotopic liver transplantation models offer some advantages over the dog models: (1) pigs are considered the most realistic choice due to the low cost, availability, and ethical reasons; (2) there is no outflow phenomenon because, different from dogs, pigs have no muscular sphincters at the confluence of suprahepatic inferior cava vein which tangle the blood flow at this level; (3) pig liver orthotopically transplanted into another animal remains fully functional even for periods of months without immunosuppressive therapy; (4) pig models offer a much closer resemblance with the human liver transplantation than dog models, because the pig liver is a firm and coherent organ, composed of eight segments (Filipponi et al., 1995) homologous to those of the human liver.

Although pig liver transplantation models are favored, both anesthesia team and surgical team are challenged by anatomical and physiological differences between human and pig. The experimental studies must be in conformity with the International Guidelines of Biomedical Research Involving Animals.

In the present chapter we focus upon anesthesia and surgical procedures used by different authors for the orthotopic liver transplantation on swine model.

2. Preoperative preparation

The importance of conducting a proper anesthesia begins with the preoperative preparation in order to avoid the occurrence of potentially lethal malignant hyperthermia and porcine stress syndrome. Thus a very gentle handling with a minimum distress for pigs must be acknowledged. Before surgical interventions, the animals should be left to adapt to the environment for 24-48 h. Some authors recommend to have the animals delivered at least 2 to 3 weeks before the experiments to get them acclimated to the personal conditions, location, and food. (Kaiser et al., 2006) The operations should be performed after a 12-24 h starvation period. During this time only ad libitum oral water intake is admitted. Brute force should be avoided. The immobilization of the pig should be conducted only by experienced staff otherwise it is stressful for both the animal and researcher.

3. Anesthesia

An anesthesia protocol is proposed: i.m. pre-anesthesia using Atropin 0.015 mg/kgc, Midazolam 2 mg/kgc, Ketamine 10 mg/kgc, i.v. (marginal ear veins) induction with Propofol 3 mg/kgc, gas maintained anesthesia with Halotane 3% - 4.5 l/min and orotracheal intubation. (Sirbu Boeti et al., 2008) Before intubation, 100% O_2 is delivered via an inhalation mask to obtain a very good oxygenation of the animal. The orotracheal intubation is quite cumbersome but can be surpassed by positioning the pig in ventral decubitus and using a laryngoscope with long blade and a mandrel. (Kaiser et al., 2006) In difficult situations, larynx and trachea are manipulated from the outside to permit passage of the 6 Fr endotracheal tube. It is important for intubation to have the swallowing reflex completely abolished. The endotracheal tube is blocked by inflating the balloon with air and fixed with a bandage. The auscultation of the chest must confirm the proper positioning of the tube. The anesthesia machine is adjusted for a tidal volume of 500 ml at a ventilation rate of 18-20 per minute. A venous line should be mounted on each ear for drug administration. A drainage tube should be passed via mouth into pig's stomach to deflate it during the operation. The anesthesia depth can be assessed by mandible relaxation, inferior-medial eye balls deviation, and corneal reflex. During the entire intervention for both donor and recipient, SpO2, heart rhythm and respiratory frequency should be monitored. Body temperature is another important parameter to check using an intrarectal probe. However, the clinical observation of the swine remains a major part of the continuous monitoring of the pig. (Kaiser et al., 2006)

Pigs are extremely sensible to medication administered during preanesthesia or anesthesia induction, being prone to developing epidermal allergic phenomenon with generalized skin rush, which may be relieved by corticoid administration. Although rare, an example of drug side effect is represented by the rapidly progressive liver decompensation with intraoperative death due to Halothane inhalation. Other inhaled anesthetics such as Isoflurane or Sevoflurane are better alternatives.

There are two main anatomical differences between human and pig with great impact on the liver transplantation technique: (1) intrahepatic parenchymal trajectory of inferior vena cava (Filipponi et al., 1995; Fondevila et al., 2010) which makes the dissection of this vein off the hepatic parenchyma impossible in pigs; (2) the existence of a very short segment of suprahepatic inferior vena cava, intimately attached to the diaphragm, which leads to difficulty in hepatic vascular reconstruction. (Sirbu Boeti et al., 2008)

Donor and recipient pigs can be operated on by the same team of surgeons. All the surgeons of the team should posses basic skills in microsurgical techniques.

4. Donor operation

The donor operation is generally performed using only an intravenous catheter placed at the start of anesthesia.

For liver harvesting, the abdomen of the donor pig is entered via a midline incision, avoiding the urethra. The liver is exposed after appropriate bilateral costal retraction, careful packing, and caudal retraction of the bowel. The liver is mobilized by dividing the falciform ligament, triangular ligament, and gastrohepatic ligament. The hepatic pedicle is exposed by moving away the small bowel using caudal and left traction of the bowel. The pedicle's elements are dissected and hepatic artery, portal vein, and common bile duct are encircled and isolated with a loop. Pedicle's elements must be dissected and divided as close as possible to the duodenum, obtaining an increased length for anastomosis. Inferior vena cava is dissected above and below the liver in order to permit its harvesting together with the whole liver. The skeletonization of the common bile duct should be avoided. The gallbladder is incised and drained if a biliary reconstruction with the cholecyst is planned. If not, an antegrade or retrograde cholecystectomy is performed. Aorta is exposed at the level of celiac trunk and iliac bifurcation on loops. The subject should receive 100 UI/Kgc of Heparine before splenic vein and aorta cannulation. The previously encircled terminal aorta is cannulated under the renal arteries for blood collection. The collected blood can be used during liver engraftment as needed. After 500 ml blood collection from the aorta, the preservative solution (e.g. lactated Ringer's solution) cooled at 4^{0} C is infused through portal cannula while the supraceliac and terminal aorta together with supra and infrahepatic vena cava are cross-clamped. Outflow of the infused solution is provided by inferior infrahepatic inferior vena cava through a slit made by cutting its wall. The liver effluent can also be allowed to drain into the thoracic cavity by cutting the diaphragm and suprahepatic inferior vena cava. Core cooling is supplemented by topical sterile ice.

The liver can be perfused not only by the portal vein alone (single) but also by both the hepatic artery and portal vein (dual). (Foley et al. 2003) Some authors found that aortic flushing shortened the operation times and proposed it for routine liver procurement even from hemodynamically stable donors. (Filipponi et al., 1996)

After core cooling, all the vascular attachments are divided. Hepatic artery is harvested with celiac trunk and a segment of abdominal aorta, after all branches of celiac trunk are divided. Portal vein should be transected near duodenum after one liter of cold preservation fluid has passed through the liver. Cranially inferior vena cava must be divided highly into the thorax maintaining a little rim of diaphragm around it. Caudally inferior cava vein is transected at the level of the right renal branch. When all vascular and peritoneal connections are transected, the liver is extracted from donor abdominal cavity. After liver harvesting the donor pig should be euthanasiated.

On the back table the fresh harvested liver is rinsed via portal infusion with 3 L, for each kg of liver mass, of cooled (4° C) preservation solution (e.g. normal saline, lactated Ringer's solution, Celsior solution (CS), an extracellular preservation solution, with Viaspan (University of Wisconsin solution, UW) (Audet et al., 2001), Collins C2 solution). UW solution can be supplemented with epidermal growth factor, insulin-like growth factor-1, nerve growth factor-beta, bactenecin, and substance P to create TF-supplemented (TFS) UW. If TFS UW is used instead of UW, hepatic function is better preserved when orthotopic liver transplantation is performed after 18 hr of static cold storage at 4° C. (Ambiru et al., 2004) OLT without cold perfusion of the donor liver is also feasible and prolonged survival of animals is possible, but the function of these organs is markedly reduced compared to the cold perfused organs. (Barbier et al., 1986) The liver is kept in the cold solution until implantation in the recipient. The donor liver is carefully prepared in order to secure any potential vascular bleeding points and adequately clean the vascular structures to facilitate anastomotic procedures. Lymphatic tissue from the pedicle is carefully removed.

5. Recipient operation

The operation on recipient can be performed with or without veno-venous bypass. (Falcini et al., 1990) The bypass can be active or passive.

The pig poorly tolerates simultaneous clamping of the liver pedicle and inferior vena cava. Pigs are sensitive to the congestion of portal vein system. Obvious intestinal mucosa injury are noticed 45 min after blockage. Another issue is the retention of blood flow in portal vein system. Having short limbs and strong gastrointestinal tract, pigs have a high blood flow in portal vein and severe congestion in portal vein system certainly leads to whole body's hemodynamic disturbances. The transplant without veno-venous bypass leads to severe hemodynamic disturbances. Hypotension occurs after more than 30 minutes and leads to immediate or late irreversible shock. (Battersby et al., 1974) Temporary clamping of the supracoeliac aorta is performed by some authors to stabilize the hemodynamic conditions during the anhepatic phase without venous bypass. If the anhepatic phase without veno-venous bypass lasts less than 30 min, temporary aortic occlusion may not be mandatory. If the anhepatic time is less than 20 min, post-reperfusion hypotension with reflex tachycardia is transient and responsive to i.v. fluid perfusion. (Fondevila et al., 2010)

In case of a Y type veno-venous bypass afferent limb is placed into the jugular vein and two efferent limbs are placed into splenic vein and inferior cava vein. Before starting vascular cannulation, 100 UI/Kgc dose of Heparine should be administered to the recipient. The vascular cannula is filed with a saline-Heparine solution to remove air bubbles. Veno-venous bypass is associated with an increased risk of bleeding, disorders of coagulation, air embolism, and venous thromboembolism. (Oike et al., 2001)

The anesthetized animal is placed on its back, the skin is prepared and the draping is made so as to allow the left cervical access to jugular veins and the midline abdominal incision. The operation begins with the dissection and cannulation of the left external jugular vein. If the external jugular vein is too thin to be cannulated, the ipsilateral internal jugular vein can be used instead. The cannula is placed through a longitudinal venotomy in the jugular vein. The cranial end of the vein is ligated and the outside end of the cannula is clamped until the introduction of the efferent limbs of the veno-venous bypass. The placement of the cannula should be done with caution to avoid all the air bubbles. After securing the afferent limb of the bypass, the abdomen of the recipient is opened via a vertical xifo-infraumbilical incision. The steps of abdominal operation are: establishment of the veno-venous bypass, hepatectomy, and engrafting of the donor liver. Prior to the mounting of the efferent limbs of veno-venous bypass, the mobilization of the liver and dissection of the elements of liver pedicle (Figure 1, 2), splenic vein (Figure 3), and inferior cava vein should be done. The technique of hepatectomy is similar to that performed on donor with special attention at the dissection of all the vessels and the bile duct near the liver in order to obtain maximal lengths of these structures needed for tension-free anastomoses.

The first efferent cannula is inserted into splenic vein via a longitudinal venotomy. The cannula is advanced maximum 3 cm toward portal vein in order to avoid the obstruction of the venous branches, especially the superior mesenteric vein. The cannula is secured in position with a simple suture. The other segment of splenic vein is ligatured at the level of the splenic hilum. The second efferent limb of the bypass is inserted into infrahepatic inferior cava vein after its complete transversal section. The cannula is advanced caudally in the inferior vena cava maximum 2 cm toward but not obstructing the right renal vein opening. The cranial stump of inferior cava vein is clamped. The cannula is fixed similar to the first one. The active circulation can be maintained by Medtronic 550 Bio-Console Pump Speed equipped with a Medtronic Bio-Pump®Plus centrifugal blood pump with flow capacity of 30 ml/kg/min. (Sirbu Boeti et al, 2008) When using vascular bypass great caution must be paid to the catheters' preparation and insertion in order to avoid air embolism and also blood clothing. For these, it is recommended to maintain all the catheters clamped until all of the veins are catheterized and their removal should be done selectively starting with portal vein and continuing with inferior vena cava, and ending with jugular vein, immediately after completing all the three venous anastomoses. It is also necessary to check all the tubes before connection by forced injection of Heparine-saline solution for the identification of the possible holes that can lead to air embolism, and maintain them filled with the same solution. In our previous study the active portal-caval jugular bypass proved to be better than the passive portal-jugular bypass. (Sirbu Boeti et al. 2008) Moreover other authors reported a low number of complications by using the active versus pasive bypass (e.g. pelvic congestion, that is the main cause for deep venous thrombosis and pulmonary emboli). (Filipponi et al., 1989; Filipponi et al., 1996, Filliponi et al., 1998)

Maintaining a good stability in pulmonary hemodynamics during anhepatic period, together with a low rate of complications if properly used, the active portal-caval jugular bypass seems to be the standard for OLT in pigs.

Regarding the engrafting technique, the most difficult problem in pigs is related to suprahepatic inferior caval vein anastomosis. The problem is raised by the fact that there is a very short segment of suprahepatic inferior caval vein. This anatomic feature determines to position the clamp on the inferior vena cava with the inclusion of a portion of the diaphragm. After transaction of inferior vena cava nearby the diaphragm, the opening of remaining vena cava to be anastomosed is kept enlarged due to the intimate connections with the diaphragmatic fibers. To overcome the incongruence between the cava vein edges two solutions can be applied.

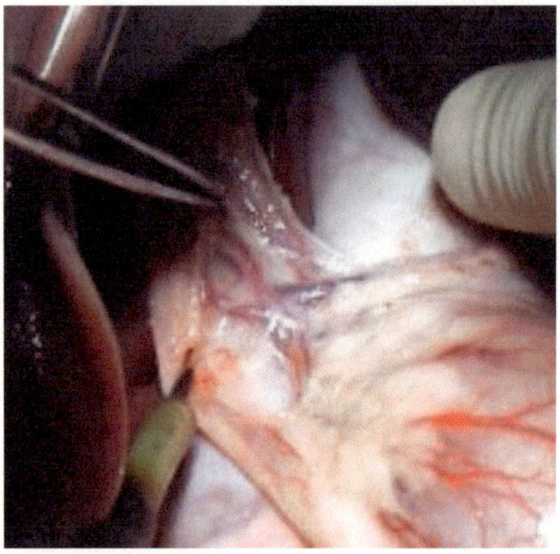

Fig. 1. Dissection of the hepatic hilum. Left, median, and right hepatic artery are identified

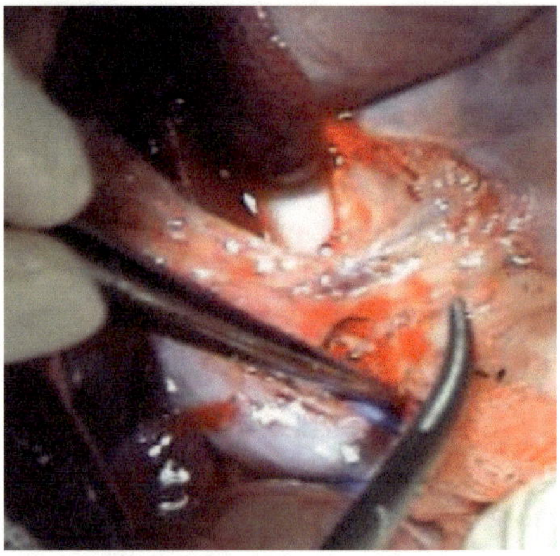

Fig. 2. Porta vein is dissected and encircled

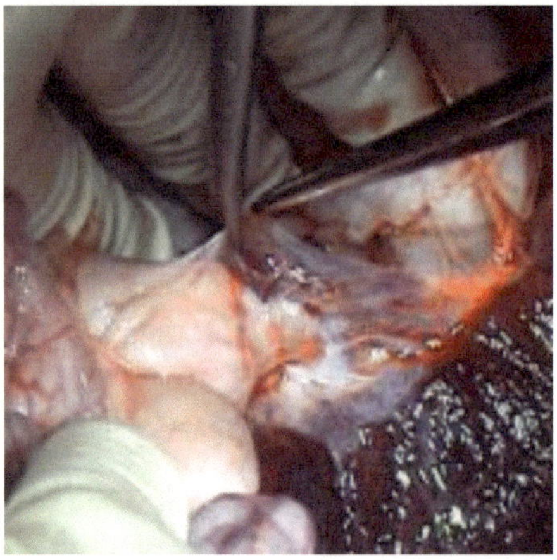

Fig. 3. The splenic vein is dissected near the splenic hilum for the introduction of one of the efferent limbs of veno-venous Y bypass

In most situations an adequate calibration of the donor inferior caval vein edge is needed. The most appropriate is the enlargement of the stump by suturing a V venous patch obtained by harvesting the liver together with a long segment of intrathoracic inferior cava vein.

The possibility to perform an end-to-end anastomosis between donor and recipient caval vein without plasty exists but it is best accomplished entering the thoracic cavity via a phrenectomy around the inferior caval vein. For this approach longer segment of the donor inferior caval vein is also needed and must be tailored by transecting it as high as possible into thorax. However this second method is cumbersome due to the difficulty of the diaphragm reconstruction and impossibility of obtaining a tight sealing of the thoracic cavity.

Immediately after declamping of the three cannula (inserted into splenic, inferior vena cava and jugular vein) and the activation of veno-venous bypass, the clamping and transection of the biliary common duct (Figure 4), hepatic artery, portal vein (Figure 5), and suprahepatic inferior vena cava (Figure 6) are done and the liver is removed. These anatomic structures should be transected near the donor's liver. After liver removal, donor's suprahepatic inferior vena cava is prepared for anastomosis by trimming the remnant liver parenchyma (Figure 7).

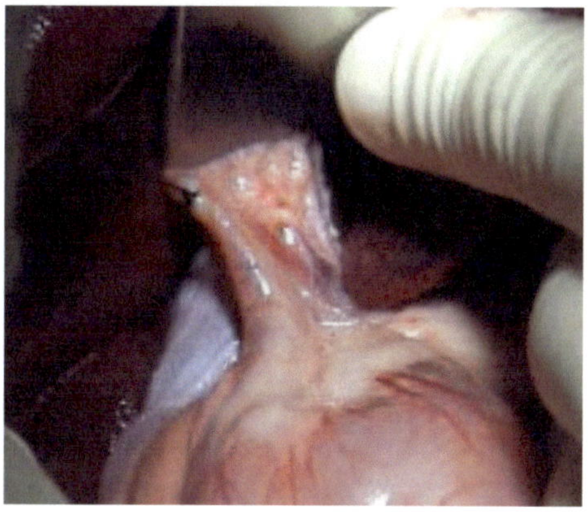

Fig. 4. Recipient's choledoch is identified and prepared to be cut between ligatures near the liver. The skeletization of the choledoch in hepatic hilum is avoided

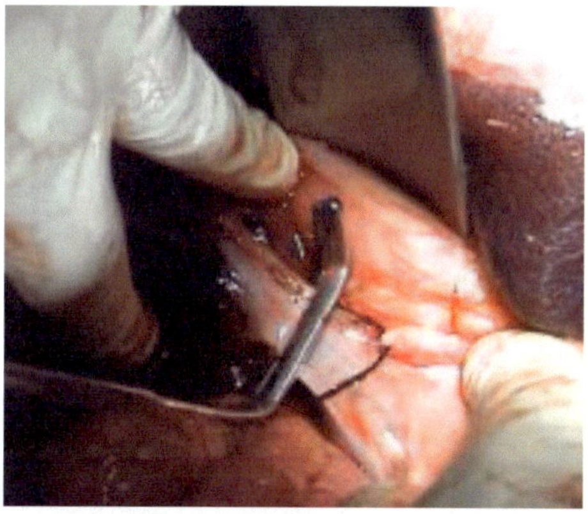

Fig. 5. Recipient's portal vein is clamped near the liver

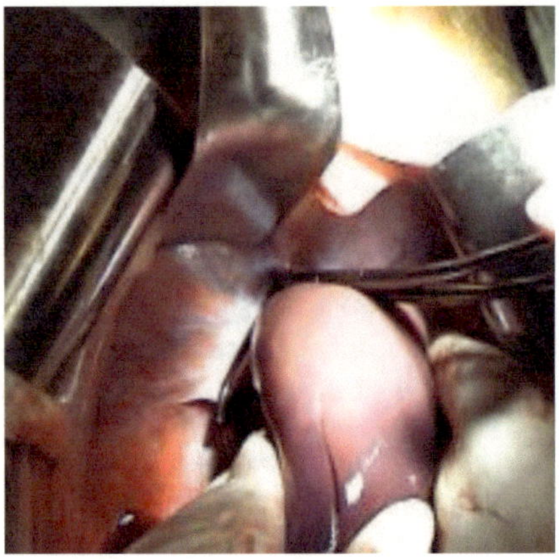

Fig. 6. Recipient's suprahepatic inferior vena cava is clamped by including the adjacent diaphragm into the clamp

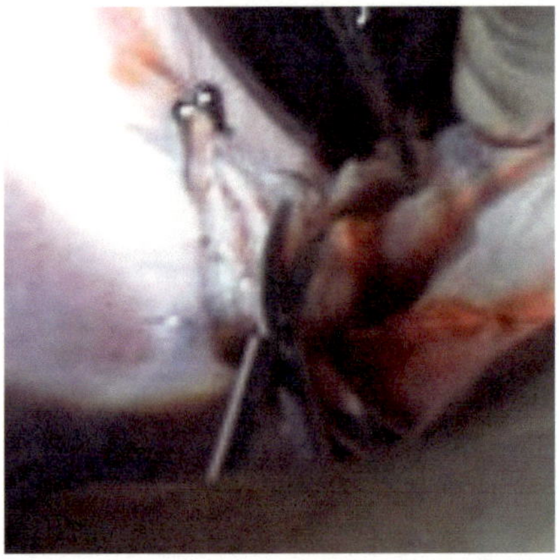

Fig. 7. Donor's suprahepatic inferior vena cava is prepared for anastomosis by removal of remnant liver parenchyma

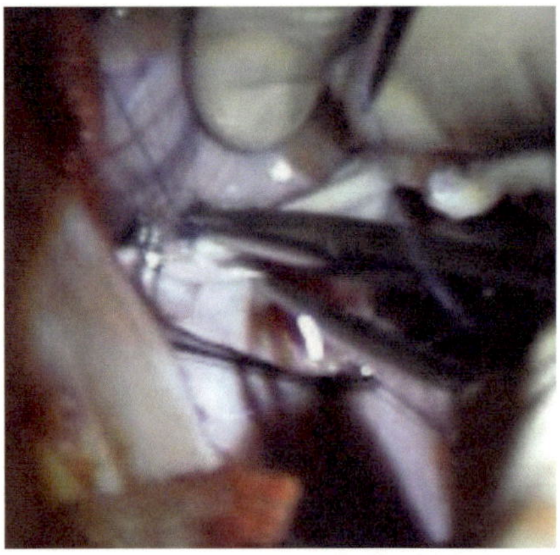

Fig. 8. Suprahepatic inferior vena cava is reconstructed in end-to-end fashion by starting the continuous suture on the left side and finishing it on the right side

Although models without the usage of bypass were described by some authors (Oike et al., 2001), our previous results were better when the bypass was used. (Sirbu Boeti et al., 2008)

After its back table preparation, the donor liver is properly placed and oriented into the right subphrenic space. The anastomoses are performed in the following order: suprahepatic inferior cava vein, portal vein, infrahepatic vena cava, arterial anastomosis, and biliary anastomosis remnant.

The end-to-end anastomoses of inferior caval vein should be made using continuous suture of 5-0 monofilament polypropylene (Prolene®, Ethicon, Inc.), starting with the left wall and finishing with the right wall (Figure 8).

While completing the suprahepatic caval anastomosis, the liver is perfused with warm lactated Ringer's solution to remove the air bubbles (Figure 9).

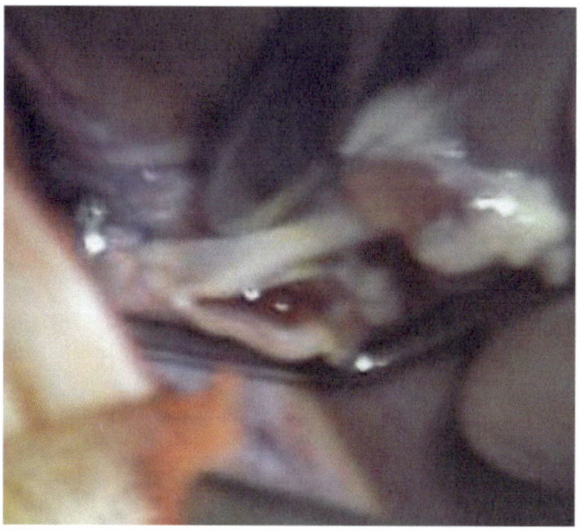

Fig. 9. The anastomosis of the suprahepatic inferior cava vein is continued on the right wall while liver is perfused with warm lactated Ringer's solution

Portal vein reconstruction is started with a continuous 5-0 monofilament polypropylene on the posterior wall (Figure 10) and is continued with the anterior wall. Before completing the anterior wall of the portal vein anastomosis, 500 ml of lactated Ringer's solution at room temperature are flushed into the liver, and after completing it portal vein clamp is removed and splenic cannula is cross-clamped. Both lactated Ringer's solution and about 250 ml of blood are let to flow out of the liver through the infrahepatic inferior vena cava stump, in order to wash-out the oxide radicals and the high potassium-containing preservation solution, and decrease the risk of hypothermic stress. It is important to tie the last suture of portal vein anastomosis leaving a growth factor of about half of the diameter of the anastomosis. Thus stenosis of portal vein is avoided on long term animal survivals. Before performing the infrahepatic inferior vena cava anastomosis, the tightness of suprahepatic vena cava (Figure 11) and portal anastomosis is verified (Figure 12).

After the suprahepatic inferior cava vein and portal vein are declamped, reperfusion of the liver is re-established (Figure 13). The infrahepatic inferior caval vein of the donor liver is clamped proximal the right renal vein and the vena cava cannula is withdrawn in order to perform the anastomosis with the inferior vena cava (Figure 14, 15) of the recipient. The anastomosis is performed with continuous suture of 5-0 monofilament polypropylene.

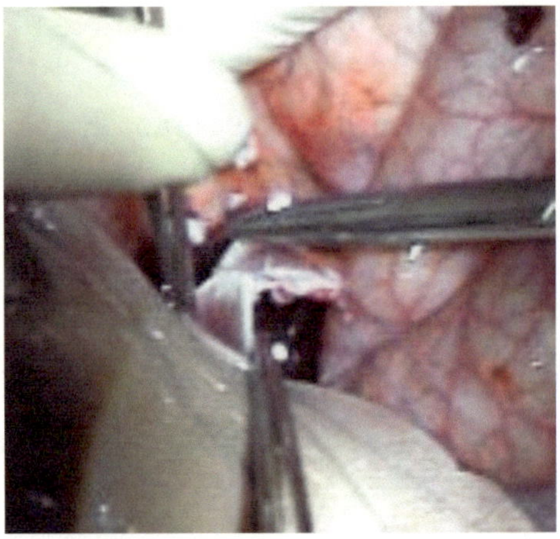

Fig. 10. Reconstruction of the portal vein starting with a continuous suture of the posterior wall

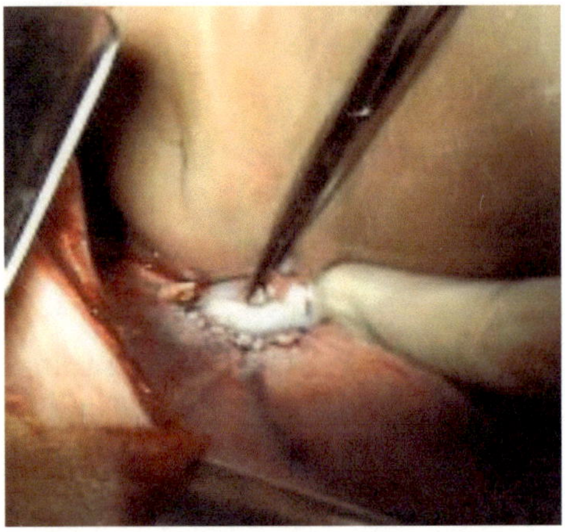

Fig. 11. Check-up of suprahepatic inferior caval vein anastomosis

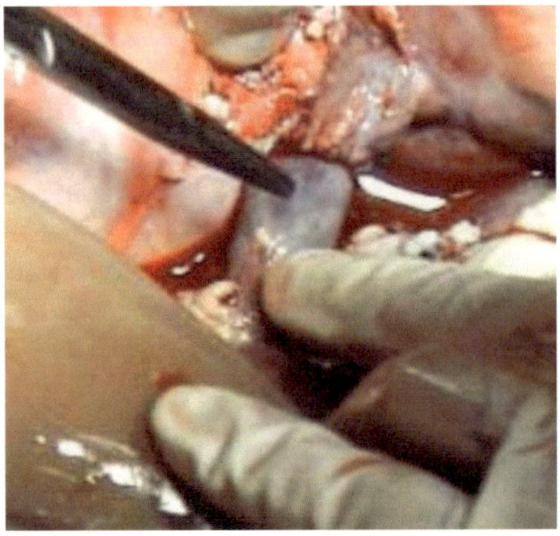

Fig. 12. Check-up of portal vein anastomosis

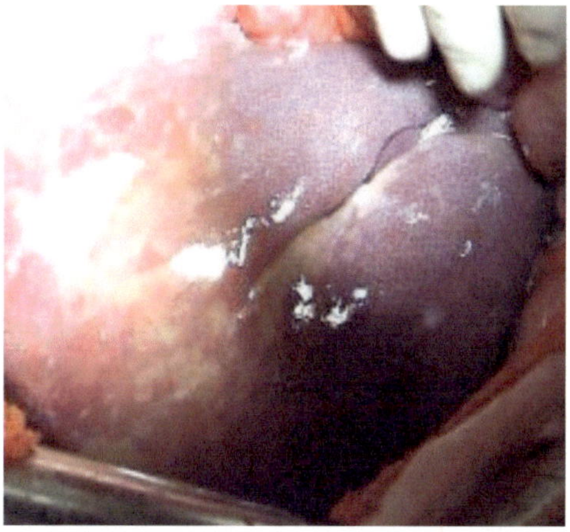

Fig. 13. The aspect of the graft at the moment of reperfusion

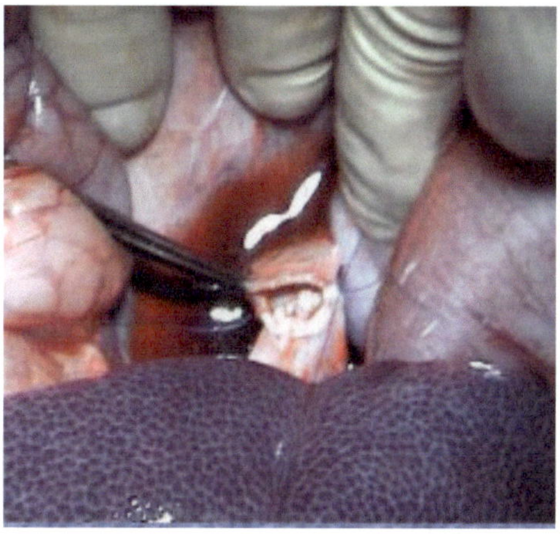

Fig. 14. The donor's infrahepatic inferior cava vein is anastomosed end-to-end to the recipient's homolog vein first performing a continuous suture on the posterior wall

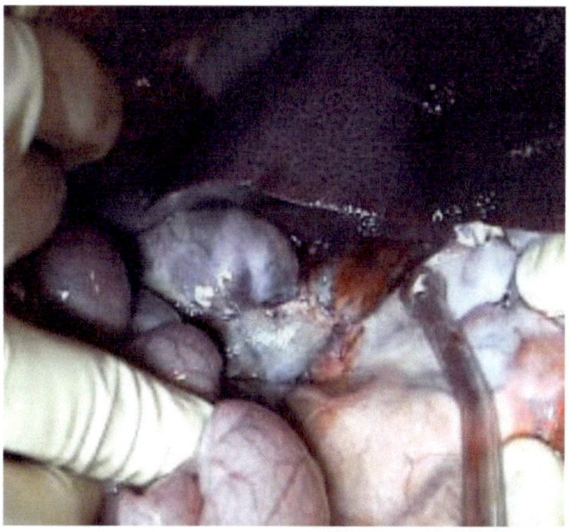

Fig. 15. The infrahepatic inferior cava vein anastomosis is checked for bleeding sites

After revascularization of the liver, the role of the anesthesiologist is crucial in dealing with reperfusion syndrome. For this it is necessary to monitor the pulmonary pressure, central venous pressure and cardiac index using Swan-Ganz catheter fixed on the right cephalic vein. (Filliponi et al., 1998) No vasoconstrictive drugs are recommended to correct postreperfusion arterial hypotension. Only fluids to correct volemia should be used instead.

During hypothermia of a liver to be transplanted, a large quantity of K+ and H+ accumulates, which may cause cardiac arrhythmia at revascularization. To preclude the reperfusion syndrome, the metabolites and potassium ions entering into systemic circulation can be removed from the graft by liver flushing. Before doing the portal revascularization of the donor livers, a washout via both the portal vein and hepatic artery can be performed with saline serum (Arias et al., 1987) or polygeline solution (Haemaccel) (Arias et al., 1990). The liver can also be washed only via portal vein with 500 ml warm (37° C) lactated Ringer's solution at room temperature before finishing the vein anastomosis. Then approximately 250-500 ml of recipient's blood are allowed to drain through the intrahepatic inferior vena cava after finishing the portal anastomosis. (Sirbu Boeti et al., 2008) During all the warm perfusion time the suprahepatic cava is maintained clamped and the washing fluids (lactated Ringer's solution and blood) are aspirated through the infrahepatic inferior caval vein stump. This fact also contributes to the controlled heating of the liver before including it into the circulatory system. The procedure of liver warm reperfusion was inspired by previous studies made on rats. (Takei & et al., 1991; Xu et al., 1992)

When the liver transplantation is performed without by-pass, the warm flush with lactated Ringer's solution is performed before rather than after vascular clamping in the recipient. Flushing the graft with the vena cava and portal vein clamped add several more minutes of splanhnic venous stasis, leading to an even greater release of cytokines and inflammatory mediators upon the restoration of flow. (Fondevila et al., 2010) An extracorporeal circulation (ECC) equipped with a polyacrylonitrile dialyzer (PAN) between the previously anastomized inferior vena cava (IVC) below the liver and the jugular vein is a solution used to entrap and thus preclude the K+ to enter the systemic circulation. (Marino & De Luca, 1985) Some authors consider that metabolic acidosis can be avoided by administration of sodium bicarbonate before declamping and corrections of alterations in serum electrolytes. (Torres et al., 2008)

Immediately after declamping of suprahepatic inferior vena cava and portal vein with subsequent revascularization of the liver, the reperfusion syndrome must be readily recognized and controlled. Swine hemodynamic status during anhepatic phase was analyzed by different authors. (Fondevila et al. 2010; Heuer et al., 2010; Torres et al., 2008)

In the unfortunate case of intraoperative sudden death of the recipient the operation should be continued with the aim of improvement of surgical techniques.

The hepatic artery of the pig has a 1.5-2.5 mm caliber which makes its suturing difficult. Hepatic artery can be reconstructed using microsurgical techniques under a magnification of 6.5 X. The donor's artery is adequately tailored to avoid tension or kinking. Vascular edges are obliquely sectioned or "fish mouth" shaped, for obtaining a larger caliber and protecting the arterial anastomosis from thrombosis and stenosis. The arterial stumps should be washed with Papaverine solution (1 vial in 15 ml of warm saline). A minimum resection of the adventitia is intended, removing only the fragments hanging outside the edges of the vessel. The end-to-end microsurgical anastomosis of the proper hepatic arteries of the donor and recipient can be executed according to 0-180° technique with separate 8-0 or 9-0 monofilament stitches. (Sirbu Boeti et al., 2008) At the end of the anastomosis there is no need for the patency test. The arterial reconstruction can also be made using an aortic graft sutured end-to-side to the infrarenal aorta (Figure 16). (Oike et al., 2001; Oldhafer et al., 1993) The cuff technique can also be used for arterial reconstruction. (Monden et al., 1982) A technique of orthotopic liver transplantation in the pig was described in which the main feature is the accomplishment of vascular anastomoses by the use of the Vogelfanger NRC vascular suturing instrument. The advantage of this instrument was the rapid accomplishment of safe leak-proof anastomoses. (Barron et al. 1975)

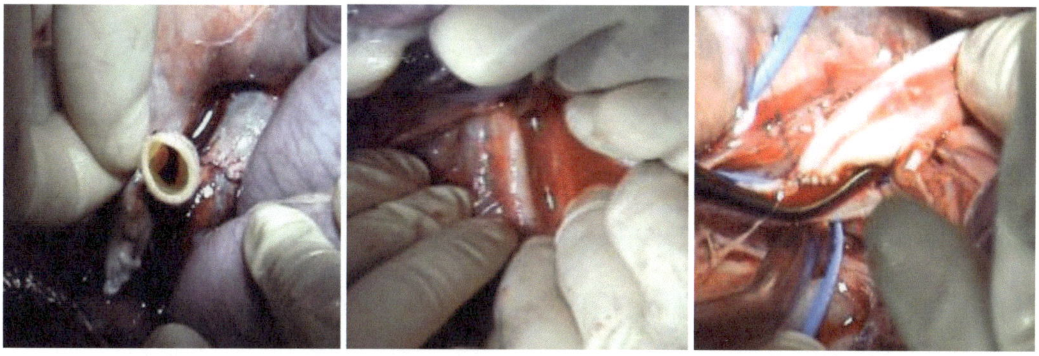

Fig. 16. Arterial reconstruction using an aortic graft. A. Back bleeding in the aortic graft. B. Identification of infrarenal abdominal aorta. C. End-to-side arterial anastomosis between donor's aortic graft and recipient's infrarenal aorta

Regarding the biliary reconstruction, some authors suggest choledocho-choledochostomy to be the most appropriate. The common biliary duct is wide enough to permit a safe anastomosis with 6-0 polydioxanone (PDS®, Ethicon, Inc.) suture. If a silastic tube is introduced in the open ends of the donor's and recipient's common bile duct, no sutures are necessary because the apposition is accomplished by securing the silastic tube with two ligatures which are then tied to one another. (Fondevila et al., 2010) Choledocho-jejunostomy with a Roux-Y-loop, choledocho-duodenostomy, cholecysto-jejunostomy with a Roux-Y loop (Oike et al., 2001) and cholecysto-duodenostomy can also be chosen for the biliary reconstruction. If the donor's gallbladder is preserved, a cholecysto-gastrostomy is very facile to be performed (Figure 17). However choledocho-choledochostomy is preferred to the biliary-duodenal anastomosis to avoid postoperative cholangitis and also to the biliary-jejunal anastomosis to avoid the danger of intestinal obstruction, which is highly common in pigs. (Lempinen et al., 1971) External biliary drainage is another alternative. (Oldhafer et al., 1993)

When an end-to-end anastomosis of the bile duct is performed for orthotopic liver allotransplantation, 70% of the subjects develop jaundice at the end of the first week after transplantation. (Battersby et al., 1975) However the jaundice is generally a result of transient rejection and usually resolves spontaneously without immunosuppression. (Battersby et al., 1975)

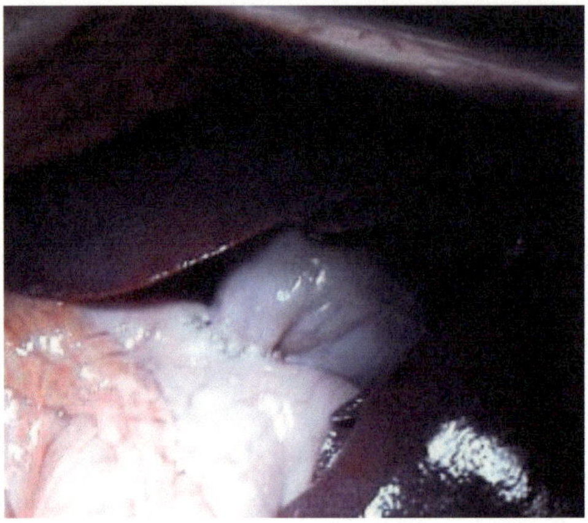

Fig. 17. Cholecysto-gastrostomy performed with continuous 6-0 PDS suture

6. Conclusions

The orthotopic liver transplantation models on swine are straightforward and reproducible and offer surgeons and researchers the opportunity to perform and study liver transplantation in conditions similar to clinical practice.

7. References

Ambiru, S.; Uryuhara, K.; Talpe, S.; Dehoux, J.P.; Jacobbi, L.; Murphy, C.J.; McAnulty, J.F. & Gianello, P. Improved survival of orthotopic liver allograft in swine by addition of trophic factors to University of Wisconsin solution. *Transplantation*, Vol.77, No.2, (January 2004), pp:302-319. ISSN 0041-1337

Arias, J.; Aller, M.A.; Fernandez-Cordero, X.; Estebanez, E.; Jimenez, G.; Enterria, F.G; Brandau, D. & Duran, H. Portal and arterial washout after hypothermic preservation of the pig liver: prevention of hyperkalaemia after revascularization. *Int Surg*, Vol.72, No.3, (July 1987), pp:134-140. ISSN 0020-8868

Arias, J.; Aller, M.A.; Lorente, L.; Rodriguez, J.C.; Fernandez, X.; Brandau, D.& Duran, H. Washout of the pig liver with Haemaccel after hypothermic preservation. *Int Surg*, Vol.75, No.2, (April 1990), pp:78-83. ISSN 0020-8868

Audet, M.; Alexandre, E.; Mustun, A.; David, P.; Chenard-Neu, M.P.; Tiollier, J.; Jaeck, D.; Cinqualbre, J.; Wolf, P.& Boudjema, K. Comparative evaluation of Celsior solution versus Viaspan in a pig liver transplantation model. *Transplantation*, Vol.71, No.12, (June 2001), pp:1731-1735. ISSN 0041-1337

Barbier, P.A.; Luder, P.J.; Wagner, H.E.; Barbier, A. & Mettler, D. Orthotopic liver transplantation in pigs without cold perfusion of the donor liver. Evaluation by quantitative liver function tests. *Eur Surg Res*, Vol.18, No.5, (May 1986), pp:293-301. ISSN 1421-9921

Barron, P.T.; Vogelfanger, I.J. & Waddell, W.G. Orthotopic liver transplantation utilizing a vascular stapling instrument. *Br J Surg*, Vol.62, No.6, (June 1997), pp:438-440. ISSN 1365-2168

Battersby, C.; Egerton, W.S.; Balderson, G.; Kerr, J.F. & Burnett, W. Early jaundice after pig liver transplantation. *Aust N Z J Surg*, Vol.45, No.2, (May 1975), pp:209-213. ISSN 1445-2197

Battersby, C.; Hickman, R.; Saunders, S.J. & Terblanche, J. Liver function in the pig. The effects of 30 minutes' normothermic ischaemia. *Br J Surg*, Vol.61, No.1, (January 1974), pp:27-32. ISSN 1365-2168

Calne, R.Y.; Yoffa, D.E.; White, H.J. & Maginn, R.R. A technique of orthotopic liver translantation in the pig. *Br J Surg*, Vol.55, No.3, (March 1968), pp:203-206. ISSN 1365-2168

Cannon, J.A. Organs (communication). *Transplant Bull*, (1956), 3:7.

Cordier, G.; Garnier, H.; Clot, J.P.; Camplez, P.; Gorin, J.P.; Clot, P.; Rassinier, J.P.; Nizza, M. & Levy, R. [Orthotopic liver graft in pigs. 1st results]. *Mem Acad Chir (Paris)*, Vol.92, No.27, (November 1966), pp:799-807. ISSN 1634-0647

Falcini, F.; Martini, E.; Marsili, M.; Benassai, C.; Fabbri, L.P.; Tanini, R.; Linden, M.; Simoncini, R.; Filipponi, F. & Cataliotti, L. Veno-venous bypass in experimental liver transplantation: portal-jugular versus caval-portal-jugular. *G Chir* 1990; 11:206-210. ISSN 0391-9005

Filipponi, F.; Falcini, F.; Marsili, M. & Boncinelli, S. A new perfusion system for the treatment of isolated pig liver damaged by warm ischemia. *Int J Artif Organs*, Vol.13, No.4, (April 1990), pp:257-258. ISSN 0391-3988

Filipponi, F.; Leoncini, G.; Campatelli, A.; Bagnolesi, A.; Perri, G.; Romagnoli, P. & Mosca, F. Segmental organization of the pig liver: anatomical basis of controlled partition for experimental grafting. *Eur Surg Res* 1995; Vol.27, No.3, (March 1995), pp:151-157. ISSN 1421-9921

Filipponi, F.; Oleggini, M.; Romagnoli, P.; Fossati, N.; Pardini, P. & Mosca, F. Exclusively aortic cold flushing for liver procurement from hemodynamically stable donors. An experimental study in the pig. *G Chir*, Vol.17, No.1-2, (January 1996), pp:59-63.

Filipponi, F.; Trivella, M.G.; Oleggini, M.; Pardini, P.; Meacci, L.; Bellissima, G.; Solari, R.; Porcelli, F.; Lucchetti, A.L.; Pardini, E. & Mosca, F. Surgical research in orthotopic liver transplantation: experiences in the pig model. *G Chir*, Vol.17, No.4, (April 1996), pp:201-209.

Filipponi, F.; Boggi, U.; Della Capanna, S.; Carmellini, M.; Meacci, L. & Mosca, F. 1998. Surgical research on orthotopic liver transplantation: Tuscany experience in the pig model. In: *Liver transplantation: from laboratory to clinic*, Filiponi F, pp:12-71, Guido Gnocchi Editore (Ed.), ISBN 9781928649045, Napoli

Foley, D.P.; Vittimberga, F.J.; Quarfordt, S.H.; Donohue, S.E.; Traylor, A.N.; MacPhee, J.; McLaughlin, T.; Ricciardi, R.; Callery, M.P. & Meyers, W.C. Biliary secretion of extracorporeal porcine livers with single and dual vessel perfusion. *Transplantation*, Vol.68, No.3, (August 1999), pp:362-368. ISSN 0041-1337

Fondevila, C.F.; Hessheimer, A.J.; Flores, E.; Vendrell, M.; Munos, J.; Escobar, B.; Calatayud, D.; Taura, P.; Fuster J. & Garcia-Valdecasas J.C. Step-by-step guide for a simplified model of porcine orthotopic liver transplant . *J Surg Res*, Vol.167, No.1, (May 2011), pp: e39-45. ISSN 0022-4804

Garnier, H.; Clot, J.P.; Bertrand, M.; Camplez, P.; Kunlin, A.; Gorin, J.P.; Le Goaziou, F.; Levy, R. & Cordier, G. [Liver transplantation in the pig: surgical approach]. *C R Acad Sci Hebd Seances Acad Sci D*, Vol.260, No.21, (May 1965), pp:5621-5623. ISSN 0762-0969

Heuer, M.; Reinhardt, R.; Kneiseler, G.; Wurzinger, P.; Zou, X.; Hua, F.; Jian, F.; Paul, A. & Kaiser, G.M. Liver transplantation in swine without venovenous bypass. *Eur Surg Res*, Vol.45, No.1, (August 2010), pp:20-25. ISSN 1421-9921

Kaiser, G.M.; Heuer, M.M.; Fruhauf, N.R.; Kuhne, C.A. & Broelsch, C.E. General handling and anesthesia for experimental surgery in pigs. *J Surg Res*, Vol.130, No.1, (January 2006), pp:73-79. ISSN 0022-4804

Kaupp, H.A. & Starzl, T.E. The use of an external bypass during experimental total hepatectomy. *Surgery*, Vol.48, (August 1960), pp:330-331. ISSN 0039-6060

Marino, I.R. & De Luca, G. Orthotopic liver transplantation in pigs. An evaluation of different methods of avoiding the revascularization syndrome. *Transplantation*, Vol.40, No.5, (November 1985), pp:494-498. ISSN 0041-1337

Mieny, C.J.; Moore, A.R.; Homatas, J. & Eiseman, B. Homotransplantation of the liver in pigs. *S Afr J Surg*, Vol.5, No.3, (July 1967), pp:109-114. ISSN 0038-2361

Monden, M.; Barters, R.H. & Fortner, J.G. A simple method of orthotopic liver transplantation in dogs. *Ann Surg*, Vol.195, No.1, (January 1982), pp:110-113. ISSN 0003-4932

Moore, F.D.; Smith, L.L.; Burnap, T.K.; Dallenbach, F.D.; Dammin, G.J.; Gruber, U.F.; Shoemaker, W.C.; Steenburg, R.W.; Ball, M.R. & Belko, J.S. One-stage homotransplantation of the liver following total hepatectomy in dogs. *Transplant Bull*, Vol.6, No.1, (January 1959), pp:103-107 ISSN 0564-1217

Oike, F.; Uryuhara, K.; Otsuka, M.; Dehoux, J.P.; Otte, J.B.; Lerut, J. & Gianello, P. Simplified technique of orthotopic liver transplantation in pigs. *Transplantation*, Vol.71, No.2, (January 2001), pp:328-331. ISSN 0041-1337

Oldhafer, K.J.; Hauss, J.; Gubernatis, G.; Pichlmayr, R. & Spiegel, H.U. Liver transplantation in pigs: a model for studying reperfusion injury. *J Invest Surg*, Vol.6, No.5, (September 1993), pp:439-450. ISSN 0894-1939

Sirbu Boeti, M.P.; Romanescu, D.; Gangone, E.; Grigorie, R.; Barbulescu, M.; Elshorbagy, A.; Jemna, C.; Efrimescu, C.; Ionescu, S.; Clinciu, P.; Badea, R. & Popescu, I. Swine model of orthotopic liver transplantation. *Annals of Fundeni Hospital*, Vol.13, No.1, (January 2008), pp:3-11. ISSN 1224-3450

Takei, Y.; Marzi, I.; Kauffman, F.C. & Lemasters, J.J. Increase in survival of liver grafts after rinsing with warm Ringer's solution due to improvement of hepatic microcirculation. *Transplantation*, Vol.52, No.2, (August 1991), pp:225-230. ISSN 0041-1337

Torres, O.J.; Pantoja, P.B.; Barbosa, E.S.; Barros, C.A; Servin, E.T. & Servin, S.C. Hemodynamic alterations during orthotopic liver experimental transplantation in pigs. *Acta Cir Bras*, Vol.23, No.2, (March 2008), pp:135-139. ISSN 1678-2674

Xu, H.S.; Wang, D.J.; Pace, R.C. & Jones, R.S. Beneficial effects of prewarming the donor liver for rat liver transplantation. *Am J Surg*. Vol.163, No.1, (January 1992), pp:164-168. ISSN 0002-9610

Welch, C.S. & Welch, C.S. A note of transplantation of the whole liver in dogs. *Transplant Bull*, Vol.2, (1955), pp:54. ISSN 0564-1217

Part 4

Surgical Complications

9

Biliary Complications After Liver Transplantation

Julius Špičák and Renáta Bartáková
Institute for Clinical and Experimental Medicine in Prague
Czech Republic

1. Introduction

Despite logistical and immunological advantages, various refinements in organ procurement, surgical techniques, and postoperative management, biliary complications remain a significant cause of morbidity and even mortality after orthotopic liver transplantation (OLT). They may appear in the immediate post-liver transplant period as well as years thereafter. With respect to the generally increased patients' vulnerability after OLT, it is necessary to manage these complications promptly and effectively to prevent irreversible liver damage and threat to the recipient's life. Biliary complications cannot be considered as a single issue, even if significant. They often develop as a consequence of the underlying problems typically associated with liver transplantation in patients with immunosuppression modulating their clinical manifestations and laboratory findings. Not exceptionally, they may occur together with other complications such as primary disease recurrence, rejection, vascular lesions or cytomegalovirus (CMV) infection, and these problems may modify the management accordingly. They may also mask biliary complications contributing hugely to their varying rates reported in particular studies. To assess the individual patient comprehensively and to correctly organize the management of such a complicated case is a masterpiece of medical skill.

2. Biliary reconstruction of liver transplantation

To achieve high technical success of endoscopic treatment of biliary complications, meticulous knowledge of the anatomy of biliary reconstruction as well as knowledge of specific issues of posttransplant pathophysiology is essential. Surgical reconstruction of the biliary tree is undertaken as the final step of OLT after vascular anastomosis determining both the diagnostic and therapeutic approaches. The gallbladder interposition technique was used in the pioneering years utilizing the gallbladder as the graft conduit between the donor and recipient bile ducts. In the early reports by Starzl and Calne, the association of bile stasis with stone formation and cholangitis resulted in morbidity of up to 50% and mortality up to 30% quite fittingly referred to as the Achilles' heel of this demanding surgical technique (Lebeau et. al, 1990).

Clearly, an end-to-end duct-to-duct anastomosis is the preferred technique in most centres in recipients with healthy native bile ducts of compatible calibre as it maintains the anatomy and preserves the sphincter mechanism. Another advantage is that it provides continuity of bile ducts with the original shape allowing access and effective treatment of complications by standard endoscopic techniques. Similarly good results were obtained by other centres using a side-to-side variant. More of historical interest, the reconstruction was complemented by temporary T-tube biliary drainage with two presumed goals: to visualise the bile ducts according to demand, and to prevent anastomotic stricture formation. The results of several comparative studies differ but the second expectation has never been reliably met, and frequent leaks prevailing in T-tube groups (Davidson et al., 1999; Graziadei et al., 2006) caused that the use of the preventive T-tube drainage has been rarely employed in choledocho-choledocho reconstruction.

Roux-en-Y hepaticojejunostomy is utilized in patients with bile ducts involved by the pre-existing disease like sclerosing cholangitis, occasionally also in patients with major incompatibility in size of ducts, and is usually preferred in the case of retransplantation because of inadequate recipient duct length. Roux-en-Y was also the routine reconstruction technique in the first series of living-related, reduced graft, and split liver transplantation procedures. With increasing knowledge of the blood supply around the biliary ducts and increasing experience, duct-to-duct anastomosis has been increasingly reported in reduced grafts of living-donor transplants and split transplant even if multiple anastomoses are needed.

References	Center	Year	N	Total, %	Leaks, %	Strictures, %
Duct - to - duct anastomosis						
Lebeau	Pittsburgh	1990	193	20	2	18
O´Connor	Boston	1995	147	33	22	12
Davidson	Royal Free	1999	100	31	17	14
Alazmi	Indianapolis	2006	916	NA	NA	16
Graziadei	Innsbruck	2006	515	16	NA	16
Roux - en Y hepaticojejunostomy						
Ringer	Hannover	1989	84	24	12	2
Lebeau	Pittsburgh	1990	187	12	9	3
Living donor liver transplantation						
Tsujino	Tokyo	2006	174	30	NA	NA
Giacomoni	Milano	2006	23	48	22	26
Wojcicki	Birmingham	2006	70	26	20	4
Cardiac death donors						
Suárez	A Coruňa	2008	22	42	4	38
De Vera	Pittsburgh	2008	141	25	NA	NA
Kobayshi	Niigata	2009	63	46	29	32

Table 1. Biliary complications in various surgical anastomosis techniques

3. Manifestation and diagnosis

Manifestations of biliary complications comprise usual symptoms but often with different presentation as compared to non-transplant conditions. They involve fever, right upper quadrant pain, non-specific abdominal discomfort, and elevation of hepatic, particularly cholestatic enzymes. On the one hand, these manifestations may rapidly progress to the development of biliary peritonitis in large leaks but, more typically, they remain mild and indistinguishable from other causes of cholestasis such as hepatitis C virus (HCV) recurrence and acute rejection to mention at least two other common complications. The diagnosis comes after precise analysis of symptoms, laboratory examinations, liver biopsy and use of imaging methods. Usually, there is absence of intrahepatic bile ducts dilatation on ultrasound, particularly early after liver transplantation, even above a tight obstruction. The final step of diagnostic work-up is direct imaging by endoscopic retrograde cholangiopancreatography (ERCP) or percutaneous transhepatic cholangiography (PTC), which should be preceded by magnetic resonance cholangio-pancreatography (MRCP; Fig. 1). Nevertheless, even MRCP has its logistic limitations and the picture of ducts fully corresponds to the picture on ERCP in about 70% of cases (Wojcicki et al., 2008).

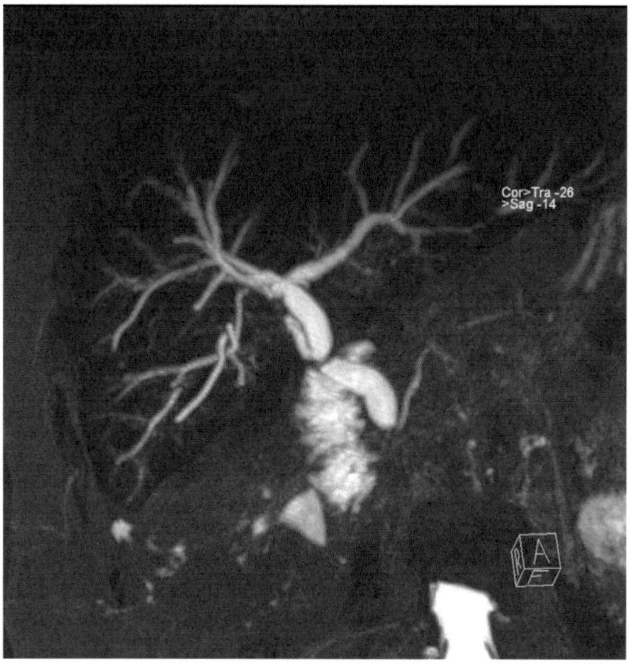

Fig. 1. Bile ducts with anastomotic stricture on MRCP

4. Classification and aetiology of biliary complications

Biliary complications comprise a wide and varied list of events with different frequency involving both direct ductal and extraluminal causes. In fact, the scope of complications corresponds to biliary problems appearing in non-transplant conditions. The difference is in the proportions and several specific aspects. The comprehensive pathogenesis of biliary complications is attributable to various factors including the rationale for selecting a particular surgical technique, ischemic damage mostly due to hepatic artery thrombosis and ischemia-reperfusion injury, immunological principles such as ABO incompatibility, CMV infection, disease recurrence in primary sclerosing cholangitis, and others. The consequent cholestasis contributes to the generally increased vulnerability after liver transplantation strongly affecting namely the outcome in patients with recurrent hepatitis C (HCV) (Katz et al., 2006; Sanni et al., 2006). Technical reasons for biliary complications comprise imperfect suture with early T-tube-related leak or anastomotic stricture, leaks from the liver surface or inadvertent bile duct injuries.

<table>
<tr><td colspan="3">Intrinsic biliary complications</td><td>Extrinsic biliary complications</td></tr>
<tr><td rowspan="6">Strictures</td><td rowspan="2">Intrahepatic</td><td>PSC recurrence</td><td>False aneurysma</td></tr>
<tr><td>Secondary cholangitis</td><td>Cystic duct mucocele</td></tr>
<tr><td rowspan="2">Peri-hilar</td><td>Ischemic</td><td>Lymphoproliferative disease</td></tr>
<tr><td>Idiopathic (ischemic-like)</td><td>Chronic pancreatitis</td></tr>
<tr><td colspan="2">Anastomotic</td><td>Recurrent/de novo cancer</td></tr>
<tr><td>Distal</td><td>Papillary dysfunction</td><td rowspan="9"></td></tr>
<tr><td rowspan="5">Leaks</td><td colspan="2">Anastomotic duct-to-duct</td></tr>
<tr><td colspan="2">Anastomotic HJA</td></tr>
<tr><td colspan="2">T-tube location</td></tr>
<tr><td colspan="2">Cut surface</td></tr>
<tr><td colspan="2">Missed segmental duct</td></tr>
<tr><td colspan="3">Stones, cast, T-tube remnant</td></tr>
<tr><td colspan="3">Haemobilia</td></tr>
<tr><td colspan="3">Recurrent sclerosing cholangitis</td></tr>
</table>

Table 2. Intrinsic and extrinsic biliary complications

5. Specific measurements before the scope is inserted

5.1 Infection prevention

After ERCP, infection remains to be a major complication occurring in about 1% of procedures overall. Several reasons may play a role. Similar to other invasive procedures, ERCP, even though rarely, may cause endocarditis in high-risk patients. Proper use of disposable accessories and utilization of standard technique can completely eliminate transmission of infection by the contaminated scope. Thanks to universally adopted measures, cases of endocarditis and nosocomial infection including hepatitis C, hepatitis B, and HIV related to endoscopy have been reported rarely in recent series. The American Heart Association recently revised their guidelines for prophylaxis of infective endocarditis, and a crucial change for endoscopic procedures is that antibiotic prophylaxis solely to prevent infective endocarditis is not recommended. Exceptions include high-risk cardiac conditions including: a prosthetic cardiac valve, a history of previous infective endocarditis, cardiac transplant recipients developing valvulopathy, patients with congenital heart disease with either uncorrected cyanosis or those with prosthetic material repair within 6 months after the procedure, or those with a residual defect. Since the enterococci making up part of the common bile duct flora in cholangitis are the invading agents in endocarditis, either amoxicillin or ampicillin should be included to the antibiotic protocol for enterococcal coverage.

The most common pathogenesis for cholangitis after ERCP is flare-up of infection already present in the bile ducts. The usual pathogens encountered in bile ducts involve Pseudomonas aeruginosa, Klebsiella spp., E. coli, Bacteroides spp., and Enterococci. The infection is precipitated by an elevated intraductal pressure when complete bile drainage has not been achieved. To eliminate these factors, it is highly recommended to aspirate bile before contrast injection and to complete endoscopic treatment (stones removal, drainage of all relevant visualised strictures). The basic principle is not to overfill the duct above the stricture, and particularly in complicated anatomy, but to fill only what can be drained. The risk factors to be considered include jaundice, previous endoscopic treatment, previous cholangitis, combined endoscopic-percutaneous procedures, transplant patients on an immunosuppressive regimen, hilar tumours, and primary sclerosing cholangitis, because the bile duct obstruction is difficult to be completely relieved. The technique of ERCP should correspond to the technique in non-transplant conditions. The role of antibiotic prophylaxis is controversial and a variety of practices exist. Several randomized controlled trials (RCTs) have been published showing reduction of bacteraemia with an inevitably limited value due to the small numbers of patients with clinical infection. No RCT has to date been conducted exclusively in transplant patients. Taken together, the general attitude to antibiotic prophylaxis is becoming more and more selective with its application only in conditions with suspected high risk. Transplant patients are exactly the case of the highest-risk group. ERCP should be attempted only in transplant patients with highly suspected biliary obstruction. If not clear from the clinical picture and other examinations, MRCP is a must. On the other hand, the finding of infection cannot be relied on absolutely. We recommend 400 mg of ciprofloxacin to be given intravenously (per oral administration is probably similarly effective) 2 hours before the procedure and to continue with the administration until complete drainage is achieved. Other options include gentamicin, quinolone, cephalosporin, and ureidopenicillin (ASGE guideline 2008; Cotton et al., 2008). In fact, most of these patients are already on an antibiotic regimen due to clinical/laboratory manifestations of infection of various organs.

5.2 Coagulopathy – bleeding disorders

After transplantation, abnormal coagulation due to liver dysfunction or anticoagulation therapy is a common concern. Other risk factors of invasive procedures include trombocytopaenia (included a haemodialysis-caused coagulation disorder) and initiation of anticoagulation therapy within three days of the invasive procedure; on the other hand, extension of previous sphincterotomy and the use of aspirin or non-steroidal anti-inflammatory drugs do not seem to raise the risk. No data dealing specifically with sphincterotomy in patients with liver disorders are available and the commonly shared opinion is that coagulopathy should be managed according to rules applied to liver biopsy. Generally, there are widely divergent opinions about the values at which abnormal coagulation indexes begin to pose a major risk for any kind of invasive procedures including endoscopic sphincterotomy. The utility of usual tests: platelet count, prothrombin time (PT)/international normalized ration (INR) in predicting bleeding risk is uncertain and generally not supported by scientific evidence. Probably more important than any laboratory parameters is to take careful medical history whether any bleeding episode after an invasive procedure has appeared in the past, and to search for any possible signs of recent bleeding. Whether the use of prophylactic blood products alters the risk of bleeding is currently unknown. However, it is commonly assumed that platelet transfusion should be considered when thrombocytes count is less than 50,000-60,000/mL and, if prothrombin time is prolonged by 4-6 seconds, then transfusion of fresh frozen plasma may bring the presumed consequent increased bleeding risk into the desired range (Rockey et al., 2009). Appropriate practice of endoscopic procedures in patients on anticoagulation or antiplatelet therapy is precisely determined in the guidelines of endoscopic societies and the conditions of post-transplant care are not specific in any way. In short, sphincterotomy should not be performed by pure cutting current. Aspirin therapy can be maintained while clopidogrel should be withheld. Adoption of all these measures cannot completely eliminate the increased risk of haemorrhage in a complex bleeding disorder accompanying liver dysfunction in the post-transplant patient. The endoscopist should actively stop any bleeding appearing immediately after sphincterotomy by local endoscopic techniques.

5.3 Sedation and anaesthesia

Several specific features of this issue after transplantation should be addressed. During comprehensive pre-transplant evaluation and post-transplant follow-up, patients are often exposed to many endoscopic procedures which may possibly make them more anxious and less tolerant. Procedures early after transplantation or in patients in generally poor condition (ASA class IV-V-E) have to be performed with the assistance of an anaesthesiologist often under general anaesthesia. Therapeutic procedures are often prolonged due to the abnormal anatomy of reconstructed bile ducts. A considerable proportion of transplant procedures is performed in alcohol abusers. Chronic alcohol use increases dose requirements for general anaesthetic, sedative or analgesic agents. This is thought to be partly because of enzyme (particularly cytochrome P-450 2E1) induction or the development of cross tolerance. If the effective doses of propofol, opioids and other drugs are increased, the patient may - quite paradoxically - become agitated, uneasily controlled and less tolerant to any disturbing procedures. The increased anaesthetic demands may exacerbate the risk of cardiovascular instability in patients suffering from cardiomyopathy and increase the risk of adverse effects of all kinds. All these consequences make endoscopic procedures extraordinarily demanding. All the administered drugs have to be precisely titrated and the patient adequately monitored. The involvement of an anaesthesiologist in all procedures presumably associated with risk is highly recommended (Chapman & Plaat, 2009).

6. Biliary complications after liver transplantation – Specific issues and their management

Basically, treatment of biliary complications does not differ from that of the identical structural entities. Nevertheless, there are several specific features which have to be considered to avoid an unexpected surprise and to obtain optimal results. These specific techniques and tricks described below are based on our constantly expanding experience with more than 700 liver transplantations and management of approximately 200 biliary complications developing in a single department. This has given us the opportunity to follow the outcome from both immediate and long-term perspective and to discuss all individual aspects with colleagues representing other specialties and involved in the transplant programme such as invasive radiologists, surgeons, and transplant hepatologists. In transplant medicine more than in non-transplant specialties, every patient is uniquely constituted and most of the conclusions and recommendations are based on observation rather than on comparative studies, which are enormously difficult to conduct.

6.1 Endoscopic sphincterotomy

The technique itself does not differ from sphincterotomy performed in other patients. Since the spontaneous motility of the bile duct is abolished due to the surgical reconstruction resulting in denervation of the biliary tree, evacuation of the contrast material cannot reliably serve as a measure of bile duct function. Even after standard-size sphincterotomy, which in a non-transplant condition be otherwise fully sufficient for what is aimed at - stent insertion or bile duct stone extraction - the cholestasis can persist. Therefore, we always recommend performing sphincterotomy to the maximal possible (safe) extent.

6.2 Anastomotic strictures

Anastomotic strictures being, together with leaks, the most common post-transplant biliary complication, are highly specific and almost unparalleled to non-transplant conditions. They are often asymmetrical with a shape that may be difficult to precisely project on x-ray due to overlap with one or two cysticus stumps. The shape of the prolonged reconstructed bile duct in the anastomotic area may resemble the letter S (Fig. 2, Fig. 3).

Given the irregular lumen of the anastomosis with cysticus stumps, it may be exceptionally uneasy to pass the guide wire through the stricture (Fig. 4). Often, several types of wire with

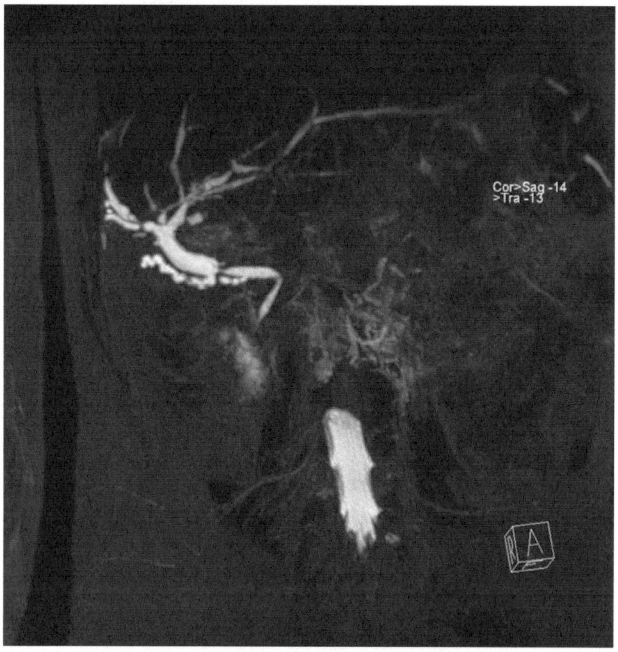

Fig. 2. S-shape of common bile duct after reconstruction on MRCP

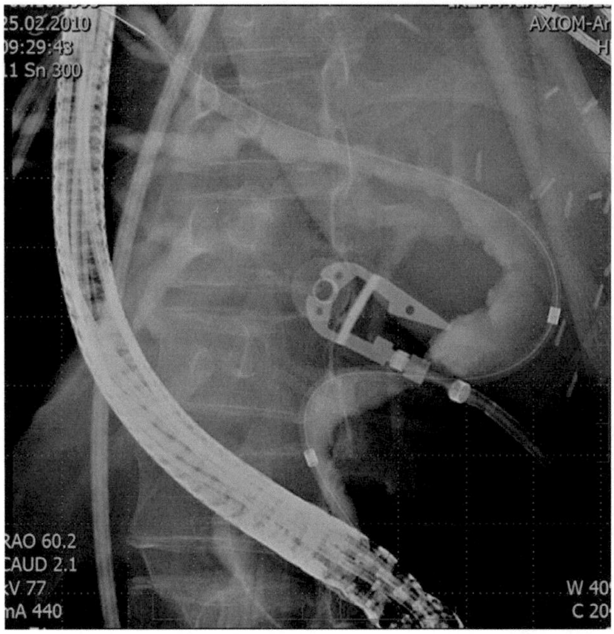

Fig. 3. S-shape of common bile duct after reconstruction on urgent ERCP

different properties in terms of diameter, flexibility/rigidity and slipperiness have to be tried. The direction of the wire tip can be enhanced by the use of an angled tip, sphincterotome or a balloon catheter.

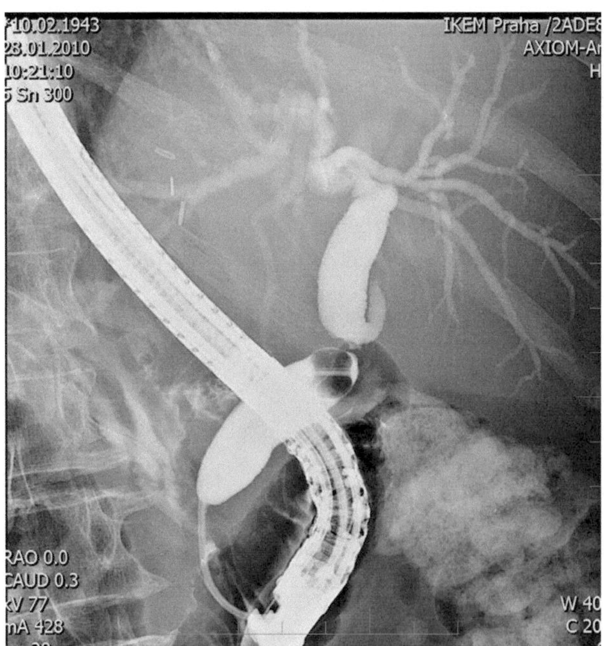

Fig. 4. Anastomotic stricture on ERCP with difficult access to common hepatic duct

Once the wire has been successfully inserted, a proper stent has to be selected. The stricture can be dilated by balloon before stenting, but we do not find it necessary if planning to insert a single stent. Both basic types of biliary stents, the Amsterdam with two flaps and the Tannenbaum with four flaps at their end are equally acceptable. The strategic principle is that a benign anastomotic stricture unlike a malignant stenosis needs not to be only bridged, but the lumen of the bile duct should to be completely reconstituted to correspond with normal anatomy. The chances for optimal remodelling of the anastomosis and the stricture seem to be higher if the diagnosis is established and treatment initiated early after transplantation and lower if a hard fibrotic stricture has already developed. If the reconstructed bile duct after liver transplantation is prolonged to form an S-shape, we select a longer stent than can be judged from the distance between the stricture and duodenum. The reason for this is that the stent passing through an S-shaped bile duct generates friction making the insertion more difficult. Should the stent be not long enough, the end may become impacted in the stricture orifice which makes it impossible to go through. On the other hand, when the curved stricture is overcome, the shape straightens and this may expel the proximal end of the stent far above the stricture, possibly above the hilar junction. This unfavourable position of the proximal end can hardly be prevented. We always place as many stents as possible according to the size of the bile ducts below and above the stricture (Fig. 5).

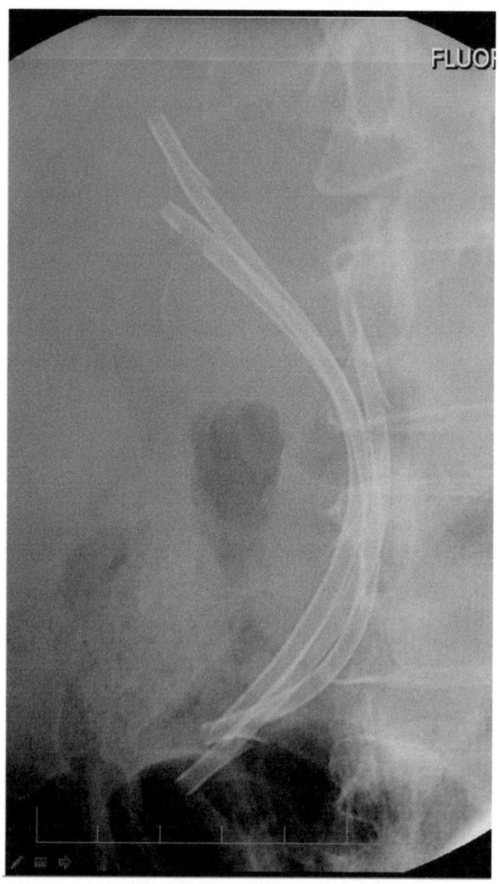

Fig. 5. Multiple biliary stents of various lengths

We use both basic techniques of multiple stents insertion: two wires prior to inserting either stent or to insert a wire along and after the first stent insertion. The optimal number and position of multiple stents are usually determined during several sessions at short one- or two-week intervals. If inserting one stent into an S-shaped bile duct with anastomotic stricture, it may adopt the curve of the bile duct, while multiple stents straighten the duct as the optimal outcome. If the first one or two inserted stents are located with their proximal end high above the stricture, we select a shorter third stent to drain the bile from various levels of the bile ducts to avoid cholestasis and debris accumulation above the stricture. A hard S-shaped bile duct may expand the stent back to the duodenum with the risk of duodenal perforation by the stent on the side opposite to the orifice. Therefore we always try to insert more stents in parallel making the expulsion less likely. We do exchange of stents at three-month intervals as recommended elsewhere, and the stents are removed usually after an interval of six months to one year. In cases where the endoscopic access has failed, the transhepatic approach follows (Fig. 6). The first plastic stent can be inserted either transhepatically or by a rendezvous transpapillary technique. The disadvantage of the single transhepatic technique is that it does not enable to insert multiple stents in one session (Holt et al., 2007; Pasha et al., 2007; Kulaksiz et al., 2008).

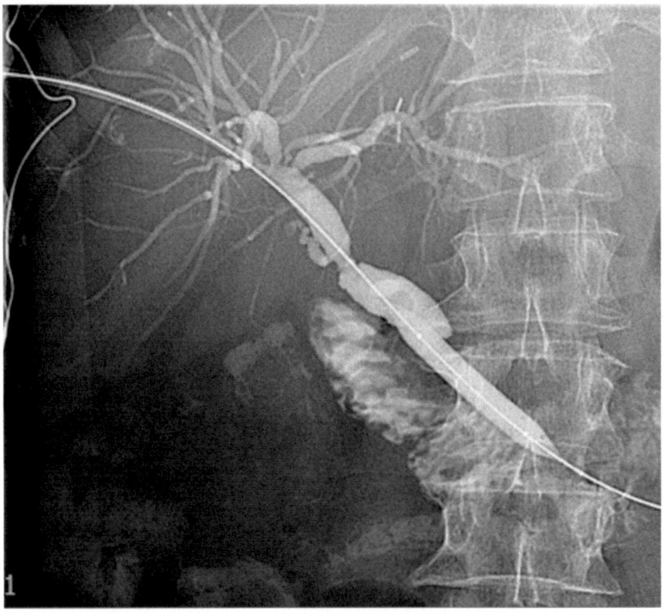

Fig. 6. Bridging of anastomotic stricture by the wire from transhepatic approach

6.3 Non-anastomotic hilar strictures (ischemic-type biliary lesions)

With an incidence in the range of between 5% and 15%, these biliary complications remain a substantial source of morbidity, graft loss, and even mortality after liver transplantation (Fig. 7). Their multifactorial origin involves various events (risk factors) including ischemia due to hepatic artery thrombosis or prolonged cold and warm ischemia, use of University of Wisconsin solution vs. histidine tryptophan ketoglutarate, ABO incompatibility, extramural pressure by lymph nodes or tumour, recurrence of the original disease or it remains obscure.

Also the altered bile composition with a significantly lower phospholipids/bile salts ratio after liver transplantation and graft steatosis may contribute to the pathogenesis of these complications (Buis et al., 2005, 2009; Pascher et al., 2005). Compared to anastomotic strictures, non-anastomotic strictures pose a higher risk of progressive disease with a severe outcome and limited graft survival. The shape of ischemic and ischemic-like strictures may change surprisingly quickly. Endoscopic treatment consists of stent insertion similar to non-transplant patients, but proper exploration and management of underlining conditions are essential. If the stricture involves the segmental branches, multiple stents bridging the strictures of all ducts are necessary. In specific conditions of malignant strictures, metallic stent insertion according to commonly shared rules is the choice. Full success of endoscopic treatment is less likely due to the location distant to the papilla making endoscopic manipulation less effective and, also, due to the various underlying conditions with different outcomes. Endoscopic treatment may be combined with the transhepatic approach if necessary. According to a recent study, percutaneous transhepatic Y-configured single-catheter stenting may enlarge the armamentarium of drainage techniques in hilar strictures (Wang et al., 2011).

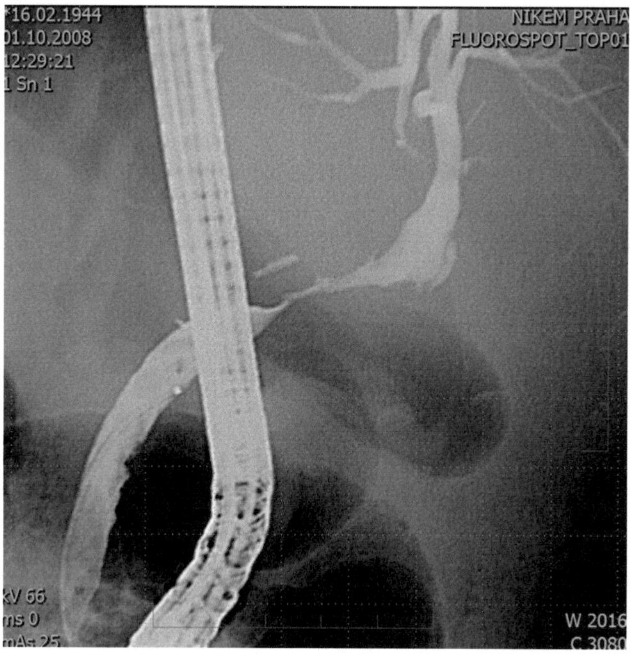

Fig. 7. Ischemic-type biliary lesion

6.4 Intrahepatic strictures

They are not unequivocally classified against non-anastomotic ischemic-type biliary lesions, and the pathogenesis shares identical principles. Wan Lee et al. classified intrahepatic stenoses into 4 groups: unilateral focal, confluence, bilateral multifocal and diffuse (Fig. 8). The success of non-surgical, either endoscopic or transhepatic interventions, is reversely related to the extent of duct involvement with a frequent need of early retransplantation (Lee et al., 2007).

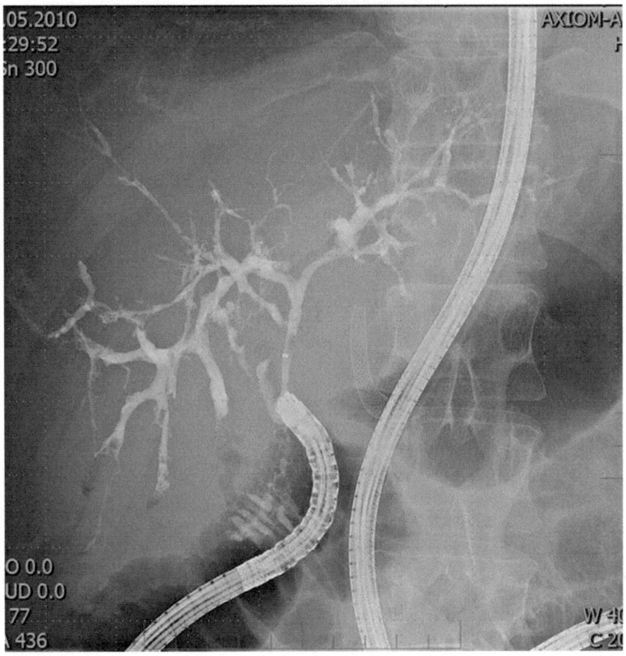

Fig. 8. Multiple intrahepatic stenoses - the recurrence of primary sclerosing cholangitis. Approach to hepatico-jejunoanastomosis with the enteroscope

6.5 Distal strictures

Strictures below the anastomosis are usually caused by chronic pancreatitis. Surprisingly, pancreatitis is often asymptomatic and cholestasis is the only manifestation of advanced pancreatic disease. Other causes include extramural pressure by malignancies, mucocele, and biloma. They can be managed in the same manner as non-transplant conditions (Pascher et al., 2005).

6.6 Papillary stenosis (sphincter of Oddi dysfunction - SOD)

Data concerning the occurrence of papillary stenosis/dysfunction after liver transplantation are less consistent compared to other specific and well defined biliary complications (anastomotic strictures, leaks). Cholestasis was observed in 3-7% of patients following T-tube clamping early after liver transplantation but, according to some authorities, it used to be transient and self-limited. Papillary stenosis may be facilitated or unmasked by liver transplantation due to the abolished bile duct spontaneous motility by duct reconstruction and denervation. On the other hand, the fact that some patients develop sphincter of Oddi dysfunction (SOD) and others do not while undergoing the same surgical procedure, is intriguing (Douzdijan et al., 1994). The embarrassment and inevitable diversity of approaches can be demonstrated on a model case: a patient developed significant cholestasis several months after liver transplantation. Biopsy excluded other causes, sonography and MRCP showed dilatation of the recipient choledochus, as confirmed by ERCP. Multiple choices were as follows: either to perform manometry or sphincterotomy, to wait, or perhaps to insert a stent and wait; if the cholestasis has resolved, the patient can be either followed only and, if it has appeared again, it would bring a strong argument for sphincterotomy. If sphincterotomy is the choice, a cut to a maximal safe extent is recommended.

6.7 Bile duct stones

While less frequent compared to leaks and anastomotic strictures, bile duct stones are still a relatively common complication after liver transplantation. Two basic categories of choledocholithiasis can be classified. Sludge or small stones usually develop as a late complication. A soft pigmented composition prevails suggesting that cholestasis and infection play a decisive role. Cholesterol supersaturation and related changes in lithogenicity are probably less important. The occurrence of stones is often associated with biliary strictures. More rarely, extensive casts completely filling biliary tree have been described. Casts usually appear relatively early after liver transplantation subsequently to prolonged ischemia resulting in severe diffuse biliary mucosal damage and defoliation. Endoscopic treatment responding to non-transplant conditions should be primarily preferred followed, alternatively, by the transhepatic approach or surgery in the case of failure. Nevertheless, the long-term outcome reflecting the underlying conditions may be limited when multiple stones or casts with diffuse bile duct damage occur (Sheng et al., 1996; Spier et al., 2008).

6.8 Post-transplant lymphoproliferative disorder (PTLD)

PTLD is a serious and complex clinicopathologic disorder that has been related to several specific factors, particularly overimmunosuppression and viral infection. The rate of PTLD is approaching 3%. The early cases are located in the liver hilum causing biliary stenosis with cholestasis. Treatment is based on several principles. The degree of immunosuppression should be reduced. Antiviral drugs have been used mostly in children. Chemotherapy has been given to patients with EBV-negative monoclonal lymphomas developing with delay after transplantation. Other options include rituximab, a chimeric anti-CD20 antibody, radiotherapy and interferon-alpha. Local biliary involvement can be relieved by stent insertion from either the endoscopic or transhepatic approach or, exceptionally, by surgery. Endoscopic treatment corresponds to the endoscopic approach to hilar strictures of other causes with a common need of transhepatic assistance. The survival is determined by the pathobiology of the PTDL with a worse prognosis in early disease similar to the prognosis of other post-transplant malignancies (Aucejo et al., 2006).

6.9 Bile leaks

Bile leaks have been reported in 1-25% of OLTs performed. They can be divided into early, defined by a time period of 1-3 months after OLT, and late leaks. Anastomotic leaks are related to technically imperfect suture, or ischemic damage of the (usually) donor bile duct (Fig. 9).

Other considered risk factors include recipient and donor age and the MELD score (Weilling et al., 2008). Bile leaks seem to be unrelated to the type of biliary duct-to-duct reconstruction. According to a recent RCT, neither end-to-end nor side-to-side choledocho-choledochostomy revealed significant differences in terms of the presentation of biliary complications. Early leakage may develop at the T-tube insertion site whenever yet typically after T-tube

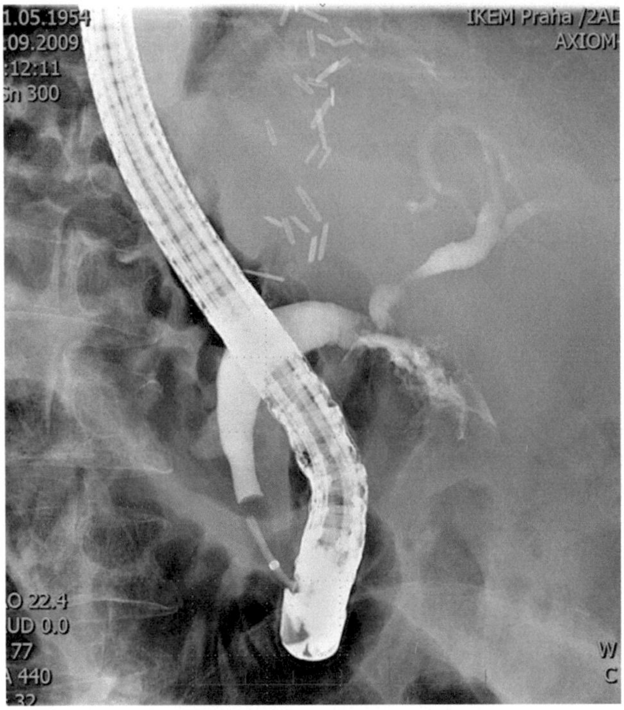

Fig. 9. Anastomotic bile leak

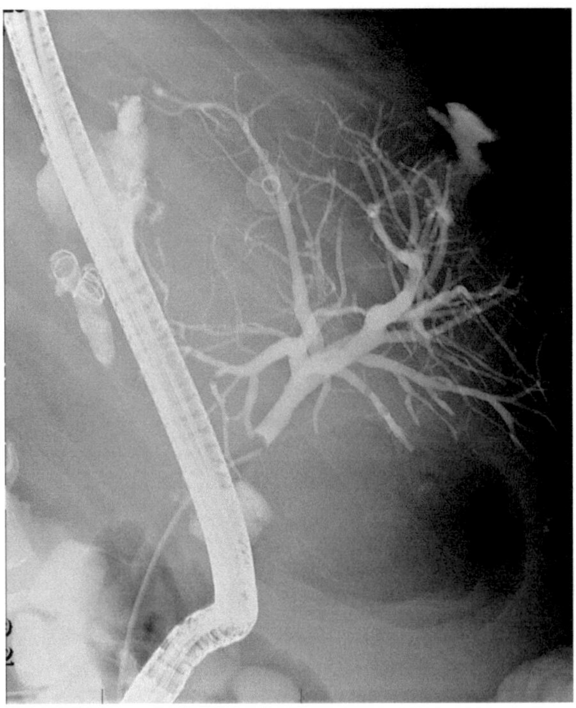

Fig. 10. Peripheral bile leak

removal, in up to 30% of procedures. The T-tube used to be inserted for a few months to maintain access to the biliary ducts and in the hope of preventing the development of a stricture at anastomosis. Other sites of leak comprise surface leaks and leaks from inadvertent bile ducts, usually after graft reduction (Fig. 10). The leaks can be treated either by stent or nasobiliary drainage insertion (after sphincterotomy). In small leaks, sphincterotomy alone may be sufficient (Skuhart et al., 1998).

6.10 Roux-en-Y anastomosis

Several small studies have focused on endoscopic treatment of patients with Roux-en-Y anastomosis, which in the past could be managed by either a standard duodenoscope or gastroscope with limited success only. Both with double- or single-balloon enteroscope, ERC is a feasible option with high success rate (Fig. 8). Limitations of this technique include the time requirement (1–2 hours) and the relatively narrow scale of accessories (Langer et al., 2009; Mönkenmüller et al., 2008).

6.11 Metal stents

The originally designed uncovered self-expanding metal stents have been shown to maintain longer patency than plastic stents in malignant strictures (Fig. 11). Nevertheless, in benign strictures, they were mostly rejected and failed due to mucosal hyperplasia and impossible removability. The advantage of covered metal stents is to prevent tissue ingrowth and removability using the snare or rat-tooth technique. In a recent study, fully

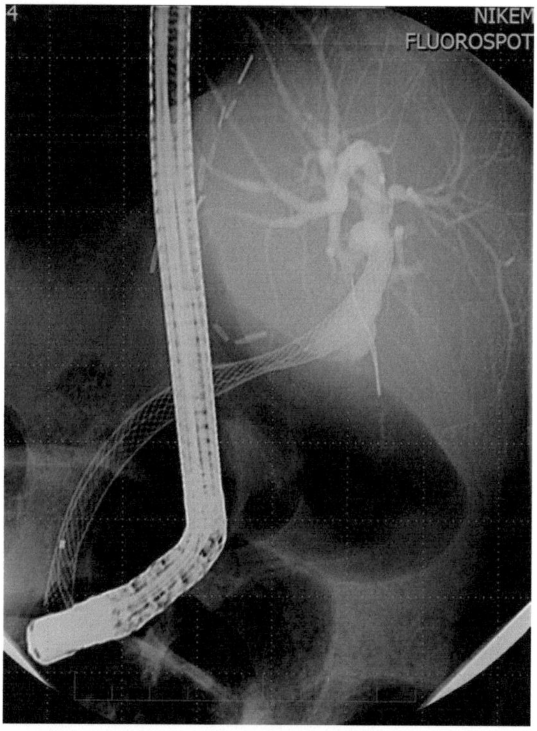

Fig. 11. Self-expanding metal stent due to ischemic-type stenosis

covered metal stents were inserted in 16 patients where plastic stent have failed. In six stents, migration occurred, nevertheless the stricture/leak resolved and a recurrent stricture developed in one patient. While a multicentre study is not easy to be designed, this is the only chance to reliably assess the potential of this modality (Costamagna et al. 2008; Kahaleh et al., 2008; Traina et al., 2009).

6.12 Living donor liver transplantation (LDLT)

The last decade has witnessed significant progress in LDLT. As compared to a whole liver transplant, the recipient of a partial graft in LDLT is faced with increased surgical complications associated with complicated hilar anastomotic variation requiring multiple biliary reconstructions. Since common biliary variations have been recognized, several types of biliary reconstructions have been developed. Both materials and type of the suture method have a major effect on the incidence biliary complications. To avoid bile duct devascularisation and consequent non-anastomotic biliary strictures, new surgical refinements have been also described. A variety of techniques have been reported to avoid injury to blood supply in LDLT. A detailed preoperative evaluation of the graft biliary system followed by an intraoperative cholangiogram through the cystic duct is a must. The optimal technique for biliary anastomosis in LDLT is still controversial. The currently most common techniques are either duct-to-duct or Roux-en-Y hepatico-jejunostomy. Since the late 1990, duct-to-duct anastomosis has been increasingly used, but the concerns regarding terms leaks and strictures seemed quite controversial. However, as the issue of LDLT is enormously complicated, prospective randomized studies are not realistic and so is not the ultimate judgment. Stenting of the anastomosis which was almost abandoned in whole liver transplantation remains another controversy in more complicating anastomoses. At this moment, several principles are universally accepted, but the type of anastomosis and possible stenting should be decided freely according to the aetiology of liver disease, duct anatomy, and type of presumed anastomosis. The endoscopist can expect greater engagement and, in the case of complicated anastomosis, a creative approach with the use of a wide range of instruments as described above (Giacomoni et al., 2006; Grande et al., 1999; Kobayashi et al., 2009; Wojcicki et al., 2006).

6.13 Donation after cardiac death donors

The increased number of patients listed for liver transplantation requires expansion of the pool of donors. To balance the donor organ shortage, livers donated after cardiac death is increasingly used. Nevertheless, both graft and patient survival rates compared to donation after brain death remain inferior, often due to biliary complications whose incidence ranges from 25% to 60%. Compared to brain death donors, in organs donated after cardiac death, ischemic cholangiopathy without hepatic artery injury frequently requires urgent retransplantation. Often there is a discrepancy between acceptable hepatocellular function and dim prognosis due to septic cholangitis. Therefore, the MELD score is useless when considering retransplantation. As a bridge, attempts of multiple endoscopic and transhepatic draining are often needed carrying the risk of other complications. Currently, the only way of minimizing the risk of cholangiopathy seems to be careful selection of young donors and cold ischemic time well below 8 hours (Feng et al., 2011; Foley et al., 2011; de Vera et al., 2009).

7. Conclusion

The high rates and wide range of biliary complications after liver transplantation remain a most important issue. The advent of new strategies and techniques, such as split- or reduced-size liver, living related liver transplantation, and non-heart beating donors incorporating new technical and pathogenetic principles will maintain the rate of complications on a significant level. Management has to arise from individual assessment of the patient with its unique complexity comprising the morphology of the lesion, presumed pathogenesis, comorbidities, and prior surgery including the patient´s preference. Analyses that consider all these factors should determine the strategy that may offer optimal profit for the patient. Management of biliary complications requires a multidisciplinary approach, in which all three main options, endoscopic, radiologic and surgical, have to be weighed one against each other. Generally, endoscopic management has to be considered as the first therapeutic option due its complexity, efficacy and safety in the majority of patients. The radiologic approach can be used alternatively in the majority of complications, preferably if there is not transluminal access to the biliary tree. Proper location of the stent by x-ray alone is more difficult to control, and multiple stents usually cannot be inserted. Both approaches can be combined. The disadvantage of these methods is the need for multiple sessions annoying the patient and increasing the risk of complications. Surgery - usually Roux-en-Y anastomosis - is a demanding technique potentially eliminating the obstruction forever. However, anastomosis obstruction and episodes of reflux cholangitis may compromise long-term outcome in up to 20% of patients. The standard therapeutic approach to biliary complications has not been uniformly defined and local expertise, usually inevitably uneven, plays an important role. The same biliary complication, i.e. extrahepatic stricture can be (and used to be) either treated by endoscopy, interventional radiology, or surgery, without significant difference in the results among the studies. A direct comparative study has not been published yet and one cannot be expected to be conducted even in the future. The diverse nature of the complications requires usual endoscopic techniques of treatment and, similar to non-transplant conditions, sphincterotomy, stent insertion with or without dilatation, and stone extraction are the most common therapeutic modalities. With the advent of new technologies like metal (semi-) covered stents and balloon enteroscopes, the range of options will enlarge. Specific issues of endoscopic procedures after liver transplantation include prevention of postprocedural cholangitis, consideration of coagulation disorders, and sedation of patients with various mental impairments.

8. References

ASGE guideline. (2008). Antibiotic prophylaxis for GI endoscopy. Gastrointestinal endoscopy, Vol.67, No.6, (May 2008), pp. 791-798, ISSN 0016-5107

Aucejo, F.; Rofaiel, G.; Miller, C. (2006). Who is at risk for post-transplant lymphoproliferative disorders (PTLD) after liver transplantation?. *Journal of Hepatology*, Vol.44, No.1, (January 2006), pp. 19-23, ISSN 0168-8278

Buis, C. I.; Hoekstra, H.; Verdonk, R. C. & al. (2006). Causes and consequences of ischemic-type biliary lesions after liver transplantation. *Journal of Hepato-Biliary-Pancreatic Surgery*, Vol.13, No.6, (November 2006), pp. 517-524, ISSN 0944-1166

Buis, C. I.; Geuken, E.; Visser, D. S. & al. (2009). Altered bile composition after liver transplantation is associated with the development of nonanastomotic biliary strictures. *Journal of Hepatology*, Vol.50, No.1, (October 2008), pp. 69-79, ISSN 0168-8278

Costamagna, G. (2008). Covered self-expanding metal stents in benign biliary strictures: not yet a "new paradigm" but a promising alternative. *Gastrointestinal endoscopy*, Vol.67, No.3, (March 2008), pp. 455-457, ISSN 0016-5107

Cotton, P. B.; Connor, P.; Rawls, E. & al. (2008). Infection after ERCP and antibiotic prophylaxis: a sequential quality-improvement approach over 11 years. *Gastrointestinal endoscopy*, Vol.67, No.3, (March 2008), pp.471-475, ISSN 0016-5107

Davidson, B. R.; Rai, R.; Kurzawinski, T. R. & al. (1999). Prospective randomized trial of end-to–end versus side-to-side biliary reconstruction after orthotopic liver transplantation. *The British Journal of Surgery*, Vol.86, No.4, (April 1999), pp. 447-452, ISSN 0007-1323

De Vera, E. M.; Lopez- Solis, R.; Dvorchik, I. & al. (2009). Liver transplantation using donation after cardiac death donors. Long-term follow-up from a single center. *American Journal of Transplantion: official journal of the American Society of Transplantation and the American Society of Transplant Surgeons*, Vol.9, No.4, (April 2009), pp. 773-781, ISSN 1600-6143

Douzdijan, V.; Abecassis, M. M.; Johlin, F. C. & al. (1994). Sphincter of Oddi Dysfunction following liver transplantation. Screening by bedside manometry and definitive manometric evaluation. *Digestive diseases and sciences*, Vol.39, No.2, (February 1994), pp. 253-256, ISSN 0163-2116

Feng, X. N.; Ding, C. F.; Xing, M. Y. & al. (2011). Technical aspects of biliary reconstruction in adult living donor liver transplantation. *Hepatobiliary & Pancreatic Diseases International: HBPD INT*, Vol.10, No.2, (April 2011), pp. 136-142, ISSN 1499-3872

Foley, D. P.; Fernandez, L. A.; Leverson, G. & al. (2011). Biliary complications after liver transplantation from donation after cardiac death donors: an analysis of risk factors and long-term outcomes from a single center. *Annals of Surgery*, Vol.253, No.4, (April 2011), pp. 817-825, ISSN 1528-1140

Giacomoni, A.; Lauterio, A.; Slim, A. Q. & al. (2006). Biliary complications after living donor adult liver transplantation. *Transplant international: official journal of the European Society for Organ Transplantation*, Vol.19, No.6, (June 2006), pp. 466-473, ISSN 0934-0874

Grande, L.; Pérez-Castilla, A.; Matus, D. & al. (1999). Routine use of the T-tube in the biliary reconstruction of liver transplantation: is it worthwhile?. *Transplantion proceedings*, Vol.31, No.6, (September 1999), pp. 2396-2397, ISSN 0041-1345

Graziadei, I. W.; Schwaighofer, H.; Koch, R. & al. (2006). Long-term outcome of endoscopic treatment of biliary strictures after liver transplantation. *Liver transplantation: official publication of the American Association for the Study of Liver Diseases and the International Liver Transplantation Society*, Vol.12, No.5, (May 2006), pp. 718-725, ISSN 1527-6465

Holt, A. P.; Thorburn, D.; Mirza, D. & al. (2007). A prospective study of standardized nonsurgical therapy in the management of biliary anastomotic strictures complicating liver transplantation. *Transplantation*, Vol.84, No.7, (October 2007), pp. 857-863, ISNN 0041-1337

Chapman, R.; Plaat, F. (2009). Alcohol and anaesthesia. *Continuing Education in Anaesthesia, Critical Care and Pain*, Vol.9, No.1, (February 2009), pp. 10-13, ISSN 1743-1816

Kahaleh, M.; Behm, B.; Clarke, B. W. & al. (2008). Temporary placement of covered self-expandable metal stents in benign biliary strictures: a new paradigm?. *Gastrointestinal endoscopy*, Vol.67, No.3, (March 2008), pp. 446-454, ISSN 0016-5107

Katz, L. H.; Mor, E.; Brown, M. & al. (2006). Recurrent hepatitis C virus disease after liver transplantation and concurrent biliary tract complications: poor outcome. *Clinical transplantion*, Vol.20, No.4, (August 2006), pp. 465-470, ISSN 0902-0063

Kobayashi, T.; Sato, Y.; Yamamoto, S. & al. (2009). Long-term follow-up study of biliary reconstructions and complications after adult living donor liver transplantation: feasibility of duct-to-duct reconstruction with a T-tube stent. *Transplantation proceedings*, Vol.41, No.1, (February 2009), pp. 265-267, ISSN 0041-1345

Kulaksiz, H.; Weiss, K. H.; Gotthardt, D. & al. (2008). Is stenting necessary after balloon dilation of post-transplantation biliary strictures? Results of a prospective comparative study. *Endoscopy*, Vol.40, No.9, (September 2008), pp. 746-751, ISSN 1438-8812

Langer, F. B.; Györi, G. P.; Pokorny, H. & al. (2009). Outcome of hepaticojejunostomy for biliary tract obstruction following liver transplantation. *Clininical transplantion*, Vol.23, No.3, (July 2009), pp. 361-367, ISSN 0902-0063

Lebeau, G.; yanaga, K.; Marsh, J. W. & al. (1990). Analysis of surgical complications after 397 hepatic transplantations. *Surgery, Gynecology & Obstetrics*, Vol.170, No.4, (April 1990), pp. 317-322, ISSN 0039-6087

Lee, H. W.; Suh, K. S.; Shin, W. Y. & al. (2007). Classification and prognosis of intrahepatic biliary stricture after liver transplantation. *Liver transplantation: official publication of the American Association for the Study of Liver Diseases and the International Liver Transplantation Society*, Vol.13, No.12, (December 2007), pp. 1736-1742, ISSN 1527-6465

Mönkemüller, K.; Bellutti, M.; Neumann, H. & al. (2008). Therapeutic ERCP with the double-balloon enteroscope in patients with Roux-en-Y anastomosis. *Gastrointestinal endoscopy*, Vol.67, No.6, (May 2008), pp. 992-996, ISSN 0016-5107

Pasha, S. F.; Harrison, M. E.; Das, A. & al. (2007). Endoscopic treatment of anastomotic biliary strictures after deceased donor liver transplantation. Outcomes after maximal stent therapy. *Gastrointestinal endoscopy*, Vol.66, No.1, (July 2007), pp. 44-51, ISSN 0016-5107

Pascher, A.; Neuhaus, P. (2005). Bile duct complications after liver transplantation. *Transplant international: official journal of the European Society for Organ Transplantation*, Vol.18, No.6, (June 2005), pp. 627-642, ISSN 0934-0874

Rockey, D. C.; Caldwell, S. H.; Goodman, Z. D. & al. (2009). Liver biopsy. *Hepatology*, Vol.49, No.3, (March 2009), pp. 1017-1044, ISSN 1527-3350

Sanni, A.; Asher, J.; Wilson, C. & al. (2006). Predisposing factors for biliary complications following liver transplantation. *Transplantion proceedings*, Vol.38, No.8, (October 2006), pp. 2677-2678, ISSN 0041-1345

Sheng, R.; Ramirez, C. B.; Zajko, A. B. & al. (1996). Biliary stones and sludge in liver transplant patients: a 13-year experience. *Radiology*, Vol.198, No.1, (January 1996), pp. 243-247, ISSN 0033-8419

Shuhart, M. C.; Kowdley, K. V.; McVicar, J. P. & al. (1998). Predictors of bile leaks after T-tube removal in orthotopic liver transplant recipients. *Liver transplantation: official publication of the American Association for the Study of Liver Diseases and the*

International Liver Transplantation Society, Vol.4, No.1, (January 1998), pp. 62-70, ISSN 1074-3022

Spier, B. J.; Pfau, P. R.; Lorenze, K. R. & al. (2008). Risk factors and outcomes in post-liver transplantation bile duct stones and casts: A case-control study. *Liver transplantation: official publication of the American Association for the Study of Liver Diseases and the International Liver Transplantation Society*, Vol.14, No.10, (October 2008), pp. 1461-1465, ISSN 1527-6465

Suárez, F.; Otero, A.; Solla, M. & al. (2008). Biliary complications after liver transplantation from Maastricht category-2 non-heart-beating donors. *Transplantation*, Vol.85, No.1, (January 2008), pp. 9-14, ISSN 0041-1337

Traina, M.; Tarantino, I.; Barresi, L. & al. (2009). Efficacy and safety of fully covered self-expandable metallic stents in biliary complications after liver transplantation: a preliminary study. *Liver transplantation: official publication of the American Association for the Study of Liver Diseases and the International Liver Transplantation Society*, Vol.15, No.11, (November 2009), pp. 1493-1498, ISSN 1527-6465

Wang, M. C.; Li, X.; Song, S. & al. (2011). Newly designed Y-configured single-catheter stenting for the treatment of hilar-type nonanastomotic biliary strictures after orthotopic liver transplantation. *Cardiovascular and interventional radiology*, (June 2011), Epub ahead of print, ISSN 1432-086X

Welling, T. H.; Heidt, D. G.; Englesbe, M. J. & al. (2008). Biliary complications following liver transplantation in the model for end-stage liver disease era: effect of donor, recipient and technical factors. *Liver transplantation: official publication of the American Association for the Study of Liver Diseases and the International Liver Transplantation Society*, Vol.14, No.1, (January 2008), pp. 73-80, ISSN 1527-6465

Wojcicki, M.; Silva, M. A.; Jethwa, P. & al. (2006). Biliary complications following adult right lobe ex vivo split liver transplantation. *Liver transplantation: official publication of the American Association for the Study of Liver Diseases and the International Liver Transplantation Society*, Vol.12, No.5, (May 2006), pp. 839-844, ISSN 1527-6465

Wojcicki, M.; Milkiewicz, P.; Silva, M. (2008). Biliary tract complications after liver transplantation: a review. *Digestive Surgery*, Vol.25, No.4, (July 2008), pp. 245-257, ISSN 1421-9883

10

Biliary Complications in Liver Transplantation

Ilka de Fatima Santana Ferreira Boin, Fernando Romani de Araujo,
Elaine Cristina de Ataide, Anaisa Portes Ramos and Ciro Garcia Montes
Unit of Liver Transplantation – State University of Campinas – Unicamp
Brazil

1. Introduction

Orthotopic Liver Transplantation (OLT) is the only treatment capable to reverse end-stage chronic liver disease, and is also indicated for the treatment of hepatocellular carcinoma, acute liver failure and a series of metabolic disorders caused by liver dysfunction, even those that do not course with cirrhosis. The evolution of surgical techniques, the proper selection of potential recipients, perioperative and ICU care, and better organ preservation solutions and immunosuppressive medications currently available, greatly increase success rates and survival after liver transplantation. Despite these many advances liver transplantation continues to have a high number of postoperative complications, with significant morbidity and mortality. These include biliary complications, that because of their high incidence have been called the Achilles' heel of liver transplantation. In initial reports the complication rates in the biliary tree range from 34 to 50%, with mortality reaching up to 30% of transplanted patients. In more recent series these complications have been reduced to 10 from 30% and associated mortality to about 10% (Welling et al. 2008).

Biliary complications can occur both in the area of the anastomosis or be intrahepatic. The forms of biliary fistula or stenosis are different not only in clinical presentation and treatment, but also in the period in which they occur. The association with vascular complications, arterial thrombosis specifically, makes treatment even more complicated. The incidence following transplants with living donors is greater, given the wide anatomical variation and smaller size of bile ducts in this situation.

2. Types of biliary reconstruction

Biliary anastomosis is the final step in a liver transplant, being performed after the completion of vascular reconstruction and graft reperfusion. [Figure 1] The technique of end-to-end duct-to-duct anastomosis is the widely accepted standard, although some controversy exists on whether or not the bile duct T-tube drains should be used. [Table 1] This type of reconstruction has the advantage of maintaining the physiological mechanism of biliary excretion and be easily accessible by endoscopy, which is very useful in the case of anastomotic or intrahepatic biliary complications. There are reports of some groups that vary this form of reconstruction with side-to-side anastomosis, in order to enlarge the anastomosis, thus trying to prevent stenosis (O'Connor et al. 1995).

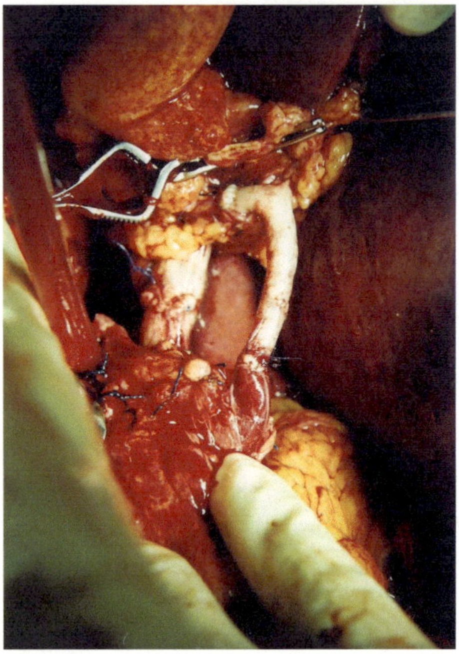

Fig. 1. Identification of patients' biliary tract for duct-to-duct anastomosis after vascular anastomosis and graft reperfusion

The choice for Roux-en-Y hepaticojejunostomy is an exception in transplants with deceased donors. It is indicated when there is some anomaly in the recipient bile duct, such as obstruction, atresia, sclerosing cholangitis, or large size difference between the donor and recipient bile ducts. In the case of living donor transplantation or the use of spit liver, hepaticojejunostomy has been considered the standard, due to the small size, anatomical variation and the presence of multiple ducts to be drained.

Types of Biliary Reconstruction With or without T-tube drains
Duct-to-Duct: End-to-End Side-to-Side
Roux-en-Y Hepaticojejunostomy

Table 1. Types of biliary reconstruction

In right lobe living donor liver transplantation (LDLT) there are several reports of duct-to-duct anastomosis, and this type of reconstruction is already well accepted. In the case of left lobe LDLT there is still a tendency to perform Roux-en-Y hepaticojejunostomy in published reviews. However, there are reports of successful transplants carried out with multiple duct-to-duct anastomosis for drainage of various liver segments, which uses the right and left recipient hepatic branch ducts, or sometimes even the cystic duct to obtain the drainage path for reconstruction (Azoulay et al. 2001).

3. Bile duct drainage

In the firsts series of liver transplantation bile duct drainage with the use of T-tubes was performed routinely. The aim was to decompress the bile flow and reduce pressure on the anastomosis, allowing greater control over the excretory function of the liver and easy access for performing contrasted studies of the biliary tree during the postoperative period. [Figure 2] The presence of T-tube drains in the area of anastomosis prevents the formation of cicatricial stenosis, ensuring a minimum diameter molded into the drain.

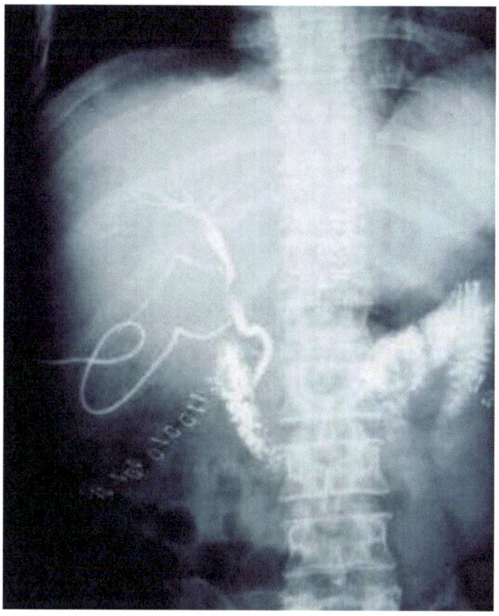

Fig. 2. T-tube drain cholangiography with short, anastomotic type stricture

The occurrence of various complications related to T-tube drain and its removal led to questioning of its real benefit. The occurrence of bile leaks after the drain removal occurs in up to 15% of cases. When added to other complications such as obstruction, displacement and cholangitis, complications directly related to the drain reach between 10 and 22% of patients (Gantxegi et al. 2011).

The use of immunosuppressive drugs and high-dose corticosteroids in liver transplantation delays fibrogenesis, preventing the formation of a fibrous path around the drain, which justifies such a high number of complications. Several attempts to reduce these numbers have been tried, such as using rubber tubes instead of silicone ones and late removal of the drain, between 4 to 6 months post transplant. A prospective randomized trial in the late '90s demonstrated objectively that duct-to-duct anastomosis without bile duct T-tube drains was possible, with lower complication rates and cost-effectiveness (Verran et al. 1997).

Currently, the use of bile duct drains after deceased donor liver transplantation (DDLT) is carried out selectively. In the case of partial liver transplants, either by LDLT or split DDLT, bile duct T-tube drain has the advantage of relieving the pressure in the biliary tree, preventing fistula formation in the liver cut surface. Because of this, drain use is still more frequent in this type of transplantation.

4. Types of biliary complications

Occurrence of fistulas and stenosis account for about 80% of all biliary complications, and the remaining 20% are due to less frequent causes, such as extrinsic compression, hemobilia, mucoceles, and obstructions caused by biliomas, stones, biliary sludge or nematodes.

These complications are related to a number of factors such as technical errors, thrombosis or stenosis of the hepatic artery, recurrence of underlying disease and ischemic-type lesions. In case of partial liver grafts there is also the risk of inadvertent injury during duct dissection and section of hepatic parenchyma, leading to cicatricial strictures or fistulas, and the risk of bile leak in the cut surface (Noujaim et al. 2003).

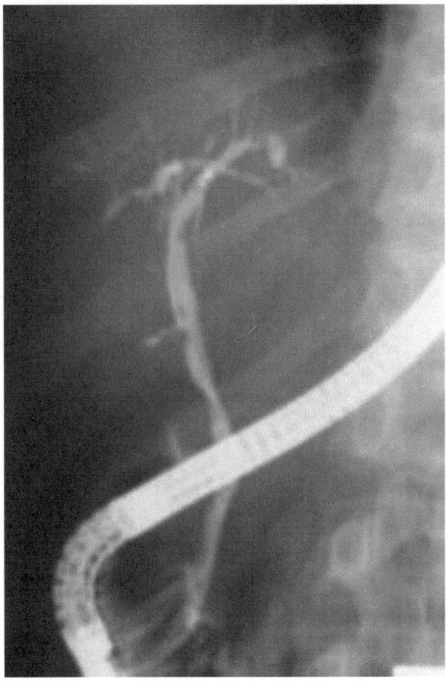

Fig. 3. Endoscopic Retrograde Cholangiography with short segmental stricture

The type of injury varies according to etiology. In case of technical errors in the anastomosis confection single and short extrahepatic stenosis is the rule. [Figure 3] Because of the peculiarities of biliary tree vasculature, in a radial manner, the excessive dissection of the duct in the recipient or in the graft may lead to ischemia in the anastomosis area, resulting in necrosis and fistula or late cicatricial retraction. [Figure 4]

Strictures of the ischemic type are characterized by multiple areas of stenosis within the liver, interspersed with areas of dilation. The main cause of this type of injury is the occurrence of stenosis and thrombosis of the hepatic artery. However several other factors may be involved, such as prolonged cold and hot ischemia periods, poor preservation of the graft, delayed arterialization of the liver, recurrence of underlying disease, and toxicity of drugs and immune-mediated injury. Among the causes immune-mediated chronic rejection, ABO incompatibility and cytomegalovirus infection must be remembered. It is also suggested that the presence of bile salts in contact with the epithelium during cold ischemia period is toxic, leading to autolysis of the mucosal lining. So the practice of washing the biliary tract with saline before arterial clamping and cold perfusion of the graft during the donor's removal procedure can prevent this type of complication.

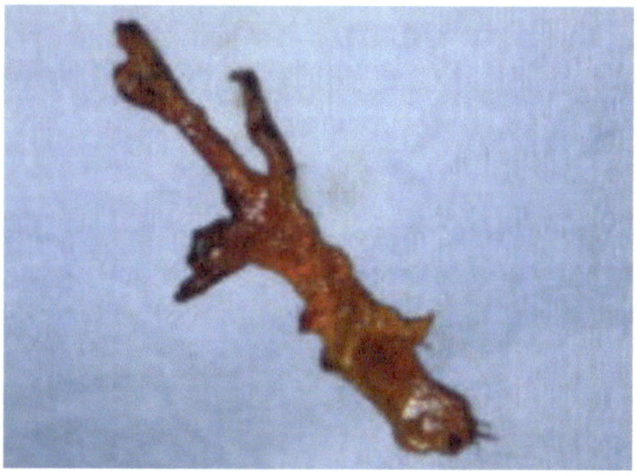

Fig. 4. Necrotic biliary tree

5. Clinical presentation

Most biliary complications occur early after liver transplant, with 60% occurring in the first six months postoperatively. The clinical presentation can be very varied, ranging from jaundice or bile leaks through abdominal drains to unspecific pictures of worsening liver tests and infections.

The presence of bile in abdominal drain in early postoperative is diagnosis of fistula, but is not always present. Formation of biliomas or choleperitonitis may occur even without significant clinical manifestations, a fact due to immunosuppression and high doses of corticosteroids used in the initial postoperative phase.

The occurrence of postoperative cholestasis is a common signal for a series of complications, not to specific abnormalities in the biliary tree. Common causes of cholestasis include acute cellular rejection, liver graft dysfunction, preservation injury, medication toxicity, recurrence of viral hepatitis, vascular thrombosis or stenosis of the hepatic artery and portal vein, ascending cholangitis, or simply be due to severe sepsis.

Changes in postoperative evolution of a transplanted patient such as detection of altered liver function tests or clinical deterioration with development of sepsis should be investigated with specific protocols to detect the most common complications. The performance of Doppler ultrasound examination is a good initial measure, because it allows the evaluation of arterial and portal blood flow, presence of bile ducts dilation and assessment of liver parenchyma for its surface and texture, and also is a good initial method to identify liver abscesses and biliomas or extrahepatic collections. The absence of dilatation of the bile ducts should not be a factor sufficient to preclude the existence of complications such as biliary strictures, as there are several related cases of significant stenosis that do not course with biliary dilation. This can be explained by the presence of greater peri-duct fibrosis in transplanted livers.

When suspicion of biliary complications cannot be ruled out by the initial screening or when persistent cholestasis occurs even after exclusion of acute and chronic rejection or viral hepatitis recurrence a more detailed evaluation of the biliary tract should be performed.

Magnetic Resonance Imaging (MRI) Cholangiography allows detailed images of the biliary tract anatomy, with identification of areas of narrowing, presence of gallstones and bile leakage points, and is a good method for diagnosis and treatment planning. Endoscopic Retrograde Cholangiography (ERCP) and Percutaneous Transhepatic Cholangiography (PTC) allow not only the diagnosis of biliary lesions but also their treatment, either with endoscopic sphincterotomy, placement of biliary drains and external naso-biliary catheters or direct manipulation of lesions, with stricture dilation and passage of various types of biliary prostheses.

The strong association of biliary injury with the occurrence of hepatic artery thrombosis or stenosis should be remembered. Research with angio-CT or MRI should be performed whenever there is suspicion after the initial screening with Doppler ultrasound.

6. Biliary fistulas

Bile leaks usually occur in the early period after liver transplantation. Its presentation can be very variable, from a bile leak from abdominal drains to biliomas formation without further clinical repercussions, until the occurrence of diffuse choleperitonitis and sepsis.

Bile leak incidence varies between 0.5 and 20% and is often related to technical error in the biliary anastomosis. Its origin can be in the anastomosis itself or in areas of injury to the bile duct during dissection. Devascularization of end bile ducts in the area of anastomosis due to excessive dissection can progress to necrosis of the duct and fistula formation. In cases of partial liver grafts, from LDLT or split DDLT, there may be damage to the ducts on the cut surface of the parenchyma, leading to fistula formation.

The initial goal of treatment is to control sepsis. Percutaneous ultrasound or CT-guided drainage of biliomas can be performed. In cases of massive leaks and choleperitonitis it could be necessary to perform laparotomy. The definitive treatment of fistulas depends on the type of transplant performed, as well as the form of biliary reconstruction and the placement or not of T-tube drain in the biliary tract.

In transplants performed with whole liver grafts from deceased donors, fistulas originate almost exclusively from the anastomosis. Other less frequent causes are due to common bile duct injuries during dissection or fistula originating from areas of laceration in liver parenchyma due to prior trauma. In transplants performed with partial liver grafts, due to LDLT or split DDLT, fistulas originating from intra-parenchymal ducts or from the cut surface area of liver section have major significance.

When reconstruction is performed with duct-to-duct anastomosis ECPR treatment is usually the first option. [Figure 5] The performance of sphincterotomy and biliary stenting often induces the closure of fistulas in most cases, with mean treatment duration ranging from 60 to 90 days according to some series (Londono et al. 2008). Another option is the passage of naso-biliary tubes, with the advantage of easy access to perform contrast-enhanced studies of the biliary tract. When a T-tube drain is left during the transplantation procedure simply opening the drain should be sufficient to resolve the fistula. Surgery, as a definitive treatment, is usually indicated only in case of failure of the initial endoscopic treatment, in this case the conversion of the anastomosis to hepaticojejunostomy to be resolutive.

In fistula occurring after reconstruction with Roux-en-Y hepaticojejunostomy the treatment is more complicated. This type of anastomosis is virtually inaccessible by endoscopy, forcing early surgery indication. The reconfiguration of the anastomosis is usually effective for the resolution of this picture. One controversial option is to perform a jejunostomy stoma, to allow endoscopic access to the anastomosis if necessary in the future. This stoma could be closed a few months after resolution of symptoms.

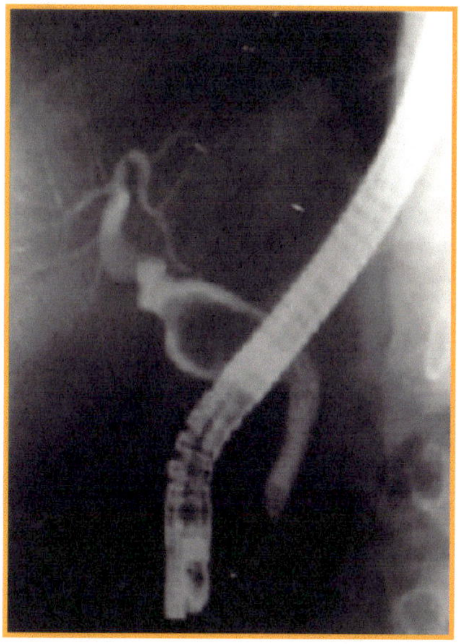

Fig. 5. Bile leak in duct-to-duct anastomosis

Fistulas originating after removal of biliary drains are also initially treated with endoscopic papillotomy. Primary surgical indication to suture the drain hole, allows faster resolution of the fistula, but with higher associated morbidity.

The occurrence of bile leaks leads to significant morbidity and mortality after orthotopic liver transplantation. Although not altering the function or long-term survival of the liver graft after its resolution, it is a risk factor for the occurrence of cicatricial stenosis.

7. Biliary strictures

The occurrence of biliary strictures after liver transplantation has declined over the years due to improved surgical materials, better organ preservation and postoperative care. Incidence of up to 40% initially reported fell from 5 to 15% in recent reviews. In LDLT it still occurs in about 30 to 35%, according to published series (Renz et al. 2004). While the vast majority of stenosis occur within the first year after transplantation, with peak incidence between 5 and 8 months, it is known that the incidence is progressively increased with longer follow-up periods. The early occurrence of stenosis is related to technical conditions, such as improper suture materials, tension at the anastomosis and duct size difference between recipient and donor. Late presenting strictures are usually related to ischemic or immunologic events or inadequate organ preservation.

Strictures can be of two types, anastomotic or non-anastomotic. Strictures that occur in the region of the anastomosis are influenced by local factors and are usually short and unique. [Figure 6] The incidence appears to be greater after the completion of Roux-en-Y hepaticojejunostomy than after duct-to-duct anastomosis. The use of T-tube bile drains seems to have a protective effect on the occurrence of stenosis, while the occurrence of fistula is an independent risk factor for stricture development.

Risk factors for Biliary Strictures	
Anastomotic	Suture technique Bile leaks Bile duct dissection

Ischemic type	Hepatic artery Thrombosis
	Prolonged cold ischemia period
	Prolonged arterialization time
	Donor related:
	    Age
	    High dose vasoactive drugs
	    Cardiac arrest
	Immune-mediated:
	    Chronic ductopenic rejection
	    ABO incompatibility
	Bile salts toxicity
	Infection
	    Citomegalovirus
	    Viral hepatitis recurrence

Table 2. Risk factor for biliary stricture

Strictures of late onset usually are related to ischemic or immunological events. The ischemic causes may be related or not to hepatic artery thrombosis, other causes being long cold or hot ischemia period, prolonged graft arterialization time, removal of the organ after donor cardiac arrest, excessive use of vasoactive drugs or high age of the donor. Root causes are mostly alo-immune ABO incompatibility, chronic ductopenic rejection, recurrence of underlying disease such as sclerosing cholangitis and autoimmune hepatitis, bile salts toxicity to the epithelium, recurrent viral hepatitis and cytomegalovirus infection (Suarez et al. 2008). These types of stenosis, classified as ischemic type, usually are long, multiple, interspersed with areas of dilation and can occur both intra and extra hepatic. [Table 2]

There may be asymptomatic presentation or only with vague symptoms like fatigue, itching and jaundice. The change in liver function markers, such as elevated bilirubin, gamma-glutamyl transferase, alkaline phosphatase and serum aminotransferases should raise suspicion for biliary stenosis or obstructions.

Doppler ultrasound evaluation should be performed to evaluate the presence of hepatic blood flow. If stenosis or artery obstruction is suspected, complete evaluation by angiography or angio-MRI should be performed.

The assessment of biliary obstruction by ultrasonography has poor accuracy in transplanted patients and is not a reliable marker of good biliary drainage. The sensitivity for detection of obstructions varies from 40 to 65%, with a high number of false negatives. The biliary tree in transplanted livers may not dilate, even in the presence of significant obstruction. This is explained by the possible presence of peri-ductal fibrosis that can occur in these patients.

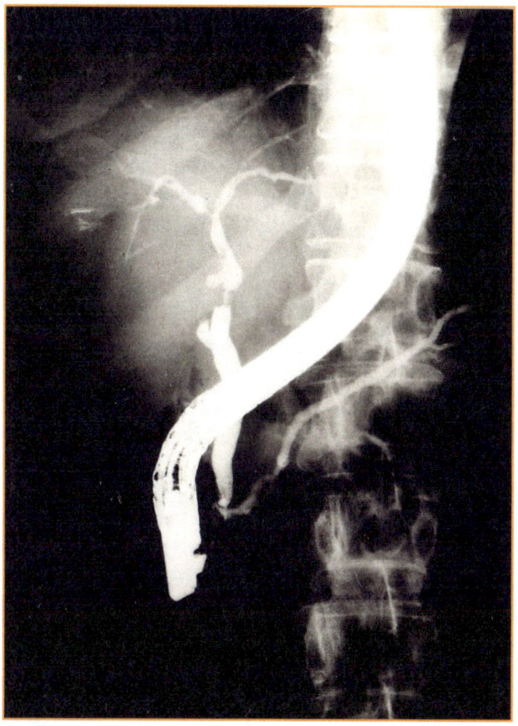

Fig. 6. Anastomitic type biliary stricture, shown in ERCP

The gold standard test for the detection of biliary strictures is cholangiography, both when percutaneous or endoscopic. This test allows proper identification of the cause of obstruction to bile flow and allows therapeutic measures, such as stone removal, dilation and biliary stent insertion. The preference is for performing endoscopic procedure (ERCP) because it is less invasive, with lower bleeding or fistula risk when compared with percutaneous procedure (PTC). The existence of anastomosis in Roux-en-Y is an impediment to the conduct of endoscopic procedure. Although there are series that could demonstrate factual ERCP using ballon-enteroscopy or through previously made stomas, this is not usually available in clinical practice. When ERCP is not possible or when it is not adequate PTC could be tried.

The performance of MRI-cholangiography shows results comparable to ERCP in diagnostic aspect. In a prospective trial, MRI-cholangiography achieved 95% accuracy and 98% sensitivity, when compared to ERCP. The lack of therapeutic capability is a major drawback of the method, serving as an intermediate examination prior to invasive procedures in interventional radiology.

Treatment of biliary obstruction is time consuming, requiring multiple interventions and with high risk of relapse. The initial therapeutic option is interventional radiology procedures, endoscopic or percutaneous whenever possible. Dilation of strictures with balloon dilators when performed alone has a long-term success rate of only 40%. The placement of biliary prostheses, ranging between 7 and 10fr increases the effectiveness to about 75%. Studies with the placement of multiple parallel plastic stents solved up to 90% of cases of strictures (Williams & Draganov, 2009). The procedure should be repeated at regular intervals to prevent obstruction of the stents and cholangitis. Intervals of three to six months are well accepted, but the carrying out of more aggressive treatments at intervals of two weeks, has shown good results.

Recurrence of stenosis is the rule, with multiple procedures being needed to settle the case, with treatment periods ranging from one to two years. The use of self-expandable metal stents seems to allow a longer period of symptom relief, with need of fewer procedures, but there are still not many published results (Kusano et al. 2005).

Endoscopic treatment failure leads to the need for a surgical approach. In cases of anastomotic stenosis the resolution and prognosis are good. If the primary reconstruction is duct-to-duct anastomosis, the procedure is the conversion to Roux-en-Y hepaticojejunostomy. If the obstruction occurs on a previously performed enteric bypass the anastomosis should be reconfigured. In selected cases, some services choose to make a jejunostomy stoma to allow access to future possible endoscopic interventions in the biliary tree, if needed.

Ischemic stenosis type has a worse prognosis and lower resolvability even with surgical treatment. The failure to obtain adequate biliary drainage has a strong association with decreased graft survival. Patients with unresolved biliary strictures evolve to liver failure, with up to 30 to 50% progressing to death or retransplantation, despite continuous endoscopic and percutaneous drainage (Yazumi et al. 2006).

Retransplantation is indicated especially in cases associated with arterial thrombosis, or in cases that progress to cirrhosis secondary to chronic biliary obstruction. The mortality associated with this procedure is significantly higher than in the first transplant (Verdonk et al. 2006).

8. Other complications

In addition to fistulas and strictures, several other forms of complications can occur in the bile ducts after liver transplantation. Obstruction of the biliary tract by extrinsic causes, bleeding and recurrence of pre-existing diseases are most common (Wojcickia et al. 2008).

Extrinsic compression of the bile ducts can occur by several factors, such as hepatic hilar lymph nodes, recurrence of hepatic neoplasms, compression by other anatomical structures such as the hepatic artery and pseudoaneurysms, and because of mucoceles. Treatment of this type of compression can be with interventional radiology stenting or Roux-en-Y hepaticojejunostomy in refractory cases.

Mucocele of the cystic duct stump is infrequent, occurring when the donor cystic duct is blindly sutured to the anastomosis. The accumulation of mucus produced by the biliary epithelium leads to expansion of this segment, with compression of the common bile duct. The prevention of this complication should be performed by complete excision of the cystic duct of the donor or by section of the septum and communication of both ducts before the anastomosis. Cholangiography with typical findings of external compression and thinning of the distal bile duct make the diagnosis. The treatment is excision of the cystic duct remnant and biliary bypass with hepaticojejunostomy.

Cases of jaundice and dilatation of the distal bile duct without an obstructive factor identified on cholangiography may be due to sphincter of Oddi or ampullary dysfunction.

This variation can occur in up to 3% of transplanted patients and is justified due to denervation of autonomic plexus during the surgery. Although the diagnosis can only be confirmed with duodenal papilla manometry, the resolution after endoscopic papillotomy strongly supports this hypothesis.

The occurrence of spontaneous hemobilia is rare after liver transplantation and may occur due to rupture of pseudoaneurysms of the hepatic artery. Bleeding is more common after invasive procedures such as liver biopsies and percutaneous transhepatic cholangiography, in these cases with an incidence of 2%. The clinical presentation is of upper gastrointestinal bleeding and the diagnosis made by endoscopy. In cases of major bleeding or lack of spontaneous resolution arteriography with selective embolization of the responsible branches should be performed. Endoscopic retrograde cholangiography may be indicated for the removal of blood clots and passage of biliary stent.

Recurrent disease after liver transplant may be up to 20% of patients with autoimmune hepatitis, primary biliary cirrhosis and sclerosing cholangitis. The development of multiple biliary strictures can occur and are often difficult to differentiate from ischemic injury. In patients with confirmed diagnosis of sclerosing cholangitis prior to liver transplantation, biliary reconstruction is done preferably by Roux-en-Y hepaticojejunostomy, aiming for the prevention of recurrent disease in the receptor distal common bile duct remnant. Duct-to-duct anastomosis has been performed selectively in patients who show no signs of stenoses or inflammation in the distal bile duct during the transplant. However, a recent multicenter review showed higher risk of stenosis and lower graft survival rates in patients with primary sclerosing cholangitis undergoing duct-to-duct anastomosis compared to those submitted to Roux-en-Y hepaticojejunostomy (Welling et al. 2008).

9. Experience at unit of liver transplantation – Unicamp

Between September/1991 and May/2011 528 orthotopic liver transplants from deceased donors were conducted. Follow-up period ranged from 1 month to 19 years.

The type of biliary reconstruction used was end-to-end duct-to-duct anastomosis in 477 patients (90.4%). Biliary T-tube drains were used in only 17 patients (3.5%). Patients undergoing Roux-en-Y hepaticojejunostomy represented 9.6% of the total (51 patients). [Table 3]

We identified 95 cases of complications in the biliary tract, representing an incidence of 17.9%, consistent with the literature. Among these complications 86.3% were stenosis and 13.7% were bile leaks. The association of arterial thrombosis with biliary complications was

Type of Reconstruction	Number	(%)
Duct-to-Duct	447	(90,4%)
with T-tube	17	(3,2%)
without T-tube	460	(87,2%)
Roux-en-Y Hepaticojejunostomy	51	(9,6%)
Total	528	(100%)

Table 3. Biliary reconstruction at Unit of Liver Transplantation - Unicamp

consistent with recent reports published by various centers, with 32.6% of all leaks and strictures due to ischemic events.

The analysis of incidence of complications in relation to the type of reconstruction employed had a slightly higher complication rate of 21.5% in the group undergoing hepaticojejunostomy against 17.6% in the group with duct-to-duct anastomosis. The highest incidence of fistulas was observed after Roux-en-Y reconstruction, 36.4% versus 10.8%. But the small number of patients undergoing this type of anastomosis precluded a more detailed analysis. [Table 4]

Type of Reconstruction	Duct-to-Duct		Hepaticojejunostomy		Total	
Complications	84/477	(17,6%)	11/51	(21,5%)	95/528	(17,9%)
Bile Leaks	9	(1,9%)	4	(7,8%)	13	(2,4%)
Strictures	75	(15,7%)	7	(13,7%)	82	(15,5%)
Artery Thrombosis	28/84	(33,3%)	3/11	(27,2%)	31/95	(32,6%)

Table 4. Complications incidence related to reconstruction technique

Complications after duct-to-duct anastomosis were initially treated with endoscopic retrograde cholangiography (ERCP) in 72.6% of cases, and in about 35% of the patients this was the only treatment employed. [Figure 7] Reference to percutaneous cholangiography (PTC) was restricted in this group, in only 3.5%. Surgical treatment had to be carried out in 54% of these patients, including percutaneous drainage, laparotomy for peritonitis and sepsis and hepaticojejunostomy anastomosis conversion. [Table 5]

In the group with Roux-en-Y bileo-enteric shunt, indication of initial surgical treatment was approximately 64% and in about 20% of cases percutaneous cholangiography was performed. The main indication for surgery as initial treatment in this group is consistent with the difficulty in addressing this anastomosis by interventional radiological techniques.

Retransplant was indicated in approximately 8% of patients with biliary strictures, all of which were associated with hepatic artery thrombosis. In 85% of these patients, other forms of treatment had been tried before retransplantation. The cumulative mortality of patients undergoing retransplantation was 50%.

Treatment	Duct-to-Duct		Hepaticojejunostomy		Deaths	
ERCP	61	(72,6%)	0	-	16	(26,2%)
PTC	3	(3,5%)	2	(18,2%)	2	(40%)
Surgery	46	(54,7%)	7	(63,6%)	9	(17%)
Retransplant	6	(7,1%)	2	(18,2%)	4	(50%)
Total	84		11		26	(27,4%)

Table 5. Treatment of biliary complications at Unit of Liver Transplantation - Unicamp

The group undergoing combined surgical and endoscopic treatment showed the highest resolution rate of the complications, achieved in 75% of the cases. Despite the various forms of treatment employed, the mortality from biliary complications remained high, 27.4%, consistent with the data in the literature.

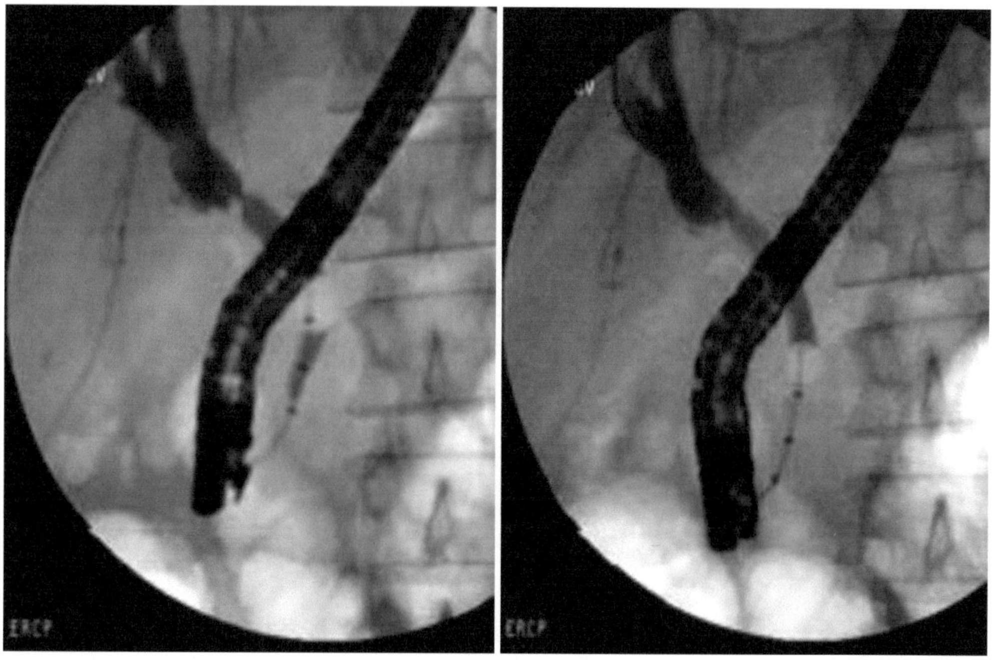

Fig. 7. Endoscopic treatment of biliary stricture. Left: Pre-procedure cholangiography with short segmental stricture. Right: Radiological control after stent placement

10. Conclusions

Several advances in the care of patients undergoing liver transplantation have increased the survival of grafts and recipients. Despite this, the complications arising in the bile ducts are still of great importance to its incidence, difficulty of treatment, morbidity and mortality.

The proper technical care in the anastomosis confection and in the selection of donors, organ preservation, reduction in the ischemic period and arterialization time are the best ways to prevent this type of complication. A fact demonstrated by the lower incidence and the increasing role of hepatic artery thrombosis in the development of biliary complications as the transplant teams gain more experience.

The diagnosis and treatment of biliary leakage and stenosis depend on a large number of imaging and interventional procedures. So the care of such patients should be individualized, depending on experience and availability of local resources.

11. References

A. Gantxegi, M. Caralt, I. Bilbao, L. Castells, J.L. Lázaro, L. Llopart, I. Díez, C. Dopazo, G. Sapisochín, M. Pérez, and R. Charco Evolution of Biliary Complications After Liver Transplantation: A Single European Series Transplantation Proceedings, 43, 745–748 (2011)

Azoulay D, Marin-Hargreaves G, Castaing D, Rene A, Bismuth H: Duct-to-duct biliary anastomosis in living related liver transplan- tation. *Arch Surg* 2001;136:1197–1200.

Emmanuelle D Williams, Peter V Draganov Endoscopic management of biliary strictures after liver transplantation *World J Gastroenterol* 2009 August 14; 15(30): 3725-3733

Kusano T, Randall HB, Roberts JP, Ascher NL: The use of stents for duct-to-duct anastomoses of biliary reconstruction in ortho- topic liver transplantation. *Hepatogastroenterology* 2005;52:695–699.

Londono MC, Balderramo D, Cardenas A. Management of biliary complications after orthotopic liver transplantation: the role of endoscopy. *World J Gastroenterol* 2008; 14: 493-497

Maciej Wojcickia, Piotr Milkiewicza, b Michael Silvac: Biliary Tract Complications after Liver Transplantation: *A Review Dig Surg* 2008;25:245–257

Noujaim HM, Gunson B, Mayer DA, Mirza DF, Candinas D, Buckels JA, McMaster P, de Ville de Goyet J: Worth continuing doing ex situ liver graft splitting? A single-center analysis. *Am J Transplant* 2003;3:318–323.

O'Connor TP, Lewis WD, Jenkins RL: Bili- ary tract complications after liver transplantation. *Ann Surg* 1995;130:312–317.

Renz JF, Emond JC, Yersiz H, Ascher NL, Bu- suttil RW: Split-liver transplantation in the United States. Outcome of a national survey. *Ann Surg* 2004;239:172–181.

Scotte M, Dousset B, Calmus Y, Conti F, Houssin D, Chapuis Y: The influence of cold ischemia time on biliary complications fol- lowing liver transplantation. *J Hepatol* 1994; 21:340–346.

Suarez F, Otero A, Solla M, Arnal F, Lorenzo MJ, Marini M, Vazquez-Iglesias JL, Gomez M: Biliary complications after liver trans- plantation from Maastricht category-2 non-heart-beating donors. *Transplantation* 2008; 85:9–14.

Testa G, Malago M, Valentin-Gamazo C, Lindell G, Broelsch CE: Biliary anastomosis in living related liver transplantation using the right liver lobe: Techniques and compli- cations. *Liver Transpl* 2000;6:710–714.

Verdonk RC, Buis CI, Porte RJ, Van der Jagt EJ, Limburg AJ, Van den Berg AP, Slooff MJ, Peeters PM, de Jong KP, Kleibeuker JH, Haagsma EB: Anastomotic biliary stric- tures after liver transplantation: causes and consequences. *Liver Transpl* 2006;12:726– 735.

Verran DJ, Asfar SK, Ghent CN, Grant DR, Wall WJ: Biliary reconstruction without T- tubes or stents in liver transplantation: re- port of 502 consecutive cases. *Liver Transpl Surg* 1997;3:365–373.

Welling TH, Heidt DG, Englesbe MJ, Magee JC, Sung RS, Campbell DA, Punch JD, Pelletier SJ. Biliary complications following liver transplantation in the model for end-stage liver disease era: effect of donor, recipient, and technical 35 factors. *Liver Transpl* 2008; 14: 73-80

Welling TH, Heidt DG, Englesbe MJ, Magee JC, Sung RS, Campbell DA, Punch JD, Pelletier SJ: Biliary complications following liv- er transplantation in the model for end-stage liver disease era: effect of donor, recipient, and technical factors. *Liver Transpl* 2008;14: 73–80.

Yazumi S, Yoshimoto T, Hisatsune H, Hasegawa K, Kiola M, Tada S, Uenoyama Y, Yamauchi J, Shio S, Kasahara M, Ogawa K, Egawa H, Tanaka K, Chiba T: Endoscopic treatment of biliary complications after right-lobe living-donor liver transplantation with duct-to-duct biliary anastomosis. *J Hepatobiliary Pancreat Surg* 2006;13:502– 510.

11

Ischemic Type Biliary Lesions

Dennis Eurich, Daniel Seehofer and Peter Neuhaus
Charité Campus Virchow / General, Visceral and Transplant Surgery / Berlin, Germany

1. Introduction

Liver transplantation (LT) is an established therapy for end-stage liver disease based on a substantial progress in surgical and immunological management of concomitant post-transplant phenomena. Apart from rejection and HCV-recurrence, the development of biliary strictures is one of the most serious complications observed after LT significantly affecting graft and patient survival [1, 2]. Frequently compared to Achilles foot, the dynamics of post-transplant biliary restitution may determine the overall transplant success and play the role of a critical step after LT. Post-transplant complications in the biliary system occur in 10-50% with significant mortality in up to 19% and re-transplantation rates of 6-12.5% [3-6]. Early post-transplant biliary complications are predominantly related to technical aspects of the operation regarding the insufficiency of bile duct anastomosis, biliary leaks or anastomotic stenosis [7]. One third of all biliary complications occur later than first two months after LT affecting intrahepatic integrity on donor side and functionality of distal parts of the biliary tree in the recipient including the bile duct anastomosis and the ampulla of Vater [1, 2, 8]. In contrast to the anastomotic strictures, which can be successfully treated endoscopically or surgically, non-anastomotic strictures represent a significant therapeutic problem [9, 10]. Non-anastomotic strictures of the bile duct may develop in up to 20% of all LTs. Untreated stricture-associated complications may lead to cholestasis, severe graft dysfunction, cholangiosepsis, secondary cirrhosis and even death [6, 8, 11, 12]. Non-anastomotic strictures may be classified according to their etiology into strictures related to PSC-recurrence (primary sclerosing cholangitis), strictures occurring due to vascular complications in case of a manifest hepatic artery thrombosis as ischemic biliary lesions (IBL), strictures occurring after prolonged ischemia (e.g. successfully treated hepatic artery thrombosis) and strictures occurring without an obvious vascular complication. In the presence of a macroscopically obviously undisturbed perfusion they are described as so-called ischemic type biliary lesions (ITBL). The occurrence of biliary lesions after primarily successful LT justifies the necessity to introduce ITBL as an independent pathologic entity. In spite of a certain descriptive inaccuracy, the terms "non-anastomotic strictures", "intrahepatic biliary strictures" and "ischemic type biliary strictures" are usually used as synonyms for post- transplant strictures, diffuse dilatations and segmental ectasia of the biliary tract as a result of inflammation and fibrotic remodeling (figs. 1 and 2) [13]. Due to terminological diversity, the incidence of ITBL significantly varies among published studies between 1.4 and 26% [1, 5, 14]. The diagnosis "ITBL" may be made only after the exclusion of vascular (IBL) and immunologic pathologies (PSC-recurrence and chronic ductopenic rejection) [1]. As a diagnosis of exclusion, ITBL is regarded as a serious transplant complication and a notable graft disease, undeniably deserving scientific attention.

1.1 Anatomical aspects of the biliary tract

Biliary tract is a complex network of ductal structures beginning with Hering-canals, merging into major ducts and finally into intestine in a highly coordinated manner [15, 16]. Apart from conductive functions, the biliary epithelium demonstrates morphological heterogeneity, which depends upon functional requirements [17]. The ability to undergo phenotypic changes, to participate in inflammatory processes and even to behave as liver progenitor cells underlines the uniqueness of cholangiocytes under physiological conditions [15, 18]. In contrast to parenchymal blood supply of liver sinusoids via portal vein and hepatic artery, biliary tree predominantly depends on the integrity of the hepatic artery and periductal plexus being more vulnerable to transplant-related disrupted blood supply and immunologic processes justifying the metaphoric comparison to Achilles foot [19, 20].

1.2 Biliary tract reconstruction

One of the most important surgical steps and goals during LT is the reconstruction of the biliary tract and the restitution of its function. The most widely employed reconstructive techniques are choledocho-choledochostomy (with or without T-tube) performed in patients with uncomplicated anatomy and intact distal segment of the biliary tract including functioning sphincter Oddi and Roux-en-Y hepatico-jejunostomy, which is usually reserved for cases with intrinsic damage to the biliary system (e.g. PSC) and technically difficult anastomosis (e.g. re-transplantation, living donor LT) [6, 21, 22]. Underlying liver disease, size of biliary tracts of the donor and the recipient, anatomic aspects, prior surgery on the biliary duct and surgeon preference may influence the choice of the reconstructive technique [23].

2. Non-anastomotic strictures: Morphology

Chronic disturbance of bile flow, accompanied by inflammatory processes, may lead to the development of irregular strictures, dilatations and sequestrations of the biliary tree (figs 1 and 2). Bacterial ascension, causing cholangitis, cholangiohepatitis and cholangiosepsis, may forward the progression of ITBL. Macroscopically, ITBL is classified according to the localization of pathological alterations in three groups (type-I: extrahepatic; type-II: intrahepatic; type-III: intra- and extrahepatic), which may determine the severity of the disease, its course and therapeutic options. Inflammation and remodeling represent the functional backbone of ITBL-development. Presence of intracellular cholestasis, abundance of lymphocytes and granulocytes and proliferation of new bile ducts represent the microscopic picture of ITBL, hardly differing from biliary pathologies with unrelated etiologies [24]. Remodeling processes result in the formation of connective tissue. Degree, localization and duration of inflammation determine the extent of the disease. Resulting in a "scar" and the perpetuation of bile flow obstruction, inflammation and progression of biliary damage may promote secondary alterations and forward extensive fibrogenesis and tissue remodelling of the graft parenchyma [25]. Finally, graft atrophy and the reduction of functional reserve may develop, compromising the result of an initially successful LT.

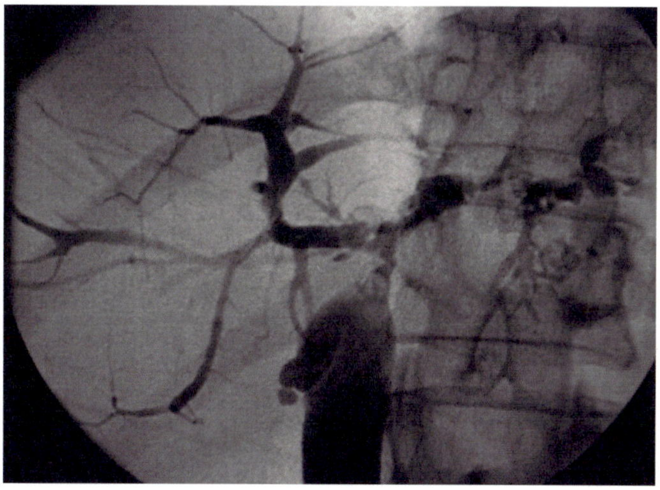

Fig. 1. Cholangiograph. Illustration of central stenosis at the level of distal right and left ductus hepatici, diffuse biliary strictures and dilatations in the left lobe, cholestasis in the right lobe. ITBL developed within the first post-transplant year

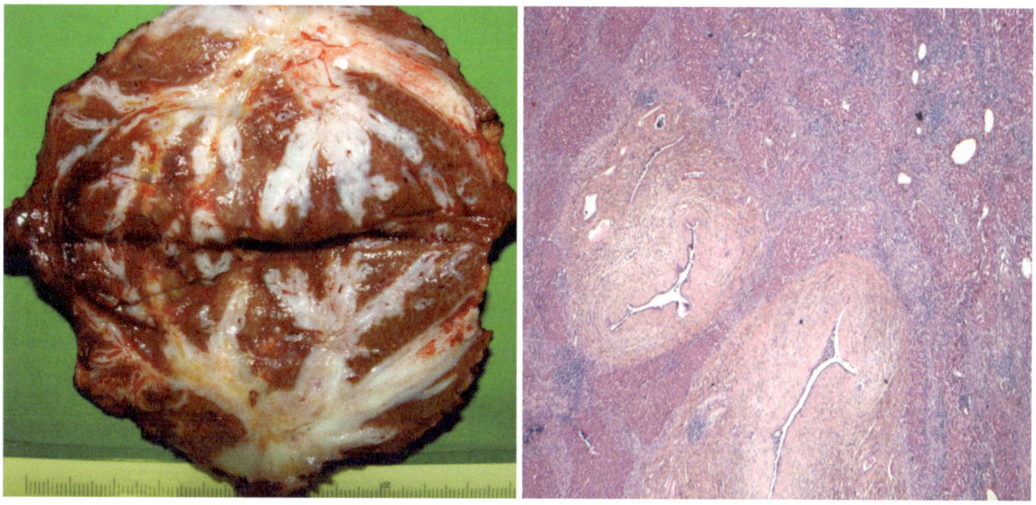

(A) (B)

Fig. 2. (A) Resected graft with ITBL (left liver lobe). Macroscopically evident atrophy of liver parenchyma with broad peribiliary shroud of connective tissue (B) Microscopic view of the same graft depicting a profound periductular inflammation (lymphocytes, granulocytes), connective tissue and remaining islets of liver parenchyma

Significant morphological similarities are observed in a non-transplant setting as well: in patients with HIV-associated cholangiopathy as vanishing bile duct-syndrome, sclerosing cholangitis and shock-liver [1, 26]. In summary, chronic inflammation caused by any noxious effectors may lead to the uniform picture described above. Frequently, significant difficulties arise in the attempt of differentiation between recurrent PSC and ITBL in the graft. Morphologically these entities may present identical pictures [1].

Variables		
Donor	Age (years)	older than 60
	Size	small-for-size
	LT-mode	living donor
Stage of liver disease	Child & Pugh	C > A or B
Surgery	Solution	UW > HTK
	Perfusion mode	retrograde caval
		gravity arterial perfusion
	Periductal tissue	little
	Reconstructive technique	hepatico-jejunostomy
Ischemic factors	Cold and warm ischemia	prolonged
	Reperfusion injury	not assessable
	Periductal plexus	altered
	Re-arterialization	present
Cholangial pressure & bile toxicitiy	External bile drainge	no T-tube
	Bile acids	high bile-to-phospholipid ratio
Immunologic factors	ABO-system	incompatible
	Immunosuppression	Low level
	Rejection	chronic / ductopenic
	Autoimmune disease	PSC, PBC, AIH
	Co-infection	CMV
	Genetic variants	CCRdelta32, Mdr-2

Table 1. Suspected risk factors for the development of ITBL

3. Pathophysiology

The process of ITBL-development is not clearly understood yet. ITBL seems to be a polygenic disease, influenced by a whole variety of confounders. Currently identified risk factors may be divided into four major pathogenetic columns: peri-operative ischemia (including preserving solution), immunologic damage, toxicity of bile salts and epidemiological confounders [1, 27]. The degree and relation of the functional impact among risk factors are not fully investigated. Hereby, ischemic injury seems to be the most important factor including cold and warm ischemia during transplantation, disturbed blood flow in the peribiliary plexus resulting from an inappropriate procurement of the donor liver with little periductal tissue, and hypoxemia during the postoperative period [12, 27]. Immunological injury including ABO-incompatibility, rejection, pre-existing liver disease with autoimmune component, CMV-Infection, immunosuppressive medication and chronic rejection also seem to play a role in the development of the non-anastomotic strictures [1, 27, 28]. Moreover, bile fluid has been shown to be toxic for the vulnerable biliary epithelium of the graft [29]. Although biliary strictures have been reported to be more frequent in transplant patients with hepatico-jejunostomy, they may occur, disregarding the type of biliary tract reconstruction [6, 30]. Finally, factors related to epidemiology (older donor age, advanced stage of pre-transplant liver disease) and donation (preservation solution, perfusion technique) also seem to be relevant in the pathogenesis of ITBL [1, 27, 31]. Table 1 summarizes currently known risk factors.

4. Diagnostics

The diagnosis of non-anastomotic lesions or ITBL is made by clinical presentation, exclusion of evident vascular complications, histological pattern and cholangiography as gold standard either by ERC (endoscopic retrograde cholangiography) or by PTC (percutaneous transhepatic cholangiography) [1, 2, 32]. Increased expertise in diagnostic and therapeutic ERC in transplant-related liver diseases has been demonstrated to be a safe and effective tool. Therefore ERC has been suggested to be the primary method for diagnosis and treatment of most transplant-related biliary complications except for acute surgical complications (broad insufficiency of biliary duct anastomosis) [33]. The diagnosis "ITBL" is made when typical signs of segmental strictures and dilatations appear on the cholangiography (fig. 1, 3, 4).

4.1 Clinical aspects

Characteristic and disease-specific aspects of clinical presentation do not exist. Symptoms reflect cholestasis and subsequent infective tendency ranging from unspecific discomfort in the right abdomen, elevated temperatures, shivering and jaundice. Clinical presentation of ITBL-patients may cover the whole range of complaints and symptoms originating from the biliary tract. Classical symptoms are pruritus, jaundice and fever. Untreated ITBL may lead to cholangiosepsis, graft insufficiency and patient death [27]. Clinically, ITBL closely resembles liver diseases with chronic inflammation of the biliary tract (PSC, SSC, cholangitis) [1].

4.2 Laboratory

Although laboratory parameters are frequently normal or only slightly elevated, alkaline phosphatase (AP), gamma glutamyltransferase (γ-GT) and bilirubin may indicate pathological processes in the biliary tree. Biochemical results do not reliably reflect early stages of the disease and easily be misinterpreted as normal or acceptable in the post-transplant setting. Highly sensitive but not disease-specific, laboratory parameters are, nevertheless, helpful as a non-invasive tool and their deviation is frequently the first sign perceived in the outpatient setting of most follow-up programs. Cholestatic profile with leukocytosis usually indicates complicated biliary pathology. Clinical symptoms and pathological laboratory findings may necessitate hospitalization and the initiation of further diagnostic procedures [32].

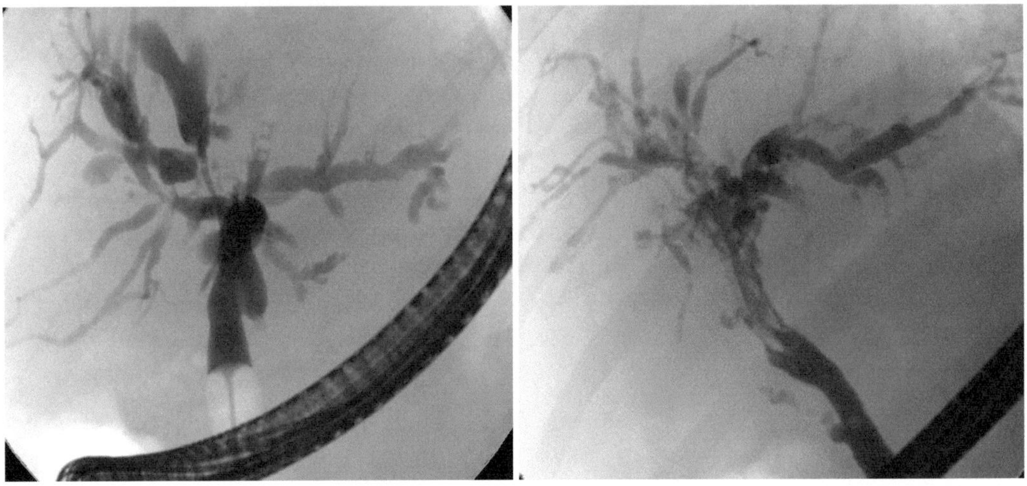

(A) (B)

Fig. 3. (A) Cholangiograph (ERC): Illustration of central stenosis at the level of distal right and left ductus hepatici, diffuse biliary strictures and dilatations in the left lobe and cholestasis in the right lobe. (B) Cholangiograph (ERC): Diffuse strictures and dilatations nearly in the entire biliary tree

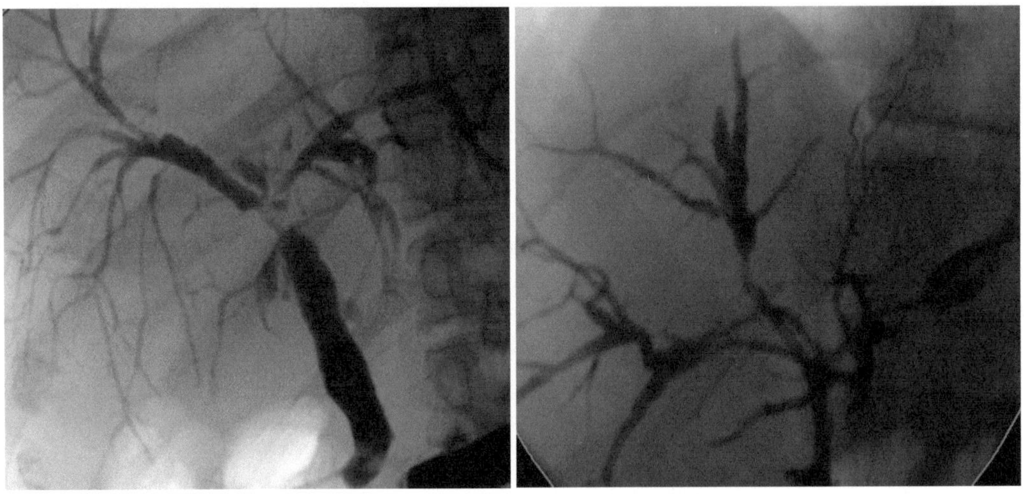

(A) (B)

Fig. 4. (A) Cholangiograph (ERC): Central stenosis and proximal cholestasis in both graft lobes (B) Cholangiograph (ERC): Relevant strictures close to the biliary bifurcation with dilatations in both graft lobes

4.3 Radiology

Radiological examination is the most important column in ITBL-diagnostics comprising conventional X-ray performed during ERC or PTC and indirect imaging methods: ultrasound, computer tomography (CT) and magnetic resonance cholangiography (MRC).

4.3.1 Ultrasound

As a safe and easily accessible tool, ultrasound examination including Doppler-mode is definitely helpful and routinely performed to rule out vascular causes for biliary dysfunction. In contrast to early changes, advanced stages of ITBL may well be assessed by ultrasound, revealing dilatations, stenosis and sediment, which predispose to the development of secondary complications regarding infection and disease progression. However, morphologic differences between naive liver and graft must be considered. Due to a higher stiffness of the graft, dilatations caused by strictures tend to appear more slowly and less distinctly in the affected biliary tract and may remain invisible or mistaken for normal conditions on a routine ultrasound examination.

4.3.2 Conventional cholangiography

Cholangiography is usually performed by ERC as the method of choice, if technically possible in the absence of contra-indications [9, 32]. Based on the classical endoscopic examination of the upper digestive tract, the goal of ERC is the visualization of the biliary tract by a selective instillation of contrast agent through the sphincter Oddi (fig. 3, 4). As a rather invasive diagnostic method, ERC should be performed with maximal accuracy, in order to avoid frequently observed pancreatitis, which is a potentially severe iatrogenic complication [34]. In contrast to the usually easily assessable biliary tract, if reconstructed as standard choledochocholedochostomy, endoscopic cholangiography is impossible with the majority of patients with hepatico-jejunostomy [32]. Occasionally, ERC may be feasible in patients with short efferent loops of hepatico-jejunal anastomosis if examined by experienced endoscopists. In most cases, cholangiography must be performed percutaneously as transhepatic punction and instillation of contrast fluid in the biliary system (fig. 6) [2, 35]. Elevated pressure and subsequent dilatation of the biliary tract may facilitate the examination. In spite of high effectiveness, transhepatic punction may cause graft damage, bleeding and injury of adjacent abdominal organs. Therefore, maximal accuracy and caution are required when applying this method. Simultaneous diagnostic and therapeutical options are the major advantages of conventional cholangiography (ERC or PTC).

4.3.3 Computer tomography (CT)

CT-scan may accurately visualize graft perfusion using contrast agent and biliary pathology regarding the localization, structural changes and secondary complications (abscess, atrophy). In spite of frequent incapability to detect short segment stenosis without pre stenotic dilatations, full-blown ITBL can easily be diagnosed by this method [32, 36]. In general, CT is considered to be a reliable diagnostic tool.

4.3.4 Magnetic resonance cholangiography (MRC)

MRC is a reliable noninvasive technique to visualize the biliary anastomosis and depict biliary strictures after LT (fig. 5) [37]. MR-cholangiography has been shown to be an accurate imaging technique to non-invasively detect biliary complications in patients especially in patients with bilio-enteric anastomosis with high positive and negative predictive values [32, 38]. However, no direct therapeutical options are available during this procedure. Non-invasiveness and significant risk reduction for side events are major advantages of MRC. Further progress in MRC-processing may increase the potential to complement or even replace conventional cholangiographic methods [32].

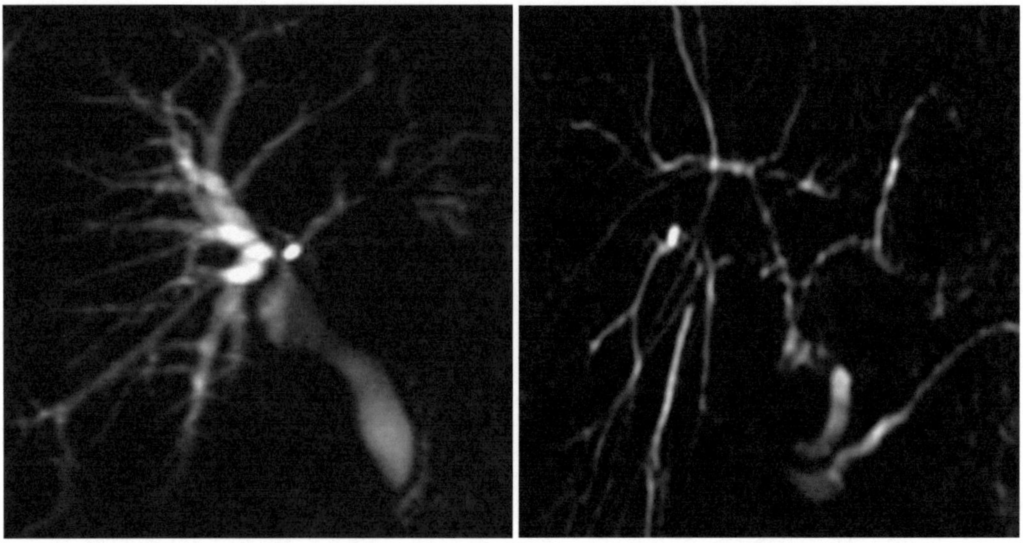

(A) (B)

Fig. 5. (A) Cholangiograph (MRC): Central strictures and proximal diffuse dilatation (B) Cholangiograph (MRC): Diffuse strictures and dilatations of the entire biliary tract

5. Therapy

Early identification of high risk patients for ITBL-occurrence may help to initiate necessary therapeutical steps and possibly prevent disease progression. The goal of ITBL-treatment implies the reduction of morbidity and mortality among the diseased transplant population. Previously, surgery including re-transplantation of the diseased liver had been thought to be the leading therapeutical option for ITBL-patients [39]. Modern ITBL-treatment strategy comprises a multimodal approach and an excellent cooperation between departments of radiology, endoscopy and surgery (fig. 6) [2, 10, 25]. In most cases the treatment of strictures is performed conservatively by endoscopic or transhepatic dilatation [24, 33, 40]. Supportive measures should comprise antibiotic prophylaxis and treatment with ursodesoxycholic acid [2].

5.1 Endoscopic and transhepatic treatment

Most of the ITBL-patients are currently treated by the endoscopic or percutaneous placement of stents and balloon dilatation [32, 33, 40]. However, significantly different success rates are observed depending upon the localization and occurrence of the strictures. Anastomotic strictures are usually easier to treat than intrahepatic lesions. Early non-anastomotic strictures demonstrate higher success rates than strictures appearing later than three months after LT [41-43]. Endoscopic and transhepatic treatment options are limited in patients with impaired liver function similarly to the diagnostic procedure. Complication rates (bleeding, pancreatitis) are reported to be 3.4% for PTC and up to 7% for endoscopic treatment [44].

5.2 Surgery

Surgical intervention may still be required in patients who do not respond to dilatative treatment or in patients with circumscribed localization of the strictures either in the extrahepatic biliary tree or resectable graft lobe [2, 33, 39]. Endoscopic or radiological dilatation of strictures has been shown to be ineffective in some patients, who may profit from surgical treatment [10]. Therefore, reconstructive surgical approach should be reserved to ITBL patients not responsive to endoscopic or trans-hepatic interventions [2].

5.2.1 Resection

Sufficient evidence exists about beneficial effects of partial graft resection, resection of biliary bifurcation and performance of hepatico-jejunostomy in liver transplant recipients with anatomically limited biliary damage, thus avoiding re-transplantation and preserving scarce donor organs [25, 45, 46]. In spite of higher vulnerability of the graft and a certain reluctance, graft resection in ITBL-patients with a sufficient graft function is possible and comparable to common liver surgery.

5.2.2 Re-transplantation

In spite of encouraging progress in interventional non-surgical ITBL-treatment, and achievements in graft resection, up to 50% of patients with non-anastomotic strictures still require re-transplantation of the liver [30, 43, 47, 48]. Re-transplantation of the liver is supposed to be the definitive therapy of graft damage being the last resort of therapeutical options. Unfortunately, survival rates after re-transplantation are significantly lower than after first LT. In technically more complicated re-transplant setting, cold ischemia and MELD-score have been shown to be associated with higher mortality rates [49]. Prevention of re-transplantation should be aspired as the goal of ITBL-treatment, especially in the era of organ shortage.

In summary, ITBL-treatment may require an unpredictable amount of patience regarding the strategy, performance and follow-up. Exemplarily, more than two dozens of dilatative interventions and one graft resection (left hemihepatectomy) have been reported in one case of successful ITBL-treatment, preventing re-transplantation of the liver (fig. 6) [25].

6. Prevention

The principle of ITBL-prevention focuses on the major pathogenic factors mentioned above and should be considered in the peri-operative period as far as possible. Hereby, allocation, preservation, reduction of ischemia, reconstructive techniques and adequate immunosuppression seem to be very important. Once, immunological effects were claimed to cause spasms in hepatic arteries, resulting in hypoxemia of the bile duct system [50]. Currently, the mechanism of the disease is considered to be multifactorial. Immunological injury including ABO-incompatibility, rejection, pre-existing disease with autoimmune component, CMV-Infection and chronic rejection also seem to play a role in the development of the non-anastomotic strictures [12, 47]. Finally the toxicity of the bile fluid has been shown to be relevant in the pathogenesis of ITBL [51]. In summary, the development of ITBL is influenced by a whole range of donor, recipient, technical and immunological factors.

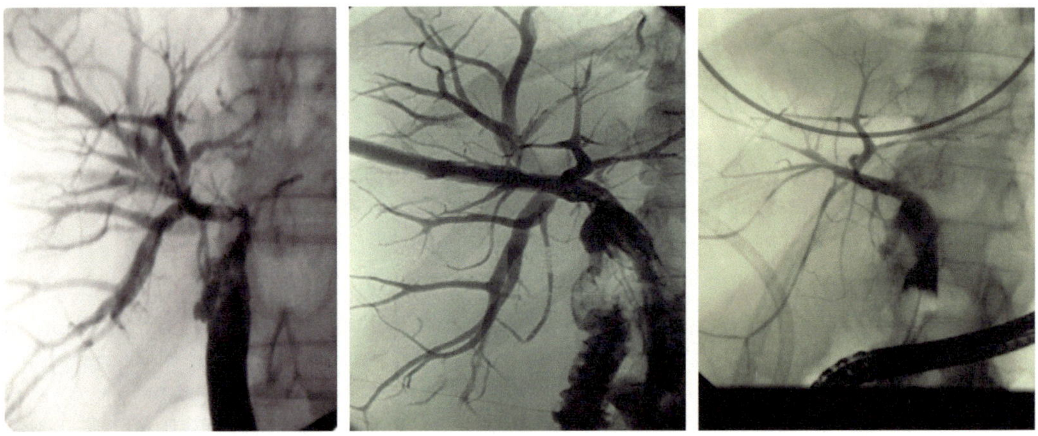

(A) (B) (C)

Fig. 6. (A) ERC after left hemihepatectomy in a patient with ITBL after LT for HCV-induced cirrhosis demonstrating a significant stenosis of the right hepatic duct and proximal dilatations (B) PTC via Yamakawa-drain of the same patient during the dilatative treatment (C) ERC after the completion of treatment depicting acceptable conditions in the right biliary tree

6.1 Ischemic time

Several studies have demonstrated a significant correlation of ITBL-incidence with ischemic time before reperfusion. In spite of controversial discussion, cold ischemic time especially of more than 10 hours may affect the development of ITBL [1, 12, 52]. Analogously, re oxigenation and warm ischemia time also seem to be involved in the pathogenesis of the disease [27, 53]. Moreover, delayed re-arterialization of the graft may favor the occurrence of ITBL [2, 43, 54]. Therefore, the time period between explantation and reperfusion should be as short as possible under an adequate preserving temperature.

6.2 Epidemiologic aspects

The use of donor organs particularly older than 60 years is associated with ITBL [1, 31]. Furthermore, patients with advanced liver disease before transplantation seem to be more likely to develop ITBL compared to lower Child and Pugh-stages [1]. Deteriorated pre-operative status, early biliary complications and "small-for-size" transplantation are currently suspected to contribute to the occurrence and progression of ITBL [55]. Further potential confounders regarding the recipient (age, gender) do not seem to play a significant role in the pathogenesis of ITBL [1]. Interestingly, the incidence of ITBL seems to be higher in patients undergoing living-donor-liver-transplantation of the right lobe [14, 56]. A differentiated selection of donor and recipient simply based on epidemiological data might help to avoid the accumulation of predisposing factors.

6.3 Reconstructive technique

In spite of ischemia reduction in LDLT-recipients, the increased susceptibility may be explained by the difference of biliary reconstruction, which is performed as hepatico-jejunostomy compared choledocho-choledochostomy in patients receiving whole organs. Bacterial ascension leading to cholangitis may negate the expected advantage of reduced cold ischemia time [55, 57]. Thus, the main advantages of choledocho-choledochostomy comprise the integrity of anatomic barrier regarding the reflux of intestinal flora to a great extent, better technical feasibility than Roux-en-Y and physiological condition for an endoscopic access [35, 58]. Choledocho-choledochostomy in side-to-side-technique seems to be the most reliable reconstructive method [22, 59]. Particular attention should be paid to periductal tissue. The integrity of the periductal vascular plexus must be guaranteed.

6.4 Preservation and perfusion

Among the two commonly used preservation solutions, the UW-solution (University of Wisconsin) has been shown to increase the risk of ITBL-occurrence compared to the less viscous HTK-solution [1, 60, 61]. Furthermore, retrograde graft perfusion via vena cava seems to exhibit a negative effect on the development of ITBL, whereas, additional back-table arterial graft perfusion lowers the risk of ITBL [1, 62]. Regular gravity arterial perfusion has been suspected to be insufficient to flush the arterial system of the biliary tract completely [1]. All inflammatory active and potential fibrogenic blood compounds should be removed before transplantation. Therefore, additional arterial pressure perfusion preferably with a HTK-solution should be performed [1].

6.5 Toxicity of the bile

Bile acids may exhibit their toxic potential on vulnerable cholangiocellular epithelium and therefore, be relevant in the pathogenesis of ITBL. In contrast to hydrophilic bile salts, hydrophobic compounds are cytotoxic [29, 63]. Prolonged warm ischemia is associated with the formation of an unfavorable bile salt-to-phospholipid ratio subsequently contributing to bile duct injury [51]. The exposure of biliary epithelium to toxic bile compounds can be minimized by the careful retrograde flushing of the bile duct with perfusion solution during liver explantation, strictly avoiding bile duct ligation [27].

6.6 Genetic aspects

Highly variable rates of functional impairment suggest the existence of endogenous risk compounds both in natural and post-transplant settings of the disease. The maximal capacity to produce different levels of cytokines in response to noxious stimulation has been shown to be under genetic control and differs among liver graft recipients. Chemokine receptor 5delta32 polymorphism has been suggested to increase the incidence of ITBL and to reduce patient survival [64]. As demonstrated in a rat model, genetic polymorphisms of the multidrug resistance protein 2 (Mdr-2), which is involved in the regulative processes of bile fluid composition, may negatively affect bile salt to phospholipid ratio, and contribute to cholangiocellular vulnerability [27]. Although, the exact mechanism is not yet understood in detail, both, donor and recipient genetics may interact. The expression of disease-related effectors may be individual and tissue dependant [65]. In spite of the pathogenetic heterogeneity, the role of genetic variants in the development of ITBL should be investigated in large scale multi-center trials regarding diagnostic, therapeutic and predictive values. Currently, no conclusion can be made considering ITBL-management.

6.7 External bile drainage

Internal or external drainage of the bile in the early postoperative period may have an impact on the development of non-anastomotic strictures [34]. Although the external bile drainage via T-tube is currently a subject of controversy, T-tube insertion has been demonstrated to reduce the risk for ITBL in several randomized studies and recent a meta-analysis [23, 34, 66-69]. T-tube may prevent the occurrence of ITBL and potentially reduces long-term morbidity especially regarding late strictures [34, 67]. The arterial perfusion of the biliary tract, which is at risk in transplant setting, remains one of the most important determinants of ITBL. Manipulations on ligamentum hepatoduodenale may affect the function of sphincter Oddi and result in discoordinated motility of the biliary tract. [6, 33]. Sphincter spasms may contribute to bile flow obstruction as demonstrated by elevated intra-biliary pressure after LT, which has been observed to be twice as high (up to 20mm H_2O) as in livers without dyskinesia of the biliary tract (10mm H_2O) (unpublished data). Elevated intra-biliary pressure may aggravate blood supply, which is predominantly maintained by periductal arterial plexus [20, 70]. Any kind of tools, which are capable of pressure reduction (intra-operative insertion of T-tube, pre-transplant sphincterotomy) should be regarded as helpful methods for ITBL-prevention. Moreover, T-tube has been demonstrated to prevent bile leakage in split-liver transplantation via pressure reduction [71]. Therefore, T-tube should be used in biliary tract reconstruction as side-to-side choledocho-choledochostomy during LT, in order to avoid the negative effect of elevated pressure and theoretically increased toxic impact of bile acids [59, 66].

6.8 Immunological aspects

Although a rejection is likely to induce significant damage in the biliary tree, no clear evidence is currently available about the role in the development of ITBL except for chronic ductopenic rejection [1, 2]. Compared to sinusoidal liver parenchyma, cholangiocytes are more vulnerable and seem to have less potential for regeneration [15]. Triggered by insufficient immunosuppression, immune complexes may induce inflammatory and fibrotic processes in tiny arteries of the biliary tract, thus forwarding ischemic damage [47, 72, 73]. Unfortunately, only inconsistent data are currently present regarding the role of immunosuppression mode and CMV-infection in the development of ITBL [1, 2]. Therefore, these factors should be re-evaluated in larger cohorts based on multi-center concepts. In contrast to patients transplanted due to virally or metabolically induced liver disease, the immunosuppression in patients with autoimmune component should be sufficient and preferably stronger according to current standards, in order to prevent rejection processes. ABO-incompatibility should be completely avoided because the antigens of the blood-type system may also be expressed on biliary epithelium and serve as immunologic target for preformed blood group antibodies.

7. Conclusion and future prospective

The development of non-anastomotic strictures in the biliary tract after LT is a serious post-transplant complication, potentially compromising the initial success of the surgical treatment of patients with advanced liver disease. ITBL represents a post-transplant biliary disease, which cannot be explained by vascular damage or PSC-recurrence. Due to a strong similarity to ischemia-induced biliary injury, and ischemia-reperfusion injury, disrupted or disturbed microcirculation seems to be the main pathogenic column. Most probably, ITBL develops in a highly individual manner from ischemic injury acquired in the peri-operative period predominantly before LT in spite of the restored arterial blood supply. The integrity of arterial perfusion separates ischemia-related strictures from IBL, playing a central role in the definition of the disease. In spite of the significant correlation between ITBL-incidence and pre-transplant ischemia, current definition of ITBL, based on radiological evidence of an undisturbed graft perfusion, does not depict the actual extent of ischemic damage. The assessment of ischemia- and reperfusion-related alterations should be therefore performed at the cellular level. Moreover, additive ischemic damage caused by thrombosis of the hepatic artery, occurring in about 10%, may contribute to the total cellular hypoxygenation. Not assessable pathogenic effect of prolonged ischemia in patients after a successful thrombectomy and restitution of blood supply may increase the risk for the development of ITBL in spite of formally intact vascular status. Unfortunately, current definition of ITBL does not allow a clear categorization of this subpopulation. Remarkable similarities of ITBL and PSC or biliary pathologies in non-transplant setting resulting from chronic inflammation, fibrotic remodeling with a secondary loss of organ function seem to be uniform. Although patients transplanted due to PSC may also develop ITBL, no diagnostic method can definitively guarantee the differentiation between ITBL and PSC-recurrence. Therefore, the relatively high chance of misclassification regarding patient cohorts undergoing statistical analysis of etiologic risk factors including epidemiologic aspects may explain differences in ITBL-incidence reported in the literature [10, 74]. After the exclusion of PSC-patients and managed post-transplant vascular complications the incidence of ITBL is supposed to be much lower than 20% [27, 40, 47, 75]. Recent analysis performed in a homogenous cohort after the exclusion of patients with prolonged re-arterialization and PSC-recurrence, seems to reflect the incidence of ITBL (3.9%) most accurately [1]. Therefore, a precise and uniform definition of the disease, awareness of risk factors and potential confounders may help to understand the mechanism of ITBL-development, prevent its occurrence and progression, select and initiate an adequate treatment. Any progress in the understanding of the development and clinical course of post-transplant biliary strictures should be welcome at a time of donor organ shortage.

8. References

[1] Heidenhain C, Pratschke J, Puhl G, Neumann U, Pascher A, Veltzke-Schlieker W et al. Incidence of and risk factors for ischemic-type biliary lesions following orthotopic liver transplantation. Transpl Int; 23:14- 22.

[2] Pascher A, Neuhaus P. Bile duct complications after liver transplantation. Transpl Int 2005;18:627-642.

[3] Jeffrey GP, Brind AM, Ormonde DG, Frazer CK, Ferguson J, Bell R et al. Management of biliary tract complications following liver transplantation. Aust N Z J Surg 1999;69:717-722.

[4] Koivusalo A, Isoniemi H, Salmela K, Edgren J, von Numers H, Hockerstedt K. Biliary complications in one hundred adult liver transplantations. Scand J Gastroenterol 1996;31:506-511.
[5] Li S, Stratta RJ, Langnas AN, Wood RP, Marujo W, Shaw BW, Jr. Diffuse biliary tract injury after orthotopic liver transplantation. Am J Surg 1992;164:536-540.
[6] Greif F, Bronsther OL, Van Thiel DH, Casavilla A, Iwatsuki S, Tzakis A et al. The incidence, timing, and management of biliary tract complications after orthotopic liver transplantation. Ann Surg 1994;219:40- 45.
[7] Moser MA, Wall WJ. Management of biliary problems after liver transplantation. Liver Transpl 2001;7:S46-52.
[8] Lewis WD, Jenkins RL. Biliary strictures after liver transplantation. Surg Clin North Am 1994;74:967-978.
[9] Hintze RE, Abou-Rebyeh H, Adler A, Veltzke W, Langrehr J, Wiedenmann B et al. [Endoscopic therapy of ischemia-type biliary lesions in patients following orthotopic liver transplantation]. Z Gastroenterol 1999;37:13-20.
[10] Thethy S, Thomson B, Pleass H, Wigmore SJ, Madhavan K, Akyol M et al. Management of biliary tract complications after orthotopic liver transplantation. Clin Transplant 2004;18:647-653.
[11] Porayko MK, Kondo M, Steers JL. Liver transplantation: late complications of the biliary tract and their management. Semin Liver Dis 1995;15:139-155.
[12] Guichelaar MM, Benson JT, Malinchoc M, Krom RA, Wiesner RH, Charlton MR. Risk factors for and clinical course of non-anastomotic biliary strictures after liver transplantation. Am J Transplant 2003;3:885-890.
[13] Ludwig J, Batts KP, MacCarty RL. Ischemic cholangitis in hepatic allografts. Mayo Clin Proc 1992;67:519-526.
[14] Nakamura T, Tanaka K, Kiuchi T, Kasahara M, Oike F, Ueda M et al. Anatomical variations and surgical strategies in right lobe living donor liver transplantation: lessons from 120 cases. Transplantation 2002;73:1896-1903.
[15] Strazzabosco M, Fabris L. Functional anatomy of normal bile ducts. Anat Rec (Hoboken) 2008;291:653- 660.
[16] Roskams TA, Theise ND, Balabaud C, Bhagat G, Bhathal PS, Bioulac-Sage P et al. Nomenclature of the finer branches of the biliary tree: canals, ductules, and ductular reactions in human livers. Hepatology 2004;39:1739-1745.
[17] Crawford AR, Lin XZ, Crawford JM. The normal adult human liver biopsy: a quantitative reference standard. Hepatology 1998;28:323-331.
[18] Sell S. Heterogeneity and plasticity of hepatocyte lineage cells. Hepatology 2001;33:738-750.
[19] Abt P, Crawford M, Desai N, Markmann J, Olthoff K, Shaked A. Liver transplantation from controlled non- heart-beating donors: an increased incidence of biliary complications. Transplantation 2003;75:1659- 1663.
[20] Kono NNakanuma Y. Ultrastructural and immunohistochemical studies of the intrahepatic peribiliary capillary plexus in normal livers and extrahepatic biliary obstruction in human beings. Hepatology 1992;15:411-418.
[21] Neuhaus P, Platz KP. Liver transplantation: newer surgical approaches. Baillieres Clin Gastroenterol 1994;8:481-493.

[22] Nuno J, Vicente E, Turrion VS, Pereira F, Ardaiz J, Cuervas V et al. Biliary tract reconstruction after liver transplantation: with or without T-tube? Transplant Proc 1997;29:564-565.

[23] Paes-Barbosa FC, Massarollo PC, Bernardo WM, Ferreira FG, Barbosa FK, Raslan M et al. Systematic review and meta-analysis of biliary reconstruction techniques in orthotopic deceased donor liver transplantation. J Hepatobiliary Pancreat Sci;18:525-536.

[24] Abou-Rebyeh H, Veltzke-Schlieker W, Radke C, Steinmuller T, Wiedenmann B, Hintze RE. Complete bile duct sequestration after liver transplantation, caused by ischemic-type biliary lesions. Endoscopy 2003;35:616-620.

[25] Eurich D, Seehofer D, Veltzke-Schlieker W, Neuhaus R, Neumann U, Neuhaus P. Successful endoscopic and surgical management of non-anastomotic biliary strictures after liver transplantation - case report. Ann Transplant 2009;14:47-51.

[26] Hindupur S, Yeung M, Shroff P, Fritz J, Kirmani N. Vanishing bile duct syndrome in a patient with advanced AIDS. HIV Med 2007;8:70-72.

[27] Buis CI, Hoekstra H, Verdonk RC, Porte RJ. Causes and consequences of ischemic-type biliary lesions after liver transplantation. J Hepatobiliary Pancreat Surg 2006;13:517-524.

[28] Urbani L, Mazzoni A, Bianco I, Grazzini T, De Simone P, Catalano G et al. The role of immunomodulation in ABO-incompatible adult liver transplant recipients. J Clin Apher 2008;23:55-62.

[29] Hertl M, Hertl MC, Kluth D, Broelsch CE. Hydrophilic bile salts protect bile duct epithelium during cold preservation: a scanning electron microscopy study. Liver Transpl 2000;6:207-212.

[30] O'Connor TP, Lewis WDJenkins RL. Biliary tract complications after liver transplantation. Arch Surg 1995;130:312-317.

[31] Serrano MT, Garcia-Gil A, Arenas J, Ber Y, Cortes L, Valiente C et al. Outcome of liver transplantation using donors older than 60 years of age. Clin Transplant;24:543- 549.

[32] Zoepf T, Maldonado-Lopez EJ, Hilgard P, Dechene A, Malago M, Broelsch CE et al. Diagnosis of biliary strictures after liver transplantation: which is the best tool? World J Gastroenterol 2005;11:2945-2948.

[33] Pfau PR, Kochman ML. Endoscopic management of biliary tract disease. Curr Opin Gastroenterol 1999;15:448-453.

[34] Weiss S, Schmidt SC, Ulrich F, Pascher A, Schumacher G, Stockmann M et al. Biliary reconstruction using a side-to-side choledochocholedochostomy with or without T-tube in deceased donor liver transplantation: a prospective randomized trial. Ann Surg 2009;250:766-771.

[35] Hisatsune H, Yazumi S, Egawa H, Asada M, Hasegawa K, Kodama Y et al. Endoscopic management of biliary strictures after duct-to-duct biliary reconstruction in rightlobe living-donor liver transplantation. Transplantation 2003;76:810-815.

[36] Quiroga S, Sebastia MC, Margarit C, Castells L, Boye R, Alvarez-Castells A. Complications of orthotopic liver transplantation: spectrum of findings with helical CT. Radiographics 2001;21:1085-1102.

[37] Pecchi A, De Santis M, Gibertini MC, Tarantino G, Gerunda GE, Torricelli P et al. Role of magnetic resonance imaging in the detection of anastomotic biliary strictures after liver transplantation. Transplant Proc;43:1132-1135.

[38] Collettini F, Kroencke TJ, Heidenhain C, de Bucourt M, Renz D, Schott E et al. Ischemic type biliary lesions after ortothopic liver transplantation: diagnosis with magnetic resonance cholangiography. Transplant Proc;43:2660-2663.
[39] Schlitt HJ, Meier PN, Nashan B, Oldhafer KJ, Boeker K, Flemming P et al. Reconstructive surgery for ischemic-type lesions at the bile duct bifurcation after liver transplantation. Ann Surg 1999;229:137-145.
[40] Rizk RS, McVicar JP, Emond MJ, Rohrmann CA, Jr., Kowdley KV, Perkins J et al. Endoscopic management of biliary strictures in liver transplant recipients: effect on patient and graft survival. Gastrointest Endosc 1998;47:128-135.
[41] Thuluvath PJ, Atassi TLee J. An endoscopic approach to biliary complications following orthotopic liver transplantation. Liver Int 2003;23:156-162.
[42] Jagannath S, Kalloo AN. Biliary Complications After Liver Transplantation. Curr Treat Options Gastroenterol 2002;5:101-112.
[43] Colonna JO, 2nd, Shaked A, Gomes AS, Colquhoun SD, Jurim O, McDiarmid SV et al. Biliary strictures complicating liver transplantation. Incidence, pathogenesis, management, and outcome. Ann Surg 1992;216:344-350; discussion 350-342.
[44] Boraschi P, Braccini G, Gigoni R, Sartoni G, Neri E, Filipponi F et al. Detection of biliary complications after orthotopic liver transplantation with MR cholangiography. Magn Reson Imaging 2001;19:1097-1105.
[45] Guckelberger O, Stange B, Glanemann M, Lopez-Hanninen E, Heidenhain C, Jonas S et al. Hepatic resection in liver transplant recipients: single center experience and review of the literature. Am J Transplant 2005;5:2403-2409.
[46] Filipponi F, Vistoli F, Urbani 1 L, Mosca F. Extended right hepatectomy as graft-saving option in non- anastomotic biliary strictures after liver transplantation. Hepatogastroenterology 2002;49:1679-1681.
[47] Rull R, Garcia Valdecasas JC, Grande L, Fuster J, Lacy AM, Gonzalez FX et al. Intrahepatic biliary lesions after orthotopic liver transplantation. Transpl Int 2001;14:129-134.
[48] Sanchez-Urdazpal L, Gores GJ, Ward EM, Maus TP, Buckel EG, Steers JL et al. Diagnostic features and clinical outcome of ischemic-type biliary complications after liver transplantation. Hepatology 1993;17:605-609.
[49] Zhu ZJ, Rao W, Sun JS, Cai JZ, Deng YL, Zheng H et al. Liver retransplantation for ischemic-type biliary lesions after orthotopic liver transplantation: a clinical report of 66 cases. Hepatobiliary Pancreat Dis Int 2008;7:471-475.
[50] Nakamura K, Murase N, Becich MJ, Furuya T, Todo S, Fung JJ et al. Liver allograft rejection in sensitized recipients. Observations in a clinically relevant small animal model. Am J Pathol 1993;142:1383-1391.
[51] Yska MJ, Buis CI, Monbaliu D, Schuurs TA, Gouw AS, Kahmann ON et al. The role of bile salt toxicity in the pathogenesis of bile duct injury after non-heart-beating porcine liver transplantation. Transplantation 2008;85:1625-1631.
[52] Sanchez-Urdazpal L, Gores GJ, Ward EM, Hay E, Buckel EG, Wiesner RH et al. Clinical outcome of ischemic-type biliary complications after liver transplantation. Transplant Proc 1993;25:1107-1109.
[53] Noack K, Bronk SF, Kato A, Gores GJ. The greater vulnerability of bile duct cells to reoxygenation injury than to anoxia. Implications for the pathogenesis of biliary strictures after liver transplantation. Transplantation 1993;56:495-500.

[54] Sanchez-Urdazpal L, Gores GJ, Ward EM, Maus TP, Wahlstrom HE, Moore SB et al. Ischemic-type biliary complications after orthotopic liver transplantation. Hepatology 1992;16:49-53.
[55] Kasahara M, Egawa H, Takada Y, Oike F, Sakamoto S, Kiuchi T et al. Biliary reconstruction in right lobe living-donor liver transplantation: Comparison of different techniques in 321 recipients. Ann Surg 2006;243:559-566.
[56] Trotter JF, Wachs M, Everson GT, Kam I. Adult-to-adult transplantation of the right hepatic lobe from a living donor. N Engl J Med 2002;346:1074-1082.
[57] Ikegami T, Taketomi A, Soejima Y, Yoshizumi T, Shimada M, Maehara Y. Characteristics of biliary reconstruction using a T-tube as compared with other methods in left-lobe adult living-donor liver transplantation. J Hepatobiliary Pancreat Surg 2008;15:346-347.
[58] Ishiko T, Egawa H, Kasahara M, Nakamura T, Oike F, Kaihara S et al. Duct-to-duct biliary reconstruction in living donor liver transplantation utilizing right lobe graft. Ann Surg 2002;236:235-240.
[59] Neuhaus P, Blumhardt G, Bechstein WO, Steffen R, Platz KP, Keck H. Technique and results of biliary reconstruction using side-to-side choledochocholedochostomy in 300 orthotopic liver transplants. Ann Surg 1994;219:426-434.
[60] Canelo R, Hakim NS, Ringe B. Experience with hystidine tryptophan ketoglutarate versus University Wisconsin preservation solutions in transplantation. Int Surg 2003;88:145-151.
[61] Buis CI, V 1 erdonk RC, Van der Jagt EJ, van der Hilst CS, Slooff MJ, Haagsma EB et al. Nonanastomotic biliary strictures after liver transplantation, part 1: Radiological features and risk factors for early vs. late presentation. Liver Transpl 2007;13:708-718.
[62] Heidenhain C, Heise M, Jonas S, Ben-Asseur M, Puhl G, Mittler J et al. Retrograde reperfusion via vena cava lowers the risk of initial nonfunction but increases the risk of ischemic-type biliary lesions in liver transplantation--a randomized clinical trial. Transpl Int 2006;19:738-748.
[63] Geuken E, Visser D, Kuipers F, Blokzijl H, Leuvenink HG, de Jong KP et al. Rapid increase of bile salt secretion is associated with bile duct injury after human liver transplantation. J Hepatol 2004;41:1017- 1025.
[64] Moench C, Uhrig A, Lohse AW, Otto G. CC chemokine receptor 5delta32 polymorphism-a risk factor for ischemic-type biliary lesions following orthotopic liver transplantation. Liver Transpl 2004;10:434-439.
[65] Eurich D, Boas-Knoop S, Ruehl M, Schulz M, Carrillo ED, Berg T et al. Relationship between the interleukin-28b gene polymorphism and the histological severity of hepatitis C virus-induced graft inflammation and the response to antiviral therapy after liver transplantation. Liver Transpl;17:289-298.
[66] Riediger C, Muller MW, Michalski CW, Huser N, Schuster T, Kleeff J et al. T-Tube or no T-tube in the reconstruction of the biliary tract during orthotopic liver transplantation: systematic review and meta- analysis. Liver Transpl;16:705-717.
[67] Randall HB, Wachs ME, Somberg KA, Lake JR, Emond JC, Ascher NL et al. The use of the T tube after orthotopic liver transplantation. Transplantation 1996;61:258-261.
[68] Vougas V, Rela M, Gane E, Muiesan P, Melendez HV, Williams R et al. A prospective randomised trial of bile duct reconstruction at liver transplantation: T tube or no T tube? Transpl Int 1996;9:392-395.

[69] Rabkin JM, Orloff SL, Reed MH, Wheeler LJ, Corless CL, Benner KG et al. Biliary tract complications of side-to-side without T tube versus end-to-end with or without T tube choledochocholedochostomy in liver transplant recipients. Transplantation 1998;65:193-199.

[70] Scanga AEKowdley KV. Management of biliary complications following orthotopic liver transplantation. Curr Gastroenterol Rep 2007;9:31-38.

[71] Wojcicki M, Silva MA, Jethwa P, Gunson B, Bramhall SR, Mayer D et al. Biliary complications following adult right lobe ex vivo split liver transplantation. Liver Transpl 2006;12:839-844.

[72] Oguma S, Belle S, Starzl TE, Demetris AJ. A histometric analysis of chronically rejected human liver allografts: insights into the mechanisms of bile duct loss: direct immunologic and ischemic factors. Hepatology 1989;9:204-209.

[73] Ludwig J, Wiesner RH, Batts KP, Perkins JD, Krom RA. The acute vanishing bile duct syndrome (acute irreversible rejection) after orthotopic liver transplantation. Hepatology 1987;7:476-483.

[74] Sanchez-Bueno F, Robles R, Ramirez P, Acosta F, Rodriguez JM, Lujan J et al. Hepatic artery complications after liver transplantation. Clin Transplant 1994;8:399-404.

[75] Feller RB, Waugh RC, Selby WS, Dolan PM, Sheil AG, McCaughan GW. Biliary strictures after liver transplantation: clinical picture, correlates and outcomes. J Gastroenterol Hepatol 1996;11:21-25.

12

Minimal Invasive (Endovascular and Percutaneous) Treatment of Post Liver Transplantation Complications in Pediatrics

Ghazwan Kroma, Jorge Lopera and Rajeev Suri
University of Texas Health Science Center at San Antonio
USA

1. Introduction

Liver transplantation is the only potentially curative treatment for patients with end-stage liver disease or unresectable primary hepatic tumors. Biliary atresia accounts for approximately 40% of liver transplant performed in children in the United State (Carter et al, 2006). Intra-hepatic cholestasis and inborn metabolic errors resulting in cirrhosis constitute the second most common group. Progressive liver failure and finally acute liver failure following hepatitis or drug toxicity represent a small referral group.

First human liver transplantation was performed by Starzl in 1963 at the University of Colorado Health Science Center on a three years old patient with biliary atresia and the patient died before the completion of the surgery (Starzl et al, 1963). First successful liver transplantation was performed in 1967 on an eighteen months old patient with malignant liver tumor and the patient survived for 400 days before she succumbed from disseminated malignancy (Carter et al, 2006). Survival after pediatric liver transplantation has improved significantly in recent decades because of the advances in surgical techniques, immunosuppressive therapy, and peri-operative care (Jain et al, 2002). Pediatric liver transplant recipients also have benefited from major technologic advances in diagnostic and interventional radiology. Radiology has acquired a key role in both pediatric and adult liver transplantation programs because it allows early detection and prompt treatment of post-transplantation vascular and nonvascular complications, helping to improve graft and patient survival and obviating surgical revision or repeat transplantation in most cases (Amesur & Zajko, 2006; Rose et al, 2001; Sze & Esquivel, 2002). Various interventional radiology procedures may be applied during the follow-up of pediatric liver transplant recipients to detect and diagnose graft disease and to treat vascular and biliary complications. The interventional radiology procedures most commonly used in this context include percuntaneous and transjugular liver biopsies for the diagnosis of graft disease; angioplasty and stent placement for the treatment of vascular stenosis or occlusion; biliary drain placement for the treatment of biliary strictures; coil embolization and stent graft placement for the treatment of pseduoaneurysm and artriovenous fistulas. Brief description of the surgical technique for split liver transplantation, the technical considerations involved in interventional radiology procedures, the expected results, and the possible complications are described in details in this chapter.

2. Surgical technique for split liver transplantation

Reduced liver technique or split liver transplantation represents a major advance in liver transplantation that significantly reduced the waiting period for liver transplantation.

Most pediatric liver transplantations are performed today by using left lateral segmental (II&III) transplantation or so called split liver transplantation (Fig. 1), a technique that accommodates the needs of pediatric patients without depleting the pool of organs available for adult patients with excellent patient and graft survival rate (90 and 87% respectively) (Deshpande et al, 2002) . Radiologist should be familiar with the surgical techniques used in the transplantation such as Piggy back technique for the anastomosis between the inferior vena cava of the recipient and the hepatic veins of the graft, end to end or interposition conduit for the hepatic arterial and the portal venous anastomosis, and Roux-en-y technique for the hepaticojejunostomy biliary anastomosis (Fig. 2).

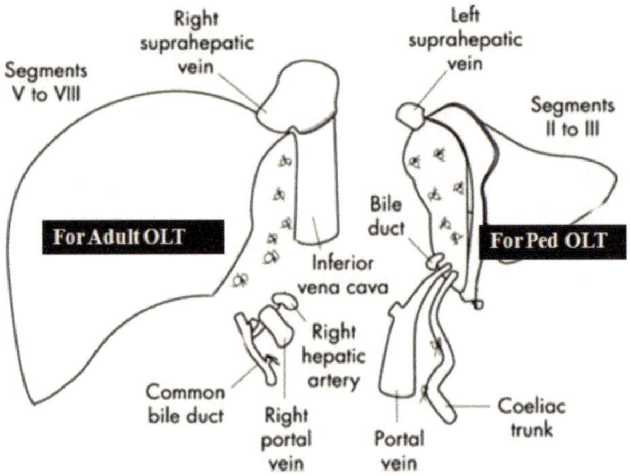

Fig. 1. Schematic diagram of split liver to provide two grafts from single donor, left lateral segment for a child and the right lobe for an adult recipient

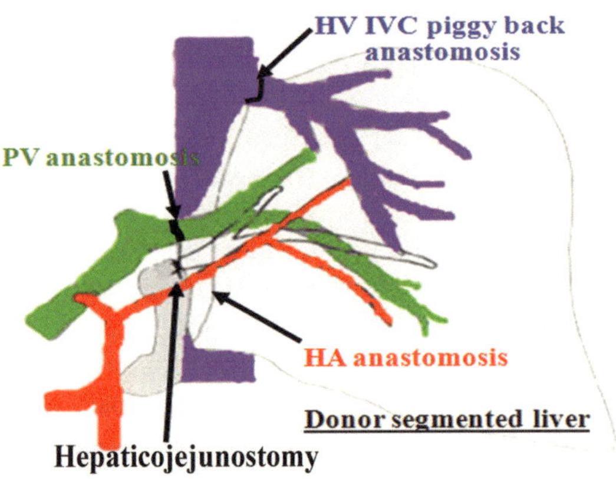

Fig. 2. Schematic diagram illustrating orthotopic segmental liver transplantation. Piggy back hepatic vein to IVC anastomosis. Hepatic arteries and portal veins end to end anastomosis. Roux-en-y hepaticojejunostomy biliary anastmosis

3. Imaging spectrum and image-guided procedures for the management of complications after split liver transplantation

3.1 Organ rejection

Organ rejection develops in about 50% of patients, but improved immunosuppressive medications permit successful management of this problem in most cases (Zalasin et al, 1998). The ultrasound appearances of acute rejection are nonspecific, and the only identifiable abnormality is heterogeneity of the liver parenchyma, which may, however, have other causes (Crossin et al, 2003; Marder et al, 1989; Zalasin et al, 1998). The role of imaging consists of excluding these other possible causes, which can manifest with clinical signs and symptoms similar to those of acute rejection (Crossin et al, 2003). The diagnosis of acute rejection, one of the most serious complications following liver transplantation, is established by graft biopsy and histologic study (Nghiem, 1998).

3.1.1 Percutaneous liver biopsy

Percutaneous ultrasonography (US)-guided random liver biopsy is frequently requested after pediatric liver transplantation. Any alteration in liver function test results that cannot be explained on the basis of findings at diagnostic imaging requires a liver biopsy to exclude organ rejection. US guidance of biopsy is necessitated by the small volume of the transplanted liver, especially in split-liver transplantation, and the need to avoid perforating the bowel, other adjacent organs, and important intrahepatic vascular structures. If a coagulation defect is present (eg, platelet count of less than 50 × 1000 per microliter, prothrombin activity less than 50% of the normal level), patients receive an infusion of platelets, fresh frozen plasma, or both. If the presence of massive perihepatic ascites make liver biopsy infeasible, a percutaneous drainage catheter might be placed first to eliminate the ascites. The use of a coaxial technique in pediatric patients also has been described. In this procedure, a coaxial sheath is used to inject slurry of microfibrillar collagen into the needle tract to reduce the risk of bleeding after biopsy (Hoffer, 2000). An antibiotic is administered prophylactically before the procedure. Core biopsies are performed by using an 18-gauge needle and monitored anesthesia care with additional local anesthesia administered at the site selected for puncture. An anterior approach is usually the only one possible in patients with a split-liver transplant. After the biopsy, manual compression is applied to the puncture site for ten minutes. Possible major complications of percutaneous liver biopsy are bleeding, hemobilia, arterioportal fistula, and infection; these have been reported in 4.6% of pediatric patients who have undergone the procedure (Amaral et al, 2006).

3.1.2 Transjugular liver biopsy

The transjugular approach is widely used for random liver biopsies in adult patients with massive perihepatic ascites, severe coagulopathy, or both because it is associated with a lower rate of bleeding complications than is percutaneous biopsy (Furuya, 1992). The transjugular technique incurs a lower risk of hemorrhage because a biopsy specimen is acquired through the hepatic vein and any bleeding from the puncture site remains within the vascular space. In addition, if there are clinical signs of portal hypertension, the hepatic vein pressure gradient can be measured during the transjugular biopsy procedure. The use of combined US and Fluoroscopic guidance during transjugular hepatic biopsies in pediatric patients has been reported to help reduce the risk of capsule perforation (Habdank, 2003). Complications of this biopsy procedure, which have been reported in 3%-11% of cases, include subcapsular hematoma, intraperitoneal bleeding, Subclavian artery puncture, pneumothorax, and hemothorax (Furuya, 1992; Kaye et al, 2000; Habdank, 2003). Transjugular random liver biopsy with catheterization of the right hepatic vein also has been reported in pediatric whole-liver transplant recipients (Habdank, 2003). Prophylactic antibiotics are routinely administered before the biopsy procedure, and an infusion of platelets or fresh frozen plasma is administered if coagulation defects are present. The small size of the liver in pediatric patients with a left lateral transplant and patient weight of less than 15 kg are considered relative contraindications to the procedure.

3.2 Vascular complications and treatment

Vascular complications that occur after pediatric liver transplantation are associated with high rates of morbidity, graft loss, and mortality (Sieders et al, 2000). These complications may involve the hepatic artery, hepatic vein, portal vein, or inferior vena cava. Most vascular complications appear within 3 months after transplantation. Clinical manifestations vary from mildly elevated values on hepatic function tests to fulminant hepatic failure (Bergey et al, 1998; Furuya, 1992; Hasegawa et al, 2002; Hoffer, 2000). Because their clinical manifestations often are indistinguishable from those of biliary complications, graft rejection, graft dysfunction, and infection, imaging is necessary for diagnosis. Color Doppler US, Multidetector computed tomography (CT), and magnetic resonance (MR) imaging all are useful for the diagnosis and follow-up. US is the primary screening modality used for the detection of vascular complications and imaging by Doppler US starts intra-operatively, in the ICU and twice daily for the first three days. The normal Doppler US parameters should include hepatopetal (toward the liver), pulsatile, low resistant flow in the hepatic artery with systolic velocity of more than 30 cm/s (fig. 3a), hepatopetal flow in the portal vein with velocity of at least 10 cm/s (fig. 3b) and phasic hepatofugal (outward the liver)

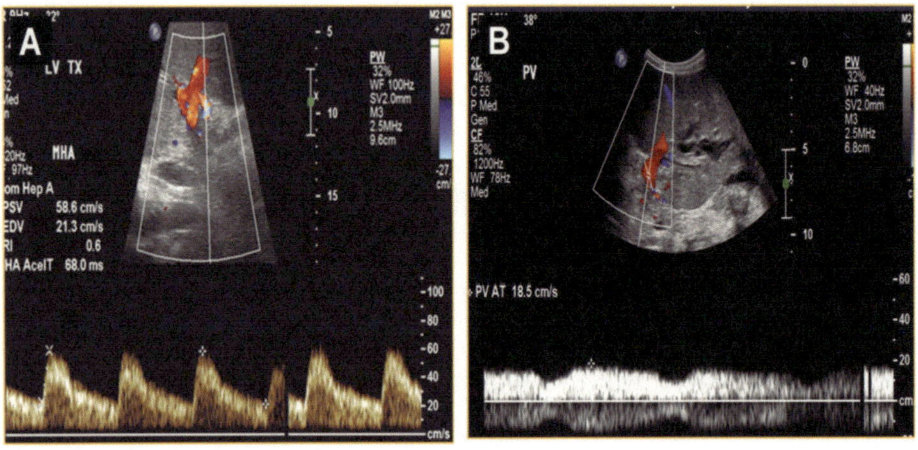

Fig. 3. Normal Doppler US study of the hepatic artery and portal vein after liver transplantation. (A) Pulsatile, low resistant hepatopetal flow in hepatic artery with velocity of 58.6 cm/s. (B) Phasic hepatopetal flow in portal vein with velocity of 18.5 cm/s

flow in the hepatic veins. MR angiography is performed to confirm abnormalities demonstrated at US or in patients in whom the US study is suboptimal. CT.scan is less frequently used today in this patient population due to the concern about the high radiation dose associated with it. Conventional vascular studies are currently reserved for endovascular treatment of these complications.

3.2.1 Hepatic artery stenosis

Hepatic artery stenosis occurs in 11%-20% of patients who have undergone pediatric liver transplantation (Moray, 2005). Most hepatic artery stenosis arise at the anastomosis site within 3 months after transplantation and are due to the small caliber of the arteries or to arterial injury by a vascular clamp during transplantation. However, nonanastomotic stenosis may occur in cases of graft rejection or necrosis. Early diagnosis and intervention may help to reduce ischemic damage to the graft, consequent bile duct damage, and progression to hepatic artery thrombosis. Doppler US is the imaging modality of choice for diagnosis and follow-up. The reported sensitivity of Doppler US for the detection of hepatic artery stenosis is 80%-90% (Abbasoglu et al, 1997; Crossin et al, 2003; Kok et al, 1998). Spectral broadening and focal accelerated velocity greater than 2 m/sec (Crossin et al, 2003; Nghiem et al, 1996; Platt et al, 1997) at the site of arterial anastomosis indicate stenosis. However, the site of narrowing is often difficult to identify by US due to overlying bowel gas especially in conduit graft, and the diagnosis is usually made on the basis of the Doppler US findings obtained distal to the stenosis. Intrahepatic arterial waveforms distal to the stenosis display a tardus parvus pattern with a decreased resistive index (<0.5) and prolonged acceleration time (80 msec) (Fig. 4a) (Dodd et al, 1994; Platt et al, 1997; Vignali et al, 2004). Associated turbulences distal to the stenosis are commonly observed at color Doppler US (Crossin et al, 2003; Platt et al, 1997). A tardus parvus pattern may be a normal finding during the first 72 hours after transplantation due to edema at the anastomotic site (Kok et al, 1998). In these cases, serial US will reveal a normal waveform 3-4 days after transplantation. MR angiography offers an alternative noninvasive technique for confirming the stenosis and for better evaluation of the anastomosis and the entire hepatic artery (Ito et al, 2000; Vignali et al, 2004). Conventional arteriography is currently reserved for endovascular treatment of the stenosis (Boraschi& Donati, 2004; Vignali et al, 2004). Early hepatic artery stenosis (less than two weeks post transplantation) should be treated surgically because endovascular treatment has the risk of suture line rupture. The use of percutaneous transluminal angioplasty with or without stent placement to treat hepatic artery stenosis in adult and pediatric liver transplant recipients have been reported (Hashikura et al, 2001; Kok et al, 1998; Nghiem et al, 1996). Possible complications that have been described include dissection, pseudoaneurysm, and rupture of the hepatic artery. When Doppler US or MRA findings are suggestive of hepatic artery stenosis, hepatic arteriography is performed by using a transfemoral approach and a standard 4-F angiographic catheter with monitored anesthesia care or general anesthesia. A coaxial microcatheter is then advanced through the stenosis, and the trans-stenotic pressure gradient is measured. If a significant pressure gradient is present (>10 mm Hg), angioplasty is performed. Before angioplasty, 0.2 mg nitroglycerin and 100 IU heparin per kilogram of body weight are infused into the hepatic artery to reduce the risks of spasm and thrombosis. A 6-F guiding catheter is inserted, and a balloon catheter is advanced over a 0.018- or 0.014-inch stiff wire. The balloon diameter varies in accordance with the diameter of the hepatic artery (Figs. 5&6). Procedural success is defined as the reduction or absence of stenosis at arteriography, accompanied by a significant reduction of the trans-stenotic pressure gradient. Angioplasty is technically successful in about 80% of the cases with restenosis rate of 30-60%. The long-term patency of stents is unknown; for this reason, stent placement in pediatric patients is recommended only if angioplasty fails or if complications such as hepatic artery dissection or rupture ensue. Doppler US is performed the day after the procedure to obtain baseline measurements of the intra and extrahepatic arterial resistive index (RI) and systolic acceleration time for comparison with follow up measurements (Fig. 4c).

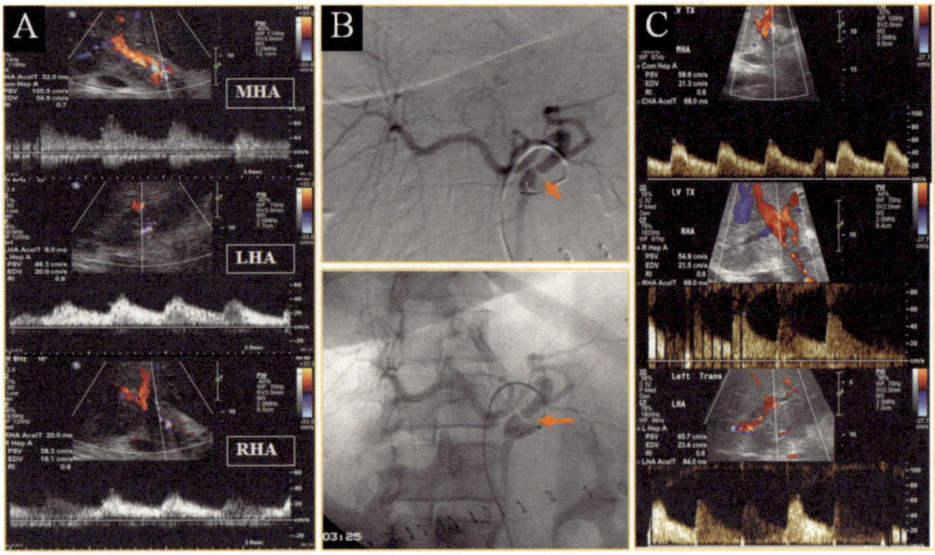

Fig. 4. Early hepatic arterial stenosis (Surgically treated). (A) Doppler US performed day 5 post liver transplant shows tardus parvus waveform and low acceleration times in the right, left and main hepatic arteries. (B) Catheter angiogram, subtracted and un-subtracted images, confirms the stenosis at the proper hepatic artery. (C) post surgical revision follow up Doppler US reveals normal hepatic arteries wave forms

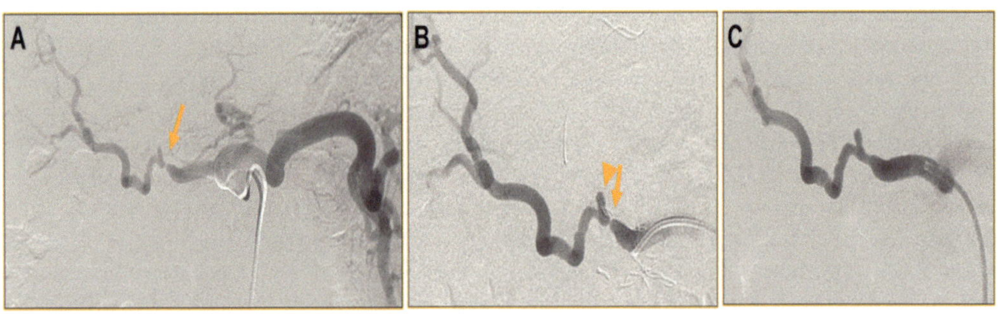

Fig. 5. (A) Celiac angiogram demonstrates sever stenosis at the anastomosis (arrow). (B) Hepatic artery stenosis (arrow) confirmed with selective proper hepatic angiogram with a small outpouching due to a ligated gastrodoudenal artery (arrowhead). (C) Post angioplasty with no significant residual stenosis

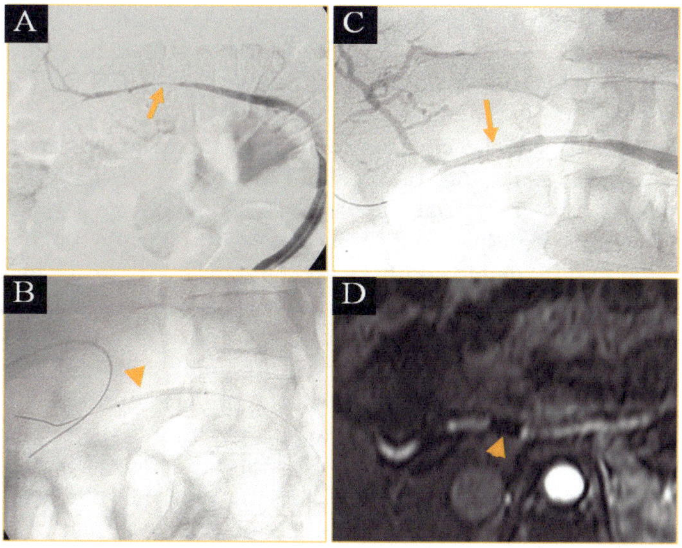

Fig. 6. Hepatic artery stenosis treated with stent. (A,B,C) angiogram of the aorta-hepatic artery conduit with persistent severe stenosis (arrow in A) in the proper HA. As stenosis persists after angioplasty (arrowhead in B), it was treated with a 4 x 20 mm balloon expandable stent (arrow in C). Stenosis is resolved in post stenting angiogram (C).
(D) Follow up MRA demonstrates stent artifact in the proper hepatic artery with adequate flow proximal and distal to the stent

3.2.2 Hepatic artery thrombosis

In the past, hepatic artery thrombosis was the most common and dreads vascular complication of orthotopic liver transplantation, with a prevalence of 4%–12% in adult recipients, a prevalence of up to 40% in children, and a mortality rate of 50%–58% (Mazzaferro et al, 1989). Microsurgical techniques have improved these results, and the prevalence of hepatic artery thrombosis during the first thirty days after transplantation has been reduced to approximately 5% in whole liver transplantation (Settmacher et al, 2000). However, hepatic artery thrombosis is more common in split or living donor liver transplantation (Ghobrial et al, 2000; Hashikura et al, 2001; Katyal et al, 2000). Associated risk factors include prolonged cold ischemia time of the donor liver, previous orthotopic liver transplantation, significant differences in caliber between the donor and recipient hepatic arteries, an interposition conduit for the anastomosis, small donor or recipient vessels, acute rejection, ABO blood type incompatibility, and cytomegalovirus infection (Crossin et al, 2003; Dodd, 1995; Vivarelli et al, 2004). As in hepatic artery stenosis, clinical manifestations vary considerably, ranging from mild elevation of liver enzyme levels to delayed bile leak, bile duct stricture or ischemic changes, or fulminant hepatic necrosis (Ametani et al, 2001; Dodd et al, 1994; Ito et al, 2000). Patency of the hepatic artery is vital for long-term survival of the graft because this artery is the sole blood supply to the biliary epithelium of the transplanted liver, unlike in a native liver (Crossin et al, 2003; Kaneko et al 2004). As a result, complete occlusion of the hepatic artery results in infarction or necrosis of the liver parenchyma and may lead to fulminant hepatic failure in the early post-transplantation period. Doppler US allows correct identification of hepatic artery thrombosis in up to 90% of cases (Crossin et al, 2003; Garcı´a-

Criado et al, 2003; Glockner & Forauer 1999; Nghiem et al, 1996). At doppler US examination, there is usually complete absence of both proper hepatic and intrahepatic arterial flow (Chong, 2004; Kok T et al, 1998; Nghiem et al, 1996). The initial doppler waveform of the hepatic artery may be normal, with follow-up doppler US images showing a progressive decrease in systolic and diastolic flow, followed by absent diastolic flow, dampening of the systolic peak, and, finally, total loss of the hepatic waveform (Nolten & Sproat, 1996). After thrombosis, arterial collateral vessels can develop, especially in children, and intrahepatic flow may be identified. Nevertheless, the intra-hepatic arterial waveform will display a tardus parvus pattern with an acceleration time greater than 80 msec and a resistive index less than 0.5 (Chong, 2004; Crossin et al, 2003; Dodd, 1995). Therefore, a complete absence of flow in the main hepatic artery and a tardus parvus pattern in the intrahepatic branches of the hepatic artery are highly suggestive of hepatic artery thrombosis and should be confirmed with other imaging techniques (Hall et al, 1990). MR angiography is a useful and noninvasive method for evaluating the patency of the hepatic artery and may play an important role in identifying patients who require hepatic angiography (Glockner et al, 2000; Ito et al, 2000). When thrombosis is present, MR angiography accurately demonstrates the location of the thrombus by showing arterial opacification up to the thrombus, abrupt cutoff of the hepatic artery at the thrombus, and lack of opacification of distal branches (Fig. 7a) (Glockner et al, 2000; Ito et al, 2000).

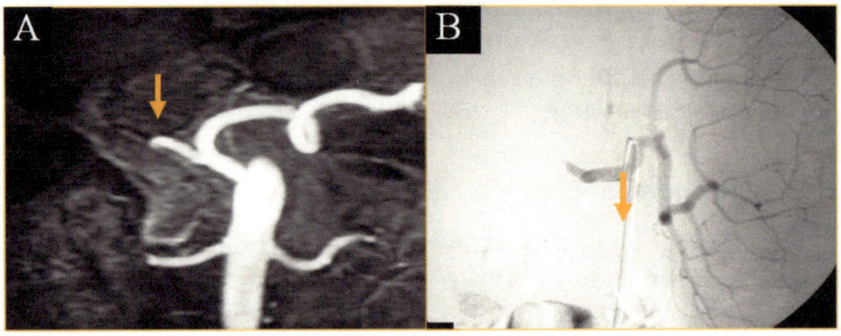

Fig. 7. Hepatic artery thrombosis (A) MRA demonstrating common hepatic artery (arrow) visualized to the level of the anastomosis, and complete occlusion of the hepatic artery beyond the anastomosis. (B) Selective celiac angiogram confirms hepatic artery thrombosis

Angiography is useful when fibrinolytic endovascular therapy is indicated (Fig. 7b). With early diagnosis, thrombectomy and revision of the transplant can be used to salvage the graft. Thrombolysis has high risk of hemorrhage in early hepatic artery thrombosis, especially if associated with liver infarction. If occlusion occurs at a late stage, the graft may survive with the support of portal venous flow, but there may be necrosis of the bile duct epithelium and consequent biliary strictures or leaks (Chong, 2004; Lorenz et al, 2001). Late hepatic artery thrombosis can be treated safely with thrombectomy, fibrinolysis, angioplasty and stenting Fig. 8.

3.2.3 Hepatic artery pseudoaneurysms (HAP)

Hepatic artery pseudoaneurysm is a rare complication after liver transplantation seen mostly at the donor-recipient anastomosis and less often at the ligation site of the gastrodoudenal artery and those are likely related to infection, technical failure or biliary leakage. Intrahepatic pseudoaneurysm can also be seen and may be related to percutaneous biliary procedures or liver biopsies. Mycotic hepatic artery pseudoaneurysm can fistulize to the portal vein or bilary tree and presents with hemobilia, gastrointestinal bleeding or hemoperitoneum. Endovascular treatment may be performed by transcatheter or percutaneous coil embolization or exclusion of the pseudoaneurysm with covered stent (Figs. 9&10). Surgical excision and revascularization using bypass graft can also be performed.

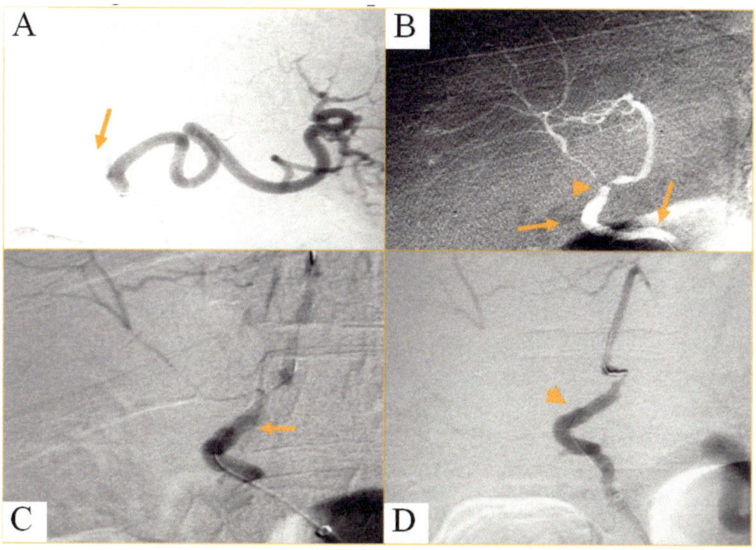

Fig. 8. Management of late hepatic artery thrombosis (A) Pre- and (B) Post-thrombolysis hepatic angiograms demonstrating recanalization of the hepatic artery (arrow). Sever stenosis (arrowhead) is seen at the hepatic artery bifurcation. (C) The stenosis was angioplastied with a 5 x 20 mm balloon (arrow) with no residual stenosis seen in the final angiogram (D)

3.2.4 Hepatic vein stenosis\thrombosis

Hepatic vein stenosis with resultant outflow insufficiency is a major postoperative complication that leads to graft failure in 5% of pediatric liver transplant recipients; most often in those with a partial liver graft (Buell et al, 2002) and Piggy back hepatic venous anastomosis. Hepatic veins stenosis usually produce hepatic congestion, refractory ascites and alteration of liver function test results. Transjugular or transfemoral angioplasty or metallic stent placement usually is selected as the first-line treatment for this complication (Cheng et al, 2005; Lorenz et al, 2006). In pediatric patients, balloon dilation is the preferred treatment choice because the long-term patency of metallic stents is unknown and repeat transplantation is always possible. Metallic stent placement should be reserved for the treatment of persistent hepatic vein stenosis that is unresponsive to multiple angioplasties. The persistence of a pressure gradient of more than 5 mm Hg between the hepatic vein and the right atrium after several angioplasties is an indication for metallic stent placement (Lorenz et al, 2006). Good technical and clinical success rates are reported after hepatic veins angioplasty and stenting with patency rates ranging from 70% at 3 months to 50% at 36 months (Lorenz et al, 2006). Long term patency may require repeated interventions. In adult and pediatric patients in whom transjugular or transfemoral recanalization of the stenotic or occluded hepatic vein stenosis has failed, the use of a percutaneous transhepatic approach or a combined transhepatic-transjugular approach has been reported (Kubo et al, 2006; Miraglia et al, 2007). For the transhepatic approach, preprocedural drainage of ascites and postprocedural embolization of the transhepatic tracts are, in our opinion, mandatory to reduce the risk of bleeding. Hepatic vein stenosis usually occurs at the anastomosis site; less frequently, an intrahepatic stenosis is found that is likely due to injury of the hepatic vein during a previous surgical or percutaneous procedure (eg, biopsy or biliary catheter placement). Treatment is performed with angioplasty or metallic stent placement (Fig. 11). Doppler US should be performed the day after the procedure for a baseline evaluation of the hepatic vein velocity and flow spectrum, which are compared with the findings at follow up Doppler US evaluations. Imaging follow-up is performed every 3 months in the first post procedural year or at any occurrence of ascites or any alteration in liver function test results,

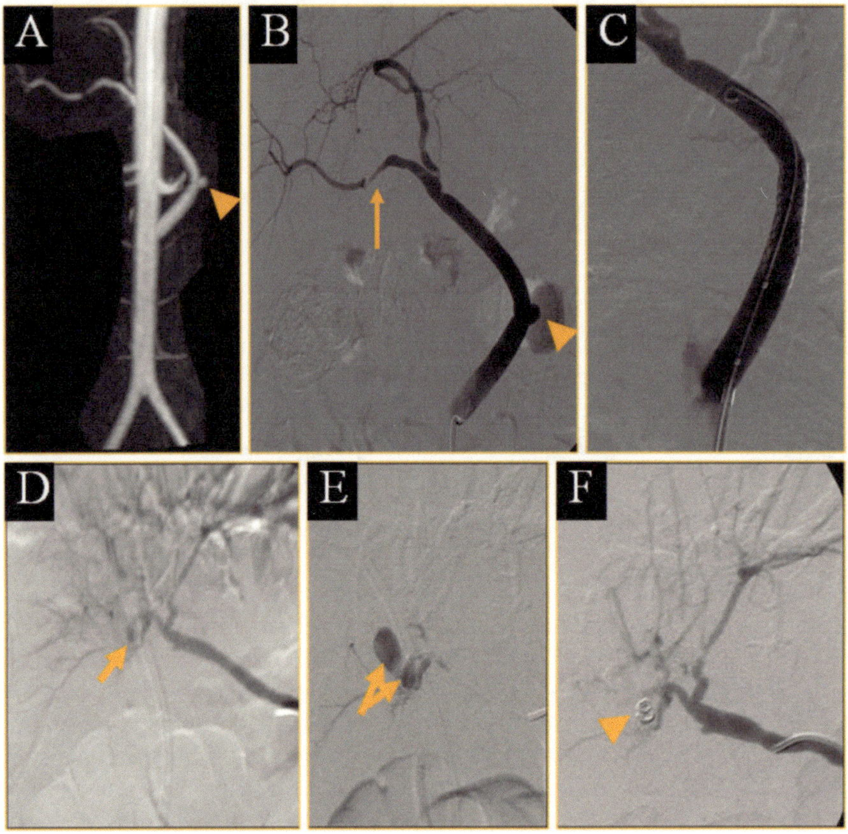

Fig. 9. Management of hepatic artery pseudoaneurysms (HAP). (A,B,C) Extrahepatic aneuryusm: (A) MRA and (B) graft hepatic angiogram revealing an outpouching (HAP) at the lateral aspect of the graft (arrowhead). (C) After stent graft deployment, angiogram reveals no further filling of the Pseudoaneurysm. (D,E,F) Intrahepatic HAP s/p ERCP (D&E) catheter angiography shows a bilobed collection of contrast from the right hepatic artery (arrow) in this patient with hemobilia. (F) Post-coil embolization (arrowhead), no filling of the HAP is seen

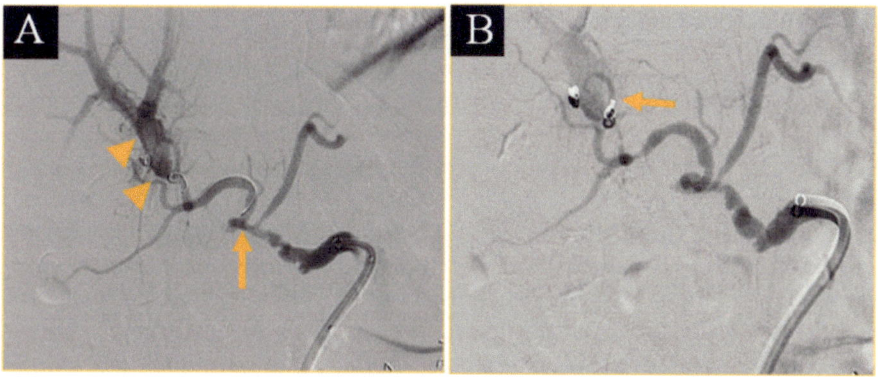

Fig. 10. Management of hepatic arteriovenous fistula. (A) Right hepatic angiogram reveals filling of the portal vein (arrowhead) and the hepatic artery (arrow) at the same time. (B) Post coil embolization reveals minimal filling of the fistulous communication (arrow)

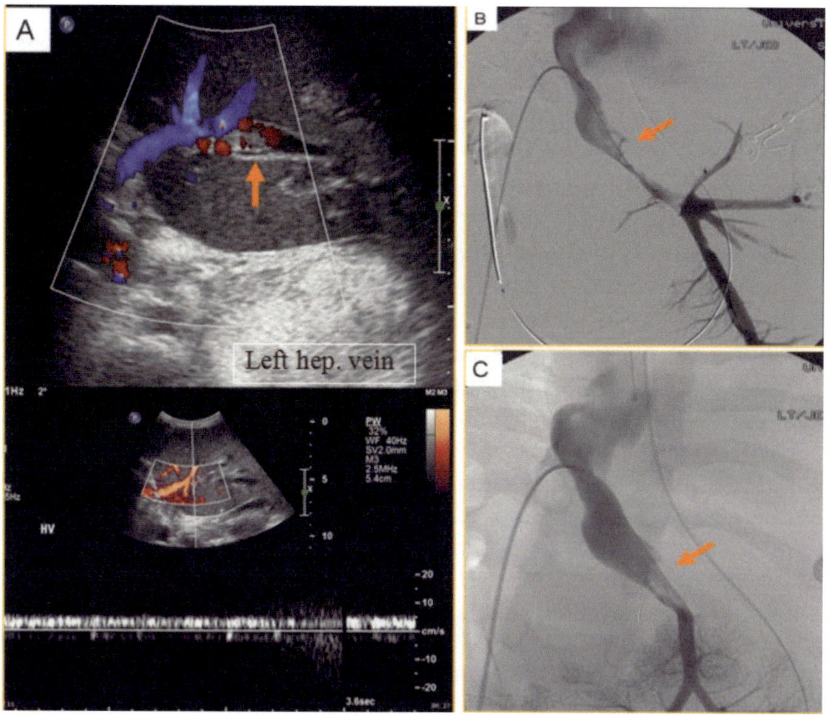

Fig. 11. Management of hepatic vein stenosis\thrombosis. (A) Doppler US reveals thrombus in the left hepatic vein (arrow) with abnormal monophasic flow. (B) Hepatic venogram reveals patent hepatic veins-IVC anastomosis and non-occlusive thrombus (arrow) in the hepatic vein confluent. (C) After local thrombolysis, thrombectomy and venoplasty, improved flow with residual thrombus (arrow)

both being suggestive of stenosis recurrence. If clinical or imaging signs of recurrent stenosis are present, hepatic vein phlebography with trans-stenotic pressure gradient measurement is recommended.

3.2.5 Inferior vena cava stenosis\thrombosis

Inferior Vena Cava (IVC) stenosis is more common in the pediatric population, especially among recipients of partial liver transplants, including living donor liver transplants, reduced-size liver transplants, and split liver transplants (Carnevale et al, 2004; Egawa et al, 1997). IVC stenosis may occurs acutely secondary to an anastomotic size discrepancy or suprahepatic caval kinking from organ rotation. Delayed caval stenosis may occur secondary to fibrosis, a chronic thrombus, or neointimal hyperplasia (Carnevale et al, 2004; Katyal et al, 2000). Clinical manifestations include pleural effusions, hepatomegaly, ascites, and lower extremity edema. A significant suprahepatic caval stenosis may result in reversed flow or absence of phasicity in the hepatic veins (Crossin et al, 2003). Nevertheless, monophasic waveforms are not specific for hepatic vein stenosis (Chong, 2004). A monophasic flat waveform with a relatively low average peak velocity in the hepatic vein (mean, 11 cm/sec) is a common finding. Sometimes, graft growth and twisting are causes of IVC pseudostenosis (Ametani et al, 2001), which may increase or disappear depending on the patient's posture. Hemodynamically significant IVC stenosis can be differentiated from pseudostenosis on the basis of the presence of features of Budd-Chiari syndrome and Doppler velocity measurements. IVC stenosis and hepatic vein stenosis may manifest as Budd-Chiari syndrome, with hepatomegaly, ascites, reversed flow or absence of phasicity in the hepatic veins, and reversed flow in the portal vein (Buell et al, 2002; Crossin et al, 2003; Katyal et al, 2000). Contrast-enhanced CT is useful in demonstrating congestive changes in the liver parenchyma as a manifestation of blocked outflow but is of little help in depicting the stenosis itself (Ametani et al, 2001; White et al, 2004). Coronal MR imaging is useful in determining the extent of IVC stenosis and associated anomalies (Ito et al, 2000). Frequently, cavogram is required to confirm the stenosis. Pressure gradient measurements can help distinguish physiologically significant lesions from pseudostenoses (Carnevale et al, 2004). Treatment includes IVC recanalization, balloon angioplasty and stent placement (Fig. 12). Color Doppler US performed after the interventional procedure is also useful in confirming the restoration of normal hepatic venous flow by demonstrating a multiphasic waveform and an objective increase in flow velocity (Huang et al, 2004; Totsuka et al, 2004). Ascites usually disappears rapidly after the procedure. IVC thrombosis is a rare occurrence. It tends to occur at the superior and inferior caval anastomoses. Risk factors include technical problems during transplantation, use of intravascular catheters, and compression of vessels by a fluid collection. Color Doppler US may reveal obvious vessel narrowing or an echogenic intraluminal thrombus with absence of flow. At MR angiography, IVC thrombosis is seen as an intraluminal defect. Coronal imaging is useful for determining the extent of IVC thrombosis (Chong, 2004; Glockner et al, 2000).

3.2.6 Portal vein stenosis

Portal vein stenosis has been reported to occur as a postoperative complication in 4%–8% of pediatric liver transplant recipients (Ueda et al, 2005). It occurs more frequently in reduced-size liver transplantation than in whole liver transplantation owing to the limited length of the portal vein that can be obtained from the donor (Unsinn et al, 2003). A difference in caliber between donor and recipient portal veins is normal and can be helpful in locating the portal venous anastomosis. An echogenic shelf like ring can often be seen at the anastomotic site. These findings should not be misinterpreted as a stenosis. At gray-scale US, portal vein

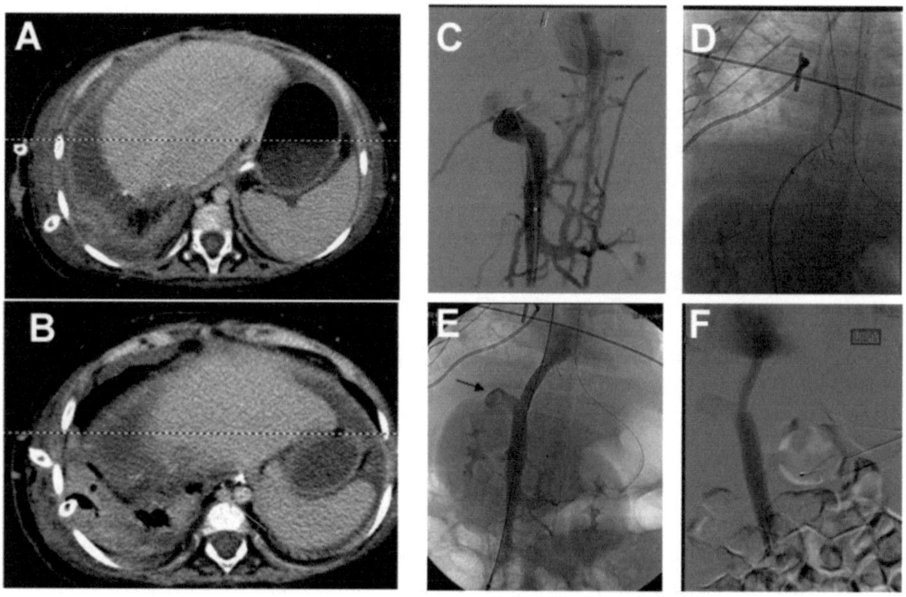

Fig. 12. Managment of IVC occlusion. (A&B) CT.scan of the upper abdomen demonstrating absence of the suprahepatic IVC in (A) and congested azygus vein (arrow) in B. (C) Initial cavogram confirms the occlusion of the IVC with opacification of the azygus system. (D&E) Successful recanalization and stenting of the IVC. The arrow in E points to the piggyback stump. (F) Follow up cavogram after six months confirms the patency of the stented IVC

stenosis is diagnosed when a reduction of the vessel lumen of 50% or more is observed (Fig. 13) at the site of narrowing relative to the prestenotic area, or when the caliber of the vessel is 2.5 mm or less at the site of narrowing (Boraschi & Donati, 2004; Crossin et al, 2003; Glockner & Forauer, 1999). Color Doppler US shows focal color aliasing at the vascular anastomosis. At pulsed doppler US, the waveform shows a systolic velocity greater than 20 m/sec or a velocity in the stenotic segment that is three to four times greater than that in the prestenotic segment. A poststenotic jet with a velocity between 1 and 3 m/sec is a characteristic finding (Crossin et al, 2003; Nghiem et al, 1996; Stell et al, 2004). MR angiography can provide excellent visualization of portal vein stenosis (Fig. 13). Portography helps confirm the presence of the stenosis, and a pressure gradient may be obtained to determine the hemodynamic significance of the stenosis (Nghiem, 1996).Clinical symptoms of hemodynamically significant portal vein stenosis are related to portal hypertension and include bleeding from varices, splenomegaly, and ascites. Percutaneous transhepatic angioplasty is considered the standard treatment for portal vein stenosis. The placement of metallic stents also has been reported for treatment of recurrent or nonresponsive elastic stenosis (Funaki et al, 2000; Zajko et al, 1994). In the largest patient series for which data are available, a very good patency rate of 100% was found at 46 months after treatment with angioplasty and metallic stent placement (Funaki et al, 2000). A transhepatic puncture of the portal vein is performed with a 21-gauge needle while using US for guidance. An introducer system is advanced over an 0.018-inch nitinol wire to the portal branch and then exchanged for a 6-F vascular sheath over a 0.035-inch wire. The trans-stenotic pressure gradient is measured by using a 5-F hydrophilic catheter. Before balloon dilation, a bolus of heparin

(100 IU/kg) is administered intravenously to reduce the risk of thrombosis during balloon induced occlusion. Technical success is represented by resolution of the stenosis on a follow-up portogram and by a significant reduction in the trans-stenotic pressure gradient (Fig. 14). The persistence of a pressure gradient of more than 5 mm Hg has been considered an indication for metallic stent placement (Funaki et al, 2000). Coil or gelfoam embolization of transhepatic needle tracts can be done to reduce the risk of bleeding. Doppler US should be performed on the day after the procedure for baseline evaluation of the portal vein velocity and flow spectrum. If findings at doppler US or clinical signs are suggestive of stenosis recurrence, MRI can be performed to confirm the findings before percutaneous intervention is repeated.

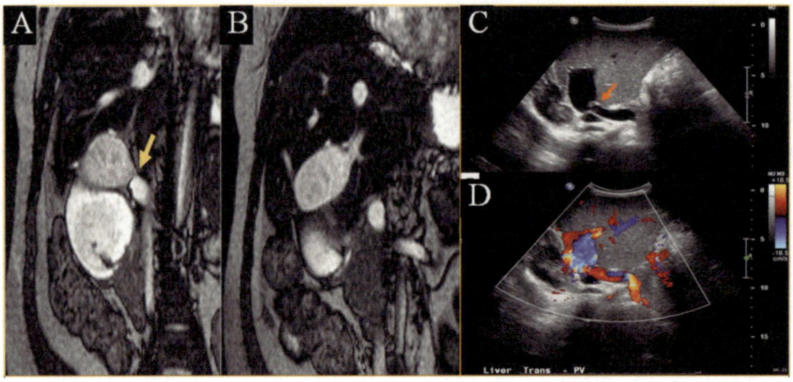

Fig. 13. Portal vein stenosis. (A&B) MRA reveals moderate stenosis (arrow) of the main portal vein. (C&D) US and color US shows portal vein stenosis and turbulent flow

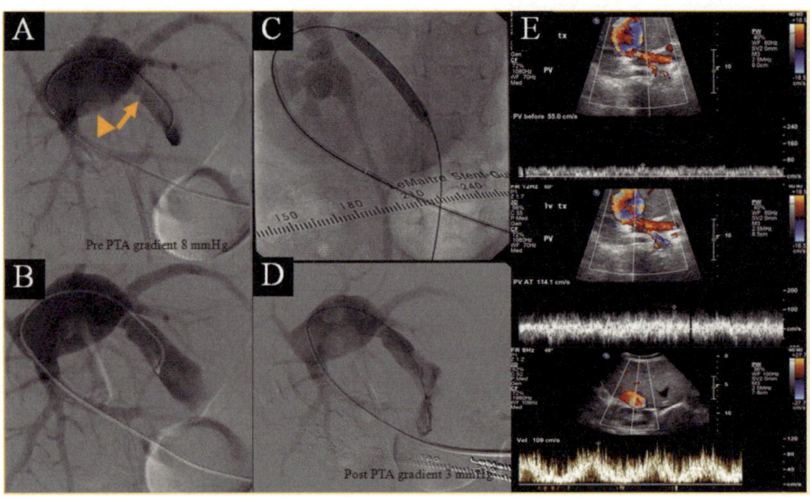

Fig. 14. Angioplasty of portal vein (PV) stenosis. (A&B) Percutaneous portogram reveals saccular dilatation of the portal vein (arrowhead) and moderate stenosis at the PV anastomosis (arrow) with an 8 mm pressure gradient noted. (C&D) Post venoplasty with 6 x 40 mm balloon, mild residual stenosis is noted with gradient drop to 3 mm Hg indicating successful treatment. (E) follow up US demonstrates improved velocities and decrease in the spatial gradient across the stenosis

3.2.7 Portal vein thrombosis

Portal vein thrombosis occurs more frequently in reduced size liver transplantation, mostly involving the main extrahepatic portal segment. Risk factors include surgical difficulties, decreased portal venous inflow; the presence of portosystemic shunts before transplantation; prior splenectomy; excessive vessel redundancy; and use of the venous conduits, most commonly cryopreserved iliac veins (Buell et al, 2002; Hashikura et al, 2003; Nghiem, 1998). Clinical manifestations include new-onset massive ascites, variceal bleeding, elevated values on hepatic function tests, splenomegaly, hepatic failure, and lower extremity edema (Buell et al, 2002; Millis et al, 1996). An acute thrombus is frequently anechoic and may be imperceptible on gray-scale US images and the portal vein appears normal. In these cases, color flow and spectral doppler analysis will show no detectable flow within the portal vein (Langnas et al, 1991; Nghiem, 1998). Vessel narrowing or an echogenic luminal thrombus with no Doppler flow may also be seen (Nghiem et al, 1996). Partial portal vein thrombosis may appear as a nonocclusive filling defect at US. Resultant luminal narrowing can be mistaken for portal vein stenosis at gray-scale, spectral, and color doppler US (Funaki et al, 2000; Langnas et al, 1991). Occasionally, reversed flow in the intrahepatic branches may be observed in patients with portal vein thrombosis with complete absence of flow in the main portal vein. This finding is due to arterioportal shunts that develop soon after the thrombosis. Care should be taken to avoid making a false-negative diagnosis (Nghiem, 1996, 1998; Stell et al, 2004). MR venography can provide an excellent visualization of portal vein thrombosis and can facilitate the differentiation of thrombosis from slow flow (Stafford-Johnson et al, 1998; Unsinn et al, 2003). At contrast material–enhanced CT, portal vein thrombosis is seen as a low-attenuation filling defect (Ametani et al, 2001; Garcı´a-Criado et al, 2003; Unsinn et al, 2003). Portal vein stenosis with thrombus formation in the immediate postoperative period is quickly diagnosed with Doppler US and is managed surgically. Treatment of portal vein thrombosis may include mechanical thrombectomy, segmental portal vein resection, percutaneous thrombolysis and stent placement, or balloon angioplasty (Fig. 15) (Holbert et al, 1995; Rossi et al, 2004). However, when the thrombus extends to the periphery of the intrahepatic portal venous branches, it can no longer be treated with balloon dilation or thrombolysis, and the patient must undergo repeat transplantation (Ametani et al, 2001). Thus, early diagnosis of portal vein thrombosis before formation of a complete thrombus is important. Occasionally, portal vein thrombosis is

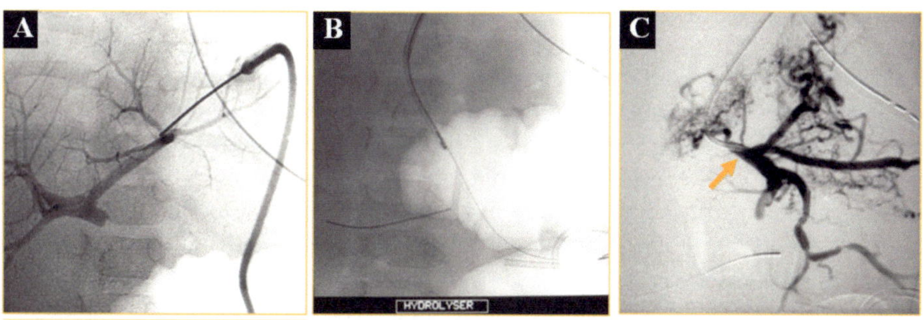

Fig. 15. Portal vein thrombosis. (A) Percutaneous portogram reveals occlusion of the main portal vein. (B) The portal vein was recanalized and thrombectomy was performed. (C) Post recanalization portogram reveals patent mesenteric veins (arrow) with filling of collateral varices

detected in patients with normal allograft function and no portal hypertension. In these patients, sufficient hepatopetal collateralization has developed to maintain adequate venous flow (Holbert et al, 1995; Unsinn et al, 2003). A cavernomatous transformation is the usual finding at Doppler US in these cases.

3.3 Biliary complications imaging and treatment

Biliary complications are the most common complications following pediatric liver transplantation estimated to involve 20%–40% of pediatric liver transplant recipients, more frequently seen in children who have undergone reduced-size transplantation. Most biliary complications develop during the first 3 months after pediatric liver transplantation, but strictures and stones may develop months or years later. Complications include anastomotic leakage and stenosis with bile duct dilatation; intrahepatic bile duct stones, sludge, or debris; and biloma. These complications are related to the surgical method of biliary reconstruction and to prolonged cold ischemia time, immunologic reactions, hepatic artery thrombosis, ABO blood group system incompatibility between donor and recipient, and cytomegalovirus infection (Ametani et al, 2001). Non-anastomotic strictures are probably caused by hepatic arterial insufficiency from either stenosis or thrombosis. These ischemic arterial events may result in bile duct strictures or leaks, increasing the risk of cholangitis, sepsis, and abscess (Boraschi & Donati, 2004; Glockner & Forauer, 1999). The blood supply to the recipient CBD is rich because of collateral flow, whereas the vascularity of the donor duct and the proximal intrahepatic ducts is derived solely from the reconstructed hepatic artery. Biliary disease should be suspected in a post-transplantation patient who presents with elevated values on hepatic function tests, jaundice, fever, or abdominal pain (Lorenz et al, 2001; Vitellas & Guttikonda, 2002). The clinical manifestations of biliary complications often are indistinguishable from those of vascular complications, graft rejection, graft dysfunction, and infections. Although US is commonly performed to screen for biliary complications, the false-negative rate is high; therefore, negative findings at US do not suffice to exclude biliary complications. MRCP can be used as a non-invasive imaging tool to confirm US findings. Percutaneous trans-hepatic cholangiography can depict the type, location, and severity of biliary complications, allowing treatment in many cases.

3.3.1 Anastomotic biliary strictures

Anastomotic biliary strictures are a common problem after pediatric liver transplantation, with a reported incidence of 10%–35% (Lallier et al, 1993; Heffron et al, 1992). Such strictures are usually related to scar tissue and retraction at the suture site. Untreated biliary strictures are associated with high morbidity and mortality. Because hepatico-jejunostomy with Roux-en-Y reconstruction is the most common type of biliary anastomosis in pediatric liver transplant recipients, endoscopy is rarely feasible and percutaneous intervention is usually the only treatment approach possible. Percutaneous treatment of biliary strictures in pediatric liver transplant recipients is considered safe and effective, and in most cases obviates surgical revision of the affected anastomoses (Lorenz et al, 2005; Schwarzenberg et al, 2002). Possible complications of percutaneous transhepatic cholangiography include hemobilia, intra- or extrahepatic hematoma, and fever with bacteremia; a cumulative incidence of 10.8% is reported for these complications in the pediatric population (Lorenz et al, 2005). Among 35 pediatric liver transplant recipients who underwent percutaneous treatment of biliary strictures, the reported success rate was 34% after a single course of therapy and 60% after repeat percutaneous therapy, with a median follow-up period of 4.5 years (Sunku et al, 2006). Suspicion about the presence of a biliary stricture may be aroused by one or more of the following findings, clinical manifestations such as fever or cholangitis; biochemical indicators such as increased levels of alkaline phosphatase, direct bilirubin, and transaminases; biliary duct dilatation observed at US, CT, or MR imaging; and liver biopsy with histologic findings indicative of cholestasis due to biliary obstruction. Biliary strictures may be present also in the absence of ductal dilatation (Berrocal et al, 2006). Some investigators have reported better sensitivities (80%-100%) when using MR cholangiography for the detection of biliary obstruction (Kitazono et al, 2007; Norton et al, 2001). However, in pediatric patients, deep sedation or general anesthesia is necessary during MR cholangiography and adds considerably to the cost of management; for this reason, MR cholangiography is not generally used as a screening modality in children. It does afford a global evaluation of the ductal anatomy, a capability that might be especially helpful when planning the placement of a biliary drainage catheter in a patient with two separate hepaticojejunostomies and a nondilated bile duct, because it allows avoidance of puncture of a hepatic segment with a normal bile duct. As an alternative, hepatobiliary scintigraphy with technetium 99m Mebrofenin iminodiacetate could be performed, with a segmental delay in clearance of the radiotracer being suggestive of a biliary stricture. Percutaneous transhepatic cholangiography is performed to confirm clinical, histologic, or imaging evidence of biliary strictures. Percutaneous transhepatic cholangiography is performed with monitored anesthesia care, spontaneous respiration, and additional local anesthesia. Intravenous antibiotic prophylaxis is administered before the procedure. If coagulation defects (platelet count $< 50 \times 1000/\mu L$, prothrombin activity $< 50\%$) are present, the patient receives an infusion of platelets, fresh frozen plasma, or both. Percutaneous transhepatic cholangiography is usually performed with a subxiphoid approach by using a 20-gauge needle positioned in a peripheral bile duct with US and fluoroscopic guidance. If the cholangiogram shows an anastomotic stricture, the biliary tree is catheterized by using an introducer system over a nitinol wire; the stricture is crossed, when possible, with 0.035- or 0.038-inch hydrophilic wire, and a transanastomotic biliary catheter (diameter range, 5–6.6 F) is placed with side holes above and below the stricture (Fig. 16).

The catheter is left in place to allow external gravity drainage for at least 1 day. If the patient has no fever or cholangitis the day after the procedure, the catheter is clamped to allow internal drainage. Diagnostic cholangiography and the first session of balloon dilation of the anastomosis are performed on different days to reduce the risk of sepsis. The first session of balloon dilation is usually performed 1 week after cholangiography, with a 5-F or 6-F sheath and with a balloon size ranging from 5 mm to 7 mm at a pressure of 6–11 atm. The balloon size selected is usually 1 mm larger than the diameter of the intrahepatic bile duct above the stricture. In every session, trans-anastomotic balloon dilation should be performed three times, 10 minutes each. A transanastomotic biliary catheter is placed after every session of dilation, with the catheter size ranging from 6 to 12 F, according to the diameter of the anastomosis. The antibiotic infusion is repeated 6 hours after the procedure. A minimum of three separate sessions of biliary anastomotic dilations are performed, followed by a cholangiographic evaluation, and if necessary, further sessions of dilation every 4–6 weeks. At each session of dilation, the size of the balloon catheter is increased by 1 mm, until a maximum diameter of 10 mm is reached. The drainage catheter is finally removed when

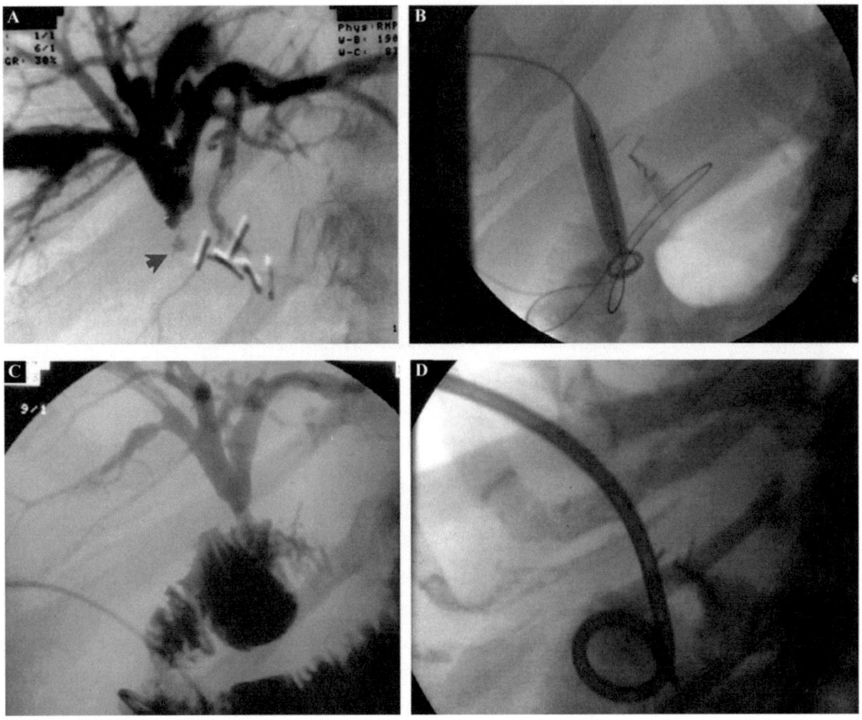

Fig. 16. Anastomotic biliary stricture. (A) Percutaneous cholangiogram demonstrating dilated biliary ducts with total occlusion of the hepatico-jejunostomy (arrow). (B) Successful recanalization and a balloon cholangioplasty of the biliary anastomosis. (C) Final cholangiogram demonstrated patent anastomosis with contrast drained into the jejunum. (D) Internal\external biliary drain placed across the anastomosis

cholangiography performed through a sheath depicts resolution of the stricture and a good transanastomotic bile flow, which is defined as a complete passage of contrast material from the bile duct to the bowel loop within three minutes after injection. Biliary manometry or clinical trial using a capped "end-hole" catheter proximal to the treated duct or anastomosis can also be performed to determine the treatment success and the resolution of the anastomotic biliary stricture (Scott et al, 1998). In up to 41% of left lateral split-liver transplant recipients, the ducts for segments II and III are separately anastomosed to the jejunum (Broelsch et al, 1991). In these patients, biliary strictures may develop in one or both anastomoses (Fig. 17 a&b). For this reason, it is mandatory to know the number of hepaticojejunostomies present in a patient before performing percutaneous transhepatic cholangiography. In partial liver transplant recipients with an occlusive anastomotic biliary stricture that is not traversable with standard interventional radiology techniques, sharp percutaneous recanalization of the hepaticojejunostomy may be performed using a long needle, thus obviating surgery (Miraglia et al, 2007) (Fig. 17 C&D).

3.3.2 Intrahepatic biliary strictures and bilomas

Intrahepatic biliary strictures are usually related to chronic transplant rejection or arterial insufficiency caused by hepatic artery stenosis or thrombosis. A single focal stricture or multiple or combined intrahepatic and anastomotic strictures may be present (Fig. 18). Percutaneous treatment of intrahepatic biliary strictures is usually performed with the same techniques used for anastomotic biliary strictures; however, a recurrence rate of 90% was reported in a long-term follow-up study of intrahepatic strictures (Sunku et al, 2006).

Intrahepatic bilomas develop in the presence of arterial insufficiency due to hepatic artery stenosis or thrombosis or because of ABO incompatibility. Bilomas frequently are infected by gram-negative organisms that enter via the biliary anastomosis from the gastrointestinal tract. Percutaneous drainage of intrahepatic bilomas usually is performed with US guidance and is mandatory to reduce the risk of sepsis and graft loss (Hoffer et al, 1988).

3.3.3 Bile leakage

Postoperative bile leakage is a complication that usually occurs within few weeks after pediatric liver transplantation. Bile may leak from the bile duct anastomosis or from the resection margin in a split-liver transplant. Nonanastomotic leaks are usually associated with hepatic artery thrombosis.

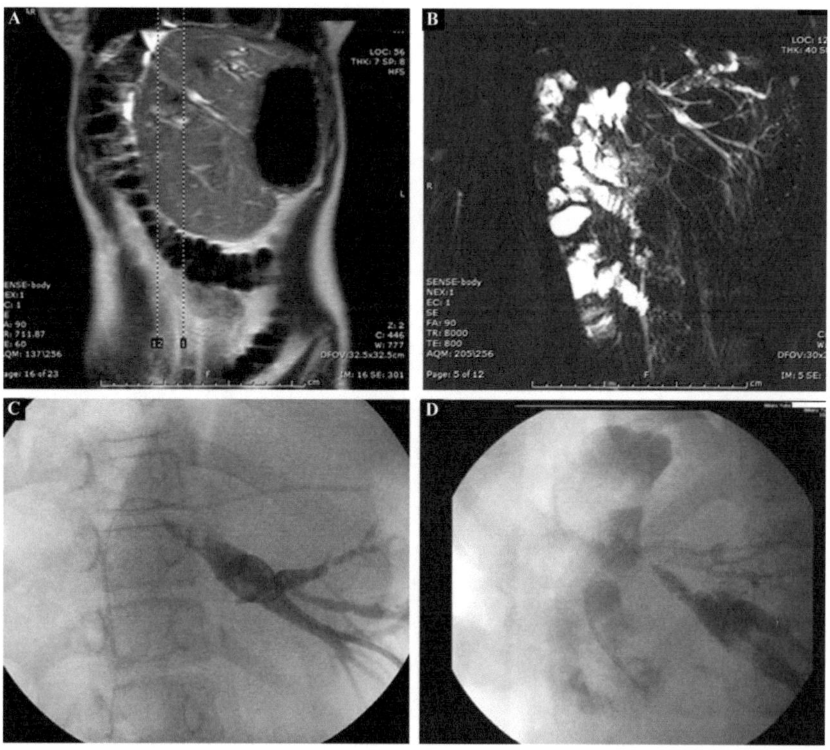

Fig. 17. Sharp recanalization of occlusive hepatico-jejunostomy. (A&B) MRI coronal images and MRCP demonstrating two separate heptico- jejunostomy with multiple filling defects in the superior bile duct. (C) Cholangiogram demonstrated external drain in the lower segmental bile duct with total occlusion of the inferior anastomosis, a plastic stent is noted across the superior anastomosis. (D) S/p sharp recanalization of the inferior anastomosis with the contrast drained through the anastomosis into the jejunum

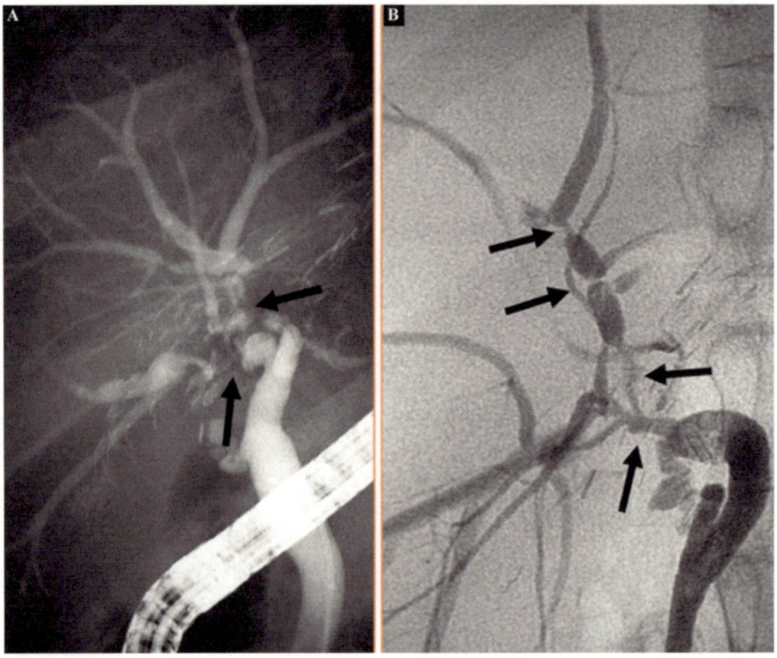

Fig. 18. Ischemic biliary duct injuries. (A) Intra-hepatic biliary ducts stenosis seen by ERCP cholangiogram. (B) Combined intra-hepatic and anastomotic biliary stricture

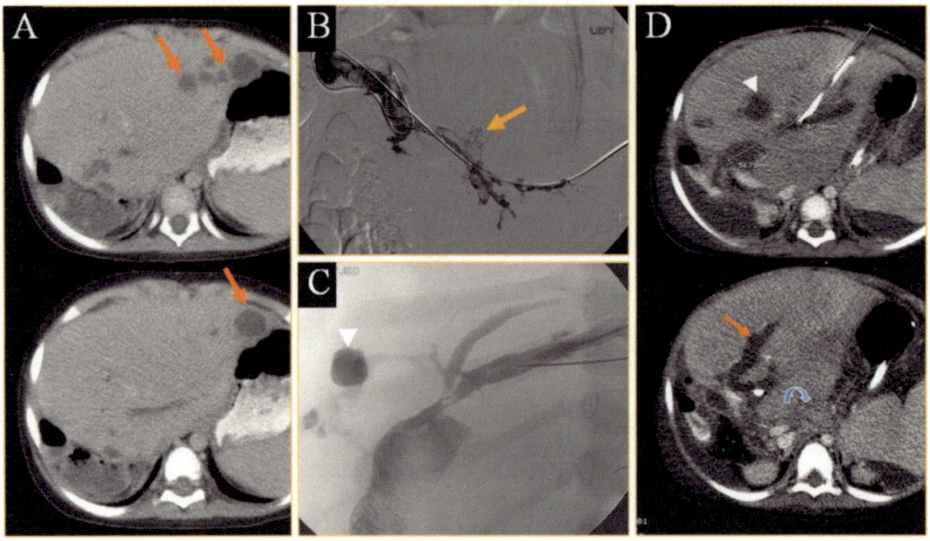

Fig. 19. (A) CT showing multiple bilomas (arrows). (B) Percutanous cholangiogram reveals irregular and dilated bile ducts (arrow) consistent with ischemic injury due to hepatic artery thrombosis. (C) Percutaneous cholangiogram in different duct reveals a small biloma (arrowhead). (D) Follow up CT of the abdomen reveals resolving bilomas with draining catheter in site (arrow). Retroperitoneal lymphadenopathy (curved arrow) consistent with post transplant lymphoproliferative disorder (PTLD)

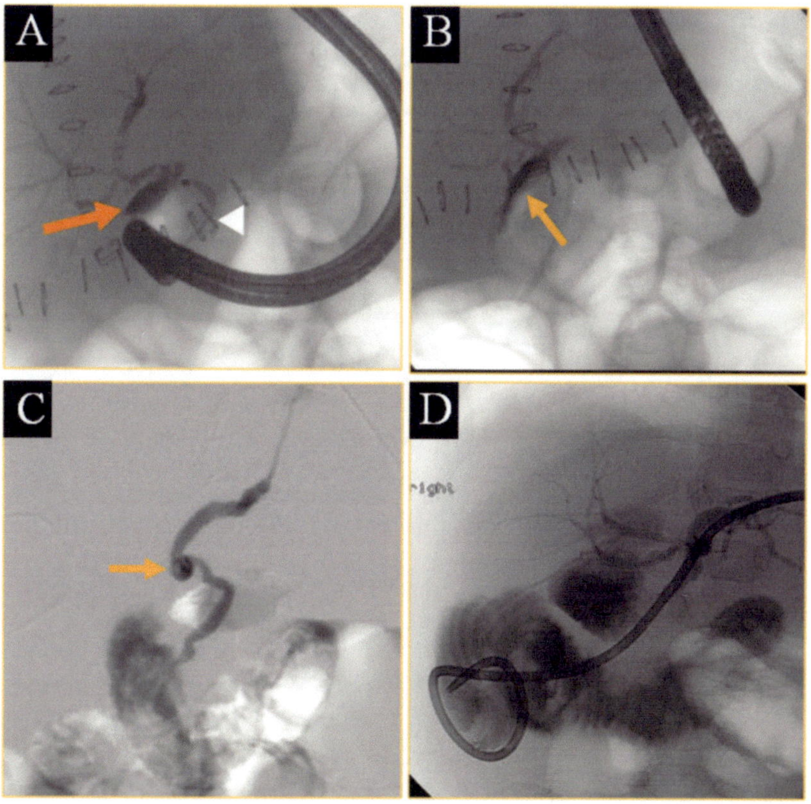

Fig. 20. (A&B) ERCP demonstrating bile leakage from CHD (arrow in A) and stricture at the distal CBD (arrowhead). Plastic stent is placed through the scop (arrow in B). (C) Percntaneous cholangiogram after the removal of the internal stent revealing a kink and narrowing at the CBD anastomosis (arrow). (D) 6.5 Fr internal\external drainage catheter was placed

Another possible site of leakage is the T-tube insertion in patients with a choledocho-choledochal anastomosis. Small leaks usually resolve spontaneously; whereas large ones are associated with significant morbidity and occasional mortatlity, thus require treatment. Clinical manifestation of bile leak vary, and can be presented as fever, abdominal pain, fluid and electrolyte depletion, fat malabsorption, and the possibility of sepsis or bleeding due to hilar vascular erosion. The bile extravasates into the peritoneal cavity or forms a perihepatic fluid collection. These fluid collections are usually well depicted at US. Percutaneous drainage catheters are placed with US guidance to drain these large bile collections. Bile leak can be confirmed by hepatobiliary scintigraphy with Technitum 99m Mebrofenin iminodiacetate. Recently, MR cholangiography performed with specific contrast agents has proved useful in the diagnosis of small bile leaks (Akin et al, 2004; Vitellas & Guttikonda, 2002). Adult patients who have undergone endoscopic or percutaneous transhepatic treatment for large bile leaks have experienced good outcomes obviating surgical repair in most cases (Akin et al, 2004; Kok et al, 1996). In pediatric liver transplant recipients, percutaneous transhepatic cholangiography and biliary catheter placement may be attempted for the treatment of large bile leaks from anastomoses only if the bile duct and the jejunal loop have not completely separated. A modified multipurpose drainage catheters can be placed in the intrahepatic biliary ducts crossing the leaking anastomosis into the distal bowel loop by adding holes proximally to reduce the contact between the bile and the anastomotic lesion and thereby facilitate the repair process Fig. (20). Surgical revision often is necessary or strongly recommended if cholangiography shows complete separation of the bile duct from the jejunal loop.

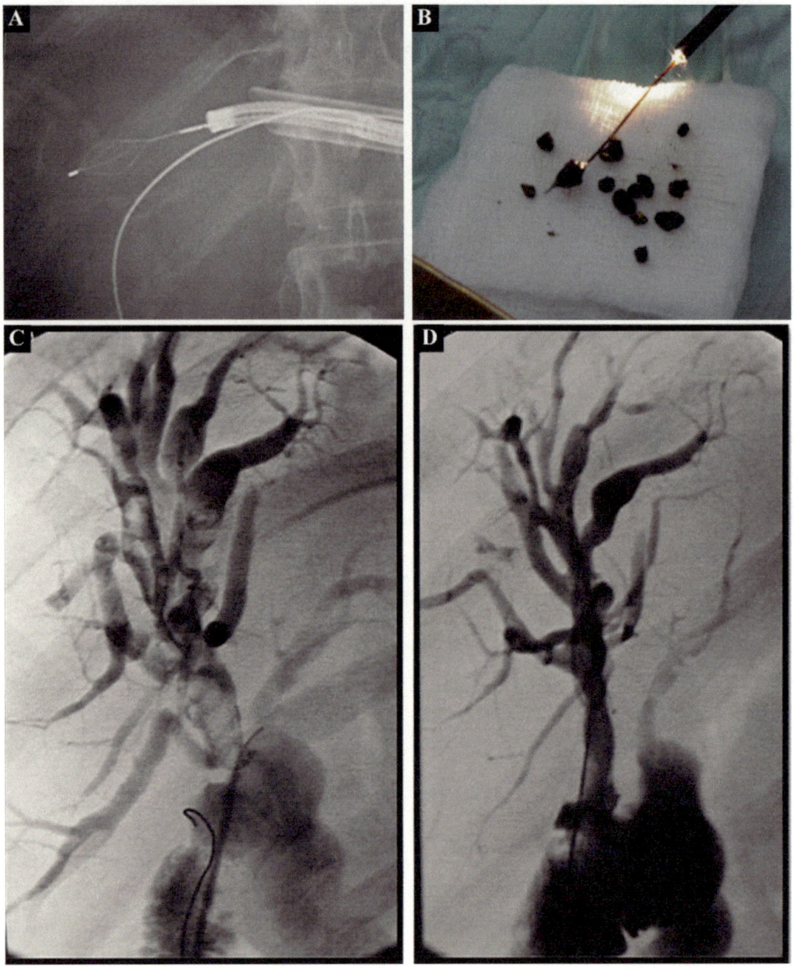

Fig. 21. Percutaneous retrieval of biliary stones. (A) a basket inserted co- axially with the cholangioscope through a large percutaneous access sheath to the left hepatic duct. (B) On table mage shows the retrieved stones. (C and D) pre and post stone retrieval cholangiogram demonstrated successful treatment with no residual stone and resolution of the biliary duct dilatation

3.3.4 Bile duct stones

Although stones and sludge occur only infrequently after transplantation, they are associated with high morbidity. Several factors can lead to the formation of biliary stones and sludge. Cyclosporine can alter the bile composition, inducing crystal formation, which results in biliary sludge and stone formation (Fulcher & Turner, 1999). Other causes include retained stones within the graft or stones formed secondary to bile stasis from biliary strictures. Biliary stones are well depicted with US and MR imaging (Kok et al, 1996; Laghi et al, 1999; Linhares et al, 2004). Interventional procedures may be useful for obviating surgery in these patients (Lorenz et al, 2005). Biliary stone removal can be performed through the percutaneous access to the involved bile duct and the stone can be retrieved using a basket or can be fragmented into small pieces using small forceps to drain with the bile into the intestine Fig. (21).

4. Conclusion

Liver transplantation is the ultimate treatment for children with end-stage liver disease. The application of reduced-size transplantation and the development of living related donor partial liver transplantation have expanded the donor pool, which, however, has in turn increased the risk for vascular and biliary complications. Imaging studies are extremely important for early diagnosis of post-transplantation complications because the clinical manifestations of these complications are frequently nonspecific and vary widely. Doppler US plays the leading role in the postoperative evaluation of pediatric patients. It is the imaging tool of choice for initial screening for biliary, arterial, and venous complications and is helpful in determining the next logical imaging test to confirm these complications. Current MR imaging techniques, including MR angiography and MR cholangiography, may provide a comprehensive evaluation of the transplanted liver; reveal abnormalities of vascular structures, bile ducts, and liver parenchyma; and depict extrahepatic tissues. If available, MR imaging should be used when US is inconclusive. CT is a valuable complement to US in the evaluation of complications involving the hepatic parenchyma as well as extrahepatic sites, especially the thorax. A number of complications can be corrected by using interventional radiologic techniques. Advances in minimally invasive, image-guided percutaneous and endovascular techniques of various vascular and nonvascular complications of liver transplantation, have led to improved Graft and patient survival and have obviated surgical revision or repeat transplantation in most cases.

5. References

Abbasoglu O., Levy MF., Vodapally MS., et al. (1997) Hepatic artery stenosis after liver transplantation: incidence, presentation, treatment, and long term outcome. *Transplantation*; 63:250–255.

Akin EB., Vitellas KM., Rajab A., et al. (2004) Magnetic resonance cholangiography with mangafodipir trisodium (Teslascan) to evaluate bile duct leaks after T-tube removal in liver transplantation. *J Comput Assist Tomogr*; 28:613–616.

Amaral JG., Schwartz J., Chait P., et al. (2006) Sonographically guided percutaneous liver biopsy in infants: a retrospective review. *AJR Am J Roentgenol*; 187(6):W644–W649.

Amesur NB & Zajko AB. (2006) Interventional radiology in liver transplantation. *Liver Transpl*; 12(3): 330–351.

Ametani F., Itoh K., Shibata T., Maetani Y., Tanaka K & Konishi J. (2001) Spectrum of CT findings in pediatric patients after partial liver transplantation. *Radio-Graphics*; 21:53–63.

Bergey EA., Sane SS., Kaye RD., Redd DC & Towbin RB. (1998) Pediatric transvenous liver biopsy. *J Vasc Interv Radiol*; 9(5):829–832.

Berrocal T., Parrón M., Alvarez-Luque A., Prieto C & Santamaría ML.(2006) Pediatric liver transplantation: a pictorial essay of early and late complications. *RadioGraphics*; 26(4):1187–1209.

Boraschi P& Donati F. (2004) Complications of orthotopic liver transplantation: imaging findings. *Abdom Imaging*; 29:189–202.

Broelsch CE., Whitington PF., Emond JC., et al. (1991) Liver transplantation in children from living related donors. Surgical techniques and results. *Ann Surg*; 214(4):428–437; discussion 437–439.

Buell JF., Funaki B., Cronin DC., et al. (2002) Long-term venous complications after full-size and segmental pediatric liver transplantation. *Ann Surg*; 236(5): 658–666.

Carnevale FC., Borges MV., de Paula Pinto R ., Oliva JL ., de Castro Andrade W & Maksoud JG. (2004) Endovascular treatment of stenosis between hepatic vein and inferior vena cava following liver transplantation in a child: a case report. *Pediatr Transplant*; 8:576–580.

Carter A, Beth., Kilic, Murat., Karpen, Saul & Goss, John. (June 13, 2006) History of Pediatric liver Transplantation, In: *Emedicine*, 2/19/2007, Available from: http://www.emedicine.com/ped/topic2840.htm

Cheng YF., Chen CL., Huang TL., et al. (2005) Angioplasty treatment of hepatic vein stenosis in pediatric liver transplants: long term results. *Transpl Int*; 18(5):556–561.

Chong WK. (2004) Ultrasound evaluation of liver transplants. *Abdom Imaging*; 29:180–188.

Crossin JD., Muradali D & Wilson SR. (2003) US of liver transplants: normal and abnormal. *RadioGraphics*; 23:1093– 1114.

Deshpande RR .,Bowles MJ., Vilca- Melendez H., et al. (2002) Result of split liver transplantation in children. *Ann Surg*; 236:248-53.

Dodd GD., Memel DS., Zajko A.,; Baron RL & Santaguida LA. (1994) Hepatic artery stenosis and thrombosis in transplant recipients: Doppler diagnosis with resistive index and systolic acceleration time. *Radiology*; 192:657–661.

Dodd GD. (1995) What is the tardus parvus spectral Doppler waveform and what is its usefulness in the detection of hepatic or renal artery stenosis? *AJR Am J Roentgenol*; 165:1299–1300.

Egawa H., Inomata Y., Uemoto S., et al. (1997) Hepatic vein reconstruction in 152 living-related donor liver transplantation patients. *Surgery*; 121: 250–257.

Fulcher AS & Turner MA. (1999) Orthotopic liver transplantation: evaluation with MR cholangiography. *Radiology*; 211:715–722.

Funaki B., Rosenblum JD., Leef JA., et al. (2000) Percutaneous treatment of portal venous stenosis in children and adolescents with segmental hepatic transplants: long-term results. *Radiology*; 215(1):147–151.

Furuya KN., Burrows PE., Phillips MJ & Roberts EA. (1992) Transjugular liver biopsy in children. *Hepatology*; 15(6):1036–1042.

Ghobrial RM., Yersiz H., Farmer DG., et al. (2000) Predictors of survival after in vivo split liver transplantation. *Ann Surg*; 232:312–323.

Garcı´a-Criado A., Gilabert R., Salmero´n JM, et al. (2003) Significance of and contributing factors for a high resistive index on Doppler sonography of the hepatic artery immediately after surgery: prognostic implications for liver transplant recipients. *AJR Am J Roentgenol*; 181:831–838.

Glockner JF & Forauer AR. (1999) Vascular or ischemic complications after liver transplantation. *AJR Am JRoentgenol*; 173:1055–1059.

Glockner JF., Forauer AR., Solomon H., Varma CR & Perman WH. (2000) Three-dimensional gadoliniumenhanced MR angiography of vascular complications after liver transplantation. *AJR Am J Roentgenol*; 174:1447–1453.

Habdank K., Restrepo R., Ng V., et al. (2003) Combined sonographic and fluoroscopic guidance during transjugular hepatic biopsies performed in children: a retrospective study of 74 biopsies. *AJR Am J Roentgenol*; 180(5):1393–1398.

Hall TR., McDiarmid SV., Grant EG., Boechat MI & Busuttil RW. (1990) False-negative duplex Doppler studies in children with hepatic artery thrombosis after liver transplantation. *AJR Am J Roentgenol*; 154:573–575.

Hasegawa T., Sasaki T., Kimura T., et al. (2002) Successful percutaneous transluminal angioplasty for hepatic artery stenosis in an infant undergoing living-related liver transplantation. *Pediatr Transplant*; 6(3): 244–248.

Hashikura Y., Kawasaki S., Terada M., et al. (2001) Longterm results of living-related donor liver graft transplantation: a single-center analysis of 110 transplants. *Transplantation*; 72:95–99.

Heffron TG., Emond JC., Whitington PF., et al. (1992) Biliary complications in pediatric liver transplantation. A comparison of reduced-size and whole grafts. *Transplantation*; 53(2):391–395.

Hoffer FA., Teele RL., Lillehei CW & Vacanti JP. (1988) Infected bilomas and hepatic artery thrombosis in infant recipients of liver transplants: interventional radiology and medical therapy as an alternative to retransplantation. *Radiology*; 169(2):435–438.

Hoffer FA. (2000) Liver biopsy methods for pediatric oncology patients. *Pediatr Radiol*; 30(7):481–488.

Holbert BL., Campbell WL & Skolnick ML. (1995) Evaluation of the transplanted liver and postoperative complications. *Radiol Clin North Am*; 33: 521–540.

Huang TL., Chen TY., Tsang LL., et al. (2004) Hepatic venous stenosis in partial liver graft transplantation detected by color Doppler ultrasound before and after radiological interventional management. *Transplant Proc*; 36:2342–2343.

Ito K., Siegelman E., Stolpen A & Mitchell D. (2000) MR imaging of complications after liver transplantation. *AJR Am J Roentgenol*; 175:1145–1149.

Jain A., Mazariegos G., Kashyap R., et al. (2002) Pediatric liver transplantation. A single center experience spanning 20 years. *Transplantation*; 73(6): 941–947.

Kaneko J., Sugawara Y., Akamatsu N., et al. (2004) Prediction of hepatic artery thrombosis by protocol Doppler ultrasonography in pediatric living donor liver transplantation. *Abdom Imaging*; 29: 603–605.

Katyal S., Oliver JH 3rd., Buck DG & Federle MP. (2000) Detection of vascular complications after liver transplantation: early experience in multislice CT angiography with volume rendering. *AJR Am J Roentgenol*; 175:1735–1739.

Kaye R., Sane SS & Towbin RB. (2000) Pediatric intervention: an update—part II. *J Vasc Interv Radiol*; 11(7): 807–822.

Kitazono MT., Qayyum A., Yeh BM., et al. (2007) Magnetic resonance cholangiography of biliary strictures after liver transplantation: a prospective doubleblind study. *J Magn Reson Imaging*; 25(6): 1168–1173.

Kok T., Slooff MJ., Thijn CJ., et al. (1998) Routine Doppler ultrasound for the detection of clinically unsuspected vascular complications in the early postoperative phase after orthotopic liver transplantation. *Transpl Int*; 11:272–276.

Kok T., Van der Sluis A., Klein JP., et al. (1996) Ultrasound and cholangiography for the diagnosis of biliary complications after orthotopic liver transplantation: a comparative study. *J Clin Ultrasound*; 24:103–115.

Kubo T., Shibata T., Itoh K., et al. (2006) Outcome of percutaneous transhepatic venoplasty for hepatic venous outflow obstruction after living donor liver transplantation. *Radiology*; 239(1):285–290.

Laghi A., Pavone P., Catalano C., et al. (1999) MR cholangiography of late biliary complications after liver transplantation. *AJR Am J Roentgenol*; 172: 1541–1546.

Langnas AN., Marujo W., Stratta RJ., Wood RP & Shaw BW. (1991) Vascular complications after orthotopic liver transplantation. *Am J Surg*; 161:76–83.

Lallier M., St-Vil D., Luks FI., Bensoussan AL., Guttman FM & Blanchard H. (1993) Biliary tract complications in pediatric orthotopic liver transplantation. *J Pediatr Surg*; 28(9):1102–1105.

Linhares MM., Gonzalez AM., Goldman SM., et al. (2004) Magnetic resonance cholangiography in the diagnosis of biliary complications after orthotopic liver transplantation. *Transplant Proc*; 36:947–948.

Lorenz JM., Denison G., Funaki B., Leef JA., Van Ha T & Rosenblum JD. (2005) Balloon dilatation of biliary- enteric strictures in children. *AJR Am J Roentgenol*; 184:151–155.

Lorenz JM., Funaki B., Leef JA., Rosenblum JD &Van Ha T. (2001) Percutaneous transhepatic cholangiography and biliary drainage in pediatric liver transplant patients. *AJR Am J Roentgenol*; 176: 761–765.

Lorenz JM., Van Ha T., Funaki B., et al. (2006) Percutaneous treatment of venous outflow obstruction in pediatric liver transplants. *J Vasc Interv Radiol*; 17(11 pt 1):1753–1761.

Lorenz JM., Denison G., Funaki B., et al. (2005) Balloon dilatation of biliary-enteric strictures in children. *AJR Am J Roentgenol*; 184(1):151–155.

Marder DM., DeMarino GB., Sumkin JH & Sheahan DG. (1989) Liver transplantation rejection: value of the resistive index in Doppler ultrasound of hepatic arteries. *Radiology*; 173:127–129.

Mazzaferro V., Esquivel CO., Makowka L., et al. (1989) Hepatic artery thrombosis after pediatric liver transplantation: a medical or surgical event? *Transplantation*; 47:971–977.

Miraglia R., Luca A., Marrone G., et al. (2007) Percutaneous transhepatic venous angioplasty in a two-yr-old patient with hepatic vein stenosis after partial liver transplantation. *Pediatr Transplant*; 11(2): 222–224.

Millis JM., Seaman DS., Piper JB., et al. (1996) Portal vein thrombosis and stenosis in pediatric liver transplantation. *Transplantation*; 62:748–753.

Miraglia R., Luca A., Maruzzelli L., et al. (2007) Percutaneous recanalization of an occluded hepatico-jejunostomy, using Colapinto needle, in a two-yr-old patient after partial liver transplantation. *Pediatr Transplant*; 11(6):676–679.

Moray G., Boyvat F., Sevmiş S., et al. (2005) Vascular complications after liver transplantation in pediatric patients. *Transplant Proc*; 37(7):3200–3202.

Nghiem HV. (1998) Imaging of hepatic transplantation. *Radiol Clin North Am*; 36:429–443.

Nghiem HV., Tran K., Winter TC 3rd., et al. (1996) Imaging of complications in liver transplantation. *RadioGraphics*; 16:825–840.

Nolten A & Sproat IA. (1996) Hepatic artery thrombosis after liver transplantation: temporal accuracy of diagnosis with duplex US and the syndrome of impending thrombosis. *Radiology*; 198:553–559.

Norton KI., Lee JS., Kogan D., et al. (2001) The role of magnetic resonance cholangiography in the management of children and young adults after liver transplantation. *Pediatr Transplant*; 5(6):410–418.

Platt JF., Yutzy GG., Bude RO., Ellis JH & Rubin JM. (1997) Use of Doppler sonography for revealing hepatic artery stenosis in liver transplant recipients. *AJR Am J Roentgenol*; 168:473–476.

Rose SC., Andre MP., Roberts AC., et al. (2001) Integral Role of interventional radiology in the development of a pediatric liver transplantation program. *Pediatr Transplant*; 5(5):331-338.

Rossi C., Zambruni A., Ansaloni F., et al. (2004) Combined mechanical and pharmacologic thrombolysis for portal vein thrombosis in liver-graft recipients and in candidates for liver transplantation. *Transplantation*; 78:938–940.

Schwarzenberg SJ., Sharp HL., Payne WD., et al. (2002) Biliary stricture in living-related donor liver transplantation: management with balloon dilation. *Pediatr Transplant*; 6(2):132–135.

Scott J. S., John L. C., Keith D. L., Gunnar B. L., Sally E, M & Anthony C. V. (1998) The biliary manometric perfusion test and clinical trial--long-term predictive value of success after treatment of bile duct strictures: ten-year experince *J Vasc Interv Radiol*; 9(6):976-85.

Settmacher U., Stange B., Haase R., et al. (2000) Arterial complications after liver transplantation. *TransplInt*; 13:372–378.

Sieders E., Peeters PM., TenVergert EM., et al. (2000) Early vascular complications after pediatric liver transplantation. *Liver Transpl*; 6(3):326–332.

Stafford-Johnson DB., Hamilton BH., Dong Q., et al. (1998) Vascular complications of liver transplantation: evaluation with gadolinium-enhanced MR angiography. *Radiology*; 207:153–160.

Starzl TE., Marchiaro TL., et al. (1963) Homotransplantation of the liver in humans. *Surg Gynecol Obstet*; 117: 659-64.

Stell D., Downey D., Marotta P., et al. (2004) Prospective evaluation of the role of quantitative Doppler ultrasound surveillance in liver transplantation. *Liver Transpl*; 10:1183–1188.

Sze DY & Esquivel CO. (2002) The role of interventional radiology in a pediatric liver transplant program. *Pediatr Transplant*; 6(1):1–4.

Sunku B., Salvalaggio PR., Donaldson JS., et al. (2006) Outcomes and risk factors for failure of radiologic treatment of biliary strictures in pediatric liver transplantation recipients. *Liver Transpl*; 12(5):821–826.

Totsuka E., Hakamada K., Narumi S., et al. (2004) Hepatic vein anastomotic stricture after living donor liver transplantation. *Transplant Proc*; 36:2252- 2254.

Ueda M., Egawa H., Ogawa K., et al. (2005) Portal vein complications in the long-term course after pediatric living donor liver transplantation. *Transplant Proc*; 37(2):1138–1140.

Unsinn KM., Freund MC., Ellemunter H., et al. (2003) Spectrum of imaging findings after pediatric liver transplantation. II. Posttransplantation complications. *AJR Am J Roentgenol*; 181:1139-1144.

Vignali C., Bargellini I., Cioni R., et al. (2004) Diagnosis and treatment of hepatic artery stenosis after orthotopic liver transplantation. *Transplant Proc*; 36:2771–2773.

Vitellas KM & Guttikonda S. (2002) Hepatic transplant complicated by hepatic artery thrombosis and bile duct necrosis: case report and potential application of contrast-enhanced MR cholangiography following intravenous mangafodipir trisodium in the emergency room setting. *Emerg Radiol*; 9:106–109.

Vivarelli M., Cucchetti A., La Barba G., et al. (2004) Ischemic arterial complications after liver transplantation in the adult: multivariate analysis of risk factors. *Arch Surg*; 139:1069–1074.

White SA., Al-Mukhtar A., Lodge JP & Pollard SG. Progress in living donor liver transplantation. *Transplant Proc*; 36:2720–2726.

Zajko AB., Sheng R., Bron K, Reyes J., Nour B & Tzakis A. (1994) Percutaneous transluminal angioplasty of venous anastomotic stenoses complicating liver transplantation: intermediate-term results. *J Vasc Interv Radiol*; 5(1):121–126.

Zalasin S., Shapiro RS., Glajchen N & Stancato- Pasik A. (1998) Liver transplant rejection: value of hepatic vein Doppler waveform analysis. *Abdom Imaging*; 23:427–430.

Part 5

Nonsurgical Complications

13

Renal Dysfunction and Liver Transplantation

Naglaa Allam
National Liver Institute, Menoufeyia University, Egypt

1. Introduction

Liver transplantation, whether living donor (LDLT) or deceased donor (DDLT), is currently the treatment of choice for patients with advanced liver disease. While initially the focus was on acceptable short-term survival, currently the efforts are aimed at improving long-term prognosis. Thus, focus is now on the quality of life after liver transplantation, as well as prediction and management of conditions related to morbidity and mortality in long-term survivors. Renal dysfunction is an important problem in this scenario. Both acute (ARD) and chronic renal dysfunctions (CRD) develop frequently after liver transplantation and can seriously jeopardize postoperative patient survival.

Acute kidney injury is one of the most common complications of liver transplantation. It occurs more frequently in those who have hepatorenal syndrome at the time of liver transplantation. Acute renal dysfunction has been associated with an 8-fold increase in mortality risk, prolonged intensive care unit stay and a greater risk for infectious complications. In the subgroup of patients who develop acute renal failure and survive, 80% to 90% regain some degree of renal function, whereas the rest develop permanent renal dysfunction. Chronic renal dysfunction, not only has implications in terms of an increased demand on resources, but is also significantly associated with a higher patient mortality rate.

In order to minimize the occurrence of ARD and CRD thereafter, it is vital to define the possible preoperative, intraoperative and postoperative risk factors. In this review, we discuss the various definitions, diagnostic tools, predictors of renal dysfunction after liver transplantation together with discussion of specific causes of renal dysfunction. This information will be useful in developing strategies for preventing the development or progression of renal dysfunction in liver transplant recipients, especially in view of the current availability of nonnephrotoxic immunosuppressive drugs.

2. Assessment of renal function prior to transplantation

With broadening of the inclusion criteria for liver transplantation, the majority of liver transplant recipients have some impairment of renal function prior to transplantation and most have clinically apparent renal insufficiency at some time in the posttransplant period. Among those with renal impairment at the time of transplant are patients whose renal failure is due to the same underlying process that caused the liver disease (hepatitis B, hepatitis C, analgesic overdose, amyloidosis, autoimmune disease), patients with underlying parenchymal renal disease from diseases such as diabetes and hypertension, and other patients in whom the functional renal impairment is caused by the liver failure itself and its complications. The latter group may have manifestations ranging from mild sodium retention to oliguric renal failure termed hepatorenal syndrome (HRS) (Smith, 2006).

For both prognostic and therapeutic reasons it is important to *assess the level of renal function* in patients being considered for liver transplantation and to determine if there is any reversible component. Also given organ shortage it should be essential to determine which patients will experience progressive and severe renal dysfunction after liver transplantation (Burra et al., 2009).

2.1 Methods of measurement of renal function

The most commonly used markers of glomerular filtration rate (GFR), blood urea nitrogen (BUN) and serum creatinine (Scr), have limitations that should be kept in mind, especially in the setting of liver transplantation. Because **urea** is generated by the liver from the metabolism of protein and ammonia, both malnutrition and poor hepatic function may cause a falsely low BUN that can lead to an overestimation of GFR. Conversely, corticosteroids, bleeding (particularly in the gastrointestinal tract), and renal hypoperfusion cause higher BUN levels than one would expect for a given level of GFR (Cholongitas et al., 2007 a).

Also current diagnostic paradigms for acute kidney injury are limited by reliance on **serum creatinine (Scr)**, which is affected by age, gender, nutrition and the amount of muscle mass which may render the values inaccurate. Thus, most patients with endstage liver disease with decreased muscle mass may have a misleadingly low Scr. In addition, elevations in Scr may occur several days after the actual injury (Fieghen et al., 2009). Also, a number of medications (including trimethoprim) inhibit the secretion of creatinine, so that when these medications are used, Scr may rise without any true change in GFR (Cholongitas et al., 2007). Furthermore, creatinine is both filtered and secreted by the nephron, so that its clearance is an overestimate of GFR. It should also be noted that the relationship between the serum creatinine and GFR is not linear; at high levels of GFR, the Scr is insensitive to large changes in GFR, while at low levels of GFR, small changes in GFR cause large changes in serum creatinine (Mariat et al., 2004). A problem, not often recognized is that measurement of Scr suffers from a variety of interferences (Cholongitas et al., 2007 b) and absence of international standard for measurement (Seronie-Vivien et al., 2005). Serum creatinine is usually measured by the Jaffè method, but this is prone to interference, for example, from protein, ketones and bilirubin. Hence, hyperbilirubinemia often impacts on the measurement of Scr in endstage liver disease population (Owen et al., 2006). These findings can result in an underestimation of renal function.

Despite the above limitations, the endogenous creatinine clearance from a timed urine collection or as calculated from the Cockcroft–Gault formula {(140- age)/Cr × (weight in kg/72) (× 0.85 for females)} (Cockcroft and Gault, 1976) remains the most common measure of GFR (Lewandowska & Matuszkiewicz-Rowinska, 2011). If a timed urine collection is performed, the amount of creatinine excreted in 24 hours should be 12–25 mg/kg body weight as a crude test for completeness of the collection. Because of the variability in the accuracy of timed collections performed by outpatients, and the excellent correlation of the Cockcroft–Gault calculation with timed creatinine clearance measurements under controlled conditions, a timed collection may be necessary only for a baseline creatinine clearance and to measure protein excretion. It can then be repeated only as necessary to confirm abrupt or unexpected changes in the serum creatinine (Smith, 2006). However, it should be noted that there is some debate concerning the use of the Cockcroft-Gault equation to estimate GFR (Gonwa et al., 2004). This formula may be inaccurate and pick up small differences in GFR that are statistically significant but clinically irrelevant. Although GFR calculations often overestimate GFR measurements (Poge et al., 2005), even using the best formulas available, the Cockcroft-Gault equation has been used in many published studies and was widely used in clinical practice (Burra et al., 2009).

Modification of diet in renal disease (MDRD) equation (Levey et al., 1999) is another method that is considered more accurate than other formulas to measure GFR in patients with intact kidney function. MDRD equation: GFR = 170 x [Serum creatinine]-0.999 x [Age]-0.176 x [0.762 if patient is female] x [1.180 if patient is black] x [BUN]-0.170 x [Albumin] + 0.318. Most often, the formula, excluding urea and albumin (four variables), is used to calculate GFR, as it is as accurate as the original six-variable formula (Levey et al., 2006). Neither these formulas nor calculation of creatinine clearance from a 24-hour urine collection has been well studied or validated in patients with decompensated cirrhosis. Preliminary data suggest that the MDRD equation is more precise in liver transplant (LT) patients than other renal formulas, but the MDRD equation actually underestimates GFR measured by the gold standard of iothalamate clearance. There are now online calculators that provide a convenient way to estimate GFR (e.g. http://nephron.com/gi-bin/MDRDSIdefault.cgi) (Fabrizi et al., 2010). However, in LT recipients, even the best performing equation, the six-variable MDRD equation, provides an estimate that is within 30% of the actual GFR only two-thirds of the time (Gonwa et al., 2004).

Ideally, renal function can be estimated through the use of inulin, (125I) iothalamate, or 51Cr-EDTA clearance methods, but these are costly and often impractical. Many nuclear medicine departments perform isotopic GFR measurements based on the decay of the plasma level of an injected radiolabeled GFR marker over a few hours (Mariat et al., 2004). However the cost of the radiolabeled GFR markers and the precautions needed in handling them make these tests expensive.

2.2 Diagnosis of pre-transplant kidney dysfunction

Patients with cirrhosis are candidates to develop acute renal failure from different causes; each of them requiring specific treatments. In cirrhotic patients with ascites, pre-renal failure (42%) and acute tubular necrosis (ATN) (38%) represent the most common forms of acute renal failure while hepatorenal syndrome (HRS) is somewhat less frequent (20%) (Fasolato et al., 2007). Approximately 18% will develop HRS at 1 year and 39% at 5 years (Terra et al., 2005). However, it may be difficult to identify the cause and start the appropriate treatment (Moreau and Lebrec, 2003). The different causes of acute renal failure in cirrhotics are discussed below. Table 1 shows the differential diagnosis of the causes that are most commonly encountered during preparation for liver transplant.

2.2.1 Hepatorenal syndrome

Patients with end-stage liver disease may exhibit a spectrum of functional renal impairment from mild sodium retention and clinically inapparent reduction in GFR, to an oliguric state with severe intrarenal vasoconstriction, avid sodium conservation, and very low GFR referred to as hepatorenal syndrome (Eckardt, 1999). In almost half the cases of HRS, one or more precipitating factors may be identified, including bacterial infections (57%), gastrointestinal hemorrhage (36%), and large volume paracentesis (7%) (Fasolato et al., 2007). The hallmark of HRS is intense renal vasoconstriction with predominant peripheral arterial vasodilation. Kidney histology is normal (Wadei et al., 2006).

HRS is a diagnosis of exclusion, requiring the absence of sepsis and nephrotoxic agents, less than 500 mg/day of protein excretion and no microhaematuria, an ultrasound showing no evidence of obstruction or parenchymal renal disease, and a lack of improvement of serum creatinine (<1.5mg/dl) with cessation of diuretic therapy and plasma volume expansion (albumin 1 g/kg upto max. of 100g/day) (*New International Ascites Club's diagnostic criteria of hepatorenal syndrome* (Salerno et al., 2007). If the syndrome persists, acute tubular necrosis may result. Thus, the urine sodium concentration is less than 10 meq/L early in the process, but as tubular ischemia occurs, the urine sodium rises, clouding the diagnostic issue.

2.2.2 Volume depletion induced renal dysfunction

Prerenal failure usually occurs in patients with decompensated cirrhosis. These patients already have significant circulatory dysfunction characterized by low arterial pressure, renal vasoconstriction and decreased renal blood flow; but they have no or only mild reduction in GFR. Volume depletion further decreases renal blood flow and induces a marked decline in GFR which may be rapidly reversible if the underlying cause is corrected (Moreau and Lebrec, 2003). Ten to twenty percent of patients with gastrointestinal hemorrhage have hypovolemic shock on admission. This true hypovolemia is one cause of prerenal azotemia. A retrospective study showed that 5% of patients with cirrhosis hospitalised for acute upper gastrointestinal hemorrhage had early renal failure that lasted less than 7 days after index bleeding (Cardenas et al., 2001). Patients admitted for hemorrhage may also develop prerenal failure due to other causes such as bacterial infection (Cardenas et al, 2001).

True hypovolemia and subsequent renal failure may also result from vomiting, diarrhea, glycosuria or diuretic treatment used to mobilize ascites.

2.2.3 Severe sepsis

Patients with cirrhosis are susceptible to bacterial infections, in particular spontaneous bacterial peritonitis (SBP). Septic shock and subsequent prerenal azotemia occurs in 10% of patients with SBP. At the onset of SBP, 20-40% of patients have renal failure without shock (Moreau and Lebrec, 2006). Thirty percent of those admitted for SBP or for another bacterial infection develop type 1 HRS during hospitalization (Terra et al., 2005).

2.2.4 Drugs

NSAIDS

Cyclo-Oxygenase (COX)-derived vasodilator prostaglandins protect renal perfusion in patients with cirrhosis and ascites. Hence administration of non-selective non-steroidal anti-inflammatory drugs (NSAIDs) (i.e., drugs that can inhibit cyclooxygenase-1 (COX-1)) and cyclooxygenase-2) in cirrhotic patients may lead to marked renal hypoperfusion and subsequent prerenal failure following COX inhibition induced by non-selective NSAIDs. It was also shown that COX-2 inhibitors, like non-selective NSAIDs, may also induce prerenal failure in patients with cirrhosis and ascites (FitzGerald and Patrono, 2001).

Antibiotics

Patients with cirrhosis and ascites are predisposed to aminoglycoside nephrotoxicity, the reported incidence of which (32%) is much higher than that found by other investigators in the general population (3–11%). Aminoglycoside nephrotoxicity is associated with a marked deterioration in renal function (Cabrera et al., 1982). Patients with decompensated cirrhosis are prone to develop this complication, since they frequently have impaired renal blood flow and glomerular filtration rates, and renal accumulation of aminoglycosides is greater with renal impairment (Moore et al., 1984).

2.2.5 Contrast induced nephropathy

This is defined as impairment of renal function subsequent to the administration of contrast media in the absence of any other cause. Contrast induced nephropathy (CIN) is diagnosed when there is an increase in serum creatinine concentration of > 0.5 mg/dl or a relative increase of > 25% from the baseline within 72 hrs after contrast media administration (Barrett and Parfrey, 1994).

Pre-existing renal dysfunction and diabetes mellitus are the two most important risk factors for CIN. The incidence of CIN is less than 2% when basal creatinine is less than 1.6 mg/dl and increases to 12-29% when above 1.6 mg/dl and to 38% when above 2.0 mg/dl. The presence of more than one risk factor increases the risk to develop CIN by many folds (Liu et al., 2005). The incidence of CIN also rises with increase in the volume of the contrast media. It is less than 2% when patients receive less than 125 ml of contrast media compared with 19% in patients receiving more than that volume. Peri-procedural hydration is regarded as a simple and effective means to prevent CIN. Results of a large number of clinical trials go in favour of post-procedural acetylcystine which is a free radical scavenger and precursor of antioxidant glutathione (Tepel et al., 2006). Recovery occurs in the majority of cases within 2–3 weeks; few patients require dialysis for recovery (Barrett & Parfrey, 1994).

2.2.6 Intrinsic renal failure

2.2.6.1 Viral hepatitis and associated glomerular diseases

Viral infections such as hepatitis B (HBV) and C (HCV) are well-known to induce concomitant severe hepatic and renal injuries with ultimate endstage renal disease. The most common clinical presentation in both cases is the nephrotic syndrome with a slowly progressive decline in renal function (Lai & Lai, 1991 and Johnson et al., 1994a). The proteinuria remits spontaneously in a minority of patients, but may also recur. The degree of proteinuria appears to correlate with viremia as spontaneous remission of the glomerulopathy is usually associated with clearance of viral antigens from the blood. The mechanisms whereby different viral infections induce distinct glomerular lesions and/or systemic complications have not been fully elucidated. Circulating and most likely in situ immune complexes involving viral antigens and host anti-viral antibodies have been implicated in hepatitis B- associated membranous glomerulonephropathy (Pham et al., 2005).

HCV-related glomerulonephritis

Hepatitis C has been associated most closely with mesangiocapillary glomerulonephritis (Bursten & Rodby, 1993, Johnson et al., 1993 & Johnson et al., 1994b). Many of the patients with chronic HCV and mesangiocapillary glomerulonephritis also have hypocomplementemia, cryoglobulinemia (the cryoprecipitates contain HCV-RNA), and rheumatoid factors (IgM antibodies directed against anti-HCV antibodies). Other symptoms and signs of mixed cryoglobulinemia such as skin lesions, arthritis, and neuropathy may not be present. Indeed, even the hepatitis associated with the renal disease may be asymptomatic and the transaminases may be normal (Johnson et al., 1994b). Less commonly, non-cryoglobulinemic mesangiocapillary glomerulonephritis, focal and segmental glomerulosclerosis, mesangial proliferation with IgA deposition, fibrillary and immunoactoid glomerulopathies occur (Dore et al., 2007). A purely membranous glomerulonephritis has also been reported in patients with HCV, and may have a different pathogenesis (Stehman-Breen et al., 1995). McGuire et al performed kidney biopsies at the time of liver transplantation in 30 patients with HCV-related cirrhosis and a median creatinine of 1.4 mg/dL; immune complex glomerulonephritis was reported in 83% of the patients (McGuire et al., 2006).

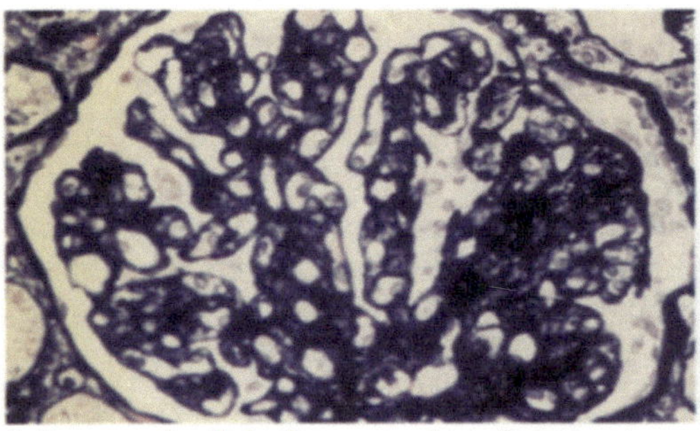

A. Increased cellularity, expansion of mesangium, Thickening & splitting of capillary walls

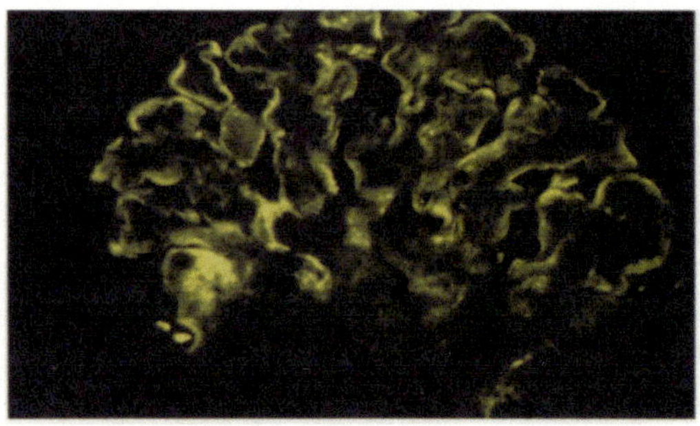

B. Capillary wall deposits of Ig G

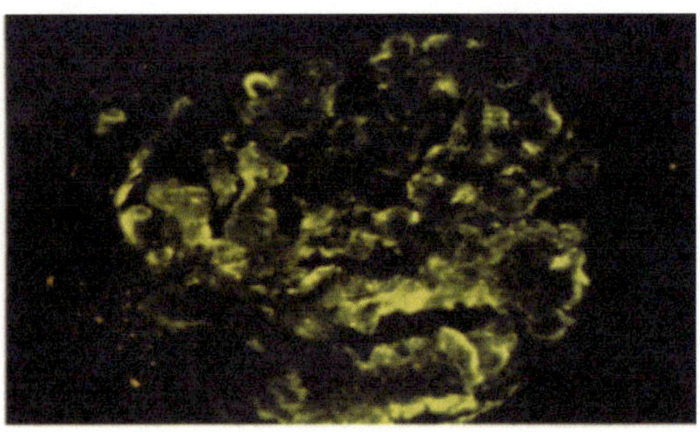

C. Capillary wall deposits of IgM

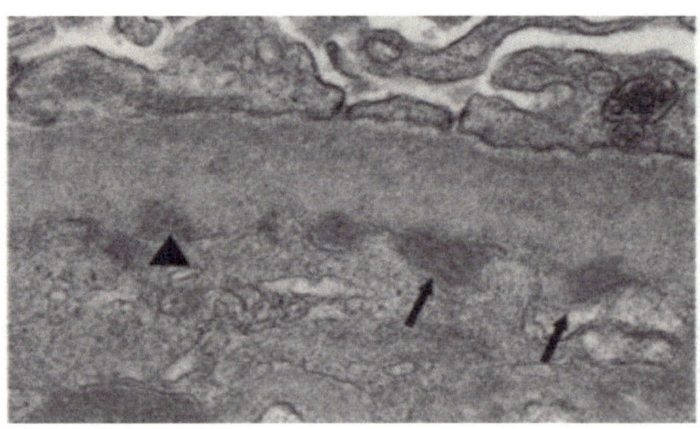

D. EM of glomerular capillary: subendothelial immune deposits as tactoids (arrows) & microtubules (arrowheads) characteristic of cryoglobuinns

Fig. 1. Renal Biopsy specimen from a patient with Hepatitis C (Johnson et al., 1993)

HBV-related glomerulonephritis

HBV-related glomerulonephritis is more often found in children. Membranous glomerulonephritis is the most common form of HBV-related glomerulonephritis, but mesangiocapillary glomerulonephritis, mesangial proliferative glomerulonephritis, focal segmental glomerulosclerosis, IgA nephropathy and minimal change disease have all been described. In addition, in patients with HBV-associated polyarteritis nodosa, a variety of histologic patterns have been documented (Lai & Lai, 1991). Immune complexes of hepatitis B surface, core, and e antigens as well as antibodies together with complement components have been demonstrated in glomerular basement membrane and mesangium. HBV antigens have been localized in the glomeruli using immunofluorescent antibodies, electron microscopy, and molecular techniques. HBeAg has been consistently associated with capillary basement membrane deposits (membranous form of glomerulopathy), while HBsAg is more closely associated with deposits in the mesangium (Lai and Lai., 1991; Takekoshi et al., 1991).

Liver disease tends to be mild in patients who present with HBV-related glomerulonephritis. Disease remission is especially evident after HBeAg seroconversion. A significant percent of adults (30%) may progress to renal failure and as many as 10% will require maintenance dialysis (Bhimma et al., 2002).

2.2.6.2 Renal disease associated with poor hepatic function

Patients with poor hepatic function of any cause may develop parenchymal renal disease manifested by nonnephrotic proteinuria, microscopic hematuria, and reduced GFR. The most common histologic picture is a mesangiopathic glomerulonephritis with deposition of IgM and often IgA, perhaps because of impaired clearance by the liver. It has not been proved that these immune complexes are the cause of the renal disease (Smith, 2006).

	Prerenal Azotemia	**Acute tubular Necrosis**	**Hepatorenal Syndrome**	**Primary Nephropathy**
Urine sodium	<10 mEq/L	>30 mmol/L	<10 mmol/L	>30 mmol/L
Urine to plasma creatinine ratio	>30:1	<20:1	>30:1	<20:1
Proteinuria	<100mg	<500mg	<500mg	Variable

Table 1. Differential Diagnosis of Acute renal failure in advanced liver disease. (Eckardt, 1999)

Renal failure post liver transplantation

Renal insufficiency, whether acute renal failure (ARF) or chronic kidney disease (CKD), is a common complication after liver transplantation and represents a major cause of morbidity and mortality following LT (Yalavarthy et al., 2007).

3. Acute renal failure

3.1 Epidemiology

Acute renal failure (ARF) is one of the most common complications of liver transplantation (LT), with a variable incidence rate in different studies. The incidence of acute kidney injury (AKI) has been reported to vary between 17% to 95% post-liver transplantation (Bilbao et al.,

1998, Lima et al., 2003). The difference in the incidence reported may be due in part to the large difference in the criteria used to define ARF.

Campbell et al., 2005 and Lebrón Gallardo et al., 2004 used a value of serum creatinine above 1.5 mg/dl as diagnostic of acute Kidney injury (AKI) and reported an incidence as high as 64%. On the other hand, Junge et al, 2006, reported a relatively low incidence of 11.9% and defined AKI post-LT as serum creatinine of 2.5 mg/dl in the first week only. Actually the incidence rate of post-LT ARD differs even in the same center when variable definitions are used. Barri and colleagues, 2009 conducted a study on 1050 patients who underwent LT, using changes in serum creatinine from baseline as the main marker for acute kidney injury (AKI). They used three different definitions to diagnose post-LT AKI. Defining AKI as a rise in serum creatinine of >0.5 mg/dL resulted in the highest incidence of AKI (78%). The second definition of AKI was a rise in serum creatinine of >1 mg/dl and this resulted in an incidence of AKI 46%. When AKI was defined as a rise of serum creatinine of >50% from baseline to above 2 mg/dl, the lowest incidence of AKI (14%) was found (Barri et al., 2009). Hence, these variations in definitions cause difficulties in comparing different studies and demonstrate the need for a consensus in the diagnosis of acute renal disease after LT.

3.2 Definition of acute renal failure

Several researchers have evaluated the problem of renal impairment post-LT but it is difficult to meaningfully compare these studies as a series of different definitions are used (Cabezuelo et al., 2002).

To address this issue, RIFLE classification was introduced in 2002. RIFLE is an acronym for *risk* of renal dysfunction, injury to the kidney (ARI), *failure* of the kidney (ARF), *loss* of kidney function and *end-stage kidney disease* (Table 2). It was later modified and is functioning as AKIN (Acute Kidney Injury Network) classification since 2005 (Table 3). The AKI term includes a wide range of renal dysfunction, starting with a very early and discrete renal failure with minimal changes in the serum creatinine level (*stage 1, Risk*), through moderate changes (*stage 2, Injury*), to an advanced renal failure (*stage 3, Failure*), often requiring renal replacement therapy (Bellomo et al., 2004 & Mehta et al., 2007). Two additional stages (*Loss of function* and *Endstage- renal-disease*) were introduced in order to classify cases of a partial or total and permanent loss of renal function. Some studies used these criteria to determine the incidence of ARF post-LT. Kundakci reported that AKD occurred in more than half of LTs postoperatively. AKI occurred in 64 (57%) LTs with risk, injury, and failure frequencies of 19%, 11%, and 28%, respectively (Kundakci et al., 2010). Zhu et al reported that postoperatively, AKI was found in 60% of patients. According to the AKIN criteria, it was: stage 1 - in 30%, stage 2 - in 13%, and stage 3 - in 17% of the individuals (Zhu et al., 2010).

AKIN classification was introduced with great enthusiasm, but soon proved to be of little use. Its main disadvantages include undersensitivity and no reference to aetiology or pathophysiology of AKI. Thus, it does not distinguish between the prerenal azotemia and a real injury of the renal parenchyma. Serum creatinine level and eGFR based on it are not useful parameters in the early diagnostics of AKI. First of all, the increase in creatinine level occurs late, after a few days, with an injury of more than 50% of the renal parenchyma.

Moreover, it is influenced by too many factors of creatinine synthesis and secretion in the renal tubules. In patients with graft dysfunction, these indicators are even less reliable, because of malnutrition and - frequently observed in these patients - high levels of serum bilirubin which interferes with creatinine measurements and causes a significant reduction in serum creatinine level (Cholongitas et al., 2007a).

Risk	Increase of serum creatinine 1.5-2 times baseline	Less than 0.5ml/kg/hr for >6hrs
Injury	Increase of serum creatinine 2-3 times baseline	Less < 0.5ml/kg/hr for >12hrs
Failure	Increase of serum creatinine of > 3 times baseline	<0. <0.3ml/kg/hr for >24hrs or anuria>12hrs
Loss	Persistent need for RRT for >4 weeks	
End-stage	Persistent need for RRT for >3 months	

Table 2. Risk, Injury, Failure, Loss of Kidney Function, End-stage (RIFLE) Kidney Disease classification (Mehta et al., 2007)

Acute Kidney Injury			**Recovery**
Stage1	**Stage 2**	**Stage 3**	Loss of function>4 weeks but <3 months
Rise in serum creatinine ≥0.3 mg/dl or Increase to ≥150% to 200% (1.5-fold to 2-fold) from baseline.	Increase in serum creatinine to > 200%- 300% (> 2-fold to 3-fold) from baseline.	Increase in serum creatinine to > 300% (> 3-fold) from baseline, or serum creatinine ≥4.0 mg/dl with an acute increase of at least 0.5 mg/dl.	End-stage renal failure >3 months
Urine output < 0.5 ml/kg/hour for > 6 hrs.	Urine output < 0.5 ml/kg/hour for > 12 hrs.	Urine output < 0.3 ml/kg/hr for 24 hrs, or anuria for 12 hrs.	Death

Table 3. Classification/staging system for acute kidney injury modified from RIFLE criteria. (Bellomo et al., 2004)

3.3 Aetiology and risk factors of acute kidney injury after liver transplantation

In order to apply protective strategies to minimize the occurrence of acute renal dysfunction (ARD) and chronic renal dysfunction thereafter, it is vital to define risk factors for ARD and manage properly as early as possible (Barri et al., 2009).

The evaluation of predictive factors for renal failure that occurs postoperatively has been the matter of several investigations. Clinical studies evaluating these risk factors have yielded variable results. Although the risk factors for AKI are often multifactorial and difficult to establish, they can be linked to three distinct time frames in relation to the liver transplant: the pretransplant (pre-LT), intraoperative, and post-LT periods as follows: pre-transplant (HRS, pre-transplant kidney dysfunction, high bilirubin concentrations), intra-operative (hemodynamic instability, intraoperative bleeding), and postoperative factors (contrast nephropathy, acute tubular necrosis secondary to ischemic or toxic agents, liver allograft dysfunction, multiple antibiotic use, reoperations especially re-transplantation). Actually the most common cause of ARF early after LTx is ischemic acute tubular necrosis, followed later by cyclosporine toxicity and sepsis (Fabrizi et al., 2010).

Preoperative	Intraoperative	Postoperative
Pretransplant renal dysfunction Hepatorenal syndrome High MELD score Preexisting Diabetes mellitus Hypertension Hyponatremia	Hemodynamic instability during anesthesia Longer anhepatic phase Intraoperative bleeding Volume of transfused blood products Intraoperative acidosis	Hypovolemia Need for pressor amines Haemodynamic instability Perioperative volume of transfused blood products. Sepsis. Relaparotomy. Contrast nephropathy Delayed liver graft function or primary graft nonfunction Calcineurin inhibitors Drug-induced interstitial nephritis. HCV recurrence

Table 4. Risk factors for Post liver transplant Acute Renal Dysfunction (Lewandowska & Matuszkiewicz-Rowinska, 2011)

3.3.1 Pretransplant renal dysfunction

The rate of renal failure among patients awaiting liver transplantation (LT) and the waiting time for LT have increased in recent years. The introduction of the Model for End-Stage Liver Disease (MELD) score will likely further enrich the proportion of LT candidates who have renal dysfunction, as creatinine is a key component of MELD calculation. The decision to perform combined kidney/liver transplantation (CKLT) as opposed to liver transplantation alone can be difficult in patients with end-stage liver disease and recent onset renal insufficiency. Because of scarce organ resources, it is important to predict accurately which patients with pretransplant renal dysfunction will recover after LT and who will have persistent or progressive kidney disease.

**Pretransplantation serum creatinine level:* is an important predictor of post-LT survival and renal dysfunction (Brown et al., 1996, Lafayette et al.,1997, Bilbao et al., 1998, Markmann et al., 2001, Nair et al., 2002, Pawarode et al., 2003 and Campbell et al., 2005). Even relatively mild elevations in preoperative creatinine (>1.0-1.5 mg/dL) may portend poor renal function postoperatively (Lafayette et al., 1997, Bilbao et al., 1998 and Pawarode et al., 2003). Bilbao (1998), Sanchez (2004) and Yalavarthy (2007) observed that preoperative creatinine >1.5 mg/dl was predictive of the need for postoperative renal replacement therapy (RRT) and also the risk of postoperative infection. Contreras et al reported that preoperative blood urea nitrogen was also an important predictive factor for the need for renal replacement therapy post-transplant (Contreras et al., 2002). Nair et al, (2002) demonstrated that patients with an average preoperative serum creatinine of 0.8 mg/dl had a 5-year patient survival of 62% compared to a 5-year survival of only 42% in patients with a preoperative serum creatinine of 2.7 mg/dL. Organ Procurement and Transplantation Network/United Network for Organ Sharing (OPTN/UNOS) data from 1988 to 1995 demonstrated that patients with a preoperative serum creatinine >2 mg/dl had a 5-year survival of only 50%. Furthermore, patients requiring preoperative RRT had worse outcomes compared to those not requiring RRT (Jeyarajah et al., 1997).

Cause of renal disease

May also help predict posttransplantation creatinine. Certainly patients with underlying chronic kidney diseases such as *glomerulonephritis, diabetic nephropathy* would be expected to have persistently poor or worsening renal function after LT alone, particularly in the setting of calcineurin inhibitor-based immunosuppression. Sezer et al., reported that microalbuminuria is a main risk for renal function deterioration (Sezer et al., 2011). Many transplant centers have reported that a large majority of their CKLT patients underwent transplantation for chronic kidney disease. In contrast, hepatorenal syndrome (in studies from the early 1990s) demonstrated a good post-LT alone renal outcome and hence concomitant renal transplantation may be avoided. Of patients with ARF due to the hepatorenal syndrome, approximately two-thirds will recover, although recovery may be delayed 3 months or longer after LT (Yalavarthy et al., 2007). Because waiting times for liver transplantation and duration of renal dysfunction prior to transplantation have increased since then, it is possible that renal outcomes after LT alone in patients with HRS may be less favorable now.

Duration of pretransplant renal dysfunction

Bahirwani et al., 2008 showed that patients with preexisting renal dysfunction, especially if the duration is more than 12 weeks, experience a significant fall in eGFR after liver transplantation alone.

Most studies agreed on reporting the negative impact of pretransplant renal dysfunction on posttransplant renal function, regardless of the criteria that they depended upon to define the dysfunction. Lebrón Gallardo (2004), Faenza (2006) and Burra (2009), used serum creatinine; Gonwa et al., 2004 used pre-LT GFR & Kim et al., 2004 used creatinine clearance. Indeed mortality after LT is affected modestly by the presence of pretransplant acute renal failure (<2-fold increase), but increases markedly (up to 8-fold) in the face of acute renal failure posttransplant (Yalavarthy et al., 2007).

3.3.2 MELD score

The proportion of patients undergoing liver transplantation (LT) with renal insufficiency has significantly increased after the MELD era due to the fact that more patients with high serum creatinine are being transplanted and hence affecting the posttransplant kidney function (Sharma et al., 2009). An association was observed between postoperative ARF and a higher Model for End-Stage Liver Disease (MELD) score (Sanchez et al., 2004, Campbell et al., 2005, Tinti et al., 2010 and Sezer et al., 2011) and between ARF and a reduced pre-LT serum albumin (Tinti et al., 2010). No association was noted between ARF and other pre-LT parameters. The association of ARF with MELD and hypoalbuminemia may be the result of a close relationship between renal and hepatic functions among cirrhotic patients (Tinti et al., 2010). Schnitzbauer reported that time on the waiting list with endstage hepatic disease is a major risk factor associated with early posttransplant renal impairment (Schnitzbauer et al., 2010).

3.3.3 Early liver allograft dysfunction

Several studies reported that early liver allograft dysfunction is among the major risk factors associated with early posttransplant renal impairment (Fraley et al.,1998, Gainza et al., 2002, Ojo et al., 2003, Lebrón Gallardo et al., 2004, Cabezuolo et al., 2006, Yalavarthy et al., 2007 and Schnitzbauer et al., 2010). *Small-for-size (SFS) grafts*, which may lead to specific problems of delayed function or SFS syndrome (characterized by prolonged cholestasis, ascites or coagulopathy) may also aggravate the problem of post-transplant renal dysfunction. Lee et al., 2007 in their study on 248 adult patients who underwent LDLT reported a significant relationship between small-for-size grafts (GRWR < 0.8) and early postoperative renal dysfunction. Yamamoto et al., 2004 also demonstrated this relationship.

3.3.4 CNI nephrotxicity

Acute, reversible nephrotoxicity accompanying CNI therapy results from the imbalance in vasoactive substance release. The administration of CNI causes vasoconstriction of both the afferent and, to a greater degree, the efferent arterioles, which leads to a decrease in renal blood flow and glomerular filtration rate (GFR), and an increase in renal vascular resistance. In its most extreme form, there is tubular damage and a clinical picture of acute tubular necrosis, perhaps on the basis of ischemia. Kidney biopsy histopathology shows characteristic isometric vacuoles in proximal and distal tubular cells. Calcineurin inhibitors can also cause an acute form of nephrotoxicity manifested by acute renal failure in the early posttransplant period. Renal biopsy in these patients shows endothelial damage, formation of fibrin thrombi in capillary loops (Fig. 2), eosinophilic material in the walls of arterioles and small arteries, with patchy necrosis of smooth muscle cells. This lesion is histologically similar to that seen in malignant hypertension and thrombotic thrombocytopenic purpura. Indeed, thrombocytopenia sometimes accompanies this syndrome in transplanted patients (Remuzzi & Bertani, 1989).

Diagnosis of ARF

Vigilant postoperative care including not only monitoring of renal parameters, but also a thorough analysis of risk factors of renal dysfunction is vital.

3.4 Postoperative monitoring of renal parameters

At present, monitoring of the renal function bases mostly on the results of the serum creatinine level and the estimated glomerular filtration rate (eGFR rate) calculated with the use of MDRD and Cockcroft-Gault formula and on monitoring of diuresis (Cockcroft & Gault, 1976 and Levey et al., 1999).

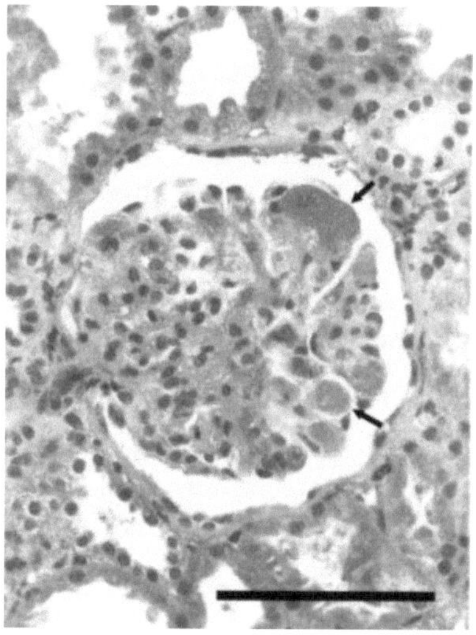

Fig. 2. Thrombotic angiopathy of cyclosporine toxicity. The arrowheads point to fibrin thrombi in the capillary loops of a glomerulus from a patient with acute cyclosporine toxicity. (Smith, 2006: Photomicrograph courtesy of David Howell)

Because of the above-mentioned limitations of AKIN criteria, it is now attempted to find new biomarkers released by the renal tubules, which (if increased in urine or blood serum) would allow for an early diagnosis of AKI or identification of a group at increased risk of AKI. The most frequently mentioned indicators of this type include: cystatin C (Biancofiore et al., 2006), NGAL (*neutrophil gelatinase-associated lipocalin*) (Portal et al., 2010), KIM-1 (*kidney injury molecule-1*) or interleukin-18 (Lewandowska & Matuszkiewicz-Rowinska, 2011).

Recently, there have been a few reports published that evaluated the usefulness of the latest methods of an early AKI assessment in post-LT patients. Portal et al. evaluated the usefulness of serum and urine NGAL level measurements in patients immediately after liver transplantation, in prognosing the risk of AKI development within the next 48 hours. A multivariate regression analysis showed two independent risk factors of AKI development: APACHE II (OR 1.64/point; 95% CI, 1.22-2.21, P=0.001) and serum NGAL level (OR 1.01/ng/ml, 95% CI, 1.00-1.02, P=0.002). When combined together (so called renal risk index), these two factors revealed the highest predictive value. Index with APACHE II score of >13 and serum NGAL level of >258 ng/ml, calculated at ≥1, showed a sensitivity of 100% and a specificity of 76% in the prediction of severe AKI [Portal et al., 2010].

3.4.1 Analysis of risk factors

Xu and colleagues, on the basis of the analysis of data from 102 patients subjected to LT, developed a predictive model of AKI incidence following LT. A multivariate analysis showed that independent risk factors of this complication included: preoperative creatinine level of >1.2 mg/dl, intraoperative diuresis of ≤60 ml/hour, intraoperative hypotension, and use of noradrenaline. They calculated the risk score as follows: [-2.128 + 1.109×

(preoperative creatinine level of >1.2 mg/dl) + 2.243 × (intraoperative diuresis of ≤60 ml/hr) + 1.542 × (intraoperative hypotension) – 2.463 × (intraoperative use of noradrenaline)]. Next, the authors studied the usefulness and predictive value of the developed formula in a prospective study including 44 patients after LT, assuming that the probability of AKI = EXP (risk score)/ [1 + EXP (risk score)]. Aiming to achieve the highest sensitivity and specificity of the indicator (75% and 93.8%, respectively), a cut-off value of –0.2 was assumed as optimal in determining the prognosis of AKI. This meant that among patients with an index value of ≥-0.2, the risk of AKI development was significantly higher than in patients with an index value of <-0.2. The model developed by the authors proved to be reliable: AKI occurred in 9 out of 11 patients from the group of high risk, and only in 3 individuals out of 33 from the low-risk group (Xu et al., 2010).

3.5 Prevention of acute renal dysfunction

To prevent acute kidney injury effectively, it is necessary to know its risk factors, to evaluate the patient in detail before liver transplantation, and to obey the rules of conduct, characteristic for all clinical situations that could lead to AKI development.

3.5.1 General measures

- thorough monitoring of the water and electrolyte balance,
- avoidance of nephrotoxic drugs,
- discontinuation of preparations inhibiting the effect of angiotensin II,
- careful dosing of other medicines, with adjustments of doses to the current renal function.

Unfortunately, despite promising results of *in vitro* and experimental studies, it was impossible to prove the protective effect of N-acetylcysteine on kidneys in that population (Hilmi et al., 2010, Sagias et al., 2010 and Jegatheeswaran & Siriwardena, 2011).

3.5.2 Modification of nephrotoxic immunosuppressive regimens

To avoid postoperative acute renal failure and/or chronic renal failure has met with variable results (Fabrizi et al., 2010). There are no data to suggest that switching from one calcineurin inhibitor to another at equipotent doses will result in less nephrotoxicity. However, as trough tacrolimus levels correlate more closely with the area under the curve of drug exposure than do trough cyclosporine levels, it may be easier to avoid calcineurin inhibitor toxicity using tacrolimus. If cyclosporine is used, the blood level drawn 2hrs post dose (C2 level) should be used to monitor therapy.

Strategies to limit CNI exposure include CNI minimization, avoidance, and withdrawal

Candidates for such a treatment would be first of all patients with impaired renal function found before transplantation. There is no well-defined protocol to prevent or minimize cyclosporine or tacrolimus nephrotoxicity.

Some centers advocate *Calcineurin inhibitor minimization* using mycophenolate mofetil or sirolimus. This may be associated with a modest increase in creatinine clearance (CrCl) and a decrease in serum creatinine (SCr) in the short term. Mycophenolate mofetil may improve renal outcomes during CNI minimization more than sirolimus. Despite improvement in

CrCl or SCr, CNI nephrotoxicity is progressive over time when CNI exposure is maintained. Persistent damage is observed on biopsies as long as the CNIs are continued.

CNI withdrawal

May be the best option by delivering CNIs during the early period of immunologic graft injury and then converting them to less nephrotoxic agents before significant renal damage occurs (Flechner et al., 2008). Late CNI withdrawal has achieved variable results, possibly because withdrawal was attempted after the kidney damage was too extensive. In a case report on 3 patients with renal function impairment who switched from CNI to sirolimus, 2 improved substantially and came off dialysis, while in 1 (whose renal dysfunction was initially milder, not severe enough to require dialysis) serum creatinine levels remained altered after switching to sirolimus (Kamar et al., 2007). Early CNI withdrawal, prior to significant kidney damage, has generally improved CrCl and markers of fibrosis, a finding also observed with sirolimus in most studies. Successful withdrawal appears to be more effective than CNI minimization. Lam et al stressed that sirolimus conversion should be initiated early since late conversion rarely improves chronic renal dysfunction (Lam et al., 2004). In fact, several studies have shown that in patients with pre-existing renal disease, sirolimus can even worsen nephrotoxicity and promote proteinuria (Bumbea et al., 2005, Letavarnier et al., 2005 and Diekmann et al., 2007).

Antibody induction with delayed CNI initiation

It has been suggested that in case of high serum creatinine levels at the time of grafting, it may be wise to delay the use of calcineurin inhibitor based immunosuppression in the immediate post-operative period (Distant & Gonwa, 1993). Polyclonal antibody (thymoglobulin) induction was used to delay CNI use and avoid renal toxicity without increasing the risk of rejection or HCV recurrence. However side-effects such as "first dose reaction" have been reported in 80% of patients. This can often be ameliorated by premedication with antipyretics and steroids. Other side-effects include thrombocytopenia, CMV infection, posttransplant lymphoproliferative disease (PTLD), serum sickness and anaphylaxis (Pillai & Levitsky, 2009).

Later, monoclonal antibody induction using basiliximab (anti-CD25 monoclonal anti-body) and alemtuzumab (anti-CD 52 antibody) was used. These antibodies remain in the circulatory system for weeks after initiation of therapy and have been used successfully with low-dose CNIs. Neuhaus (2002) and Liu (2004) reported successful use of basiliximab with less nephrotoxicity and fewer side-effects compared to the antithymocyte globulins. Also, Tzakis (2004) and Marcos (2004) showed that liver transplant recipients who received alemtuzumab induction with low dose tacrolimus had less renal toxicity than those who received standard doses of tacrolimus. The use of these antibodies may be effective to limit CNI exposure, but longer-term follow-up data are required (Flechner et al., 2008). Actually a recent study showed that induction with basiliximab resulted in 30-day and 1-year patient, graft and renal outcomes comparable with a control group receiving standard CNI-based immunosuppression. The authors concluded that antibody induction with delayed CNI should be further studied prospectively (Verna et al., 2011).Also a recent study showed that steroid-free alemtuzumab induction regimen was associated with less hypertension and rejection but with more infectious complications. Thus, the overall benefit of alemtuzumab induction in LT recipients is called into question (Levitsky et al., 2011).

CNI avoidance

The use of the so-called renal-sparing agents is still debatable. Avoidance is hampered by lack of experience and possible sirolimus-induced side effects (delay in surgical wound repair because it inhibits fibrogenesis (Montalbano et al., 2004), inducing proteinuria, anaemia, thrombocytopenia, peripheral swelling, hypercholesterolemia and gastrointestinal disorders (Vivarelli et al., 2006). Use of sirolimus with mycophenolate mofetil to avoid CNI exposure de novo has improved glomerular filtration rate for at least two years in most studies in kidney transplantation; however, experience is limited in liver and heart transplantation, and reports of delayed graft function and wound healing with sirolimus may have dampened enthusiasm for *de novo* use. There is hardly published evidence for CNI-free de novo approaches with mTOR-inhibitors in liver transplant collectives. Schnitzbauer et al are conducting a prospective, noncontrolled, two-stage study (PATRON07) on patients with serum creatinine >1.5mg/dl or eGFR < 50 ml/min at the time of transplantation. Its objective is to evaluate the feasibility of a de novo CNI-free immunosuppressive regimen based on induction therapy with basiliximab (20 mg IV day 0 and day 4 after transplantation), prednisolone 500mg during reperfusion then 1mg/kg and tapered by month 6 after LT, mycophenolate mofetil (2g/d bid), and mTOR-inhibition with sirolimus after day 10 after LT aiming at trough-levels of 4 to 10 ng/ml. The primary endpoint is defined as the incidence of steroid-resistant acute rejection within the first 30 days after liver transplantation. The authors hope that the results of PATRON07 may be the basis for a large multicenter randomized controlled trial in patients with poor renal function at the time-point of liver transplant (Schnitzbauer et al., 2010).

If CNI-free-"bottom-up" immunosuppression strategies are safe and effective, this may be an innovative concept that could improve the patient short and long-time outcome with regards to renal function, infectious complications and avoidance of over-immunosuppression after LT.

Future direction of immunosuppression: Costimulation blockade (Belatacept)

Belatacept is a soluble cytotoxic T-lymphocyte antigen-4 (CTLA-4) agent which binds CD80 and CD86 and inhibits T cell activation. Belatacept competes with the CD28 receptor on T cells which normally binds CD80 and CD86 on the antigen presenting cell as a co-stimulatory signal required for T cell activation. Belatacept is administered intravenously once a month and does not carry the renal toxicity of CNIs. Clinical trials in liver transplant patients are currently ongoing with this agent (Pillai & Levitsky, 2009).

3.5.3 Surgical technique of 'piggy back'

It is necessary to conduct further studies in order to answer the question whether the new surgical technique of 'piggy back' type will allow for a reduction of AKI incidence (Cabezuelo et al., 2003 and 2006).

3.6 Dialysis in the liver transplant patient

Around 8-17% of the patients with AKI after LT require renal replacement therapy (Lewandowska & Matuszkiewicz-Rowinska, 2011). Dialytic therapy in the immediate postoperative period requires close attention to hemodynamics and coagulation parameters.

(Smith, 2006 and Lewandowska & Matuszkiewicz-Rowinska, 2011).The most frequently used perioperative treatment methods include continuous techniques in 75% of cases, such as continuous veno-venous haemo(dia)filtration (CVVHD), dialysis of SLED type (slow low efficiency dialysis), and intermittent haemodialysis in 25% of cases. Continuous techniques are preferred for two main reasons: the patients are frequently haemodynamically unstable and remain at a significant risk of brain oedema. However, the real advantage of these methods over the applied standard haemodialysis has not been proven so far.

In the liver transplant patient with impaired hepatic clearance and renal failure, attention should be paid to the route of excretion of all pharmacologic agents given and doses adjusted accordingly. Cyclosporine, tacrolimus, prednisone, and mycophenolate mofetil are not removed by hemodialysis to any significant extent, while methylprednisolone and azathioprine (and its active metabolite mercaptopurine) are cleared partially during dialysis. Most angiotensin-converting enzyme inhibitors are dialyzable, with benazepril and quinapril being exceptions. Calcium channel blockers are generally not cleared by hemodialysis, while many of the beta-blockers (atenolol, acebutalol, metoprolol, nadalol, sotalol) are cleared. Because atenolol is primarily cleared by the kidneys, the dose to achieve a desired effect is much lower in patients with poor renal function. Metoprolol on the other hand is primarily metabolized by the liver. Metabolites of verapamil with atrioventricular (AV) node-blocking properties, but little antihypertensive effect can accumulate in patients on hemodialysis. This agent is thus best avoided in end-stage renal disease (Smith, 2006).

In some of the cases, there may appear a need for renal replacement therapy during LT procedure mostly due to hypervolemia and the risk of brain oedema (Lewandowska & Matuszkiewicz-Rowinska, 2011). Townsend et al. used intraoperative CVVHD in 41 out of 636 patients (6.4%) that they operated on. A mean time of dialysis was 258 minutes and a mean filtration rate was 1-1.5 l/h. No significant complications were observed apart from blood clotting in the dialyser (no anticoagulation was used in most of the patients) in 40% of cases. Indications included either typical, life threatening symptoms of AKI, such as overhydration or hyperkalemia, or disorders typical for this group of patients: lactic acidosis, hyponatremia, risk of brain oedema or necessity of transfusion of large volumes of blood preparations. In 78% of cases, CVVHD procedures were continued after OLT for 3-11 days (Townsend et al., 2009).

3.7 Prognosis of acute kidney injury

Acute renal failure (ARF) has been associated with an 8-fold increase in mortality risk, prolonged ventilation time and intensive care unit (ICU) stay, greater risk for infectious complications, and greater hospital costs. De Simone et al reported an in-hospital mortality rate as high as 41% for patients with ARF versus 5% for those with preserved renal function (De Simone et al., 2009). Mortality of patients who required renal replacement therapy is from 45.1% to 67% (Cabezuelo et al., 2002, Faenza et al., 2006).

Zhu and colleagues analysed retrospectively the influence of the renal function following LT on late clinical outcomes in 193 patients. Among patients with acute kidney injury (AKI), the 28-day and 1-year mortality was significantly higher than in non-AKI patients (15.5% and 25.9% *vs.* 0% and 3.9%, respectively; $P<0.5$). One-year survival of non-AKI patients was 96%, and of AKI patients in stage 1, 2, and 3- 85.5%, 84%, and 45.3%, respectively. The Cox regression analysis showed that the independent risk factors of death in the first year following the transplantation included postoperative AKI (HR 12.1; P<0.05), postoperative infection (HR 4.7; P<0.01), postoperative hypertension (HR 4.4; P<0.01), and postoperative APACHE II index of ≥10 (HR 3.6; P<0.05) (Zhu et al., 2010). Similar results were published by Gonwa et al. (2001a) and by Ishitani et al. (1993).

During the later course, renal dysfunction exerts an important influence on the quality of life of transplant recipients (Alessandria et al., 2005, Lewandowska & Matuszkiewicz-Rowinska, 2011). AKI significantly increases the risk of *development of chronic renal failure* in the late post-LT period. The risk of developing chronic renal failure after LT is approximately 20% after 5 years, associated with the use of calcineurin inhibitors and a 4-fold increased mortality risk (Sharma et al., 2009 and Schnitzbauer et al., 2010).

4. Chronic renal dysfunction

With improved survival of liver transplant recipients, chronic kidney disease has emerged as a major long-term complication after OLT (Bahirwani & Reddy, 2009). In fact, liver transplant recipients have the highest five-yr incidence of CRF of any non-renal solid organ transplant recipient; additionally, the risk of death is at least fourfold higher in patients who develop CRF (Ojo et al., 2003). Numerous studies have been performed in the last decade in order to clarify the epidemiology and clinical significance of chronic kidney dysfunction among liver recipients (Fisher et al., 1998, Brown et al., 2001, Cohen et al., 2002 & Herlenius et al., 2008).

4.1 Epidemiology of chronic renal dysfunction

The incidence of chronic kidney disease (CKD) post-Liver transplant varies widely, from 10 to 83%, most likely owing to the *lack of a standard definition* of post-transplantation chronic renal disease, *differences in the methodology* utilised to estimate renal function, and *variable periods of follow-up* (Fabrizi et al., 2010).The frequency of CKD (defined as eGFR <60 ml/min) according to recent series is listed in Table 5. However the incidence of the milder forms of renal dysfunction (GFR between ≥30 mL/min and ≤70 mL/min) is likely to be considerably higher than estimated (Fisher et al., 1998, Randhawa and Shapiro, 2005). Definitely, the incidence of CKD increases with time. The latest report on the epidemiology of CKD after liver transplantation has been offered by Lee et al (2010). A cohort of 431 recipients who underwent liver transplantation between 1997 and 2008 was included. The cumulative incidence of CKD (eGFR <60 ml/min) was 17% at 1 year, 23% at 3 years, and 27% at 5 years. Sharma et al., 2009 reported the cumulative incidence of post-LT CRF at 1, 3, and 5 years was 8%, 17% and 22%, respectively.

Authors	Frequency	Time post-LT
Lee J, et al (2010)	17.6% (76/431)	12 months
Burra P, et al (2009)	35.3% (143/406)	12 months
Kim S, et al (2004)	43.5% (27/62)	17 months
De Boccardo G, et al (2008)	62.3% (144/231)	73 months

Table 5. Epidemiology of chronic kidney disease among liver transplant recipients (CKD = eGFR <60 ml/min)

4.2 Definitions of chronic kidney disease

The most common definition used is eGFR<60ml/min. Other definitions of CKD have been used. Gonwa and colleagues, defined post-LT CRD as sustained serum creatinine >2.5 mg/dl. They reported that the combined incidence of CKD with end-stage renal disease (on RRT), was 4.3% at 5 years and 18% after 13 years of follow-up (Gonwa et al., 2001b). **Ojo et al, 2003** in a larger study analyzed the data from the Scientific Registry of Transplant Recipients for 36,849 adult patients who had LT in the United States between 1990, and 2000. The incidence of post-LT CRD was 18% at 5 years and 26% at 10 years. This study defined post-LT CRD as GFR < 29 mL/minute/1.73 m^2 or the development of end-stage renal disease, which was defined as initiation of RRT or listing for renal transplantation.

Chronic renal dysfunction, not only has implications in terms of an *increased demand on resources*, but is also significantly associated with a *higher patient mortality rate*. Hence identification of the risk factors for its development of chronic renal dysfunction after liver transplantation is crucial.

4.3 Risk factors for posttransplant chronic kidney disease

Although previously attributed largely to calcineurin inhibitor toxicity (Ojo et al., 2003, Pillebout et al., 2005), it has become clear that the onset of chronic renal failure following LT is multifactorial, and reported to be correlated with posttransplant acute renal failure (Lee et al., 2010 and Tinti et al., 2010), pre-transplant renal dysfunction (Kamath et al., 2001; Burra et al., 2009 and Tinti et al., 2011), hepatitis C status, age, female gender, diabetes mellitus, hypertension, Model for End Stage Liver Disease (MELD), pretransplant proteinuria (Lee et al., 2010), pretransplant hepatorenal syndrome, alcohol intake (Hetz et al., 2005, Pillebout et al., 2005 and Randhawa & Shapiro, 2005), smoking and dyslipidemia (Sezer et al.,2011).

4.3.1 Postoperative acute renal failure (ARF) and dialysis requirement in the post-transplantation period

Post-LT ARF was proved to be an early predictor of chronic kidney disease (CKD) in several studies (Ojo et al., 2003; Kim et al., 2004; Burra et al., 2009 and Sharma et al, 2009). Barri and his colleagues, 2009 stated clearly that the high incidence of acute kidney injury post-liver transplantation is an important risk factor for long-term renal dysfunction and its associated morbidity and mortality. Ojo et al., 2003 reported a relative risk of 2.13. In the study by Tinti and colleagues, post-LT CKD was present in 44.4% of patients with ARF in contrast to 6.7% of patients without ARF (Tinti et al., 2010). A multivariate Cox regression analysis revealed that the overall risk of CKD development (eGFR < 60 mL/min/1.73 m^2) was associated with the existence of posttransplant ARF and its severity. In fact, a recent consensus conference on acute kidney injury(AKI) suggested that since AKI is a very strong predictor of CKD, a milder definition for AKI should be used to detect this problem early and to intervene before it is severe and progresses to CRD (Barri et al., 2009).

4.3.2 Abnormal GFR at different intervals posttransplant

Sanchez et al., 2010 in a study conducted on 592 liver transplant recipients also confirmed this finding and showed that patients with GFR less than 60 ml/min per 1.73 m^2 *at month 3* post-transplant have a higher risk of developing renal failure; however, those who avoid renal failure seem to maintain renal function long-term. Kamar et al. reported the eGFR *after 6 months* was the only risk factor of renal failure for further 60±48 months. This was also a predictor of glomerular sclerosis found in 50% of glomerules in the renal biopsy performed afterwards (Kamar et al., 2011). Other studies have reported that an *abnormal GFR at 1 year* identifies patients at risk of chronic renal dysfunction (Cohen et al., 2002 & O'Riordan et al., 2006).

4.3.3 Pretransplant renal dysfunction

Impaired pre-transplantat kidney function is a prognostic indicator for chronic kidney disease (CKD) following liver transplantation, as recently highlighted by a meta-analysis of clinical, observational studies. A stratified analysis including only studies provided with baseline GFR, revealed that the summary estimate of RR and 95% CIs for occurrence of chronic renal failure after liver transplantation in patients with diminished renal function at transplantation was 2.12 (95% CI, 1.01-4.46, p=0.01) (Fabrizi et al., 2011). Even relatively mild elevations in pre-transplant creatinine >1.5 mg/dL may portend poor long term renal function. This was confirmed by many investigators (Moreno et al., 2003, Kim et al., 2004 and Burra et al., 2009). A multivariate Cox regression analysis performed by Lee et al revealed that the overall risk of CKD development was associated with low pre transplant eGFR in addition to post-transplant acute renal failure (Lee et al., 2010). In fact, Sharma et al., 2009 concluded that the estimated GFR at LT was the most important determinant of post-LT chronic renal failure. Sezer reported that after 5 years, GFR negatively correlated with initial Renal Resistive Index (r=-0.32; P<.01).

Duration of pretransplant dysfunction

Campbell (2005) suggested that duration, rather than the cause, of pretransplant renal dysfunction (pre-LT RD) is the key to predicting creatinine at 12 months after transplantation. ROC analysis among LT alone patients showed that the duration of renal disease by itself had a moderate ability to predict creatinine >1.5 mg/dL at 12 months posttransplantation (area under ROC curve = 0.71). The optimal predictive cutoff was 3.6 weeks. However they stated that they cannot at this time recommend that all patients with duration of renal disease longer than 3.6 weeks undergo combined liver kidney transplantation (CLKT) since creatinine of 1.5 mg/dL 1 year after transplantation is not necessarily high enough to justify concomitant renal transplantation. Instead they recommended that a threshold duration of renal dysfunction in combination with other predictive clinical variables (e.g height of creatinine, requirement for RRT) be prospectively investigated as an aid to clinical decision making.

Indeed for liver transplant (LT) candidates with pretransplant mild to moderate chronic renal impairment or recent-onset ARF, the decision of whether to perform LT alone or CLKT can be challenging because no single factor has been shown to be predictive of the degree of progression of chronic kidney disease following successful LT. Although Pham et al., 2007 suggested, like Campbell, that the duration of pretransplant renal dysfunction had a negative impact on posttransplant renal function outcome, Marik et al., 2006 and Sharma et al., 2009, in contrast, failed to demonstrate that the duration of pretransplant renal dysfunction was predictive of post-LT renal outcome.

4.3.4 Calcineurin inhibitors (CNI)

Chronic CNI nephrotoxicity is caused by immunological and non-immunological damage. Histopathological examination shows renal tubular atrophy with typical microcalcification, patchy fibrosis and nodular arteriolar hyalinosis. According to Mihatsch, arteriolopathy, the main symptom of CNI nephrotoxicity, is a variant of thrombotic microangiopathy with slow, subclinical course. Differentiation between arteriolar hyalinosis associated with CNI administration and arteriolar sclerosis in hypertension, diabetes, or the elderly poses a challenge. A typical feature of CNI toxicity is substitution of smooth muscle cells by hyaline deposits in the external media layer; while in arteriolar hyalinosis in other clinical situations the smooth muscle cells are intact and hyaline deposits accumulate beneath the endothelium (Mihatsh et al., 1994).

There is no precise classification to assess CNI nephrotoxicity; that is why new scales and classifications are developed in order to enhance the precision of diagnosing CNI nephrotoxicity. The new scales to evaluate CNI nephrotoxicity, like the older ones, show arteriolar hyalinosis as the most typical abnormality (Kambham et al., 2007). One histologic study reported the association of these changes with cyclosporine dose and over time. Mild arteriolar hyalinosis at six months appeared to be associated with high doses and was reversible. By comparison, at three years, irreversible severe arteriolar hyalinosis and glomerosclerosis was observed, despite decreased doses and trough levels (Nankivell et al., 2003).

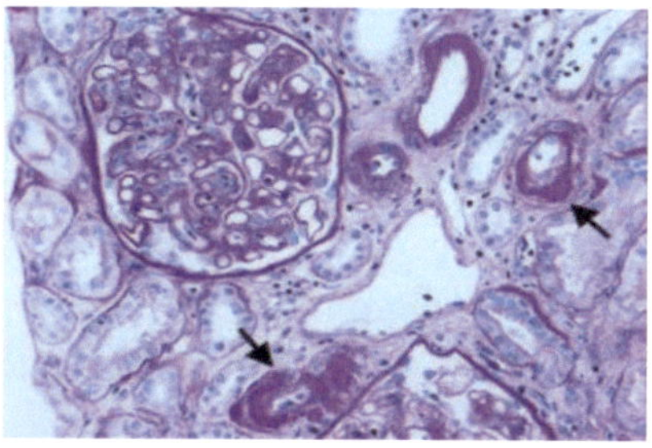

Fig. 3. Nodular hyalinosis typical of CNI (John et al., 2010)

Chronic lesions and acute nephrotoxicity in CNI treatment are caused by various mediators, including renin-angiotensin-aldosterone (RAA) system, which by activating angiotensin type 1 receptor is not only a contributory factor in renal vascular bed constriction, but also influences kidney fibrosis and aldosterone release. Activation of RAA system through CNI may cause harmful hemodynamic (vasoconstriction) and nonhemodynamic changes (via enhanced synthesis of transforming growth factor-β, vascular endothelial growth factor and enhanced renal cell apoptosis) (Friedlander, 2007). The CNI-induced TGF-β formation produces tubulointerstitial fibrosis by increased synthesis and decreased extracellular matrix degradation (Khanna et al., 2002). Administration of losartan, AT1 blocker, in transplant patients leads to a significant decrease in TGF-β serum levels and increased GFR (Campistol et al., 2001).

Recent trials have shown that aldosterone, the final product in the RAA system, may play an important role in CNI nephrotoxicity; therefore, spironolactone administration may be an effective strategy in the prevention of CNI nephrotoxicity (Perez-Rojas et al., 2007). During

CNI treatment, disturbances in nitric oxide (NO) release and NO synthase activity may generate reactive oxygen species; all of them might be involved in tubular epithelial to mesenchymal transition (Sharma et al., 2000 and Han et al., 2006). Protein kinase C (PKC-β) contributes to CNI-dependent fibrosis. It has been proved that cyclosporine administration enhanced PKC-β mRNA and protein expression; adding hispidine, a PKC-β inhibitor, inhibited TGF-β1 synthesis in proximal tubule cells (Liu, 2006).Genetic susceptibility to cyclosporine nephrotoxicity has been suggested. Cyclosporine is a substrate for the transmembrane pump P-glycoprotein. There is some evidence in animals and in vitro that decreased expression of this pump may contribute to increased cyclosporine levels, leading to nephrotoxicity. Altered protein pump expression has also been observed in association with several polymorphisms in its gene. As an example, the TT genotype is associated with decreased P-glycoprotein expression in the kidney. In a case control study of donor and recipient pairs, the TT genotype in the donor directly correlated with chronic cyclosporine nephrotoxicity in the allograft recipient. This suggests that underlying genetic factors that increase cyclosporine concentrations in the kidney may contribute to chronic nephrotoxicity (Hauser et al., 2005).

Progressive obliterative arteriolopathy and chronic interstitial fibrosis with glomerulosclerosis develop in LT recipients in a *dose-dependent* and *time-dependent* fashion and have limited potential for reversibility (Fabrizi et al., 2010).

Manifestations of Chronic calcineurin inhibitor nephrotoxicity: renal insufficiency due to glomerular and vascular disease, abnormalities in tubular function, and an increase in blood pressure (Hauser et al., 2005).

Abnormalities in tubular function include:

- hyperkalemia (due to reducing of potassium excretion both by decreasing the activity of the renin-angiotensin-aldosterone system and by impairing tubular responsiveness to aldosterone) (Tumlin and Sands, 1993).
- hypophosphatemia (due to urinary phosphate wasting) (Moz et al., 2004)
- hypercalciuria (Nijenhuis et al., 2004).
- hypomagnesemia – presumably due to drug effects on magnesium reabsorption. Hypomagnesemia has been implicated as a contributor to the nephrotoxicity associated with cyclosporine (Miura et al., 2002).

Difference between cyclosporine and tacrolimus: There are conflicting views in the literature regarding any difference in the nephrotoxic effect of either cyclosporine or tacrolimus. Many investigators did not identify any difference in the impact of either drug on the immediate postoperative kidney function (Burra et al., 2009, Dehghani et al., 2008, Kim et al., 2004 and Wei et al., 2006). On the other hand, O'Riordan et al., 2006 found a beneficial effect of tacrolimus use, compared with cyclosporine, which retarded the progression of acute renal disease to chronic renal disease. This has been previously noted by Filler et al., 2005 and Lucey et al., 2005. In contrast, a previous long-term trial comparing cyclosporine and tacrolimus in liver transplant recipients found a similar incidence of early acute renal failure and late hypertension, while late renal insufficiency was more prevalent with tacrolimus (Porayko et al., 1994). Recently, Lee and colleagues, 2010 in a multivariate Cox regression analysis revealed that the overall risk of CKD development was associated with cyclosporine more than tacrolimus.

4.3.5 Hepatitis C

Hepatitis C recurrence after transplant is almost universal. Infection with hepatitis C virus (HCV) is the leading indication for LT worldwide and one explanation for the higher incidence of renal failure in LT patients is that HCV per se and the severity of HCV recurrence are risk factors for renal dysfunction (Asfandiyar et al., 2006). The mechanism by which HCV infection may induce early renal failure is not yet fully understood. HCV infection has been associated with mesangiocapillary glomerulonephritis and cryoglobulinemia (Braun et al., 2003), conditions that have been reported in HCV+ve LT recipients (Abrahamian et al., 2000 and Kendrick et al., 1997). Immunosuppressive therapy results in an early and significant increase in HCV replication after LT (Gane et al.., 1996), which may increase the risk of glomerular damage if concurrent renal transplantation is not performed [Pascual et al., 1997]. Moreover in these series, the presence of lower GFR before transplant (although not statistically significant) and the significant higher incidence of diabetes mellitus after transplantation in HCV group, compared to non-HCV group, could be additional factors justifying the worse renal function of HCV+ve liver transplant recipients (Burra et al., 2009).

Studies have reported a different influence of hepatitis C on chronic renal dysfunction after liver transplantation. Pillebout (2005) found a strong association linking HCV infection with end-stage renal disease at biopsy, relating particularly to interferon therapy. In contrast, Burra et al., 2009 found no such association between the onset of chronic renal failure and the use of interferon before or after LT. Instead they stressed that HCV status had a negative impact on the median GFR in the first year of liver transplantation. Later on, HCV may lose this negative impact, while early stage renal failure continues to play a part in impaired renal function. Actually this study stated that HCV status, pre-LT GFR and serum creatinine levels were independent predictors of renal function a year after LT. Asfandiyar and colleagues, 2006 also demonstrated that infection with hepatitis C is an independent risk factor for chronic kidney disease as well as the relation with severity of HCV. Actually, Ojo et al., 2003, found that HCV was an independent risk factor for chronic renal dysfunction after all non-renal solid organ transplants and not just liver transplantation.

4.3.6 Glomerulonephritis

Only a few, small-sized studies on the histological features of chronic kidney disease (CKD) among LT recipients exist. In addition to histological lesions attributable to calcineurin inhibitor toxicity, a large spectrum of glomerular abnormalities was noted. Gonwa et al observed calcineurin inhibitor toxicity (n=33; 73%), non-recovered HRS (n=3; 7%), and focal segmental glomerulosclerosis (n=3; 7%) in their cohort of 45 patients who underwent kidney biopsy post-liver transplantation (Gonwa et al., 2001b). In another study by Pillebout, chronic renal failure was attributed to (i) specific chronic cyclosporine/tacrolimus arteriolopathy; (ii) typical diabetic nephropathy; (iii) acute or chronic thrombotic microangiopathy attributed to cyclosporine/tacrolimus arteriolopathy or alpha-interferon (Pillebout et al., 2005). In hepatitis B, CNI toxicity and focal segmental sclerosis, but not immune-complex disease, were revealed as significant contributors to CKD after LT (Lee et al., 2010). The question whether those cases with glomerular lesions represent de novo glomerulonephritis or progression of pre-existing disease was unanswered; only prospective studies with serial kidney biopsies can address this point (Fabrizi et al., 2010). Pre-transplant proteinuria is a significant and independent risk factor for CKD after liver transplantation, according to Lee et al., 2007 and O'Riordan et al., 2006.

4.3.7 Pre-existing comorbidities such as diabetes mellitus, hypertension

A few studies have looked at the relation between *diabetes mellitus* and *hypertension* and chronic renal dysfunction. Karie-Guigues et al., 2009 reported incidence rates of 10.5% for pre-LT hypertension and 43.4% for new-onset hypertension at one year post-transplantation. Diabetes mellitus was reported in 12.5% of the patients before LT and 19.2% developed new onset diabetes after one year of LT. They showed that neither hypertension nor diabetes (pre-transplant or de novo for both) were significantly associated with a GFR decrease at any time points after LTx. These results are in line with those previously reported by Ojo et al, 2003 for hypertension and by O'Riordan et al, 2006 for diabetes.

4.3.8 Child-pugh score and high model for end-stage renal disease (MELD) score

At 3 years after LT, GFR negatively correlated with initial Child-Pugh score (Sezer et al., 2011) and pretransplantat direct bilirubin. After 5 years, GFR negatively correlated with prothrombin time ($r=-0.29$; $P<.05$). Overall risk of CKD development (eGFR < 60 mL/min/1.73 m^2) was associated with high Child-Pugh score and high Model for End-Stage Renal Disease (MELD) score (Lee et al., 2010). Especially in recipients whose pre-operative eGFR was high (>or=60 mL/min/1.73 m^2), rapid progression of kidney disease was associated with Child-Pugh score (in addition to high tacrolimus level and posttransplant acute renal failure) (Fabrizi et al., 2011).

4.4 Prevention of CKD

Especially patients undergoing LT for HCV may benefit particularly from methods for protecting kidney function, such as:

- an optimal control of glucose metabolism,
- dyslipidemia and proteinuria, and an
- aggressive blood pressure containment treatment (Opelz et al., 1998, Randhawa and Shapiro, 2005 and Pillebout et al., 2005).
- Minimizing CNI exposure. Use of CNIs is an important contributor to CRF after liver transplant, accounting for >73% of the renal diagnoses in those patients, (Gonwa et al., 2001b) and this had led to a number of strategies to minimize CNI exposure (mentioned above).

4.5 Outcome of chronic kidney disease after liver transplantation

4.5.1 CVS morbidity/mortality

Chronic kidney disease is a known risk factor for cardiovascular morbidity/mortality in the non-transplantation setting. The Heart Outcomes and Prevention Evaluation (HOPE) study suggested that even mild renal insufficiency was a significant risk factor for a subsequent cardiovascular event (Mann et al., 2001). The Cooperative Cardiovascular project demonstrated that the mortality risk for patients with moderate renal insufficiency for myocardial infarction was three times higher than that of patients with intact kidney function (Shlipak et al., 2002). These results suggest that renal insufficiency is an independent risk factor for cardiovascular disease and should be considered in addition to other traditional risk factors. Transplant recipients are at increased risk of cardiovascular disease, and information gained in the last decade suggests that the occurrence of CKD appears to further increase the burden of cardiovascular disease among LT recipients. Therefore, the most common endpoint among LT recipients with CKD is not the need for renal replacement therapy or kidney transplantation but death secondary to cardiovascular disease (Fabrizi et al., 2010).

Calcineurin inhibitors also contribute to the development of diabetes mellitus, dyslipidemia, hypertension, and oxidative stress, all of which contribute to cardiovascular morbidity (Merville, 2005).

4.5.2 Mortality

The occurrence of CKD after liver transplantation has a major impact on post-LT mortality. Many investigators confirmed this observation. Moreno et al evaluated 289 consecutive LT patients with post-transplant follow-up longer than 6 months. Patient survival was significantly lower among LT patients with chronic renal dysfunction than in those without this complication (63% vs. 71%, p=0.024). Ojo (2003) conducted a population-based cohort analysis among 69,321 persons who received non-renal transplants (liver, lung, heart, intestine, heart-lung) in the United States between 1990 and 2000. The occurrence of CRF significantly increased the risk of death (RR, 4.55; 95% CIs, 4.38 to 4.74; P<0.0001). The 13-year survival rate in patients with end-stage renal disease posttransplant in a study performed by Gonwa et al., 2001 was only 28.2% versus 54.6% in those without posttransplant kidney disease.

Sharma (2009) evaluated retrospectively 221 adult LT recipients who had LT in the MELD era (Feb 2002-Feb 2007). In their multivariate analysis, the decrease in GFR during post-LT follow-up was the only independent predictor of post-LT mortality after adjustment for age, etiology, MELD score, and GFR at liver transplantation. The risk of post-LT patient mortality was 2.9 (1.3-6.4; p=0.008) for patients with GFR <30 versus >30-60 ml/min and 3.2 (1.19-8.67; p=0.02) for patients with GFR <30 versus>60 ml/min. Pawarode (2003) studied 172 consecutive LT recipients over a median follow-up of 72.4 months (range, 6.5 to 100.6 months). Severe renal failure was associated with significantly lower survival by Cox regression analysis (p=0.004). O'Riordan (2006) followed 230 patients after liver transplantation over 5.6 years (Irish National Liver Transplant database); the 10-year cumulative incidence of CKD stage 4 (GFR 15-29 ml/min) and 5 (dialysis or GFR <15 ml/min) was 6.1% and 2.6%, respectively. Cox regression analysis of overall patient survival suggested that the post-LT GFR < 30 ml/min was associated with a hazard ratio of 3.05 (95% CI, 1.21-7.7; p=0.02); the other independent risk factors of lower patient survival being fulminant hepatic failure and retransplantation.

Authors	Relative Risk	P
Ojo A, et al (2003)	4.55(4.38;4.74)	0.001
Pawarode A, et al (2003)	NA	0.004
O'Riordan A, et al (2006)	3.05 (1.21;7.70)	0.02
Sharma P, et al (2009)	3.2 (1.19;8.67)	0.02

Table 6. Impact of Posttransplant Chronic renal dysfunction on Mortality

5. Conclusions

- There has been abundant evidence over the last decade on the importance of kidney dysfunction among liver transplant recipients. However, still questions need to be assessed.
- Acute kidney injury (AKI) has significant prognostic implications for long-term outcomes in patients undergoing liver transplantation. Hence, every effort has to be undertaken to preserve renal function throughout all stages of patient care.
- In this review we discussed the important risk factors that negatively affect kidney function. A specially increased risk frequently exists among liver transplant recipients with pretransplant renal dysfunction.
- Diagnosis of *acute kidney injury* was also discussed. To better define acute kidney injury, new markers (e.g. neutrophil gelatinase-associated lipocalin) have become available that help to identify patients at risk for renal injury within hours of a triggering insult. Larger studies are required to validate the results. These newly established markers for injury, such as NGAL, in conjunction with improved markers for renal function will allow us to further delineate the natural course of AKI during liver transplantation.
- The occurrence of *chronic kidney disease* after liver transplantation has a major impact on mortality. Additional studies are needed to understand better the natural history of chronic kidney disease among liver transplant recipients. Strategies need to be put in place for the early detection of these individuals and then preventive measures introduced to retard the progression of chronic kidney disease.
- Hepatitis C appears to be an additional risk factor affecting renal function in the long term in liver transplanted patients. Further dedicated prospective studies aiming to evaluate the possible pathogenetic mechanism of HCV damage on long-term renal function after liver transplantation are needed. For the present time, it would be advisable to avoid combinations of risk factors for renal impairment, at least in the first year after LT in HCV+ve recipients.
- Modification of nephrotoxic immunosuppressive regimens to avoid postoperative acute renal failure and/or chronic renal failure has met with variable results. Although there is no well-defined protocol to prevent or minimize cyclosporine or tacrolimus nephrotoxicity, some centers currently advocate the use of a calcineurin-sparing protocol adjusted for the degree of renal dysfunction. Hence, the clinical evaluation of the presence of multiple risk factors for renal insufficiency and etiology of liver disease would be important to select patients who would benefit from a renal sparing regime of immunosuppression. However, dedicated large studies meticulously evaluating these renal sparing regimes in patients with risk factors for renal dysfunction are still recommended. Also trials on novel agents targeting different sites of the immune cascade and without renal toxicity are on the way. Until then, finding the balance between preserving graft function and optimizing immunosuppression while minimizing renal toxicity remains a challenge.
- Studies that incorporate renal diagnosis and other prognostic indicators (such as proteinuria) to stratify liver transplant candidates according to risk for kidney dysfunction post-liver transplant are in progress.

6. Acknowledgement

The author would like to express her thanks to: Dr Naglaa Ali Zayed, Associate Professor, Endemic Medicine Department, Cairo University. Dr Ayman AL sebaey AL Ghoraieb Assistant lecturer of Hepatology, National Liver Institute.

7. References

Abrahamian, GA; Cosimi, AB; Farrell, ML; Schoenfeld, DA; Chung, RT & Pascual M. Prevalence of hepatitis C virus-associated cryoglobulinemia after liver transplantation. (2000). Liver Transplantation, 6, 185.

Asfandiyar, S; Abouljoud, M; Kim, D; Brown, K; Yoshida, A; Arenas, J; Sherbondy, M; Divine, G & Moonka D. (2006). Influence of hepatitis C on renal function after liver transplantation. *Transplantation Proceedings*, 38, 3643–3645.

Bahirwani, R; Campbell, MS; Siropaides, T; Markmann, J; Olthoff, K; Shaked, A; Bloom, RD & Reddy, KR. (2008). Transplantation: impact of pretransplant renal insufficiency. Liver Transplantation, 14, 665-671.

Bahirwani, R & Reddy, KR. (2009).Outcomes after liver transplantation: chronic kidney disease. *Liver International*, 15, S70-S74.

Barrett, BJ & Parfrey, PS. (1994). Prevention of nephrotoxicity induced by radiocontrast agents. *New England Journal of Medicine*, 331, 1449-1450.

Barri, YM; Sanchez, Q; Jennings, W; Melton, LB; Hays, S; Levy MF & Klintmalm GB. (2009): Acute kidney injury following liver transplantation: definition and outcome. Liver Transplantation; 15, 475–483.

Bellomo, R; Ronco, C; Kellum, JA; Mehta, RL; Palevsky, P; Acute Dialysis Quality Initiative workgroup. (2004). Acute renal failure - definition, outcome measures, animal models, fluid therapy andinformation technology needs: the Second International Consensus Conference of the Acute Dialysis Quality Initiative (ADQI) Group. *Critical Care*, 8, R204–212.

Bhimma, R; Coovadia, HM; Kramvis, A; Adhikari, M & Kew, MC. (2002). Treatment of hepatitis B virus-associated nephropathy in black children. Pediatr Nephrol; 17(6):393–399.

Biancofiore, G; Pucci, L; Cerutti, E; Penno, G; Pardini, E; Esposito, M; Bindi, L; Pelati, E; Romanelli, A; Triscornia, S; Salvadorini, MP; Stratta, C; Lanfranco, G; Pellegrini, G; Del Prato, S; Salizzoni, M; Mosca, F & Filipponi, F. (2006). Cystatin C as a marker of renal function immediately after liver transplantation. Liver Transplantation, 12, 285–291.

Bilbao, I; Charco, R; Balsells, J; Lazaro, JL; Hidalgo E, Llopart L, Murio, E & Margarit, C. (1998). Risk factors for acute renal failure requiring dialysis after liver transplantation. *Clinical Transplantation*, 12, 123-129.

Braun N, Dette S, Viebahn R. Impairment of renal function following liver transplantation. (2003). *Transplantation Proceedings*, 35, 1458-1460.

Brown RS, Bombardero M & Lake JR. (1996). Outcome of patients with renal insufficiency undergoing liver or liver-kidney transplantation. *Transplantation*, 62, 1788-1793.

Brown, RS; Bombardero, M & Lake, JR. (2001). Outcome of patients with renal insufficiency undergoing liver or liver-kidney transplantation. Transplantation, 72, 1113-1122.

Bumbea, V; Kamar, N; Ribes, D; Esposito, L; Modesto, A; Guitard, J; Nasou, G; Durand D & Rostaing L. (2005). Longterm results in renal transplant patients with allograft dysfunction after switching from calcineurin inhibitors to sirolimus. Nephrology, Dialysis and Transplantation, 20: 2517-2523.

Burra, P; Senzolo, M; Masier, A; Prestele,H, Jones R, Samuel D & Villamil F. (2009). Factors influencing renal function after liver transplantation. Results from the MOST, an international observational study. *Digestive and Liver Disease,* 41,350-356.

Bursten, DM & Rodby, RA. (1993). Membranoproliferative glomerulonephritis associated with hepatitis C virus infection. *Journal of American Society of Nephrology*, 4, 1288-1293.

Cabezuelo, JB; Ramirez, P; Acosta, F, Sanchez Bueno, F; Robles, R; Pons, JA; Miras, M; Munitiz, V; Fernandez, JA; Lujan, J; Rodriguez, JM; Bru, M; Berenguer, JJ & Parrilla P. (2002). Prognostic factors of early acute renal failure in liver transplantation. *Transplantation Proceedings*, 34, 254-255.

Cabezuelo, JB; Ramirez, P; Acosta, F; Torres, D; Sansano, T; Pons, JA; Bru, M; Montoya, M; Rios, A; Sánchez Bueno, F; Robles, R & Parrilla, P. (2003). Does the surgical technique used (standard vs. Piggy Back) have an effect on development of early acute renal failure after orthotopic liver transplantation? *Transplantation Proceedings*, 35, 1913–1914.

Cabezuelo, JB; Ramirez, P; Rios, A; Acosta, F; Torres, D; Sansano, T; Pons, JA, Bru, M; Montoya, M; Bueno, FS; Robles, R & Parrilla, P.(2006). Risk factors of acute renal failure after liver transplantation. *Kidney International*, 69, 1073–1080.

Cabrera, J; Arroyo, V; Ballesta, AM; Rimola, A; Gual, J; Elena, M & Rodes, J. (1982): Aminoglycoside nephrotoxicity in cirrhosis - value of urinary beta-2-microglobulin to discriminate functional renal failure from acute tubular damage. *Gastroenterology*, 82, 97–105.

Campbell, M; Kotlyar, D; Brensinger, M; Lewis, JD; Shetty, K; Bloom, RD; Markmann, JF; Olthoff, KM; Shaked, A & Reddy, KR. (2005). Renal function after orthotopic liver transplantation is predicted by duration of pretransplantation creatinine elevation. *Liver Transplantation,* 11, 1048−1055.

Campistol, JM; Inigo, P; Larios, S; Bescos, M & Oppenheimer, F. Role of transforming growth factor-beta1 in the progression of chronic allograft nephropathy. (2001). *Nephrology Dialysis and Transplantation*, 16 (Suppl 1), 114-116.

Cardenas, A; Ginès, P; Uriz, J; Bessa, X; Salmerón, JM; Mas, A; Ortega, R; Calahorra, B; De Las Heras, D; Bosch, J; Arroyo, V & Rodés, J. (2001). Renal failure after upper gastrointestinal bleeding in cirrhosis: incidence, clinical course, predictive factors, and short-term prognosis. *Hepatology*, 34, 671-676.

Cockcroft, DW & Gault, MH. (1976). Prediction of creatinine clearance from serum creatinine. *Nephron,* 16, 31-41.

Cohen, AJ; Stegall, MD; Rosen, CB; Wiesner, RH; Leung, N; Kremers, WK & Zein NN. (2002): Chronic renal dysfunction late after liver transplantation. *Liver Transplantation*, 8, 916-921.

Cholongitas, E a; Shusang, V; Marelli, L; Nair, D; Thomas, M; Patch, D; Burns, A; Sweny, P & Burroughs AK. (2007). Review article: renal function assessment in cirrhosis - difficulties and alternative measurements. *Alimentary Pharmacology and Therapeutics,* 26(7), 969-978.

Cholongitas, E b; Marelli, L; Kerry, A; Senzolo, M; Goodier, DW; Nair, D; Thomas, M; Patch, D & Burroughs, AK. (2007).Different methods of creatinine measurement significantly affect MELD scores. *Liver Transplantation,* 13, 523–529.

Contreras, G; Garces, G; Quartin, A; Cely, C; LaGatta, MA; Barreto, GA; Roth, D & Gomez, E. (2002). An epidemiologic study of early renal replacement therapy after orthotopic liver transplantation. *Journal of the American Society of Nephrology,* 13, 228-333.

Dehghani, S; Derakhshan, A; Taghavi, A; Gholami, S; Jalaeian, H & Malek-Hosseini, SA. (2008). Prevalence and Risk Factors of Renal Dysfunction after Liver Transplant: A Single-Center Experience. *Experimental and Clinical Transplantation*, 1, 25-29.

De Boccardo, G; Kim, JY; Schiano, T; Schiano, TD; Maurette, R; Gagliardi, R; Murphy, B; Emre, S & Akalin, E. (2008). The burden of CKD in long-term liver transplant recipients. *Transplantation Proceedings*, 40, 1498-1503.

De Simone, P; Precisi, A; Petruccelli, S; Balzano, E; Carrai, P; Catalano, G; Campani, D & Filipponi, F. (2009). The impact of everolimus on renal function in maintenance liver transplantation. *Transplantation Proceedings*, 41(4), 1300-1302.

Diekmann, F; Gutierrez-Dalmau, A; Lopez, S; Cofan, F; Esforzado, N; Ricart, MJ; Rossich, E; Saval, N; Torregrosa, JV; Oppenheimer, F & Campistol JM (2007). Influence of sirolimus on proteinuria in de novo kidney transplantation with expanded criteria donors: comparison of two CNI-free protocols. *Nephrology Dialysis and Transplantation*, 22: 2316-2321.

Distant, DA & Gonwa, TA. The kidney in liver transplantation. (1993). *Journal of the American Society of Nephrology*; 4, 129.

Dore, MP; Fattovich, G; Sepulveda, AR & Realdi, G. (2007). Cryoglobulinemia related to hepatitis C virus infection. *Digestive Diseases and Science*, 52, 897-907.

Eckardt, KM. (1999). Renal failure in liver disease. *Intensive Care Medicine*, 25, 5–14.

Faenza S, Santoro A, Mancini E, Pareschi S, Siniscalchi A, Zanzani C, Pinna AD. (2006). Acute Renal Failure Requiring Renal Replacement Therapy After Orthotopic Liver Transplantation. *Transplantation Proceedings*, 38,1141–1142.

Fabrizi, F, Dixit, V, Martin, P & Messa, P. (2010). Chronic kidney disease after liver transplantation: Recent evidence. *International Journal of Artificial Organs*, 33 (11), 803-811.

Fabrizi, F; Dixit, V; Martin, P & Messa, P. (2011). Pre-transplant kidney function predicts chronic kidney disease after liver transplant: meta-analysis of observational studies. *Digestive Diseases and Science*, 56(5),1282-1289. Epub 2011 Jan 8.

Fasolato, S; Angeli, P & Dallagnese, L. (2007). Renal failure and bacterial infections in patients with cirrhosis: epidemiology and clinical features. *Hepatology*, 45, 223–229.

Fieghen, H; Wald, R & Jaber, BL. (2009). Renal replacement therapy for acute kidney injury. *Nephron Clinical Practice*. 2009, 112(4), c222-9.

Filler G, Webb NJ, Milford DV, Watson AR, Gellermann J, Tyden G, Grenda R, Vondrak K, Hughes D, Offner G, Griebel M, Brekke IB, McGraw M, Balzar E, Friman S, Trompeter R.(2005). Four-year data after pediatric renal transplantation: a randomized trial of Tacrolimus vs. cyclosporin microemulsion. *Pediatric Transplantation*, 9, 498–503.

Fisher NC, Nightingale PG, Gunson BK, Lipkin GW, Neuberger JM. (1998): Chronic renal failure following liver transplantation: a retrospective analysis. *Transplantation*, 66(1), 59-66.

Fitzgerald, GA & Patrono, C. (2001). The COXIBS, selective inhibitors of cyclooxygenase-2. *New England Journal of Medicine*, 345, 433-442.

Flechner, SM; Kobashigawa, J & Goran, Klintmalm G. (2008). Calcineurin inhibitor-sparing regimens in solid organ transplantation: focus on improving renal function and nephrotoxicity. *Clinical Transplantation*, 22(1), 1–15.

Fraley, DS; Burr, R; Bernardini, J; Angus, D; Kramer, DJ & Johnson, JP. (1998). Impact of acute renal failure on mortality in end-stage liver disease with or without transplantation. *Kidney International*, 54,518-524.

Friedlander, M. (2007). Fibrosis and diseases of the eye. *Journal of Clinical Investigation*, 117: 576-586.

Gainza, FJ; Valdivieso, A; Quintanilla, N; Zti, G; Gastaca, M; Campo, M; Lampreabe, I & Ortiz-de-Urbina, J. (2002). Evaluation of acute renal failure in the liver transplantation perioperative period: incidence and impact. *Transplantation Proceedings*, 34, 250-251.

Gane, EJ; Portmann, BC; Naoumov, NV; Smith, HM; Underhill, JA; Donaldson, PT; Maertens, G & Williams R.(1996). Long-term outcome of hepatitis C infection after liver transplantation. *New England Journal of Medicine*, 334, 815.

Gonwa TA, Mai ML, Melton LB Hays SR, Goldstein RM, Levy MF & Klintmalm GB. (2001a). Renal replacement therapy and orthotopic liver transplantation: the role of continuous veno-venous hemodialysis. Transplantation, 2001, 71, 1424–1428.

Gonwa T, Mai M, Melton L, Hays S, Goldstein R, Levy M & Klintmalm GB. (2001b). End-stage renal disease after orthotopic liver transplantation using calcineurin-based immunotherapy. *Transplantation*, 72, 1934-1939.

Gonwa, TA; Jennings, L; Mai, ML; Stark, PC; Levey, AS & Klintmalm, GB. (2004). Estimation of glomerular filtration rates before and after orthotopic liver transplantation: evaluation of current equations. *Liver Transplantation*, 10, 301–309.

Han, SY; Mun, KC; Choi, HJ; Kwak, CS; Bae, JH; Suh, SI; Park, SB; Kim, HC & Chang, EJ. (2006). Effects of cyclosporine and tacrolimus on the oxidative stress in cultured mesangial cells. *Transplantation Proceedings*, 38, 2240-2241.

Hauser, IA; Schaeffeler, E; Gauer, S; Scheuermann, EH; Wegner, B; Gossmann, J; Ackermann, H; Seidl, C; Hocher, B; Zanger, UM; Geiger, H; Eichelbaum, M & Schwab, M. (2005). ABCB1 genotype of the donor but not of the recipient is a major risk factor for cyclosporine-related nephrotoxicity after renal transplantation. *Journal of American Society of Nephrology*, 16, 1501.

Herlenius, G; Fistouris, J; Olausson, M; Felldin, M; Backman, L & Friman, S. (2008). Early renal function post-liver transplantation is predictive of progressive chronic kidney disease. *Scandinavian Journal of Gastroenterology*, 43, 344-349.

Hetz, H; Bauer, M; Lahner, D; Faybik, P; Winning, J; Ankersmit, HJ; Bacher, A & Krenn, CG. (2005). Endothelin activation and postoperative renal failure after human liver transplantation. *Liver Transplantation*, 11, 1201.

Hilmi, IA; Peng, Z; Planinsic, RM; Damian, D; Dai, F; Tyurina, YY; Kagan, VE & Kellum, JA.(2010). N-acetylcysteine does not prevent hepatorenal ischaemia-reperfusion injury in patients undergoing orthotopic liver transplantation. *Nephrology Dialysis and Transplantation*, 25, 2328–2333.

Ishitani, M; Wilkowski, M; Stevenson, W & Pruett, T. (1993). Outcome of patients requiring hemodialysis after liver transplantation. *Transplantation Proceedings*, 25:1762–1763.

Jegatheeswaran, S & Siriwardena, AK. (2011). Experimental and clinical evidence for modification of hepatic ischaemia-reperfusion injury by N-acetylcysteine during major liver surgery. *HPB* (Oxford), 13, 71–78.

Jeyarajah, DR; McBride, M; Klintmalm, GB & Gonwa, TA. (1997). Combined liver-kidney transplantation: what are the indications? *Transplantation*, 64(8), 1091-1096.

John R, Herzenberg, AM. (2010). Our approach to a renal transplant biopsy. *Journal of Clinical Pathology*, 63(1), 26-37.

Johnson, RJ; Gretch, DR; Yamabe, H; Hart, J; Bacchi, CE; Hartwell, P; Couser, WG; Corey, L; Wener, MH; Alpers, CE & Willson, R. (1993). Membranoproliferative glomerulonephritis associated with hepatitis C virus infection. *New England Journal of Medicine*, 328, 465–470.

Johnson, RJ; Willson, R; Yamabe, H; Couser, W; Alpers, CE; Wener, MH; Davis, C & Gretch, DR. (1994a). Renal manifestations of hepatitis C virus infection. *Kidney International*, 46, 1255–1263.

Johnson, RJ; Gretch, DR; Couser, WG; Alpers, CE; Wilson, J; Chung, M; Hart, J & Willson, R. Hepatitis C virus-associated glomerulonephritis. Effect of a-interferon therapy. *Kidney International* 1994(b); 46, 1700–1704.

Junge, G; Schewior, LV; Kohler, S; Neuhaus, R; Langrehr, JM; Tullius, S; Kahl, A; Frei, U & Neuhaus, P. (2006). Acute renal failure after liver transplantation: incidence, etiology, therapy, and outcome. *Transplantation Proceedings*, 38(3), 723-724.

Kamar, N; Frimat, L; Blancho, G; Wolff, P; Delahousse, M & Rostaing, L. (2007). Evaluation of the efficacy and safety of a slow conversion from calcineurin inhibitor- to sirolimus-based therapies in maintenance renal-transplant patients presenting with moderate renal insufficiency. *Transplant International*, 128–34.

Kamar, N; Guilbeau-Frugier, C; Servaiss, A; Tack, I; Thervet, E; Cointault, O; Esposito, L; Guitard, J; Lavayssière, L; Muscari, F; Bureau, C & Rostaing, L. (2011). Kidney histology and function in liver transplant patients. *Nephrology Dialysis and Transplantation*, 26(7), 2355-2361.

Kamath, PS; Wiesner, RH; Malinchoc, M; Kremers, W; Therneau, TM; Kosberg, CL; D'Amico, G; Dickson, ER & Kim, WR. (2001). A model to predict survival in patients with end-stage liver disease. *Hepatology*, 33, 464–470.

Kambham, N; Nagarajan, S; Shah, S; Li, L; Salvatierra, O & Sarwal, MM. (2007). A novel, semiquantitative, clinically correlated calcineurin inhibitor toxicity score for renal allograft biopsies. Clinical *Journal of the American Society of Nephrol*ogy, 2, 135-142.

Karie-Guigues, S; Janus, N; Saliba, F; Dumortier, J; Christophe Duvoux, C; Calmus, Y; Lorho, R; Deray, G; Launay-Vacher, V & Pageaux, GP (2009): Long-Term Renal Function in Liver Transplant Recipients and Impact of Immunosuppressive Regimens (Calcineurin Inhibitors Alone or in Combination with Mycophenolate Mofetil): The TRY Study. *Liver transplantation*, 15, 1083-1091.

Kendrick, EA; McVicar, JP; Kowdley, KV; Bronner, MP; Emond, MJ; Alpers, CE; Gretch, DR; Carithers, RL Jr; Perkins, JD & Davis CL. (1997). Renal disease in hepatitis-C positive liver transplant recipients. Transplantation, 63, 1287.

Khanna, A; Plummer, M; Bromberek, C; Bresnahan, B & Hariharan, S. (2002). Expression of TGF-beta and fibrogenic genes in renal transplant recipients with tacrolimus and cyclosporine nephrotoxicity. *Kidney International*, 62, 2257-2263.

Kim, S; Kim, H; Lee, J; Lee, SG; Kim, YS; Ahn, C; Han, JS; Kim, S; Lee, JS & Suh KS. (2004). Incidence and risk factors of renal dysfunction after liver transplantation in Korea. *Transplantation Proceedings*, 36, 2318–2320.

Kundakci, A; Pirat, A; Komurcu, O; Torgay, A; Karakayalı, H; Arslan, G & Haberal, M. (2010). RIFLE criteria for acute kidney dysfunction following liver transplantation: incidence and risk factors. *Transplantation Proceedings*, 42(10), 4171-4174.

Lafayette, RA; Pare, G; Schmid, CH; King, AJ; Rohrer, RJ & Nasraway, SA. (1997). Pretransplant renal dysfunction predicts poorer outcome in liver transplantation. *Clinical Nephrology*, 48, 159-164.

Lai, KN & Lai, FM. Clinical features and the natural course of hepatitis B virus-related glomerulopathy in adults. (1991). *Kidney International*, 40(suppl 35), S40–S45.

Lebrón Gallardo, M; Herrera Gutierrez, ME; Seller Pérez, G; Curiel Balsera, E; Fernández Ortega, JF & Quesada García, G. (2004): Risk factors for renal dysfunction in the postoperative course of liver transplant. *Liver Transplantation*, 10(11), 1379-1385.

Lee, SK; Park, JB; Kim, SJ; Choi, GS; Kim, DJ; Kwon, CH; Lee, SK & Joh, JW. (2007): Early Postoperative Renal Dysfunction in the Adult Living Donor Liver Transplantation. *Transplantation Proceedings*, 39, 1517–1519.

Lee J, Heo, N; Joo, K; Yi, N; Suh, K; Moon, K; Kim, S & Kim, Y. (2010). Risk factors for consequent kidney impairment and differential impact of liver transplantation on renal function. *Nephrology Dialysis and Transplant*ation, 25, 2772-2785.

Letavernier, E; Pe'raldi, MN; Pariente, A; Morelon, E & Legendre C (2005). Proteinuria following a switch from calcineurin inhibitors to sirolimus. *Transplantation*, 80: 1198-1203.

Levey, AS; Bosch, JP; Lewis, JB; Greene, T; Rogers, N & Roth, D. (1999). A more accurate method to estimate glomerular filtration rate from serum creatinine: A new prediction equation. *Annuals of Internal Medicine*, 130, 461–470.

Levey, AS; Coresh, J; Greene, T; Stevens, LA; Zhang, YL; Hendriksen, S; Kusek, JW & Van Lente, F. (2006). Using standardized serum creatinine values in the modification of diet in renal disease study equation for estimating glomerular filtration rate. *Annuals of Internal Medicine*, 145, 247–254.

Levitsky, J; Thudi, K; Ison, MG; Wang, E & Abecassis, M (2011). Alemtuzumab induction in non-hepatitis C positive liver transplant recipients. *Liver Transplantation*, 17(1),32-7.

Lewandowska, L & Matuszkiewicz-Rowinska, J. (2011). Acute kidney injury after procedures of orthotopic liver transplantation. *Annals of Transplantation*, Jun 30, 16(2),103-108.

Lima, EQ; Zanetta, DM; Castro, I; Massarollo, PC; Mies, S; Machado, MM & Yu L. (2003). Risk factors for development of acute renal failure after liver transplantation. *Renal Failure*, 25(4),553-560.

Liu, R; Nair, D; Ix, J; Moore, DH & Bent, S. (2005): N-acetyl cysteine for prevention of contrast induced nephropathy: a systematic review and meta-analysis. *Journal of General Internal Medicine*, 20,193–200.

Liu, Y. Renal fibrosis: new insight into the pathogenesis and therapeutics. (2006). *Kidney International*, 69, 213-217.

Lucey, MR; Abdelmalek, MF; Gagliardi, R; Granger, D; Holt, C; Kam, I; Klintmalm, G; Langnas, A; Shetty, K; Tzakis, A & Woodle, ES. (2005). A comparison of tacrolimus and cyclosporine in liver transplantation: effects on renal function and cardiovascular risk status. *American Journal of Transplantation*, 5, 1111–1119.

Mann, J; Gerstein, H; Pogue, J; Bosch, J & Yusuf, S. (2001). Renal insufficiency as a predictor of cardiovascular outcomes and the impact of ramipril: the HOPE randomized trial. Ann Intern Med, 134, 629-636.

Mariat, C; Alamartine, E; Barthelemy, JC; De Filippis, JP; Thibaudin, D; Berthoux, P; Laurent, B; Thibaudin, L & Berthoux, F. (2004).Assessing renal graft function in clinical trials: can tests predicting glomerular filtration rate substitute for a reference method? *Kidney International*, 65, 289–297.

Marik, PE; Wood, K & Starzl TE (2006): The course of type 1 hepato-renal syndrome post liver transplantation. *Nephrology Dialysis and Transplantation*, 21, 478-82.

Markmann, JF; Markmann, JW; Markmann, DA; Bacquerizo, A; Singer, J; Holt, CD; Gornbein, J; Yersiz, H; Morrissey, M; Lerner, SM; McDiarmid, SV & Busuttil, RW.

(2001). Preoperative factors associated with outcome and their impact on resource use in 1148 consecutive primary liver transplants. Transplantation, 72, 1113-1122.

McGuire, BM; Julian, BA; Bynon, JS; Cook, WJ; King, SJ; Curtis, JJ; Accortt, NA & Eckhoff, DE. (2006). Brief communication: glomerulonephritis in patients with hepatitis C cirrhosis undergoing liver transplantation. Annals of Internal Medicine, 144, 735-741.

Mehta, RL; Kellum, JA; Shah, SV; Molitoris, BA; Ronco, C; Warnock, DG & Levin, A. (2007). Acute kidney injury network: Report of an initiative to improve outcomes in acute kidney injury. *Critical Care,* 11, R31.

Merville, P. (2005). Combating chronic renal allograft dysfunction: optimal immunosuppressive regimens. *Drugs*, 65, 615.

Mihatsh, MJ; Gudat, F & Ryffel, B. (1994). Cyclosporine nephropathy. In: *Renal pathology with clinical and functional correlations.* Tischer CC & Brenner BM, eds. 1641-1681, JB Lippincott Co, Philadelphia.

Miura, K; Nakatani, T; Asai, T; Yamanaka, S; Tamada, S; Tashiro, K; Kim, S; Okamura, M & Iwao H. (2002). Role of hypomagnesemia in chronic cyclosporine nephropathy. *Transplantation,* 73,340.

Montalbano, M; Neff, GW; Yamashiki, N; Meyer, D; Bettiol, M; Slapak-Green, G; Ruiz, P; Manten, E; Safdar, K; O'Brien, C & Tzakis AG.(2004). A retrospective review of liver transplant patients treated with sirolimus from a single center: an analysis of sirolimus-related complications. *Transplantation*, 78, 264.

Moore, RD; Smith, CR; Lipsky, JJ; Mellits, ED & Lietman, PS. (1984). Risk factors for nephrotoxicity in patients treated with aminoglycosides. *Clinical Research,* 31, A251.

Moreau, R & Lebrec, D. (2003). Acute renal failure in patients with cirrhosis: perspectives in the age of MELD. *Hepatology,* 37, 233-243.

Moreau, R & Lebrec, D. (2006). The use of vasoconstrictors in patients with cirrhosis: type 1 HRS and beyond. Hepatology, 43, 385-394.

Moreno J, Cuervas-Mons V, Rubio E, Pons F, Herreros P, Turrion V, Millan I. (2003). Chronic renal dysfunction after liver transplantation in adult patients: prevalence, risk factors, and impact on mortality. *Transplantation Proceedings*, 35, 1907-1908.

Moz, Y; Levi, R; Lavi-Moshayoff, V; Cox, KB; Molkentin, JD; Silver, J & Naveh-Many, T. (2004): Calcineurin Abeta is central to the expression of the renal type II Na/Pi co-transporter gene and to the regulation of renal phosphate transport. *Journal of American Society of Nephrology,* 15, 2972-2980.

Nair, S; Verma, S & Thuluvath, P. (2002). Pre-transplant renal function predicts survival in patients undergoing orthotopic liver transplantation. *Hepatology,* 35, 1179-1185.

Nankivell, BJ; Borrows, RJ; Fung, CL; O'Connell, PJ; Allen, RD & Chapman, JR. (2003): The natural history of chronic allograft nephropathy. *New England Journal of Medicine,* 349, 2326.

Nijenhuis, T; Hoenderop, JG & Bindels, RJ. (2004): Downregulation of Ca(2+) and Mg(2+) transport proteins in the kidney explains tacrolimus (FK506)-induced hypercalciuria and hypomagnesemia. *Journal of American Society of Nephrology*; 15, 549.

Ojo, AO; Held, PJ; Port, FK; Wolfe, RA; Leichtman, AB; Young, EW; Arndorfer, J; Christensen, L & Merion, RM. (2003). Chronic renal failure after transplantation of a nonrenal organ. *New England Journal of Medicine,* 349,931.

Opelz, G; Wujciak, T & Ritz E. (1998). Association of chronic kidney graft failure with recipient blood pressure. Collaborative Transplant Study. Kidney International, 53, 217.

O'Riordan, A; Wong, V; McCormick, P; Hegarty, J & Watson, A. (2006). Chronic kidney disease post-liver transplantation. *Nephrology Dialysis and Transplantation,* 21, 2630-2636.

Owen, L; Wear, J & Keevil, BG. (2006). Validation of a liquid chromatography tandem mass spectrometry assay for serum creatinine and comparison with enzymatic and Jaffe methods. *Annals of Clinical Biochemistry,* 43, 118-123.

Pascual, M; Thadhani, R; Chung, RT; Williams, WW; Meehan, S; Tolkoff-Rubin, N; Colvin, R & Cosimi, AB. (1997). Nephrotic syndrome after liver transplantation in a patient with hepatitis C virus-associated glomerulonephritis. *Transplantation,* 64, 1073.

Pawarode, A; Fine, D & Thuluvath, P. Independent risk factors and natural history of renal dysfunction in liver transplant recipients. (2003). *Liver Transplantation,* 9, 741-747.

Perez-Rojas, J; Blanco, JA; Cruz, C; Trujillo, J; Vaidya, VS; Uribe, N; Bonventre, JV; Gamba, G & Bobadilla, NA. Mineralocorticoid receptor blockade confers renoprotection in pre-existing chronic cyclosporine nephrotoxicity. (2007). *American Journal of Physiology. Renal Physiol*ogy, 292, F131-F139.

Pham, PT; Pham, PC & Wilkinson, AH. (2007). Renal function outcomes following liver transplantation and combined liver kidney transplantation. *Natural Clinical Practice Nephrol*ogy, 3, 507-514.

Pillai, A & Levitsky, J. Overview of immunosuppression in liver transplantation (2009). *World Journal of Gastroenterology* September 14; 15(34): 4225-4233.

Pillebout, E; Nochy, D; Hill, G; Conti, F; Antoine, C; Calmus, Y & Glotz, D.(2005). Renal histopathological lesions after orthotopic liver transplantation (OLT). *American Journal of Transplantation,* 5: 1120.

Poge, UGT; Palmedo, H; Klehr, H; Sauerbruch, T &Woitas, P. MDRD equations for estimation of GFR in renal transplant recipients. (2005). *American Journal of Transplantation,* 5, 1306-1311.

Porayko, MK; Textor, SC; Krom, RA; Hay JE, Gores GJ, Richards TM, Crotty PH, Beaver SJ, Steers JL, Wiesner RH. (1994). Nephrotoxic effects of primary immunosuppression with FK-506 and cyclosporine regimens after liver transplantation. *Mayo Clinic Proceedings,* 69(2), 105-111.

Portal, AJ; McPhail, MJ; Bruce, M; Coltart, I, Slack A, Sherwood R, Heaton ND, Shawcross D, Wendon JA & Heneghan MA. (2010). Neutrophil gelatinase - associated lipocalin predicts acute kidney injury in patients undergoing liver transplantation. *Liver Transplantation,* 16, 1257–1266.

Randhawa, PS & Shapiro, R. (2005). Chronic renal failure after liver transplantation. *American Journal of Transplantation,* 5, 967.

Remuzzi, G & Bertani, T. (1989) Renal vascular and thrombotic effects of cyclosporine. *American Journal of Kidney Diseases,* 13, 261–272.

Sagias, FG; Mitry, RR; Hughes, RD; Lehec, SC; Patel, AG; Rela, M; Mieli-Vergani, G; Heaton, ND & Dhawan, A. (2010). N-acetylcysteine improves the viability of human hepatocytes isolated from severely steatotic donor liver tissue. *Cell Transplant,* 19, 1487–1492.

Salerno, Fa; Gerbes, AL; Gines, P; Wong, F & Arroyo, V. (2007): Diagnosis, prevention and treatment of hepatorenal syndrome in cirrhosis. *Gut,* 56, 1310−1318.

Sanchez, EQ; Gonwa, TA; Levy, MR; Goldstein, RM; Mai, ML; Hays, SR; Melton, LB; Saracino, G & Klintmalm, GB. (2004). Preoperative and perioperative predictors of the need for renal replacement therapy after orthotopic liver transplantation. *Transplantation,* 78, 1048-1054.

Sanchez, EQ; Melton, LB; Chinnakotla, S; Randall, HB; McKenna, GJ; Ruiz, R; Onaca N; Levy, MF; Goldstein, RM & Klintmalm, GB. (2010). Predicting renal failure after liver transplantation from measured glomerular filtration rate: review of up to 15 years of follow-up. *Transplantation*, 89(2),232-5.

Schnitzbauer, AA; Scherer, MN; Rochon, J; Sothmann, J; Farkas, SA; Loss, M; Geissler, EK; Obed, A & Schlitt, HJ. A pilot study to determine the safety and efficacy of induction-therapy, de novo MPA and delayed mTOR-inhibition in liver transplant recipients with impaired renal function. (2010). PATRON-study. *BMC Nephrology*, 11, 24.

Seronie-Vivien, S; Galteau, MM; Carlier, MC; Hadj-Aissa, A; Hanser, AM; Hym, B; Marchal, A; Michotey, O; Pouteil-Noble, C; Sternberg, M & Perret-Liaudet, A; Creatinine Working Group of the Société Française de Biologie Clinique. (2005). Impact of standardized calibration on the inter-assay variation of 14 automated assays for the measurement of creatinine in human serum. *Clinical Chemistry and Laboratory Medicine*; 43, 1227-1233.

Sezer, S; Karakan, S; Erişmiş, B; Çolak, T & Haberal, M. (2011). Risk factors for kidney impairment and differential impact of liver transplantation on renal function. Transplantation Proceedings, 43(2),609-611.

Sharma, R; Khanna, A; Sharma, M & Savin, JS. (2000). Transforming growth factor B1 increases albumin permeability of isolated rat glomeruli via hydroxyl radicals. Kidney International, 58, 131-136.

Sharma, P; Welch, K; Eikstadt, R; Marrero, JA; Fontana, RJ & Lok, AS. (2009): Renal outcomes after liver transplantation in the model for end-stage liver disease era. *Liver Transplantation*, 15, 1142–1148.

Shlipak, MG; Heidenreich, PA; Noguchi, H; Chertow, GM; Browner, WS & McClellan, MB. (2002). Association of renal insufficiency with treatment and outcomes after myocardial infarction in elderly patients. Ann Intern Med, 137, 555-562.

Smith, SR. (2006). Renal function posttransplant. In: *Medical care of the liver transplant patient*. Killenberg PG & Clavien PA, 460-472, Blackwell Publishing Ltd, ISBN-13: 978-1-4051-3032-5, UK.

Stehman-Breen, C; Alpers, CE; Couser, WG; Willson, R & Johnson, RJ. (1995). Hepatitis C virus associated membranous glomerulonephritis. *Clinical Nephrology*, 44, 141–147.

Takekoshi, Y; Tochimaru, H; Nagata, Y& Itami, N. (1991). Immunopathogenetic mechanisms of hepatitis B virus-related glomerulopathy. *Kidney International*, 40(suppl 35), S34–S39.

Tepel, M; Aspelin, P & Lameire, N. (2006): Contrast induced nephropathy-a clinical and evidence based approach. *Circulation*, 113, 1799–1806.

Terra, C; Guevara, M; Torre, A; Gilabert, R, Fernández, J; Martín-Llahí, M; Baccaro, ME; Navasa, M; Bru, C; Arroyo, V; Rodés, J & Ginès, P. (2005). Renal failure in patients with cirrhosis and sepsis unrelated to spontaneous bacterial peritonitis: value of MELD score. *Gastroenterology*, 129, 1944−1953.

Tinti, F; Umbro, I; Meçule, A; Rossi, M; Merli, M; Nofroni, I; Corradini, SG; Poli, L; Pugliese, F; Ruberto, F; Berloco, PB & Mitterhofer, AP. (2010). RIFLE criteria and hepatic function in the assessment of acute renal failure in liver transplantation. *Transplantation Proceedings*, 42(4), 1233-1236.

Tinti, F; Umbro, I; Giannelli, V; Merli, M; Ginanni Corradini, S; Rossi, M; Nofroni, I; Poli, L; Berloco, PB & Mitterhofer AP. (2011). Acute renal failure in liver transplant recipients: role of pretransplantation renal function and 1-year follow-up. Transplantation Proceedings, May,43(4),1136-1138.

Townsend, DR; Bagshaw, SM; Jacka, MJ; Bigam, D; Cave, D & Gibney, RT. (2009). Intraoperative renal support during liver transplantation. *Liver Transplantation*, 15, 73–78.

Tumlin, JA & Sands, JM. (1993). Nephron segment-specific inhibition of Na+/K+-ATPase activity by cyclosporin A. *Kidney International*,43, 246.

Tzakis AG, Tryphonopoulos P, Kato T, Nishida S, Levi DM, Madariaga JR, Gaynor JJ, De Faria W, Regev A, Esquenazi V, Weppler D, Ruiz P, Miller J. (2004). Preliminary experience with alemtuzumab (Campath-1H) and low-dose tacrolimus immunosuppression in adult liver transplantation. *Transplantation*, 77, 1209-1214

Verna, EC; Farrand, ED; Elnaggar, AS; Pichardo, EM; Balducci, A; Emond, JC; Guarrera, JV & Brown, RS Jr. (2011). Basiliximab induction and delayed calcineurin inhibitor initiation in liver transplant recipients with renal insufficiency. *Transplantation*, 91(11),1254-1260.

Vivarelli, M; Vetrone, G; Zanello, M; Barba, GL; Cucchetti, A; Lauro, A; Grazi, GL & Pinna, AD (2006). Sirolimus as the main immunosuppressant in the early postoperative period following liver transplantation: a report of six cases and review of the literature. *Transplant International*, 19,1022–1025.

Wadei, HM; Mai, ML; Ahsan, N & Gonwa, TA. (2006). Hepatorenal Syndrome: Pathophysiology and Management. *Clinical Journal of American Society of Nephrology*, 1, 1066–1079.

Wei, Y; Zhang, L; Lin, H; Li, J; Li, B; Yan, L; Wen, T, Zeng, Y & Lu, S. (2006): Factors related to post-liver transplantation acute renal failure. *Transplantation Proceedings*, 38, 2982–2984.

Xu, X; Ling, Q; Wei, Q; Wu, J; Gao, F; He, ZL; Zhou, L & Zheng, SS. (2010). An effective model for predicting acute kidney injury after liver transplantation. *Hepatobiliary Pancreatic Diseases International*, 9, 259–263.

Yalavarthy, R; Edelstein, CL & Teitelbaum, I. (2007). Acute renal failure and chronic kidney disease following liver transplantation. *Hemodialysis International*,Oct,11,Suppl 3, S7-12.

Yamamoto, S; Sato, Y; Ichida, T; Kurosaki, I; Nakatsuka, H & Hatakeyama, K. (2004). Acute renal failure during the early postoperative period in adult living-related donor liver transplantation. *Hepatogastroenterology*, 51,1815.

Zhu, M; Li, Y; Xia, Q; Wang, S; Qiu, Y; Che, M; Dai, H; Qian, J; Ni, Z; Axelsson, J & Yan Y. (2010). Strong impact of acute kidney injury on survival after liver transplantation. *Transplantation Proceedings*, 42,3634–3638.

14

Post Transplant Lymphoproliferative Disorders After Liver Transplantation

Dario Marino, Savina Maria Aversa,
Silvia Stragliotto, Fabio Canova and Caterina Boso
Department of Medical Oncology, Istituto Oncologico Veneto, IRCCS
Padova,
Italy

1. Introduction

Post-transplant lymphoproliferative disorder (PTLD) is a clearly recognized and potentially life threatening complication after solid organ or bone marrow transplantation. It comprises a spectrum of diseases ranging from infectious mononucleosis and lymphoid hyperplasia to highly aggressive lymphoma. The disease has increased clinical importance in view of the constantly rising number of organ transplant recipients and the development of more potent and specific immunosuppressive drugs.

PTLD is a relatively common malignancy after transplantation with a reported incidence ranging from 2% to 10%. It is the most common form of post-transplant malignancy after skin cancer with an overall mortality often exceeding 50%.

Registry-based reports however usually do not provide details of treatment and outcome: the existing single institution studies are largely reports and only a few studies include a significant number of patients with PTLD. Most cases of PTLD are associated with Epstein Barr virus (EBV) that leads to uncontrolled B cell proliferation in patients with a decreased function of EBV specific T cell because of immunosuppressive drugs. PTLD is not exclusively associated with EBV infection as EBV-negative PTLD, often developing late after transplantation.

Post transplant lymphomas differ from lymphomas in general population in histopathological findings, increased extranodal involvement, a more aggressive clinical course and poorer response to conventional treatment.

Treatment of PTLD consists always in reduction of immunosuppression (RI) as first step. The role of chemotherapy (CT) remains unclear. In the past it was reserved for patients in whom other treatment options have failed even if the increased toxicities from cytotoxic agents, the high susceptibility to life-threatening infections and the necessity to maintain the allograft. Actually (Rituximab Hera) most authors consider new anti CD20 monoclonal antibodies (mAB) essential for treatment or as single agent or in association with CT but there is not a definitive agreement about schedules, duration of treatment and setting of patients.

2. Pathogenesis

The appearance of PTLD is often associated with clinical or serological reactivation of Epstein Barr virus infection. Tumour tissues often contain EBV-DNA sequences and express viral protein (Purtilo DT,1980; Young L et al, 1989; Hanto DW et al, 1981). In normal individuals, host defence mechanism make EBV infection a self limited disease and B cell proliferation is controlled by specific T cell lymphocytes. The infection is however not eradicated, but persists in clinical latent form. In transplanted patients, partial suppression of T lymphocyte to prevent graft rejection, makes EBV-driven B cell proliferation uncontrolled and predispose to development of PTLD.

Several single centre studies have found that EBV seronegative patients had a 10-76 times greater incidence of PTLD than EBV seropositive recipients (Walker RC et al, 1995).

Active viral replication in immunosuppressed patients results in the expression of EBV encoded genes including oncogenes as LMP1, a gene that inhibits apoptosis by up regulating the anti-apoptotic gene BCL-2 (Kulwichit W et al, 1998).

Data suggests also that prophylactic anti-Cytomegalovirus (CMV) immunoglobulin prevent the development of early post-transplant non Hodgkin lymphoma while prophylactic treatment with antiviral drugs does not reduce the risk of PTLD (Opelz G et al, 2007).

Locker and Nalesnick (Locker J & Nalesnick M, 1989) demonstrated that monomorphic PTLDs display a strong clonal immunoglobulin rearrangement band on Southern Blotting and a c-myc gene rearrangement exhibits disease progression. Also alterations of p53 and N-ras seem to be implied in pathogenesis of PTLD. BCL 6, that encodes a transcriptional repressor gene rearranged in 35-40% of diffuse large B cell lymphoma in immunocompetent patients (Bastard C et al, 1994; Lo Coco F et al, 1994), presents frequent somatic mutations in PTLD representing probably a consistent step in the progression from a PTLD that can be controlled by a reconstituted immune system to one that will require more aggressive therapeutic intervention (Cesarman E et al, 1998).

PTLD also have genomic aberration common to lymphomas in immunocompetent patients such as gain of 8q24, 3q2718q21 and loss of 17p13.

In conclusion viral oncogenes, impaired immune system, chronic antigen stimulation and genetic aberration probably contribute together to pathogenesis of PTLD (Poirel HA et al, 2005).

3. Risk factors

The most important risk factor for PTLD development is the intensity of immunosuppression administered. Induction and rejection treatment with anti-T cell antibodies, especially OKT3 and ATG may lead to an increased risk of PTLD, as demonstrated by the higher incidence of early PTLD in hearth and hearth/lung recipient. With longer follow-up, is now evident that antibody prophylaxis increased the risk of lymphoma primarily during the first post-transplant year, whereas in subsequent years the risk is similar to that in non antibody-treated patients. Whether IL2 receptor blocking monoclonal antibody, which was introduced in the late 1990s, also increases the risk of lymphoma is of great interest. Analysis of the critical 12-months data showed that use of anti IL2 receptor antibodies was not associated with an increased risk of lymphoma (Opelz G et al, 2003).

There is no conclusive evidence that development of PTLD is associated with a single immunosuppressive agent (Gao SZ et al, 2003; Pirsch JD et al, 1997; Weisner RH et al, 1998; Younes BS et al, 2000). Also the effect of everolimus and sirolimus on PTLD development is not clear. These drugs may theoretically be associated with a lower risk as demonstrated in animal model but the lack of prospective randomized trial assessing these differences restrains any firm conclusion (Yakupoglu YK et al, 2006; Majewski M et al, 2003; Kusuki S et al, 2009).

A special category of patient at risk (10 to 50 fold increased risk) are EBV seronegative patients receiving allograft from EBV seropositive donors, leading to primary EBV infection (Walker RC et al, 1995). This is also the reason for the higher incidence of early PTLD observed in paediatric transplant recipients who often are still EBV seronegative at the time of transplantation.

A high incidence of EBV related lymphoproliferative disorders has been reported in a number of congenital immunodeficiency syndromes including severe combined immunodeficiency (SCID), ataxia teleangiectasia and Wischott Aldrich syndrome Waldmann TA et al, 1983). Acquired immunodeficiency due to HIV disease has become a major clinical problem in many parts of the world. An increased incidence of aggressive non Hodgkin lymphoma which shares many of the unusual characteristics of PTLD is a manifestation of AIDS. The introduction of the Highly Active Antiretroviral Therapy (HAART) has dramatically reduced the incidence of this life threatening manifestation of HIV.

The underlying indication for transplantation may also influence the risk for PTLD. For example Hepatitis C infection (Burra P et al, 2006) is associated with a particularly high risk of PTLD in liver transplant recipients.

Recent data also suggest Hepatitis B virus reactivation as a possible risk factor for development of PTLD(Leblond V & Choquet S, 2004; Duvoux C et al, 2002; Zhang A et al 2009).

Also patients with immunological disorders before liver transplantation receiving steroids and patient transplanted for autoimmune hepatitis seems to be at higher risk for development of PTLD (Zimmermann T et al, 2010; Shpilberg O et al, 1999)

4. Epidemiology

The incidence of PTLD after solid organ transplantation is different in children and adults and varies according to the type of organ transplanted.

The incidence is significantly higher in paediatric recipients and has been reported in 1-10% of kidney or liver transplants and 6-19 of hearth, lung and hearth and lung transplants. However the true incidence of PTLD in adult and paediatric recipients is difficult to determine with accuracy(Leblond V & Choquet S, 2004; Patel H et al, 2007).

PTLD is surprisingly uncommon (<1 %) in the setting of allogenic bone marrow transplantation in the absence of specific T-cell manipulation such as use of a monoclonal anti CD3 antibody or T cell depletion of donor marrow. The incidence of PTLD would be expected to increase with the duration of immunosuppression and few studies standardise their data on incidence for this variable. Also the lack of standardised diagnostic criteria for PTLD may reflect the wide range in incidence.

Although PTLD may occur at any time after transplantation, the risk of developing PTLD is greatest within the first year and declines over time thereafter. A report by the Transplant Collaborative Study showed the incidence of PTLD to be 224/100000 in the first year, 54/100000 in the second year and 31/100000 in the sixth year following transplantation[11].

The higher incidence of PTLD in paediatric transplant recipient is attributable in large part to the development of primary EBV infection after transplantation. EBV seronegative adults who acquire primary EBV infection after transplantation are also at increased risk of PTLD but since most adults are already EBV seropositive at the time of transplantation this is a less problem.

In both children and adult, PTLD is more common after hearth and lung transplantation than after kidney or liver transplantation. This may be because more intensive immunosuppression is used in recipient of thoracic organ. In lung recipient the large number of EBV-infected lymphocytes residing in lung transplants in the form of bronchus associated lymphoid tissue may be a contributing factor in EBV seronegative recipients.

5. Pathologic features

A standardised approach to the classification of PTLD is important to allow consistency of reporting and to enable comparison of different treatments. Histology is essential also in differentiation between rejection and PTLD involvement of the graft. The classification of PTLD currently used is based on the histopathological appearance of the tumour. PTLD can be divided into three distinct morphological groups, as reported by the World Health Organization classification of neoplastic disease of the haematopoietic and lymphoid tissues.

The first group comprises diffuse B cell hyperplasia, characterised by differentiated plasma cell and preservation of the normal lymphoid architecture. This type of PTLD is most often seen in children and young adults, usually occur within the first year following transplantation and responds well to reduction of immunosuppression (Kahan BD et al, 2000).

The second group comprises polymorphic PTLD characterised by nuclear atypia, tumour necrosis and destruction of underlying lymphoid architecture. Lesions in this group are highly polymorphic, usually monoclonal and include plasmacytes and blast form. Polymorphic PTLD is the most common type of PTLD in both children and adults and may occur at any time after transplantation.

The third group comprises monomorphic PTLD and includes high grade invasive lymphoma of B or T lymphocytes. This type of PTLD is often seen several years after transplantation and resembles non Hodgkin lymphoma. Monomorphic B cell PTLD can be further divided into diffuse large cell lymphoma and Burkitt or Burkitt like lymphoma. PTLD may also present with discordant lesions, in which different histological subtypes can be present in a single patient.

Although the association between EBV and PTLD is well established, the presence of EBV in tumour cell is not required for the diagnosis. So, according to the international classification, any lymphoma arising in the post-transplant patient is considered to be a PTLD.

At least 90% of PTLD that occur in solid organ transplant patients arise from recipient cells (Weissmann DJ et al, 1995) and the opposite apply in the case of bone marrow transplantation. Donor derived PTLD in organ transplant patient may have a predilection for the allograft (Strazzabosco M et al, 1996). Some authors have suggested that they may have a worse and some a better prognosis than recipient organ PTLD even if further studies are needed in this area (Lones MA et al, 1997; Howard TK et al, 1992).

Clinical recurrence of PTLD has been estimated to occur in approximately 5% of cases. Wu et al.[30] (Wu TT et al 1996) examined a series of 11 such patients and found that the recurrent tumours comprised a heterogeneous assortment. In some cases the recurrence was morphologically and clonally identical to the original tumour. In several cases PTLD recurred in a more aggressive form. For example, patients with mononucleosis-like PTLD could present later with polymorphic PTLD, and patients whose original disease was polymorphic PTLD might later develop one of the lymphomatous forms of PTLD.

6. Clinical presentation

The clinical presentation of PTLD is highly variable. PTLD may arise at any time after transplantation with a significantly higher risk in the first post-transplant year, especially in heart and lung recipient because of the high dose of immunosuppression. Most patients present with fever (seen in 50%), lymphadenopathy (seen in 30%) or non-specific symptoms such as tonsillitis (particularly children) and weight loss. Around 15% of patients present as an emergency with intestinal perforation (Kahan BD et al 2000) or with fulminant PTLD characterised by disseminated systemic disease that clinically resembles septic shock (Orjuela M et al, 2003). Keeping in mind that PTLD often present at extra nodal sites (Bakker NA et al, 2005), including the allograft and digestive tract, there may be early signs and symptoms that should at least include PTLD in the differential diagnosis. This is especially true for allograft involvement of PTLD. The most commonly affected extranodal site of PTLD is observed in the gastrointestinal tract (G.I.). There seem to be no relation between the time of onset and the development of PTLD in the G.I. tract (Leblond V et al, 1995). The CNS is involved in up to 30% of cases of PTLD and in many of these the disease is confined to the CNS (Maecker B et al, 2007; Penn I & Porat G, 1995). In this respect, PTLD contrasts with NHL in the general population where only around 1% of cases shows isolated CNS involvement. Skin involvement is observed in approximately 5-10% of all PTLD patients and must be differentiated by other cutaneous malignancy, given the fact that organ allograft recipients have an increased risk for the development of cutaneous malignancy such as squamous and basal cell carcinoma (Beynet DP et al, 2004). The Canadian PTLD Survey Group analysed 90 cases of PTLD occurring in 4283 solid organ transplant recipients followed over a nine-year period (Allen U et al, 2001). Approximately two thirds of patients presented with disease localised to a single site, of which only a quarter were within the lymph nodes. The remaining patients had solitary lesions at extra-nodal sites including kidney, bowel, liver, mediastinum and skin. More rarely, solitary lesions were seen in the lung, tonsils and central nervous system (CNS). In particular, CNS involvement, especially in paediatric patients seems to be a risk factor for poor prognosis (Maecker B et al, 2007). In patients presenting with multiple lesions, the lymph nodes and liver were most commonly affected. In PTLD occurring after liver transplantation abdominal findings are the most common manifestation including PTLD within liver allograft and splenic abnormalities (Wu L et al, 2001). Portal masses have also been reported presenting as lesion with mass effect and intrahepatic bile duct dilatation: they have sometimes initially been treated as abscess until the diagnosis of PTLD was made (Strouse PJ et al, 1996; Armes JE et al, 1994; Sokal EM et al, 1993). Some studies have reported rates of 50% and 30% of PTLD affecting the bowel associated with high perforation rate. So after transplantation the presence of gastrointestinal disturbance should alert the clinician to the potential diagnosis of PTLD as well as the more common complications of infection and inflammation (Starzl TE et al, 1984; Steiber AC et al, 1991). Given this myriad of nonspecific clinical signs and symptoms, often masquerading PTLD as infection or adverse drug effects or reactions, or even absence of symptoms at all, methods for early detection of PTLD in transplant recipients would be extremely valuable.

7. Diagnosis of PTLD

The diagnosis of PTLD should be based on histological examination of biopsy tissue. Excision biopsy is preferable and needle biopsy should only be performed where excision of affected tissue in not practicable, also because PTLD may contain large areas of necrosis. Cytological preparation are useful, particularly in the analysis of effusion (Lechapt-Zalcman E et al, 2001) and can provide adequate diagnostic material particularly if ancillary studies such as phenotypic, clonal and viral analysis are also performed. Tissue should be subjected to standard histology, examined for the presence of EBV by immunostaining or in-situ hybridization, cellular infiltrates characterised by relevant phenotypic markers and clonality estimated. Although it would be ideal to sample each tumour in cases of multicenter PTLD, this is seldom possible. Each tumour may represent a separate clone and the histological grade may be underestimated in multicentric cases. The surgeon run also the risk, in this case, of sampling a reactive node that may contain evidence of EBV infection, while the primary lymphomatous PTLD lies elsewhere. It is also useful consider biopsy of any lesion that respond in an atypical fashion, particularly if regression is documented in other concurrent lesion.

There is no separate staging system for PTLD and it is currently staged using the same system as non Hodgkin Lymphoma (NHL) in the normal population. Staging of the disease should include computed tomography (CT) of the abdomen and thorax and bone marrow aspiration. Fluorodeoxyglucose positron emission tomography (FDG-PET) scanning is increasingly used as an important tool in the visualization of malignant lymphoma, especially for the detection of extranodal localization and post-treatment evaluation and has shown to be superior over conventional diagnostic techniques to differentiate between residual masses as a result of vital tumour or scar tissue. Bakker et al. (Bakker NA et al, 2006) reported a cases of 12 patients whit a highly avid FDG PTLD. Additional sites of extranodal localization of PTLD not visualized on CT scanning were found in 50% of all patients. (figure 1)

Additional investigations should be performed as indicated, e.g. CT or magnetic resonance scan of the cranium and spinal cord or further gastrointestinal imaging. The presence of PTLD within the graft itself may sometimes be mistaken for acute rejection and if there is diagnostic doubt, in-situ hybridisation for EBV encoded RNA, and PCR for VDJ heavy-chain rearrangements to determine clonality may be helpful. Molecular analysis of oncogenes and tumour suppressor genes will undoubtedly play an increasingly important role in predicting behaviour even if, at present, these techniques are not widely available and few genes have been analyzed.

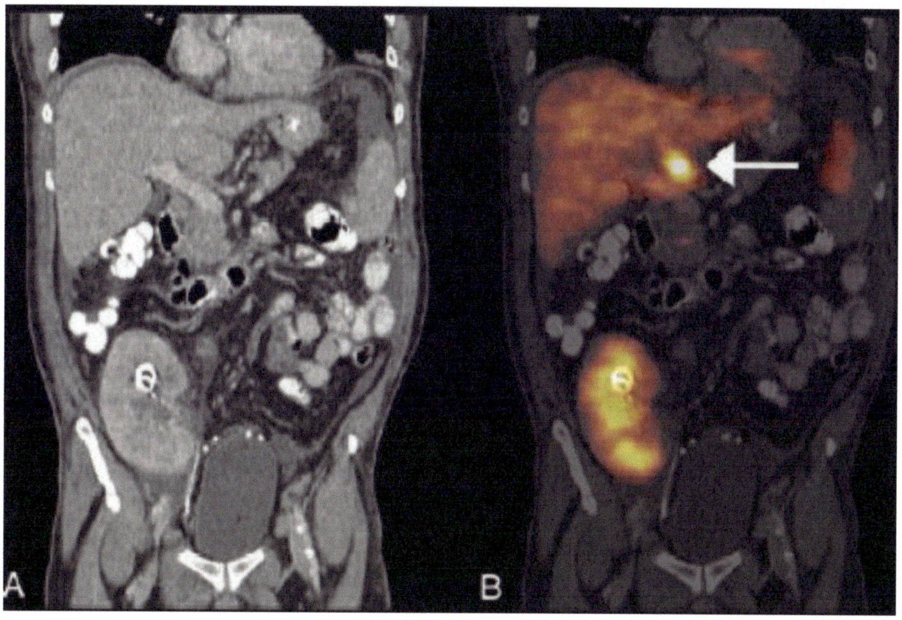

Fig. 1. Example of discordant finding. CT abdomen (A) and FDG PET fused with the same CT scan (B). Arrow indicates the histologically confirmed focal lesion with high uptake of FDG, whereas the CT scan (A) does not show any abnormalities at the site of high FDG uptake. The high uptake in the allograft, including the kidney calices and pyelum, is physiological, as is the modest uptake in liver and spleen

8. EBV DNA load monitoring after transplantation

Because elevation of EBV-DNA load in blood is considered to reflect aberrant EBV induced B-cell proliferation, much effort has been put in developing methods that might identify patients at risk for developing PTLD by measuring the amount of circulating EBV-DNA in the peripheral blood. More recently, pre-emptive strategies to prevent PTLD have been evaluated. Mc Diarmid et al. (McDiarmid SV et al, 1998) treated pre-emptively with intravenous ganciclovir 18 high-risk (donor positive for EBV serology, recipient negative for EBV serology) paediatric liver recipient and no one developed PTLD whereas they previously reported 10% incidence of post transplant lymphoproliferative disease (PTLD) in paediatric patients receiving first liver grafts and primarily immunosuppressed with tacrolimus. Despite the consensus that PTLD patients have a significantly higher EBV-DNA load compared with healthy EBV-seropositive donors or non-PTLD transplant recipients, it is still unclear which threshold values are predictive for PTLD. Many different threshold values have been reported, all with different sensitivity (60–100%) and specificity (71–100%) (Lee TC et al, 2005; Rowe DT et al, 2001; Tsai DE et al, 2002). Another limitation of EBV-

DNA load monitoring may be the observation that PTLD developing late after transplantation is not necessarily associated with EBV (negative staining for EBV in the tumour), and may therefore develop without a concomitant rise in EBV-DNA load. Indeed, there are studies showing EBV-negative PTLD developing late after transplantation without a rise in EBV-DNA load. These observations suggest that, although increased EBV-DNA load is generally considered to represent an increase in circulating EBV-positive tumour cells, these high EBV-DNA loads in reality may represent a separate population of proliferating B-cells that may have nothing to do with development of PTLD. Instead, these proliferating B-cells may only reflect a general state of decreased T-cell surveillance in the transplant recipient. In conclusion, because of the many variables that may influence the immune response of the individual transplant recipient, such as level of immunosuppression, time after transplantation, concomitant infections, type of organ transplanted, but also genetic factors, an exact cut-off value of EBV-DNA load critical for the development of PTLD in the individual patient cannot be defined. Therefore, rising EBV-DNA loads in the individual patient, instead of using a cut-off value, may be more appropriate to identify the individual patient at risk for the development of PTLD. It has been suggested that concomitant combined monitoring of EBV-DNA load and EBV-specific cytotoxic T lymphocytes (CTL) responses (the absence of which may be used as a marker for possible overimmunosuppression) might better identify the individual patient at risk for PTLD development. The positive predictive value of high EBV-DNA loads as a predictor for PTLD development might be improved with this method. Smets et al.(Smets F et al, 2002) showed that high EBV-DNA loads in patients who underwent primary EBV infection were indicative for PTLD development only if there was a low concomitant cellular immune response.

9. Clinical management

The treatment of PTLD poses a major therapeutic challenge and, although there is reasonable agreement about the overall principles of treatment no controlled studies have been undertaken and most of the recommendations result from small cohorts at single institutions.

Even if no uniform approaches to the treatment have emerged, general principles are largely shared.

- Treatment must be individualised according to clinical situation and the type of organ transplanted
- Unlike non-Hodgkin lymphoma in immunocompetent patients, PTLD can be eradicated by surgical resection
- Reduction of immunosuppression is considered the first line treatment
- Antiviral agents have showed to induce regression of disease in some cases
- Chemotherapy, traditionally considered a last resort treatment, is associated with high response rate and long progression free survival
- Rituximab has emerged as treatment of choice especially in early PTLD after failure in reduce/withdrawal immunosuppression
- Radiotherapy may be appropriate for treatment of localized PTLD together with reduction in immunosuppression

Treatment	Comments
Treatments enhancing recipient CTL function	
Reduction of immunosuppression	First line treatment for PTLD
	More likely to induce remission in early or polymorphic PTLD
Adoptive T cell therapy	Risk of graft versus host disease in case of allogenic CTLs and need for dedicated facilities. Need for growing autologous CTLs
Cytokine based therapies	
Interferon-alpha	Several case reports of successful induction of remission with reduction of immunosuppression and interferon-a
	May significantly increase the risk of organ rejection
Anti IL-6 antibodies	Promising results in phase one to two trials
Antiviral agent	Under development Acyclovir, ganciclovir
Treatments reducing tumour mass	
Surgical excision	For localized disease
	Most cases not amenable to surgical resection
Local radiation	Adjunct to surgical excision
	Treatment of choice for CNS PTLD
Chemotherapy	Used in aggressive disease
	High mortality from sepsis and toxicity
	Effective in around 2/3 of selected patients
Rituximab	Promising results when combined with reduction in immunosuppression
	Longer term results required to determine relapse rates

Table 1. Treatment of PTLD

9.1 Reduction of immunosuppression

Reduction of immunosuppression is the initial treatment in all patients with PTLD with the aim of increase antitumor activity. In EBV driven PTLD, this may partially restores CTL function resulting in an increase of EBV specific CTLs and elimination of virally infected lymphocytes, including those which constitute the tumour. The approach to reduce immunosuppressive drugs needs to be carefully individualised and will depend on the nature and extent of disease, the type of transplant recipient (life or no-life supporting graft) and the time from transplantation.

In general most clinicians adjust the corticosteroid dose to 10 mg of Prednisone daily in the hope to prevent allograft rejection. Steroids also are an important component of most chemotherapy regimen for PTLD and lymphoma in general.

A response to reduction in immunosuppression is usually seen within 2-4 weeks (Green M et al, 1999).

Reduction in immunosuppression leads to long term disease remission in 40-86% of paediatric patients and 25-63% of adults.

If PTLD develops within one year of the transplant up to 80% will respond to reducing in immunosuppression.

In contrast, after one year the response rate falls to 10% with 80% of mortality (Armitage JM et al, 1991).

9.2 The role of rituximab

PTLD is usually of B cell origin and the use of mAB to deplete B cell is a logical approach for treatment. Rituximab, a monoclonal antibody directed against CD20 antigen expressed on mature and immature B cells, results in profound and long-lasting depletion of B cell (6-8 months), together with hypogammaglobulinemia.

Rituximab is widely used in the treatment of diffuse large B cell lymphoma in immunocompetent patients with an overall survival at two years of 70% compared with 57% of patients treated with chemotherapy alone (Coiffier B et al, 2002).

Many more case reports and case series of using rituximab in PTLD are described in literature. This cases included paediatric and adult PTLD patients who underwent solid organ or bone marrow transplantations and achieved excellent results with rituximab. Most of the patients also underwent concurrent RI and some received also antiviral therapy. Many patients experienced clinical improvement within a few days after the first infusion. Most patients were treated with the standard dose of rituximab at 375 mg/m^2 once a week for four consecutive weeks. The majority of the case reports describe the use of rituximab in the early onset PTLD, but it might be effective also for patients with late onset PTLD. Gonzalez-Barca et al (Gonzalez-Barca E et al, 2004) reviewed data on 108 adult solid organ transplanted patients with PTLD including 36 patients who received rituximab. With a mean follow-up of 15 months, the OS of patients treated with rituximab was significantly better than for the whole group (76% vs. 21). In a multicenter, prospective phase II study, Oertel et al.(Oertel SH et al, 2005) treated 17 adult patients with PTLD with standard dose of rituximab. The mean follow-up time was 24 months. Overall response rate was obtained in 12 (71%) patients. Nine patients (53%) achieved complete remission (CR), with a mean duration of 17.8 months. Two patients relapsed, respectively 3 and 5 months after obtaining CR. The mean overall survival was 37 months with 11 (65%) patients alive at the end of the study. Adverse events were rare and of low grade. Patients whose tumour was EBV positive were significantly more likely to achieve CR than patients with tumors that were EBV negative. The largest prospective trial of using rituximab in PTLD was published by Choquet et al.(Choquet S et al, 2005). This multicenter, open label, European phase II trial, enrolled 63 patients with PTLD after solid organ transplantation who did not improve after reduction of immunosuppression. The study included both paediatric and adult patients who were treated with standard dose of Rituximab 375 mg/m^2 weekly for 4 weeks. Most of the PTLD cases were of relatively late onset with only 17 patients with PTLD diagnosed <1 year after their transplantation. The overall response rate after single agent rituximab was 59% with a CR rate of 42% and a partial response rate of 17%. Stable disease was observed in 3% of patients and 38% progressed during treatment. At a median follow up of 16,3 months, median progression free survival was 6.0 months. Trappe et al. (Trappe RU et al, 2007) reported the efficacy of single agent Rituximab in eight patients (seven adults, one paediatric) with PTLD relapsed or refractory to chemotherapy after failure of reduction in immunosuppression. Complete remission was obtained in three patients and partial remission in two. Patient achieving CR either remain in CR or were successfully salvaged again with single agent Rituximab. In conclusion patients treated with rituximab benefit from the short duration of such therapy in terms of response rate and less toxic effect. However, because of the high relapse rate observed in several studies, the combination of Rituximab with cytotoxic drugs is recommended to be evaluated.

9.3 Antiviral agents

Because most PTLDs arise as a consequence of EBV infection, prophylactic measures should include avoiding over-immunosuppression of the recipient such as the use of anti-lymphocyte preparations, antiviral agents, EBV vaccination, in-vitro generated EBV specific CTL lines and avoiding, in EBV seronegative recipients, transplantation with an organ from an EBV positive donor. Regression has been described following high dose acyclovir. Targeting EBV by antiviral agents has been attempted also for prophylaxis of PTLD. An alternative approach, especially in high risk recipients, is to prospectively monitor the EBV viral load after transplantation and to initiate therapy when a pre-determined threshold is exceeded. One problem with this approach is that only a minority of patients with high EBV loads develops PTLD, and some patients with EBV-positive PTLD may have a low serum viral load

9.4 Cytokine based therapy

Agents that alter the cytokine environment of the tumour to favour remission, notably interferon-α (Davis CL et al, 1998) and anti-IL-6 have been tried as adjuvant along with reduction of immunosuppression, but at present there is insufficient evidence to recommend their routine use. Interferon-α enhances T-lymphocyte cytotoxicity and has been used as an adjunct to chemotherapy to treat B cell malignancies in non-transplanted patients and in the maintenance of remission in such patients. Swinnen et al. (Swinnen LJ et al, 2008) recently reported results of a trial for treatment of PTLD starting with a defined course of RI in all patients, escalating to interferon (IFN) alpha2b, and finally to chemotherapy, in a prospective multicenter phase II study of adult solid organ transplant recipients. Reduction in immunosuppression produced no CR, progressive disease and rejection were frequent; response to IFN was rare while chemotherapy resulted in 57% durable CR. IL-6 may play a role in the development of PTLD by promoting the growth of EBV-infected B cells and increasing tumour development in EBV-immortalised cells. Serum levels of IL-6 are raised in the majority of patients with PTLD. Anti-IL-6 mAb has been used in a phase 1–2 multi-centre clinical trial in 12 patients with PTLD that was refractory to a reduction of immunosuppression (Haddad E et al, 2001). Five of the 12 patients showed a complete response with no residual tumour and three patients showed a decrease in tumour size, which in one case was sufficient to allow surgical removal of a previously unresectable tumour. Anti-IL-6, therefore, appears to be a promising adjunct in the treatment of PTLD but further studies are needed to fully assess its efficacy.

9.5 Rapamycine

Rapamycine is increasingly used as an immunosuppressive agent for solid organ transplantation. In addition to its immunosuppressive effects, it also displays anti-angiogenic and anti-tumour properties, and this make it a potentially attractive agent for patients in remission from PTLD, particularly those who develop chronic allograft rejection as a consequence of a reduction of immunosuppression. Rapamycin inhibits the growth of EBV-transformed B lymphocyte lines in-vitro by arresting cell cycle in the G1 phase (Vaysberg M et al, 2007). There are no prospective studies addressing the use of rapamycin in the treatment or prevention of PTLD.

9.6 Adoptive T cell therapy

Adoptive T cell therapy using EBV-specific CTL lines has generated considerable interest as a treatment for PTLD. Adoptive immunotherapy was initially advocated in allogenic bone marrow transplantation to control PTLD that was donor cell in origin. Donor CTL would restore immune surveillance against EBV driven proliferation and control PTLD. A potential risk was graft versus host disease due to the donor cell infusion: this risk could be reduced by selecting donor EBV-specific T cell ex vivo prior to infusion. This approach has been used with success as prophylaxis and treatment of PTLD after stem cell transplantation using CTL lines derived from the donor and specific for EBV gene products even if it is limited by the time required to generate the CTLs (weeks to months) and the expense for dedicated facilities. Haque et al (Haque T et al, 2007) presented the results of a recent multicenter clinical trial using Epstein-Barr virus-specific CTL generated from EBV-seropositive blood donors to treat patients with EBV-positive PTLD on the basis of the best HLA match and specific in vitro cytotoxicity. The response rate (complete or partial) in 33 patients was 64% at 5 weeks and 52% at 6 months. Fourteen patients achieved a complete remission, 3 showed a partial response, and 16 had no response at 6 months (5 died before completing treatment). No adverse effects of CTL infusions were observed. These results showed that allogeneic CTLs are a safe and rapid therapy for PTLD, bypassing the need to grow CTLs for individual patients. After solid organ transplantation, PTLD is usually of recipient origin and recipient derived CTLs are required for effective killing of EBV infected B cells. It is possible to generate autologous EBV-specific CTLs from recipients who were EBV seropositive prior to transplantation. However, this approach is not applicable when PTLD arises in recipients who were EBV seronegative prior to transplantation. Savoldo et al (Savoldo B et al, 2006) treated 12 patients with persisting high EBV-DNA viral load with no evidence of PTLD (6 patients) or high EBV-DNA load with previous or current clinical diagnosis of PTLD (6 patients). Ten of the 12 patients had no evidence of overt PTLD following CTLs therapy, despite being categorized at high risk because of persisting of high EBV-DNA viral load. The two remaining patients both had evidence of pre-existing PTLD and both appeared to respond to CTLs infusion.

9.7 Chemotherapy

Conventional cytotoxic chemotherapy which has been shown to be curative for many lymphomas in non-PTLD setting, has been viewed as a treatment of last resort due to very high morbidity and mortality rates. Chemotherapy is commonly used in the treatment of PTLD when reduction in immunosuppression fails to control the disease.

Various multi-drug regimens such as CHOP (cyclophosphamide, doxorubicin, vincristine, and prednisone) have been used in PTLD patients (Wasson S et al, 2006; Elstrom RL et al, 2006; Trappe R et al, 2007; Taylor AL et al, 2006; Fohrer C et al, 2006; Buadi F et al, 2007; Patel H et al, 2007; Aversa SML et al, 2008)

In spite of the high response rate up to 70%, the associated toxicity is significant and includes treatment-related deaths in about 25% of patients. The high mortality of the standard chemotherapy regimens in the PTLD population might occur because of various factors including baseline pharmacologic immunosuppression, graft dysfunction, and colonization with resistant or hospital acquired infectious organisms.

Sepsis and other complication of chemotherapy have been the major problem in some centres, while others have found refractory disease to be common.

PTLDs after liver transplantation reported in literature are most of all cases report and only few studies analyze a larger group of this disease. (Table 2)

Ben-Ari et al (Ben-Ari Z et al, 1999) reported a series of 7 patients who developed PTLD between 1988 and 1997. 2 patients with late PTLD received anthracycline based chemotherapy and actually they are alive with no recurrence of disease respectively 10 months and 24 months after the end of treatment. Another one with polyclonal tumour EBV positive, was initially treated with high dose acyclovir IV. However he progressed to monoclonalty and systemic chemotherapy (CHOP) was instituted: the patient died 7 months later after one cycle of chemotherapy of septicaemia and rapidly progressive lymphoma.

Norin et al (Norin S et al, 2004) observed, in a population of 500 consecutive recipients of liver graft, 9 cases of monomorphic PTLD, one case of polymorphic PTLD and two case of unclassifiable NHL developed at a median time from transplantation of 19,5 months (1,5-148). Chemotherapy (CHOP or VACOP-B) was used in all patients mostly upfront but in one patient 4 months after diagnosis because of lack of response to reduced immunosuppression alone. Ten patients had a complete remission, one a partial remission and one a stable disease. Six patients are alive and in complete remission more than 4 years after the lymphoma diagnosis while 6 patients died because of progression of lymphoma in three, neutropenic sepsis in two and recurrence of cirrhosis in one.

Lorenzini et al (Lorenzini S et al, 2006) described a small series of 4 monomorphic PTLD. Two were early PTLD and EBV was detected in tumour tissue. The other was late PTLD and only one presented Latent membrane protein type 1 in lymphoma tissue. In all patients the immunosuppressive regimen was reduced. All patients underwent also two consecutive cycles of Rituximab and no severe adverse events were observed during the treatment period. Two patients received chemotherapy at progression but they died despite CHOP therapy. Only one patient, with monomorphic late PTLD is alive 5 years after disease onset. In this case lymphoma remission was obtained with reduction in immunosuppression and Rituximab administration.

	Number of patients who received chemotherapy/	Chemotherapy	response	Therapy related mortality
*Ben Ari et al (102)	4/7	2 CHOP 1 Vincristine 1 MACOP-B	2 CR 2 PD	None
*Norin et al. (103)	12/12	8 CHOP 1 Epi CEBOP 1 Paclitaxel 1 VACOP B 1 BFM90 course	10 CR 1 SD 1 PD	2 neutropenic sepsis
*Lorenzini et al. (104)	4/4	2 R+CHOP 2 Rituximab	1 CR 3 PD	None
*Kremers et al. (105)	11/37	11 CHOP or BACOP 5 Rituximab	na	None
*Avolio et al. (106)	5/5	1 R+CVP 1 R+CHOP 2 CHOP 1 ABVD	3 CR 2 PD	None
*Patel et al. (107)	10/17	5 CHOP 5 Rituximab	8 CR 2 PD	None

* retrospective study
CR: complete remission; PD: progression disease; SD: stable disease; CHOP-R cyclophosphamide, doxorubicin, vincristine, prednisone, rituximab; MACOP B: Methotrexate, doxorubicin, cyclophosphamide, vincristine, prednisone, bleomycin; CEBOP: cyclophosphamide, etoposide, bleomycin, vincristine, prednisone; VACOP-B: etoposide, doxorubicin, cyclophosphamide, vincristine, prednisone, bleomycin; BACOP: bleomycin, doxorubicin, cyclophosphamide, vincristine, prednisone; CVP: cyclophosphamide, vincristine, prednisone ABVD: doxorubicin, bleomycin, vinblastine, dacarbazine.

Table 2. Chemotherapy treatment of patients with PTLD after liver transplantation

In a retrospective study by Kremers et al (Kremers WK et al, 2006), among 1206 liver transplantation recipients, 37 patients developed PTLD. Eleven received chemotherapy (CHOP-BACOP) because of stable or progressive disease despite reduction of immunosuppression. Surprisingly, survival post PTLD diagnosis was very similar both for the EBV positive and EBV negative PTLD regardless of treatment received.

Avolio et al (Avolio AW et al, 2007) treated 5 patients with PTLD after liver transplantation. Two patients with early EBV positive PTLD received three doses of R-CVP and CHOP respectively but, after an initial response, they relapsed with progression of lymphoma and rapidly died. Among the three cases of late PTLD, 2 presented a monomorphic monoclonal disease and one a Hodgkin Lymphoma. EBV was negative in one. They received soon discontinuance of immunosuppression and chemotherapy (R-CHOP-ABVD) and they are alive without evidence of disease.

In a retrospective analysis of 17 consecutive cases (6 early and 11 late disease) of PTLD associated with liver transplantation (Patel H et al, 2007), 5 patients received chemotherapy

(CHOP), 4 obtained CR and one developed progression of disease. At a median follow up of 4,25 years only 5 patients of the entire series are alive and in clinical and radiological remission.

Marino et al (Marino D et al, 2010) reported on 10 consecutive cases of PTLD after liver transplantation with seven monomorphic diseases. Chemotherapy was used in eight patients. No treatment-related mortality was observed and no patient developed graft rejection during chemotherapy. At a median follow-up period of 25 months, 6 of the 10 patients were alive and without evidence of disease.

10. Conclusion

The patients with PTLD can be treated with chemotherapy with an overall response rate of 77% obtaining a long term disease free survival.

In immunocompetent patients, Rituximab administration represents an important step in the treatment of non Hodgkin Lymphoma and currently immunochemotherapy is the gold standard for this kind of patients (Coiffier B et al, 2002; Pfreundschuh M et al, 2008).

However, Rituximab increases the risk of CMV and Aspergillus infections (Hirokawa M et al, 2007; Askoy S et al, 2007; Suzan F et al, 2001; Van der Velden WJ et al, 2006) both in immunocompetent and in post transplant immunosuppressed patients. Recent data also report an anti-rejection activity of Rituximab (Kaposztas Z et al, 2009; Mulley WR et al 2009).

In conclusion Rituximab represents a good option in the treatment of PTLD but there are few studies with small population, so the survival rate with the use of this antibody needs to be assessed together with chemotherapy administration in patients with PTLD.

11. References

Allen U, Hébert D, Moore D, Dror Y, Wasfy S; Canadian PTLD Survey Group--1998. Epstein-Barr virus-related post-transplant lymphoproliferative disease in solid organ transplant recipients, 1988-97: a Canadian multi-centre experience. *Pediatr Transplant*. 2001 Jun;5(3):198-203.

Armes JE, Angus P, Southey MC et al. Lymphoproliferative disorders of donor origin arising in patients after orthotopic liver transplantation. Cancer 1994; 74:2436-41

Armitage JM, Kormos R, Stuart RS. Post-transplantation lymphoproliferative disease in thoracic organ transplanted patients: ten years of cyclosporine based immunosuppression. J Heart Lung Transplat. 1991; 10: 877-886

Askoy S, Harputluoglu H, Kilickap S, Dede DS, Dizdar O, Altundag K, Barista I. Rituximab-related viral infections in lymphoma patients. *Leuk Lymphoma*. 2007 Jul;48(7):1307-12. Review

Aversa SML, Stragliotto S, Marino D, Calabrese F, Rigotti P, Marchini F, Gambino A, Feltrin G, Boso C, Canova F, Soldà C, Mazzarotto R and Burra P. Post-Transplant Lymphoproliferative Disorders (PTLD) after heart or kidney transplantation at a single centre: presentation and response to treatment. *Acta Haematol*. 2008;120(1):36-46. Epub 2008 Sep 16.

Avolio AW, Agnes S, Barbarino R, Magalini SC, Frongillo F, Pagano L, Larocca LM, Pompili M, Caira M, Sollazzi L, Castagneto M. Posttransplant lymphoproliferative disorders after liver transplantation: analysis of early and late cases in a 255 patient series. *Transplant Proc*. 2007 Jul-Aug;39(6):1956-60.

Bakker NA, Pruim J, de Graaf W, van Son WJ, van der Jagt EJ, van Imhoff GW. PTLD visualization by FDG-PET: improved detection of extranodal localizations. *Am J Transplant*. 2006 Aug;6(8):1984-5.

Bakker NA, van Imhoff GW, Verschuuren EA, van Son WJ, Homan van der Heide JJ, Veeger NJ, Kluin PM, Kluin-Nelemans HC. Early onset post-transplant lymphoproliferative disease is associated with allograft localization. *Clin Transplant*. 2005 Jun;19(3):327-34.

Bastard C, Deweindt C, Kerckaert JP, Lenormand B, Rossi A, Pezzella F, Fruchart C, Duval C, Monconduit M, Tilly H. LAZ3 rearrangements in non-Hodgkin's lymphoma: correlation with histology, immunophenotype, karyotype, and clinical outcome in 217 patients. *Blood*. 1994 May 1;83(9):2423-7.

Ben-Ari Z, Amlot P, Lachmanan SR, Tur-Kaspa R, Rolles K, Burroughs AK Posttransplantation lymphoproliferative disorder in liver recipients: characteristics, management, and outcome. *Liver Transpl Surg*. 1999 May;5(3):184-91.

Beynet DP, Wee SA, Horwitz SS, Kohler S, Horning S, Hoppe R, Kim YH. Clinical and pathological features of posttransplantation lymphoproliferative disorders presenting with skin involvement in 4 patients. *Arch Dermatol*. 2004 Sep; 140(9):1140-6

Buadi F, Heyeman MR, Gocke C, Rapaport A, Hakimian R, Bartlett S et al. Treatment and outcome of post-transplant lymphoproliferative disease: a single institution study. Am J Hematol. 2007 Mar;82(3):208-14

Burra P, Buda A, Livi U, Rigotti P, Zanus G, Calabrese F, Caforio A, Menin C, Canova D, Farinati F, Aversa SML. Occurrence of post-transplant lymphoproliferative disorders among over thousand adult recipients: any role for Hepatitis C infection. Eur J Gastr Hepatol.2006, 18:1065-1070

Cesarman E, Chadburn A, Liu YF, Migliazza A, Dalla Favera R, Knowles D. BCL-6 gene mutation in post-transplantation lymphoproliferative disorders predict response to therapy and clinical outcome. Blood 1998. 92: 2294-2302

Choquet S, Leblond V, Herbrecht R, et al. Efficacy and safety of rituximab in B-cell post-transplant lymphoproliferative disorders: results of a prospective multicentre phase II study. *Blood* 2005 [prepublished online 27 October 2005]

Coiffier B, Lepage E, Briere J, Herbrecht R, Tilly H, Bouabdallah R, Morel P, Van Den Neste E, Salles G, Gaulard P, Reyes F, Lederlin P, Gisselbrecht C. CHOP chemotherapy plus rituximab compared with CHOP alone in elderly patients with diffuse large-B-cell lymphoma. *N Engl J Med*. 2002 Jan 24;346(4):235-42

Davis C.L., Wood B.L., Sabath D.E., Joseph J.S., Stehman-Breen C. and Broudy V.C. Interferon-alpha treatment of posttransplant lymphoproliferative disorder in recipients of solid organ transplants, *Transplantation* 1998; 66, 1770–1779.

Duvoux C, Pageaux GP, Vanlemmens C et al. Risk factors for lymphoproliferative disorders after liver transplantation in adults: an analysis of 480 patients. Transplantation 2002; 74:1103-1109

Elstrom RL, Andreadis C, Aqui NA et al. Treatment of PTLD with rituximab or chemotherapy. Am J Transplant 2006 ;6 :569-576

Fohrer C, Caillard S, Koumarianou A, Ellero B, Woehl-Jaegle ML, Meyer C. Long-term survival in post-transplant lymphoproliferative disorders with a dose-adjusted ACVBP regimen. *Br J Haematol.* 2006 Sep; 134(6):602-12.

Gao SZ, Chaparro SV, Perloth M, Montoya J, Miller JL, Dimiceli S, Hastie T, Oyer PE, Shoroeder J. Post-transplantation Lymphoproliferative Disease in Heart and Heart-Lung Trasplant Recipient: 30 year Experience at Stanford University. J Heart Transplant 2003, 22: 505-514

Gonzalez-Barca E, Domingo-Domenech E, Gomez-Codina J, et al. First-line treatment with rituximab improves survival of patients with post-transplant lymphoproliferative disease (PTLD). *Blood* 2004; 104: Abstract No: 1406

Green M, Michaels MG, Webber SA, Rowe D, Reyes J. The management of Epstein-Barr virus associated post-transplant lymphoproliferative disorders in pediatric solid-organ transplant recipients. *Pediatr Transplant.* 1999 Nov;3(4):271-81.

Haddad E., Paczesny S, Leblond V. et al., Treatment of B-lymphoproliferative disorder with a monoclonal anti-interleukin-6 antibody in 12 patients: a multicenter phase 1–2 clinical trial, Blood 2001; 97, 1590–1597.

Hanto DW, Frizzera G, Gajl-Peczalska J, Purtilo DT, Klein G, Simmons RL, Najarian JS. The Epstein-Barr virus (EBV) in the pathogenesis of posttransplant lymphoma. Transplant Proc. 1981 Mar, 13: 756-60

Haque T, Wilkie GM, Jones MM, Higgins CD, Urquhart G, Wingate P, Burns D, McAulay K, Turner M, Bellamy C, Amlot PL, Kelly D, MacGilchrist A, Gandhi MK, Swerdlow AJ, Crawford DH. Allogeneic cytotoxic T-cell therapy for EBV-positive posttransplantation lymphoproliferative disease: results of a phase 2 multicenter clinical trial. *Blood.* 2007 Aug 15;110(4):1123-31. Epub 2007 Apr 27.

Hirokawa M, Kawabata Y, Fujishima N, Yoshioka T, Sawada K. Prolonged reactivation of cytomegalovirus infection following successful rituximab therapy for Epstein-Barr virus-associated posttransplantation lymphoproliferative disorder. *Int J Hematol.* 2007 Oct;86(3):291-

Howard TK, Klintmalm GB, Stone MJ, Cofer JB, Husberg BS, Goldstein RM, Gonwa TA Lymphoproliferative disorder masquerading as rejection in liver transplant recipients--an early aggressive tumor with atypical presentation. *Transplantation.* 1992 May;53(5):1145-7

Kahan BD, Ponticelli C, Montagnino G. Malignancy in: Kahan BD, Ponticelli C, editors. Principles and practice of renal transplantation. Martin Duniz , 2000.

Kaposztas Z, Podder H, Mauiyyedi S, Illoh O, Kerman R, Reyes M, Pollard V, Kahan BD. Impact of rituximab therapy for treatment of acute humoral rejection. *Clin Transplant.* 2009 Jan;23(1):63-73

Kremers WK, Devarbhavi HC, Wiesner RH, Krom RA, Macon WR, Habermann TM. Post-transplant lymphoproliferative disorders following liver transplantation: incidence, risk factors and survival. *Am J Transplant.* 2006 May;6(5 Pt 1):1017-24.

Kulwichit W, Edwards RH, Davenport EM, Baskar JF, Godfrey V, Raab-Traub N. Expression of the Epstein-Barr virus latent membrane protein 1 induces B cell lymphoma in transgenic mice. *Proc Natl Acad Sci U S A.* 1998 Sep 29;95(20):11963-8

Kusuki S, Hashii Y, Fukushima N, Takizawa S, Tokimasa S, Kogaki S, Ohta H, Tsuda E, Nakagawa A, Ozono K. Paediatric post-transplant diffuse large B cell lymphoma after cardiac transplantation. *Int J Hematol.* 2009 Jan 21

Leblond V, Choquet S. Lymphoproliferative disorders after liver transplantation. *J Hepatol* 2004; 40:728-735

Leblond V, Sutton L, Dorent R, Davi F, Bitker MO, Gabarre J, Charlotte F, Ghoussoub JJ, Fourcade C, Fischer A, et al. Lymphoproliferative disorders after organ transplantation: a report of 24 cases observed in a single center. *J Clin Oncol.* 1995 Apr;13(4):961-8

Lechapt-Zalcman E, Challine D, Delfau-Larue MH, Haioun C, Desvaux D, Gaulard P. Association of primary pleural effusion lymphoma of T-cell origin and human herpesvirus 8 in a human immunodeficiency virus-seronegative man. *Arch Pathol Lab Med.* 2001 Sep;125(9):1246-8.

Lee TC, Savoldo B, Rooney CM, Heslop HE, Gee AP, Caldwell Y, Barshes NR, Scott JD, Bristow LJ, O'Mahony CA, Goss JA. Quantitative EBV viral loads and immunosuppression alterations can decrease PTLD incidence in pediatric liver transplant recipients. *Am J Transplant.* 2005 Sep;5(9):2222-8.

Lo Coco F, Ye BH, Lista F, Corradini P, Offit K, Knowles DM, Chaganti RS, Dalla-Favera R. Rearrangements of the BCL6 gene in diffuse large cell non-Hodgkin's lymphoma. *Blood.* 1994 Apr 1;83(7):1757-9.

Locker J, Nalesnik M. Molecular genetic analysis of lymphoid tumors arising after organ transplantation. Am J Pathol 1989. 135:977

Lones MA, Lopez-Terrada D, Weiss LM, Shintaku IP, Said JW. Donor origin of posttransplant lymphoproliferative disorder localized to a liver allograft: demonstration by fluorescence in situ hybridization. *Arch Pathol Lab Med.* 1997 Jul;121(7):701-6.

Lorenzini S, Andreone P, Gramenzi A, Morelli C, Zinzani PL, Grazi GL, Pileri S, Baccarani M, Tura S, Bernardi M. Posttransplant lymphoproliferative disorders in liver transplanted patients: a report of four cases. *Transplant Proc.* 2006 Jun;38(5):1477-80.

Maecker B, Jack T, Zimmerman M, Abdul-Khaliq H, Burdelski M, Fucks A, Hoyer P, Koepf S, Kraemer U, Laube G, Muller-Wiefel DE, Netz H, Pohl M, Toenshoff B, Wagner HJ, Wallot M, Welte K, Melter M, Offner G and Klein K. CNS or Bone Marrow Involvemet As Risk Factors for Poor Survival in Post Transplantation Lymphoproliferative Disorders in Children After Solid Organ Transplantation. *J Clin Oncol.* 2007 Nov; 25:4902-4908

Majewski M, Korecka M, Joergensen J, Fields L, Kossev P, Schuler W, Shaw L, Wasik MA. Immunosuppressive TOR kinase inhibitor everolimus (RAD) suppresses growth of cells derived from posttransplant lymphoproliferative disorder at allograft-protecting doses. *Transplantation.* 2003 May 27;75(10):1710-7

Marino D, Burra P, Boccagni P, Calabrese F, Canova F, Trentin C, Boso C, Soldà C, Angeli P, Aversa SML. Post transplant lymphoproliferative disorders in liver transplanted patients: a single centre experience. *Anticancer Res* 2010 Jun; 30(6) 2383.91

McDiarmid SV, Jordan S, Kim GS, Toyoda M, Goss JA, Vargas JH, Martín MG, Bahar R, Maxfield AL, Ament ME, Busuttil RW. Prevention and preemptive therapy of postransplant lymphoproliferative disease in pediatric liver recipients. *Transplantation.* 1998 Dec 27;66(12):1604-11.

Mulley WR, Hudson FJ, Tait BD, Skene AM, Dowling JP, Kerr PG, Kanellis J. A single low-fixed dose of rituximab to salvage renal transplants from refractory antibody-mediated rejection. *Transplantation*. 2009 Jan 27;87(2):286-9.

Norin S, Kimby E, Ericzon BG, Christensson B, Sander B, Söderdahl G, Hägglund H. Posttransplant lymphoma--a single-center experience of 500 liver transplantations. *Med Oncol*. 2004;21(3):273-84.

Oertel SH, Verschuuren E, Reinke P, Zeidler K, Papp-Váry M, Babel N, Trappe RU, Jonas S, Hummel M, Anagnostopoulos I, Dörken B, Riess HB. Effect of anti-CD 20 antibody rituximab in patients with post-transplant lymphoproliferative disorder (PTLD). *Am J Transplant*. 2005 Dec;5(12):2901-6.

Opelz G, Daniel V, Naujokat C, Fickenscher H, Dohler B. Effect of cytomegalovirus prophylaxis with immunoglobulin or with antiviral drugs on post-transplant non Hodgkin lymphoma: a multicentre retrospective analysis. *Lancet Oncology* 2007; 8: 212-18.

Opelz G, Dohler B. Lymphoma after Solid Organ Transplantation: a collaborative Transplant Study Report. *Am J Transplant* 2003; 4:222-30

Orjuela M, Gross TG, Cheung YK, Alobeid B, Morris E, Cairo MS. A pilot study of chemoimmunotherapy (cyclophosphamide, prednisone, and rituximab) in patients with post-transplant lymphoproliferative disorder following solid organ transplantation. *Clin Cancer Res*. 2003 Sep 1;9(10 Pt 2):3945S-52S.

Patel H, Vogl DT, Aqui N, Shaked A, Olthoff K, Markmann J, Reddy R, Stadtmauer EA, Schuster S, Tsai DE. Posttransplant lymphoproliferative disorder in adult liver transplant recipients: a report of seventeen cases. *Leuk Lymphoma*. 2007 May;48(5):885-91

Penn I, Porat G. Central nervous system lymphomas in organ allograft recipients. *Transplantation*. 1995 Jan 27;59(2):240-4

Pfreundschuh M, Schubert J, Ziepert M, Schmits R, Mohren M, Lengfelder E, Reiser M, Nickenig C, Clemens M, Peter N, Bokemeyer C, Eimermacher H, Ho A, Hoffmann M, Mertelsmann R, Trümper L, Balleisen L, Liersch R, Metzner B, Hartmann F, Glass B, Poeschel V, Schmitz N, Ruebe C, Feller AC, Loeffler M; German High-Grade Non-Hodgkin Lymphoma Study Group (DSHNHL). Six versus eight cycles of bi-weekly CHOP-14 with or without rituximab in elderly patients with aggressive CD20+ B-cell lymphomas: a randomised controlled trial (RICOVER-60). *Lancet Oncol*. 2008 Feb;9(2):105-16. Epub 2008 Jan 15.

Pirsch JD, Miller J, Deierhoi MH, Vincenti F, Filo RS. A comparison of tacrolimus (FK506) and cyclosporine for immunosuppression after cadaveric renal transplantation. FK506 Kidney Transplant Study Group. *Transplantation*. 1997 Apr 15;63(7):977-83.

Poirel HA, Bernheim A, Schneider A et al. Characteristic pattern of chromosomal imbalances in post transplant lymphoproliferative disorders. Correlation with histopathological subcategories and EBV status. Transplantation 2005; 80:176-84

Purtilo DT. Epstein-Barr-virus-induced oncogenesis in immune-deficient individuals. *Lancet*. 1980 Feb 9;1(8163):300-3

Rowe DT, Webber S, Schauer EM, Reyes J, Green M. Epstein-Barr virus load monitoring: its role in the prevention and management of post-transplant lymphoproliferative disease. *Transpl Infect Dis*. 2001 Jun;3(2):79-87

Savoldo B, Goss JA, Hammer MM, Zhang L, Lopez T, Gee AP, Lin Y, Quiros-Tejeira RE, Reinke P, Schubert S, Gottschalk S, Finegold MJ, Brenner MK, Rooney CM and Heslop HE. Treatment of solid organ transplant recipients with autologous Epstein Barr virus–specific cytotoxic T lymphocytes (CTLs). *Blood*, 1 November 2006, Vol. 108, No. 9, pp. 2942-2949

Shpilberg O, Wilson J, Whiteside TL, Herberman RB. Pre-transplant immunological profile and risk factors analysis of post-transplant lymphoproliferative disease development: the resul of a nested matched case-control study. The University of Pittsburgh PTLD study group. Leuk Lymphoma 1999; 36 (1-2): 109-21

Smets F, Latinne D, Bazin H, Reding R, Otte JB, Buts JP, Sokal EM. Ratio between Epstein-Barr viral load and anti-Epstein-Barr virus specific T-cell response as a predictive marker of posttransplant lymphoproliferative disease. *Transplantation*. 2002 May 27;73(10):1603-10.

Sokal EM, Caragiozoglu T, Lamy M et al. EBV serology and EBV associated lymphoproliferative disease in paediatric liver transplant recipients. Transplantation 1993; 56:1394-8

Starzl TE, Nalesnik MA, Porter KA et al. Reversibility of lymphoma and lymphoproliferative lesion developing under cyclosporin-steroid therapy. Lancet 1984; 17:583-7

Steiber AC, Boillot O, Scotti-Foglieni C et al. The surgical implications of the posttransplant lymphoproliferative disorders. Transplant Proc 1991; 23:1477-9

Strazzabosco M, Corneo B, Iemmolo RM, Menin C, Gerunda G, Bonaldi L, Merenda R, Neri D, Poletti A, Montagna M, Del Mistro A, Faccioli AM, D'Andrea E. Epstein-Barr virus-associated post-transplant lympho-proliferative disease of donor origin in liver transplant recipients. *J Hepatol*. 1997 Apr;26(4):926-34.

Strouse PJ, Platt JF, Francis IR et al. Tumourous intrahepatic lymphoproliferative disorders in transplanted liver. Am J Roentgenol 1996;167:1159-62

Suzan F, Ammor M, Ribrag V. Fatal reactivation of cytomegalovirus infection after use of rituximab for a post-transplantation lymphoproliferative disorder. *N Engl J Med*. 2001 Sep 27;345(13):1000

Swinnen LJ, LeBlanc M, Grogan TM, Gordon LI, Stiff PJ, Miller AM, Kasamon Y, Miller TP, Fisher RI. Prospective study of sequential reduction in immunosuppression, interferon alpha-2B, and chemotherapy for posttransplantation lymphoproliferative disorder. *Transplantation*. 2008 Jul 27;86(2):215-22.

Taylor AL, Bowles KM, Callaghan CJ, Wimperis JZ, Grant JW, Marcus RE, Bradley JA. Anthracycline-based chemotherapy as first-line treatment in adults with malignant post transplant lymphoproliferative disorder after solid organ transplantation. Transplantation. 2006 Aug 15;82(3):375-81

Trappe R, Riess H, Babel N et al. Chemotherapy for refractory and relapsed post-transplant lymphoproliferative disorders (PTLD) after treatment with a single-agent rituximab. *Transplantation* 2007; 83: 912-918.

Trappe RU, Choquet S, Reinke P, Dreyling M, Mergenthaler HG, Jäger U, Kebelmann-Betzing C, Jonas S, Lehmkuhl H, Anagnostopoulos I, Leblond V, Hetzer R, Dörken B, Riess H, Oertel S. Salvage therapy for relapsed posttransplant lymphoproliferative disorders (PTLD) with a second progression of PTLD after

Upfront chemotherapy: the role of single-agent rituximab. *Transplantation*. 2007 Dec 27;84(12):1708-12

Tsai DE, Nearey M, Hardy CL, Tomaszewski JE, Kotloff RM, Grossman RA, Olthoff KM, Stadtmauer EA, Porter DL, Schuster SJ, Luger SM, Hodinka RL. Use of EBV PCR for the diagnosis and monitoring of post-transplant lymphoproliferative disorder in adult solid organ transplant patients. Am J Transplant. 2002 Nov;2(10):946-54

van der Velden WJ, Blijlevens NM, Klont RR, Donnelly JP, Verweij PE. Primary hepatic invasive aspergillosis with progression after rituximab therapy for a post transplantation lymphoproliferative disorder. Ann Hematol. 2006 Sep;85(9):621-3. Epub 2006 Jun 7.

Vaysberg M, Balatoni CE, Nepomuceno RR, Krams SM, Martinez OM. Rapamycin inhibits proliferation of Epstein-Barr virus-positive B-cell lymphomas through modulation of cell-cycle protein expression. Transplantation. 2007 Apr 27;83(8):1114-21.

Waldmann TA, Misiti J, Nelson DL, Kraemer KH. Ataxia-telangiectasis: a multisystem hereditary disease with immunodeficiency, impaired organ maturation, x-ray hypersensitivity, and a high incidence of neoplasia. *Ann Intern Med.* 1983 Sep;99(3):367-79.

Walker RC, Paya CV, Marshall WF, Strickler JG, Wiesner RH, Velosa JA, Habermann TM, Daly RC, McGregor CG. Pretransplantation seronegative Epstein-Barr virus status is the primary risk factor for posttransplantation lymphoproliferative disorder in adult heart, lung, and other solid organ transplantations. *J Heart Lung Transplant.* 1995 Mar-Apr;14(2):214-21.

Wasson S, Zafar MN, Best J, Reddy HK. Post-transplantation lymphoproliferative disorder in heart and kidney transplant patients: a single-centre experience. J Cardiovasc Pharmacol Ther. 2006 Mar;11(1):77-83

Weisner RH. A long term comparison of Tacrolimus (FK 506) versus cyclosporine in liver transplantation : a report of the US FK506 Study Group. Transplantation 1998; 66:493-499

Weissmann DJ, Ferry JA, Harris NL, Louis DN, Delmonico F, Spiro I. Posttransplantation lymphoproliferative disorders in solid organ recipients are predominantly aggressive tumors of host origin. Am J Clin Pathol. 1995 Jun;103(6):748-55

Wu L, Rappaport DC, Hanbidge A et al. Lymphoproliferative disorders after liver transplantation: imaging features. Abdom Imaging 2001; 26:200-6

Wu TT, Swerdlow SH, Locker J, Bahler D, Randhawa P, Yunis EJ, Dickman PS, Nalesnik MA. Recurrent Epstein-Barr virus-associated lesions in organ transplant recipients. Hum Pathol. 1996 Feb;27(2):157-64

Yakupoglu YK, Buell JF, Woodle S, Kahan BD. Individualization of immunosuppressive therapy. III. Sirolimus associated with a reduced incidence of malignancy. *Transplant Proc.* 2006 Mar;38(2):358-61

Younes BS, McDiarmid SV, Martin MG, Vargas JH, Goss JA, Busuttil RW, Ament ME. The effect of immunosuppression on posttransplant lymphoproliferative disease in pediatric liver transplant patients. *Transplantation*. 2000 Jul 15;70(1):94-9.

Young L, Alfieri C, Hennessy K, Evans H, O'Hara C, Anderson KC, Ritz J, Shapiro RS, Rickinson A, Kieff E, et al. Expression of Epstein-Barr virus transformation-associated genes in tissues of patients with EBV lymphoproliferative disease. *N Engl J Med.* 1989 Oct 19;321(16):1080-5.

Zhang A, Zhang M, Shen Y, Wang W, Zheng S. Clin Transplant 2009; 23(5): 756-760

Zimmermann T, Hoppe-Lotichius M, Tripkovic V, Barreiros A, Wehler T, Zimmermann A et al. Liver transplanted patients with preoperative autoimmune hepatitis and immunological disorders are at increased risk for Post Transplant Lymphoproliferative Disorders (PTLD) European J Int Med 2010; 21: 208-15

15

Post-Transplant Lymphoproliferative Disease – PTLD

Julio Cesar Wiederkehr and Barbara de Aguiar Wiederkehr
Federal University of Paraná and Hospital Pequeno Príncipe
Brazil

1. Introduction

Post-transplantation lymphoproliferative disorders (PTLD), one of the most serious complications occurring after transplantation, have been recognized as a complication of organ and cell transplantation for more than 30 years. (Starzl, 1968)

Transplantation of solid organs has been successful in large part due to the development of immunosuppressive regimens that have controlled the recipient's immune system from rejecting the allograft. By suppressing recipient T lymphocytes with cyclosporin or tacrolimus or reversing rejection with antilymphocyte agents such as ATGAM or OKT3, rejection has become a rare cause of allograft loss. (Jain et al., 2000) The "trade off" for this non-specific immunosuppression is the increased risk of the patient contracting opportunistic infections (i. e. viral, fungal and protozoal organisms) and increased risk of malignancies. (Fung et al., 2001) In 1968, lymphoid tumors were first described in transplant patients with a subgroup of these termed "pseudolymphomas" in recognition of their ability to undergo regression after reduction of immunosuppression. (Starzl et al., 1984) "post-transplant lymphoproliferative disease" (PTLD) is now a well recognized complication of solid organ transplantation and therapeutic immunosuppression. As a result, PTLD is a major concern in the post transplant period and also a very complex disease, that encompasses a spectrum of lymphoproliferative disorders that can rise from either cells of B, T or natural killers cell origin. We will focus on the B cell type lymphoproliferative disorders in this chapter. This type is by far the most common and is usually associated with Epstein-Barr virus (EBV) infection. By definition, PTLD is a heterogeneous lymphoproliferation, ranging from benign B cell hyperplasia to aggressive B cell lymphoma, that arise in the setting of bone marrow or solid organ transplantation.

2. Incidence of PTLD

The incidence of various de novo tumors can be very dramatic in the post transplant period, either in the adult or pediatric population. Post-transplantation lymphoproliferative disorders are different from lymphoproliferative disorders that occur in the general population. Although relatively uncommon, the risk of developing lymphoma after transplantation has been reported to be 28 to 49 times greater than that in the general population. (Boubenider et al., 1997) According to the Cincinnati Transplant Tumor Registry (CTTR), which has collected data on more than 6,000 patients, PTLD accounts for 16% of cancers in transplant recipients compared with 5% in the general population. However, these data are heavily skewed toward kidney transplant recipients. (Penn, 1996)

Although the incidence of PTLD has been reported to be as high as 65% after primary and 30% after reactivation EBV infection, (Birkeland et al., 1999) overall frequency ranges from 1% to 10%. Most estimates are based on relatively small transplant series from individual institutions. (Penn et al., 1998) In an analysis of tumors in 512 patients in the CTTR, PTLD comprised 52% of all tumors. There was a disproportionately high incidence of PTLD among nonrenal allograft recipients compared with renal allograft recipients (81% vs 31%) in this group of patients.

The frequency of PTLD depends on many variables such as the allograft type, for example. Kidney can correspond to 1% to 4% of incidence; heart, 2% to 10%; heart and lung, 5% to 9%; intestine, 19%. (Fizzera, 1992) The overall incidence of PTLD after liver transplantation has been quoted as 2–8.4%. (Wu et al., 2001) In the case of bone marrow recipients, the frequency is 1% to 2% excepting cases of mismatched T-cell-depleted allografts, for which the frequency has been historically as high as 24% (Shapiro et al., 1988). Innovations such as removal of B cells from the marrow allograft have reduced and in some series eliminated this complication. (Cavazzana et al., 1998) Patients who receive allogeneic hematopoietic stem cell transplants also have an approximate 1% risk of developing PTLD. (Gross et al., 1999)

Another variable that influences the incidence of PTLD is definitely the age of the recipient at the time of the transplant. The series of Ho and colleagues, 1988, highlights differences in the frequency of PTLD based on patient age at the time of transplantation. Pediatric patients have a higher frequency of PTLD in general than do adult patients receiving similar allografts, Shapiro and colleagues 1988, reported a 10.1% PTLD frequency in pediatric kidney transplant recipients compared with a 1. 2% frequency in the adult renal transplant population; 86% percent of pediatric cases and 50% of adult cases involved a transplant from an EBV-seropositive donor to an EBV-seronegative recipient. Thus, at least part of the difference in frequency between adults and children may be explained by the higher proportion of EBV-seronegative patients in the pediatric as opposed to the adult population.

In children lymphomas are by far the most common tumors, and in the adults is the second most common following skin type lesions. (Penn, 1998) In an recent study 38% and 66% of patients developed a skin cancer after 10 years and 23 years, respectively. (Penn, 1998) This incidence is far greater than in the general population older than 75 years of age (20% to 25%). Malignant lymphomas are the second most common malignancy in transplant patients reported to the CTTR, accounting for 16% of the total tumor incidence. Most lymphomas reported are of the large-cell type; 85% of these are of B-cell origin and 90% to 95% are EBV-related.

Kaposi's sarcoma (KS) accounts for 5. 7% of cancers reported to the CTTR. Both nonvisceral (59%) and visceral types (41%) arise. Mortality was higher in patients with visceral KS (53% vs 23%) and remission rates were lower (30% vs 55%). Preventive measures (ie, sunscreen, therapy for oncogenic viruses) and screening measures (ie, mammogram, Pap smear, colonoscopy) are recommended for all age- and sex-appropriate transplant recipients together with an informed approach to the reduction and/or avoidance of drugs with oncogenic potential. (Martinez, 2008)

3. Risk factors

There is a lot of work trying to identify risk factors for PTLD. Clearly, EBV seronegativity is an important factor. This situation occurs when the recipient has not been exposed to EBV virus prior to the transplant and acquires the infection on the setting of immunosuppression. This scenario is often seen in children who are typically immunological naive to the virus and then acquire the virus with the graft, usually from an adult donor who is EBV infected.

PTLD has been documented in three transplant immunosuppression eras: conventional (precyclosporine), cyclosporine, and postcyclosporine. The level of immunosuppression (ie, intensity, type, and amount) is an independent risk factor for PTLD. Ciancio and colleagues, 1997, reported on the incidence of PTLD under different immunosuppressant regimens during an 18-year period. They noted a recent increase in the incidence of PTLD with the advent of newer immunosuppressive agents. By contrast, the use of mycophenolate mofetil in a steroid-free immunosuppressive protocol with concomitant acyclovir therapy was associated with a lower incidence of primary and reactivation EBV infection and PTLD. (Birkeland, 1999)

Efforts have been made to identify a specific immunosuppression that might predispose PTLD. The introduction of calciuneurin inhibitor has been associated with an increase in the incidence of PTLD. T cell depletion regimens, especially OKT3, have also been implicated, and more recently, the use of biologics has been followed by an increase in EBV associated tumors. According to CTTR data, the average time after transplantation to the development of lymphomas was 50 months when corticosteroids and azathioprine were used; when CsA was added, this interval dropped to 13 months and when OKT3 was used it dropped to 7 months. Nevertheless, no one particular agent has proven to be associated with the development of this disease. It is more the cumulative amount and the duration of imunossupression. Prolonged or powerful immunosuppressive therapy in renal transplantation is complicated by the development of an unusually high incidence of malignancy.

As previously mentioned, there is also a range in the incidence depending on the type of organ transplanted. Whether it has to do with the lymphoid compartment that is transferred with the graft, the aloreactivity of the graft or the amount of imunossupression required in the transplant is unclear. Several studies have implicated concurrent cytomegalovirus (CMV) and/or hepatitis C infection as risk factor for the development of PTLD, but that also has remained unclear. And finally several articles have been published looking for the role of cytokine gene polymorphisms in the genesis of PTLD. (Martinez, 2010)

Reports have suggested that underlying disease may represent a risk factor for PTLD. Shpilberg and colleagues, 1999, suggest that, in liver transplant patients, underlying autoimmune disorders such as autoimmune hepatitis or primary biliary cirrhosis may predispose to PTLD. An even more striking association was reported in one series of patients who underwent liver transplantation for treatment of Langerhans cell histiocytosis (Newell et al., 1999). In this group, two thirds of patients developed PTLD. Underlying hepatitis C virus (HCV) infection was also found to be associated with a 10.5% frequency of PTLD in one series, whereas liver transplant for other diseases was associated with a 1. 7% frequency. (Hezode et al., 1999) Although patients with HCV were noted to have a higher requirement for immunosuppression with antilymphocyte antibodies, the authors observed that an increased risk remained even after this variable had been accounted for.

Risk factors for PTLD
• EBV seronegativity
• Type and duration of immunosuppression
• Type of organ transplanted
• Concurrent CMV and/or HCV infection?
• Cytokine gene polymorphisms?

Table 1. Risk factors for PTLD

4. Epstein Barr Virus (EBV)

EBV is a B lymphotrophic DNA gamma herpes virus and it infects cells through CD21, a complement receptor (CR2), using HLA class II as a co-receptor. Once infected, persists in the cell as episome in subset of latently infected memory B cells. Using this strategy the virus is very effective, as EBV infects over 90% of the population. In addition to the PTLD, this virus is known to cause infectious mononucleosis in the general population and also has a strong association with Burkitt's lymphoma, Hodgkin's lymphoma, and other tumor of epithelial origin such as nasopharyngeal carcinoma. (Snow et al., 2006)

Understanding the life cycle of EBV in a healthy person can help us in the pathogenesis of PTLD. Typically is transmitted through the saliva and infects B cells. One of two things can happen, it can set up a lytic infection where virus particles are produced and the cells are lysed and the viral particles are released to infect other cells, or it can set up a latent infection, expression of the define viral gens, including EBV Nuclear Antigen (EBNAs) and Latent Membrane Protein 1 (LMP-1) proteins. By expressing these two antigens, the cell is now able to proliferate autonomously and becoming essentially a lymphoblast. Cytotoxic T cells and NK cells control the expansion of these cells. (Cohen, 2000)

Eventually the expression of LMP-2 antigen is shutted off and the cell exists the cell cycle, goes on to a type 2 latency state, and goes through germinal center reactions and emerges as a memory B cell, where the virus persists. Occasionally the cell can reactivate the virus and produces additional viral particles or can revert into the lymphoblast-like activity.

5. Mechanisms of oncogenesis

One of most important protein involved in the genesis of these tumors is the LMP-1, the major oncogene of EBV. It has been demonstrated that it is sufficient by itself for transformation of rodent fibroblast and is also necessary for transformation of human B cells. In an infected B cell that is undergoing a latent state, LMP-1 is expressed in the membrane of the cell via an expression of multiple spanning domains. The cytoplasmic region, signaling domain, of the molecule does not have intrinsic kinase activity, but via tumor tips, C Terminal Activating Regions (CTAR1 and CTAR2), allows the recruitment of various adaptor proteins from the cell, activating a number of cellular signaling pathways. These cellular signaling pathways are responsible for the oncogenic function of the virus. (Martinez et al., 2008)

It has been shown that tumor derived LMP-1 contains unique mutations, in position 212 and 366 (Vaysberg et al., 2008). Also, the wild type form of LMP-1 expressed on the B cell induces only a transient activation, known as benign or weakly oncogenic. In contrary, tumor derived LMP-1 is able to induce activation of various proto-oncogenes. These mutations identified in tumor derived LMP-1 may account for the oncogenic function of EBV.

A number of various cytokines is produced by EBV infected B cells, and in many cases the actual viral gene itself has been identified to be responsible for inducing the production of cellular cytokine. Some of these cytokines, especially IL-10, functions as autocrine growth factor for these tumor cells.

Also, EBV is very effective at immune evasion, a characteristic that allows for the virus to coopt and borrow a number of different cellular pathways to allow it to persist and avoid detection by the immune system. (Martinez & Gruji, 2008)

6. Classification

Lymphoproliferative lesions are currently classified according to histologic parameters. Histologic findings refer to the microscopic appearance and characteristics of the tissue. Polymorphic lesions contain a proliferation of cells with varied morphologic structure, whereas monomorphic PTLDs generally contain a uniform population of cells. With the rapid progress in molecular diagnostic techniques, including DNA array technology, it is likely that the classic approach will soon be supplemented or superseded by more comprehensive molecular approaches. (Nalesnik et al., 2000)

The features of PTLD have been categorized by the World Health Organization in 1997 and revised in 2008. It classifies PTLD into four different categories. Early lesions can be the reactive plasmacytic B cell type hyperplasia or infectious mononucleosis-like syndrome. Those are often seen as consequence of a primary disease. Various types of B cells infiltrating the lesion characterize the polymorphic PTLDs, including small B cells and lymphoblast plasma cells, and those are often seen in children. The monomorphic PTLD include those that are T cell or natural killer (NK) cell origin as well as the B cell lymphomas, the most common B cell lymphomas. They usually look like diffuse large B cell lymphomas. Finally, the classic Hodgkin lymphoma type PTDL, is diagnosed as in the non-transplant patients. (Martinez, 2010)

Classification of PTLD
• Early
• Polymorphic PTLD
• Monomorphic PTLD
• Classic Hodgkin linfoma-type PTLD

Table 2. Classification of PTLD

7. Staging

The stage of PTLD represents the extent of the disease. For example, it can be local or disseminated and nodal or organ involvement. In approximately 50% of cases, multiple organs or sites are involved at the time of presentation. (Boubenider et al., 1997) The lymph nodes and GI tract are the 2 most common sites. No formal system of PTLD staging exists, and it is suggested that the standard Ann Arbor classification with Cotswold modification, which is used to stage non-Hodgkin's lymphomas, be used when possible in reporting cases. (Paya et al., 1999)

The cases are placed into one of four stages (I-IV), based upon the sites of involvement, the number of lymph node regions involved and the presence or absence of systemic symptoms or of bulky or extended disease. Apart from these four stages, there is a subclassification, in witch "E" indicates extra-nodal involvement; "A" to indicate the absence or "B" to indicate the presence of systemic symptoms (weight loss, fever, or night sweats) and "X" to denote bulky disease, which is more than 10cm in maximum dimension or involves more than one third of the chest diameter (seen on chest x-ray).

All organs known or suspected to be involved in PTLD and the evidence for their involvement (histologic, radiologic, and/or biochemical) should be recorded. The presence or absence of allograft involvement should also be explicitly stated for each case. (Preiksaitis & Keay, 2001)

Stage	**Criteria**
I	In 1 lymph region only
II	In ≥ 2 lymph regions on the same side of the diaphragm
III	In the lymph nodes, spleen, or both and on both sides of the diaphragm
IV	Extranodal involvement (eg, bone marrow, lung, liver)

Table 3. Cotswold Modification of Ann Arbor Staging of Hodgkin Lymphoma and Non-Hodgkin Lymphoma

8. Clinical presentation

Due to the complexity of the disease, clinical presentation can be quite variable, depending on the type of immunosuppression, type of organ transplanted and type of PTLD. Generalized systemic illness symptoms, such as fever, sweats, malaise, and rapid enlargement of tonsils or cervical nodes are commonly seen in PTLD patients. In some cases the nodes are involved, and sometimes it presents as a localized disease and sometimes as a disseminated disease.

The gastrointestinal tract is a common site of extra nodal disease and it can cause abdominal pain with hemorrhage and may perforate, leading to acute abdomen. Central nervous system disease may also occur causing symptoms secondary to local necrosis and tumor mass effect. However, PTLD can occur at any site. For example, isolated skin involvement has been noted, (McGregor et al., 1993) and gallbladder involvement has been observed in one case as well (Heller et al., 2000). Disease limited to the graft is a common manifestation of early PTLD. Its differentiation from acute cellular rejection in this situation is critically important. Lesions may be limited and progress slowly, or the patient may present with a fulminant, multiple-system, sepsis-like syndrome. This last form is an uncommon presentation, occurring in approximately 1% of cases (Nalesnik et al., 2000). PTLD may resemble a self-limited infection or be indistinguishable from non-Hodgkin lymphoma. An unexplained infectious syndrome in a transplant recipient should raise the suspicion of PTLD. A mononucleosis syndrome may occur early after transplantation, particularly in association with a primary EBV infection. This presentation is particularly common in the pediatric population, and indeed, in some cases it is infectious mononucleosis. Otolaryngologic symptoms and findings are often the first manifestation of PTLD in children. (Posey et al., 1999) Patients may present with tonsillitis, tonsillar necrosis, lymphadenitis, sinusitis, and otitis media. There is a tendency for more severe upper airway symptoms, including airway obstruction. It should also be noted that the underlying process in these cases, ie, infectious mononucleosis vs frank tumorous PTLD, cannot always be inferred from the clinical picture alone.

PTLD can present as early as less than a month or lately as several years after transplantation. In a series of 71 liver transplant recipients in a pediatric population the incidence of PTLD was 9.85%. The median time from the first symptoms to the initial treatment was 9. 7 days (Wiederkehr et al., 2010). In general, however, PTLD is remarkable for a short post-transplantation time of onset. In the CTTR, the latest case occurred 25 years after transplantation. As a general rule patients who presentas lateonset (>1 year) have more aggressive tumours with poorer prognosis (Molnar & Keung, 2001).

PTLDs that do not contain EBV tend to arise at a later time than those that do contain the virus. In one series, 50% of EBV-positive PTLDs arose by 6 months following transplantation, whereas the 50% mark for occurrence of EBV-negative PTLDs was not reached until 5 years after transplantation (Leblond et al., 1998). PTLDs of T-cell origin are uncommon and may also arise later in the posttransplantation course, but a case of a monoclonal T-cell tumor arising 2 months after transplantation has been described. (Kim et al., 1999)

A PTLD that occurs later is more likely to be circumscribed anatomically and to be associated with a more gradual clinical course. In this situation, extranodal disease with visceral involvement is common with gastrointestinal, pulmonary, or central nervous system (CNS) symptoms. Lymphadenopathy is painless, and atypical lymphocytes may or may not be present in the white blood cell differential count.

Most patients with PTLD present with at least 1 tumor. About two thirds of these tumors are extranodal, and about one third are nodal. (Penn, 1994) There is a tendency to involve specific sites. The gastrointestinal tract is involved in about 26% of cases and CNS in about 27% of cases (Chen et al., 1993). The allograft can also be involved. In this case, the frequency of involvement varies according to the specific type of allograft. PTLDs that arise in lung or intestinal transplant recipients involve those allografts in up to 80% of cases. The reason for this is not known. However, it is interesting that the lung and bowel are transplanted with a large indigenous lymphoid population. PTLDs that occur in patients receiving other types of allografts, such as liver and kidney, involve the allograft in about one third of cases (Cohen, 1993). In contrast, the transplanted heart is only rarely involved with these tumors (Hanasono, 1995).

9. Diagnosis of PTLD

The diagnosis of PTLD requires an awareness of the myriad appearances of this syndrome. Isolated or systemic lymphadenopathy or "lumps and bumps" that suddenly appear should include PTLD in the differential diagnosis. (Nalesnik et al., 2000) Abdominal pain, particularly with evidence of intestinal bleeding, raises the possibility of PTLD in the GI tract. In one pediatric series, diarrhea and/or gastrointestinal bleeding in the presence of active EBV infection was associated with PTLD in 43% of cases. (Cao et al., 1998) Persistent headaches or CNS symptoms suggest localization to the brain. Upper respiratory tract infections that may be associated with lymphadenopathy or that do not resolve after a course of antibiotics should raise a suspicion of PTLD.

Several laboratory assays have applicability in suggesting or supporting the diagnosis of PTLD. Badley and colleagues, 1996, demonstrated monoclonal gammopathy in 71% of transplant recipients with and in 27% of transplant recipients without PTLD. A separate study showed that PTLD developed in 9% of all transplant recipients who had monoclonal gammopathy. (Pageaux, 1998)

The gold standard is the analyses of histology of the biopsy tissue. (Dusenbery et al., 1997) The first effort is to identify the virus, usually done by looking for EBV encoded RNA (EBER) or LMP-1 with immunohistochemical stain. Clonality and phenotyping can also be done to identify the origin of the cells involved in the tumor.

The term 'PTLD' encompass the full range of EBV-related lymphoproliferative states, including benign processes. However, when not otherwise specified, PTLD should refer to the neoplastic end of the PTLD spectrum. Neoplasia should be defined by two of the following three characteristics: (1) destruction of the underlying lymph node architecture; (2) monoclonality (regardless of morphology); (3) evidence of EBV infection in the neoplastic cells. (Loren et al., 2003)

Regarding serology, it is not diagnostic of PTLD rather than a tool to identify primary infection or reactivation. Epstein-Barr viral serologic testing may be used to evaluate the presence of recent or remote infection and thus may provide indirect information relevant to the diagnostic workup for PTLD. However, a diagnosis of EBV infection, active or remote, is not synonymous with a diagnosis of PTLD. For example, one study (Smets et al., 2000) of EBV-seronegative pediatric liver transplant recipients showed an 80% conversion rate to seropositivity within the first 3 months after transplantation. Of these patients, approximately 85% were asymptomatic and only 15% developed PTLD.

Of the various serologic assays for EBV infection, IgM antiviral capsid antigen (IgM-VCA) is particularly useful in detecting active infection. In one study, IgM-VCA antiviral capsid antigen level was elevated an average of 5 days after a detectable rise in circulating EBV genomes shown by polymerase chain reaction (PCR) assay. (Bodeus et al., 1999) Quantitative estimation of the number of EBV genomes in the peripheral blood by use of the PCR assay provides a more useful correlate of the EBV infection types most likely to be associated with PTLD.

This technique was applied following the observation that patients with PTLD had early and spontaneous outgrowth of virus when peripheral blood cells were cultured in vitro. (Rooney et al., 1995) Such outgrowth does not occur in "normal" EBV-positive patients. It was subsequently shown that patients with PTLD had elevated numbers of circulating viral genomes. Hanasono and colleagues, 1995, showed that normal EBV-positive patients had less than 2,000 viral genomes per microgram of blood cell DNA, whereas the number of genomes was increased 10- to 100-fold in patients with PTLD. Rowe and colleagues found an increased risk of PTLD when the number of circulating EBV genomes exceeded 500/105 peripheral blood lymphocytes. Furthermore, regression of PTLD was associated with a decrease in the number of circulating viral genomes, indicating that this parameter also served as a useful means of monitoring therapy. (Rogers et al., 1998)

Some tests done for confirmation of diagnosis of PTLD are HE staining, which is important to determine the morphology of the tumor and the extent of infiltration and tissue architecture destruction; phenotyping of B cells, NK cells or T cells; Ki-67 which is an important marker for the proliferative index and shows how rapidly the tumor is dividing; and EBER staining to confirm the presence of the virus itself.

10. Radiographic features

CT-scans and/or MRI are usually done for staging of the disease. The range of appearances is large due to the number of possible sites. If the disease affect solid organs (liver, spleen, kidney) it can be showed as nodules with characteristic such as hypoechoic, low density on CT or as a diffuse infiltration. When the disease affects bowel, it can appear as a circumferential wall thickening, an aneurysmal dilattation, an ulceration or perforation, and even bowel obstruction. In the lung, it can appear as nodules usually homogeneous, may centrally cavitate, or as diffuse infiltration. When the object of study is the brain, must be considered characteristics similar to lymphoma in the setting of HIV infection and also necrosis and hemorrhage. Overall, nodes can appear as non-specific nodal enlargement, similar to other lymphomas. (Pickhardt et al., 2000)

The single most frequent imaging finding is lymphadenopathy within the abdomen, as expected, being the most common region involved. Previous studies have reported lymphadenopathy between 55% and 74%. (Steiber et al., 1991) Pickhardt & Siegel, 2000, reported a lower incidence of 34%, but only concentrated on intra-abdominal abnormalities.

11. Differential diagnoses

The differential diagnosis depends on the location of PTLD and is therefore broad. If the disease locates at the small bowel the differential diagnosis can be inflammatory bowel disease - especially Crohn's disease – or acute rejection. If the disease locates at the lung, metastases, infection, lymphoid interstitial pneumonia (LIP) must be considered. When located in the head and neck, infections mononucleosis or reactive nodal enlargements are diagnostic possibilities.

12. PCR monitoring for EBV DNA

EBV titers have been shown to be sensitive to adjustments of immunosuppressive therapy, and it has been suggested that immunosuppressive therapy could be reduced when a rising titer is observed, thus preempting the development of PTLD. Studies examining this have concentrated on the pediatric population where it is thought that EBV exposure occurs at

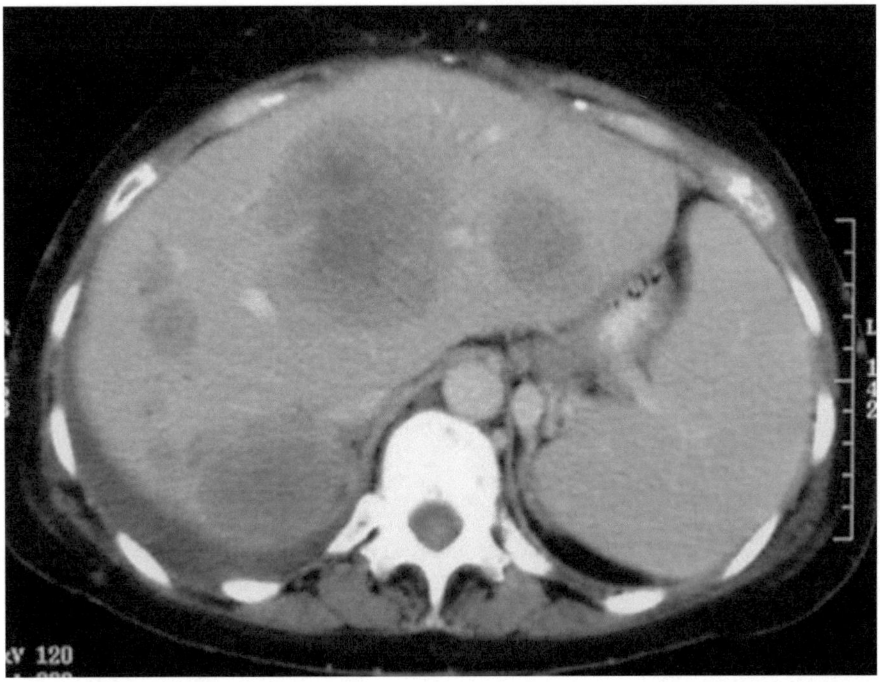

Fig. 1. CT confirmed multiple low attenuation lesions within the liver and the presence of ascites. (Dhillon et al., 2007)

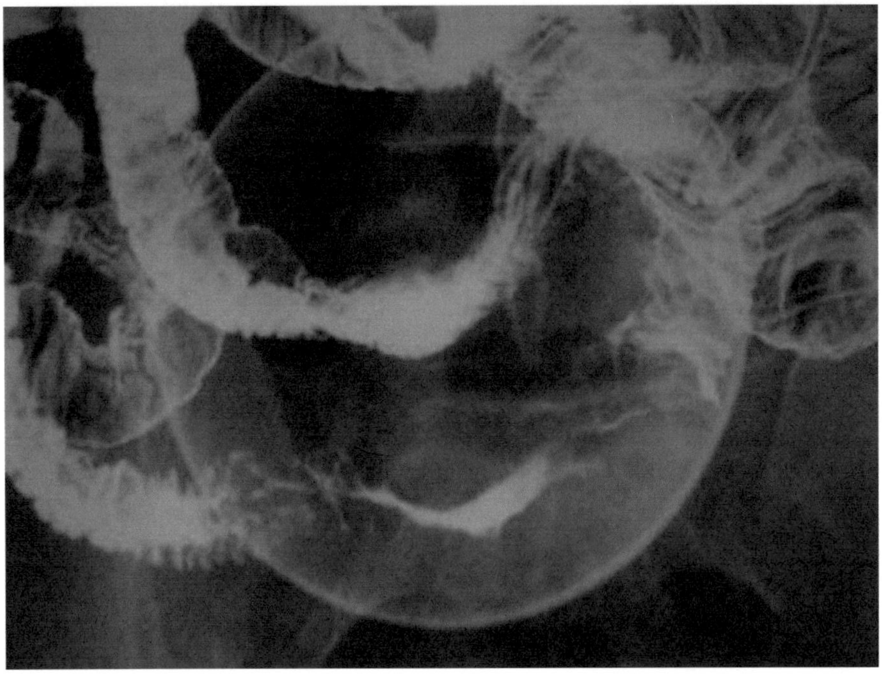

Fig. 2. Small bowel involvement: barium follow-through presenting a small bowel obstruction with an extensive stricture within the terminal ileum. (Dhillon et al., 2007)

the time of transplantation so that PTLD is most frequently observed during the first post-transplant year. (McDiarmid et al., 1998) However, in adults, there is often pre-transplant EBV immunity and this is reflected in the later development of PTLD.

In high-risk patients, such as children who are seronegative at transplant, determination of viral load throughout the post-transplant period may be useful. Increases in viral DNA can be detected months before clinical onset of PTLD. Viral load determination can also be used to monitor response to the treatment. The problem of this approach is that not all patients with PTLD will have an increase in the viral load, and only a minority of patients with high viral load will develop PTLD. Although there is no consensus on the threshold value, as well as standard methodology and compartment measured, some reports indicate 200 copies/10^5 PBMC correlates with symptomatic disease in children. (Martinez, 2010)

It has been revealed that there are subsets of patients who are chronic high load carriers, with no symptomatic or clinical disease. This is typically of patients who have undergone a primary infection and were seronegative at the time of transplant. It can also occur after asymptomatic primary infection of after EBV disease, including PTLD. (Martinez, 2010)

13. Prevention

Prophylactic treatment with antivirals, acyclovir and gancyclovir, is used in many high-risk patients. Those drugs are not effective in the context of PTLD because at that stage the virus is in a latent infection and the antivirals depend upon viral replication. One way to overcome such problem is to use arginine butyrate to re-initiate a lytic infection and combined that with antiviral drugs.

The reports that prophylactic antiviral drugs minimize PTLD risk have been somewhat unconvincing, involving very small number of patients in observational studies. Each investigator defined 'high-risk' differently: some included only patients with elevated EBV viral loads, while others included EBVnegative patients receiving organs from EBV-positive donors, or patients receiving high-dose immunosuppression or specific anti-lymphocyte therapy.

Antiviral agents (such as intravenous immunoglobulin containing neutralizing antibody or acyclovir, ganciclovir, and foscarnet) that target steps in the lytic virus cycle are sometimes used for PTLD prevention. The potential efficacy of these agents depends on the relative importance of EBV-driven lymphoproliferation (which is not influenced by these agents) and the lytic virus cycle (which is) on EBV-induced lymphomagenesis. (Preiksaiti, 2004)

However, historical comparisons of the incidence of PTLD among patients receiving and patients not receiving ganciclovir prophylaxis, either immediately after transplantation or during antilymphocyte antibody therapy, suggest that prophylactic antiviral therapy may be of some benefit (Preiksaiti, 2003). A multicenter, randomized controlled trial of CMV immunoglobulin prophylaxis in EBV-seronegative, pediatric SOT recipients was inconclusive with respect to PTLD prevention. This was likely the result of immunosuppression modification by clinicians in response to EBV load data, resulting in an overall reduction over time in the incidence of PTLD, irrespective of the prophylactic regimen used. (Green et al., 2003) Antiviral agents may have indirect benefit on PTLD risk by eliminating other viral infections, such as CMV infection, that act as cofactors in PTLD development. For this reason, the use of ganciclovir may be preferred over the use of acyclovir. Antiviral agents may also influence global immunosuppression by preventing the expression of EBV immunomodulatory proteins expressed during the lytic cycle. There is an urgent need for additional multicenter controlled trials that evaluate the efficacy of agents used alone and together for prophylaxis. (Preiksaiti, 2004)

An alternative approach to prevention employs a preemptive strategy in which intervention (usually in the form of reduction in immunosuppression and/or the use of antiviral drugs, with or without immunoglobulin) is administered in response to "trigger points," usually high EBV loads. This approach has been used in both intestinal transplant recipients and pediatric liver transplant recipients. (Green et al., 2001) Although the simultaneous use of multiple interventions makes it difficult to determine the efficacy of any single approach, the incidence of PTLD decreased in these populations, compared with historical controls, when preemptive strategies were applied. (Preiksaiti, 2004)

14. Treatment

Primary approach for of PTLD is to reduce immunosuppression in these patients. The response rate for this strategy varies from 23-100%, which in some cases places the allograft in danger for rejection, and occurs as a potential complication in 39% of the patients. It is not the ideal approach but it has been effective for some patients. Predictors of lack of response to reduction of immunosuppression include a serum LDH 42. 5 times the upper limit of normal, organ dysfunction, and multiple visceral sites of disease. (Tsai et al., 2001) In patients with life-sustaining organ transplants such as hearts, livers and lungs, reduction in immunosuppression should be more moderate and closely monitored as allograft rejection may be swift and fatal. (Loren et al., 2003)

Initial attempts to prevent PTLD in the solid-organ transplant population were focused primarily on using antiviral therapies, such as thymidine kinase inhibitors ganciclovir or acyclovir, to eradicate or control EBV for high-risk patients. These drugs inhibit the replication of other herpes viruses, such as herpes simplex and cytomegalovirus. In vivo, however, they are ineffective against EBV, because EBV survives as an episome outside of the lymphocyte's genome. In addition, these drugs do not eradicate latently infected B cells. (Crumpacker et al., 1996)

The use of humanized antibody to CD20 (anti-CD20 mAbs, Rituxan) has been shown to be effective, although there are some issues with relapse and it is restricted to CD20 positive tumors. Chemotherapy, surgery and radiation can also be used in some patients with variable outcomes. (Muchak et al., 2010)

Chemotherapy has also been used to treat PTLD, generally after patients have failed to respond to surgical excision with or without reduction of immunosuppression. Regimens are similar to those used for non-Hodgkin's lymphoma, such as CHOP and ProMACE-CytaBOM.

While chemotherapy may occasionally provide long-term relapse-free survival, it is accompanied by a high infection and mortality rate. (Mamzer-Bruneel et al., 2000)

When possible, complete surgical excision of localized disease is highly effective as well as local radiation. Localized disease treated with definitive local therapy (surgery or radiation), combined with reduction of immunosuppression, have an excellent prognosis, with PTLD-related mortality rates reported between 0 and 26%. (Davis et al., 1998)

Treatment	Response Rate (%)
Reduction immunosupression	23-100
Anti-CD20mAbs (Rituxan)	44-68
Chemotherapy	24-65
Surgery and radiation	Variable

Table 4. Therapeutic strategies for PTLD and their efficacy

Two new strategies have been shown to be of some value in the treatment of PTLD patients. One is to improve the immune system response against the virus, and a second one is to try to lower the viral load or the number of infected cells. T cell lines - CTL, specifically directed against B cell can be obtained *in vitro*. (Haque, 2002)

Attempts to establish a competent immune to control EBV-related lymphoproliferations, with immune modulators such as cytokines with or without immunoglobulins have been made. Several case series and case reports have described responses to interferon-alpha and interferon-alpha combined with intravenous IgG. (Davis, 1998) Interleukin-6, a cytokine that promotes the growth and proliferation of B cells, provides another potential target. It is difficult to assess the effectiveness of cytokine therapy as most studies utilizing these agents have also incorporated concurrent reduction in immunosuppression or antiviral agents.

Rapamycin and everolimus, mTOR inhibitors, that are antiproliferative agents may be effective in preventing PTLD. (Nepomuceno et al., 2003) Also, mTOR inhibitors provide an option of switching immunosuppression while providing some anti-tumor effect as an alternative to removal of immunosuppression. (Vaysberg et al., 2007 and Krams et al., 2008)

A promising therapeutic option to control B-cell proliferation is anti-B-cell antibody therapy. Expression of B-cell antigens is variable in PTLD, most likely because of the dysregulation by EBV infection. Nevertheless, results have been quite promising with many patients achieving longterm relapse-free survival.

15. Prognosis

Overall response and survival rates are difficult to compare because of the wide range of PTLD forms and therapies. Furthermore, crude rather than actuarial survival rates are often reported. Within these limitations, a review of relevant literature shows responses that tend to vary according to histology and stage. In two separate series, (Knowles et al., 1995 and Cohen eta l. , 1991) mortality from polymorphic and monomorphic PTLDs ranged from 0% to 20% and 67% to 87%, respectively. PTLDs with abnormalities of oncogenes or tumor suppressor genes would fit within the monomorphic category, and these abnormalities appear to augur a worse prognosis. (Knowles et al., 1995 and Locker et al., 1989) According to Cohen, 1991, it was observed that 44% of PTLD survivors had involvement of only one organ, and involvement of 3 or more organs occurred in 57% of fatal cases. Dror and colleagues considered thrombocytopenia and neutropenia to represent negative prognostic indicators and PTLD histology and stage to be marginally significant in their series. An absence of stage effect on survival was also reported in a retrospective review of 27 pediatric patients. (Donnelly et al., 1998) In this series, mortality was more closely related to the underlying procedure, with BMT and heart transplant recipients having higher mortality rates than liver and kidney transplant recipients. Gross and colleagues reported 92% mortality in PTLD arising in recipients of allogeneic hematopoietic stem cell transplants. In their series, the only responders seen were among those patients treated with interferon alpha. In a separate pediatric liver transplant series, (Praghakaran, 1999) 4 patients with B-cell lymphoma and 1 with B-cell leukemia were successfully treated with reduced immunosuppression and high-dose acyclovir alone or with this treatment followed by chemotherapy. (Praghakaran, 1999) In our series of 7 liver transplants in small children with PTLD, median age at transplantation was 35.14 months, and the mortality was 57%. (Wiederkehr et al., 2010)

The heterogeneity of these reports exemplifies the variable results seen with different treatment regimens among different centers and argues for standardized multicenter therapeutic trials against this disease. According to Nalesnik's series of 256 patients with PTLD, the overall 2-year actuarial survival is 90%, and the overall actuarial 5-year survival is 77%. (Nalesnik et al., 2000)

According to a study made by Jain et al., 2002, the actuarial patient survival rates for entire population of PTLD patients at 1, 5, 10, 15 and 20 years were 85%, 69%, 55%, 47%, and 45% respectively. In the article there was a numerical difference in survival, with women having a better survival than men but this was only evident at 10 years after PTLD diagnosis and did not reach statistical significance. Long-term survival rates for pediatric patients with PTLD were better than for adults (60% pediatric at 15 years, compared to 39% for adults). Survival in the tacrolimus group was significantly better than for cyclosporin (60% vs. 40% by 12 years). Other factors that appeared to have a positive effect on survival included single site versus multiple site. Overall, mortality due to PTLD ranges from 22% to 70%. (Levi et al., 1993 and Newell et al., 1996)

16. References

Badley AD, Portela DF, Patel R, et al. Development of monoclonal gammopathy precedes the development of Epstein-Barr virus-induced posttransplant lymphoproliferative disorder. *Liver Transplant Surg*. 1996;2:375.

Beatty, P R; Krams, S M; Esquivel, C O; Martinez, O M. Effect of cyclosporine and tacrolimus on the growth of Epstein-Barr virus-transformed B-cell lines. *Transplantation*. 1998 May 15; 65 (9) :1248-55

Birkeland SA, Andersen HK, Hamilton-Dutoit SJ. Preventing acute rejection, Epstein-Barr virus infection, and post-transplant lymphoproliferative disorders after kidney transplantation: use of aciclovir and mycophenolate mefetil in a steroid free immunosuppressive protocol. *Transplantation*. 1999;67:1209-1214.

Bodeus M, Smets F, Reding R, et al. Epstein-Barr virus infection in sixty pediatric liver graft recipients: diagnosis of primary infection and virologic follow-up. *Pediatr Infect Dis*. 1999;18:698-702.

Boubenider S, Hiesse C, Goupy C, et al. Incidence and consequences of post-transplantation lymphoproliferative disorders. *J Nephrol*. 1997;10:136-145.

Cao S, Cox K, Esquivel CO, et al. Posttransplant lymphoproliferative disorders and gastrointestinal manifestations of Epstein-Barr virus infection in children following liver transplantation. *Transplantation*. 1998;66:851.

Cavazzana-Calvo M, Bensoussan D, Jabado N, et al. Prevention of EBV-induced B-lymphoproliferative disorder by ex vivo marrow B-cell depletion in HLA-phenoidentical or non-identical T-depleted bone marrow transplantation. *Br J Haematol.* 1998;103:543-551.

Chen JM, Barr ML, Chadburn A, et al. Management of lymphoproliferative disorders after cardiac transplantation. *Ann Thorac Surg.* 1993;56:527.

Ciancio G, Siquijor AP, Burke GW, et al. Post-transplant lymphoproliferative disease in kidney transplant patients in the new immunosuppressive era. *Clin Transplant.* 1997;11:243-249.

Cohen JI. Epstein-Barr virus lymphoproliferative disease associated with acquired immunodeficiency. *Medicine.* 1991;70:137.

Cohen JI. Epstein–Barr Virus Infection. *New Engl J Med* 343:481,2000

Colby BM, Shaw JE, Elion GB, et al. Effectofacyclovir [9- (2-hydroxyethoxymethyl)guanine] on Epstein Barr virus DNA replication. J Virol 1980; 34: 560–568.

Crumpacker CS. Ganciclovir. *New Engl J Med* 1996; 335: 721–729.

Davis CL, Wood BL, Sabath DE. Interferon-alpha treat- ment of posttransplant lymphoproliferative disorder in recipients of solid organ transplants. *Transplantation* 1998; 66: 1770–1779.

Dhillon M S, J K Rai, B K Gunson et al. Post-transplant lymphoproliferative disease in liver transplantation *The British Journal of Radiology*, May 2007

Donnelly LF, Frush DP, Marshall KW, et al. Lymphoproliferative disorders: CT findings in immunocompromised children. *Am J Roentgenol.* 1998;171:725-731

Dror Y, Greenberg M, Taylor G, et al. Lymphoproliferative disorders after organ transplantation in children. *Transplantation.* 1999;67:990.

Dusenbery D, Nalesnik MA, Locker J, et al. Cytologic features of post-transplant lymphoproliferative disorder. *Diagn Cytopathol.* 1997;16:489.

Frizzera G Atypical lymphoproliferative disorders. In: Knowles DM, ed. *Neoplastic Hematopathology.* Baltimore, Md: Williams & Wilkins; 1992:459.

Fung JJ, Jain A, Kwak EJ, et al. De novo malignancies after liver transplantation: a major cause of late death. *Liver Transplant* 2001;7:S109–18.

Green M, Burroughts M, Katz B, et al. Multicenter randomized trial of CMV IVIG in the prevention of Epstein-Barr virus (EBV)/post- transplant lymphoproliferative disease (PTLD) in pediatric liver (LTx) recipients [abstract 141]. *Am J Transplant* 2003; 3 (Suppl 5):188.

Green M. Management of Epstein-Barr virus–induced post-transplant lymphoproliferative disease in recipients of solid organ transplantation. *Am J Transplant* 2001; 1:103–8.

Gross TG, Steinbuch M, DeFor T, et al. B cell lymphoproliferative disorders following hematopoietic stem cell transplantation: risk factors, treatment and outcome. *Bone Marrow Transplant.* 1999;23:251.

Hanasono MM, Kamel OW, Chang PP, et al. Detection of Epstein-Barr virus in cardiac biopsies of heart transplant patients with lymphoproliferative disorders. *Transplantation.* 1995;60:471.

Hanson MN, Morrison VA, Peterson BA, et al. Posttransplant T-cell lymphoproliferative disorders--an aggressive, late complication of solid-organ transplantation. Blood. 1996;88:3626.

Harris, A; Krams, S M; Martinez, O M. (2010). MicroRNAs as immune regulators: implications for transplantation. *Am J Transpl.* 2010; 10 (4):713-9

Haque T., PathaMRC, Gwen M, Wilkie BSca, Clare Taylor MSca, Peter L Amlot FRCPb, Parvez Murad BSca, Angela Iley BSca, Dilani Dombagoda BSca, Kate M Britton

BSca, Anthony J Swerdlow DMc and ProfDorothy H Crawford DSca. Treatment of Epstein-Barr-virus-positive post-transplantation lymphoproliferative disease with partly HLA-matched allogeneic cytotoxic T cells. *The Lancet*. 2002;9331:436-442.

Harwood JS, Gould FK, McMaster A, et al. Significance of Epstein-Barr virus status and post-transplant lymphoproliferative disease in pediatric thoracic transplantation. *Pediatr Transplant*. 1999;3:100

Heller T, Drachenberg CB, Orens JB, et al. Primary posttransplant lymphoproliferative disorder of the gallbladder in a lung transplant patient presenting with acute cholecystitis. *Transplantation*. 2000;69:668-670.

Hezode C,Duvoux C, Germanidis G, et al. Role of hepatitis C virus in lymphoproliferative disorders after liver transplantation. *Hepatology*. 1999;30:775-778

Ho M, Jaffe R, Miller G, et al. The frequency of Epstein-Barr virus infection and associated lymphoproliferative syndrome after transplantation and its manifestations in children. *Transplantation*. 1988;45:719

Jain A, Reyes J, Kashyap R, et al. Long-term survival after liver transplantation in 4,000 consecutive patients at a single center. *Ann Surg* 2000; 232: 490-500.

Kim JY, Kim CW, Ahn C, et al. Rapidly developing T-cell posttransplantation lymphoproliferative disorder. *Am J Kidney Dis*. 1999;34:e3.

Knowles DM, Cesarman E, Chadburn A, et al. Correlative morphologic and molecular genetic analysis demonstrates three distinct categories of posttransplantation lymphoproliferative disorders. *Blood*. 1995;85:552

Krams, Sheri M; Martinez, Olivia M. Epstein-Barr virus, rapamycin, and host immune responses. Current Opinion In Organ Transplantation. 2008 Dec; 13 (6) :563-8

Leblond V, Davi F, Charlotte F, et al. Posttransplant lymphoproliferative disorders not associated with Epstein-Barr virus: a distinct entity? *J Clin Oncol*. 1998;16:2052.

Levy M, Backman L, Husberg B, et al. De novo malignancy following liver transplantation: a single centre study. *Transplant Proc* 1993;25:1397–9.

Locker J, Nalesnik M. Molecular genetic analysis of lymphoid tumors arising after organ transplantation. *Am J Pathol*. 1989;135:977.

Loren A W, Porter D L, Stadtmauer E A, et al. Post-transplant lymphoproliferative disorder: a review. *Bone Marrow Transplantation* 2003 31, 145–155.

Mamzer-Bruneel MF, Lome C, Morelon E et al. Durable remission after aggressive chemotherapy for very late post- kidney transplant lymphoproliferation: a report of 16 cases observed in a single center. *J Clin Oncol* 2000; 18: 3622–3632.

Martinez AJ, Ahdab-Barmada M. The neuropathology of liver transplantation: comparison of main complications in children and adults. *Mod Pathol*. 1993;6:25.

Martinez, O M; de Gruijl, F R. Molecular and immunologic mechanisms of cancer pathogenesis in solid organ transplant recipients. *American Journal Of Transplantation*: 2008 Nov; 8 (11) :2205-11

McDiarmid SV, Jordan S, Lee GS, et al. Prevention and preemptive therapy of posttransplant lymphoproliferative disease in pediatric liver recipients. *Transplantation* 1998;66:1604.

McGregor JM, Yu CCW, Lu QL. Posttransplant cutaneous lymphoma. *J Am Acad Dermatol*. 1993;29:549.

Molnar I, Keung YK. Treatment of post-transplant lymphoproliferative disorder with rituximab and radiation in a patient with second renal allograft. *Nephrol. Dial. Transplant*. 2001;16 (10): 2114-5.

Mucha K, Foroncewicz B, Ziarkiewicz-Wróblewska B, Krawczyk M, Lerut J, Paczek L. Post-transplant lymphoproliferative disorder in view of the new WHO classification:

a more rational approach to a protean disease? *Nephrol Dial Transplant.* 2010 Jul;25 (7):2089-98.

Nalesnik MA, Jaffe R, Starzl TE, et al. The pathology of posttransplant lymphoproliferative disorders occurring in the setting of cyclosporin A-prednisolone immunosuppression. *Am J Pathol* 1988;133:173–92.

Nepomuceno, Ronald R; Balatoni, Cynthia E; Natkunam, Yaso; Snow, Andrew L; Krams, Sheri M; Martinez, Olivia M. Rapamycin inhibits the interleukin 10 signal transduction pathway and the growth of Epstein Barr virus B-cell lymphomas. *Cancer Research.* 2003 Aug 1; 63 (15) :4472-80

Newell KA, Alonso EM, Kelly SM, et al. Association between liver transplantation for Langerhans cell histiocytosis, rejection, and development of posttransplant lymphoproliferative disease in children. *J Pediatr.* 1999;131:98.

Newell K, Alonso E, Pittington P, et al. Posttranplant lymphoproliferative disease in paediatric liver transplantation. *Transplantation* 1996;62:370–5.

Newell K, Alonso E, Pittington P, et al. Posttranplant lymphoproliferative disease in paediatric liver transplantation. *Transplantation* 1996;62:370–5

Pageaux GP, Bonnardet A, Picot MC, et al. Prevalence of monoclonal immunoglobulins after liver transplantation: relationship with posttransplant lymphoproliferative disorders. *Transplantation.* 1998;65:397.

Paya CV, Fung JJ, Nalesnik MA, et al. Epstein-Barr virus-induced posttransplant lymphoproliferative disorders. *Transplantation.* 1999;68:1517.

Penn I. Cancers in cyclosporine-treated vs azathioprine-treated patients. *Transplant Proc.* 1996;28:876-878.

Penn I. De novo malignancies in pediatric organ transplant recipients. *Pediatr Transplant.* 1998;2:56-63.

Pickhardt PJ, Siegel MJ, Hayashi RJ et-al. Posttransplantation lymphoproliferative disorder in children clinical, histopathologic, and imaging features. *Radiology.* 2000;217 (1): 16-25

Pickhardt PJ, Siegel MJ. Abdominal manifestations of post- transplant lymphoproliferative disorder. *AJR Am J Roentgenol* 1998;56:1394–8.

Posey LA, Kerschner JE, Conley SF. Posttransplantation lymphoproliferative disease in children: otolaryngologic manifestations and management. *South Med J.* 1999;92:1079-1082.

Praghakaran K, Wise B, Chen A, et al. Rational management of posttransplant lymphoproliferative disorder in pediatric recipients. *J Pediatr Surg.* 1999;34:112.

Preiksaitis JK, Cockfield SM. Epstein-Barr virus and lymphoprolifer- ative disease after hematopoietic stem cell or solid organ tranplantation. In: Bowden RA, Ljungman P, Paya CV, eds. Transplant infections. 2nd ed. Philadelphia: Lippincott-Williams & Wilkins, 2003:326–49.

Preiksaitis J K, Keay S. Diagnosis and Management of Posttransplant Lymphoproliferative Disorder in Solid-Organ Transplant Recipients. *Clinical Infectious Diseases* 2001; 33 (Suppl 1):S38–46

Rogers BB, Sommerauer J, Quan A, et al. Epstein-Barr virus polymerase chain reaction and serology in pediatric post--transplant lymphoproliferative disorder: a three-year experience. *Pediatr Dev Pathol.* 1998;1:480-486.

Renard TH, Andrews WS, Foster ME. Relationship between OKT3 administration, EBV seroconversion, and the lymphoproliferative syndrome in paediatric liver transplant recipients. *Transplant Proc* 1991;23:1473–6.

Rooney CM, Loftin SK, Holladay MS, et al. Early identification of Epstein-Barr virus-associated post-transplantation lymphoproliferative disease. *Br J Haematol.* 1995;89:98.

Rowe DT, Qu L, Reyes J, et al. Use of quantitative competitive PCR to measure Epstein-Barr virus genome load in the peripheral blood of pediatric transplant patients with lymphoproliferative disorders. *J Clin Microbiol*. 1997;35:1612.

Shapiro RS, McClain K, Frizzera G, et al. Epstein-Barr virus associated B cell lymphoproliferative disorders following bone marrow transplantation. *Blood*. 1988;71:1234.

Shpilberg O, Wilson J, Whiteside TL, et al. Pre-transplant immunological profile and risk factor analysis of post- transplant lymphoproliferative disease development: the results of a nested matched case-control study: The University of Pittsburgh PTLD Study Group. *Leuk Lymphoma*. 1999;36:109.

Smets F, Bodeus M, Goubau P, et al. Characteristics of Epstein-Barr virus primary infection in pediatric liver transplant recipients. *J Hepatol*. 2000;32:100-104.

Snow, Andrew L; Lambert, Stacie L; Natkunam, Yasodha; Esquivel, Carlos O; Krams, Sheri M; Martinez, Olivia M. EBV can protect latently infected B cell lymphomas from death receptor-induced apoptosis. *Journal Of Immunology* (Baltimore, Md.: 1950). 2006 Sep 1; 177 (5) :3283-93

Snow, A L; Vaysberg, M; Krams, S M; Martinez, O M. EBV B lymphoma cell lines from patients with post-transplant lymphoproliferative disease are resistant to TRAIL-induced apoptosis. *American Journal Of Transplantation*. 2006;6:976-85

Snow, A L; Chen, L J; Nepomuceno, R R; Krams, S M; Esquivel, C O; Martinez, O M. Resistance to Fas-mediated apoptosis in EBV-infected B cell lymphomas is due to defects in the proximal Fas signaling pathway. *Journal Of Immunology*. 2001 Nov 1; 167 (9):5404-11

Starzl, T. E. In discussion of: Murray JE, Wilson RE, Tilney NL, et al. Five years' experience in renal transplantation with immunosuppressive drugs: survival, function, complications and the role of lymphocyte depletion by thoracic duct fistula. *Ann Surg*. 1968;168:416.

Birkeland SA, Andersen HK, Hamilton-Dutoit SJ. Preventing acute rejection, Epstein-Barr virus infection, and post-transplant lymphoproliferative disorders after kidney transplantation: use of aciclovir and mycophenolate mefetil in a steroid free immunosuppressive protocol. *Transplantation*. 1999;67:1209-1214.

Starzl TE, Nalesnik MA, Porter KA, et al. Reversibility of lymphomas and lymphoproliferative lesions developing under cyclosporin-steroid therapy. Lancet 1984;17:583–7.

Steiber AC, Boillot O, Scotti-Foglieni C, et al. The surgical implications of the posttransplant lymphoproliferative disorders. Transplant Proc 1991;23:1477–9.

Vaysberg, M; Hatton, O; Lambert, SL; Snow, AL; Wong, B; Krams, SM; and Martinez, OM. Tumor-derived Variants of Epstein-Barr Virus Latent Membrane Protein 1 Induce Sustained Erk Activation and c-Fos. *J Biol Chemistry*, 283:36753-36585, 2008.

Vaysberg, M; Lambert, S L; Krams, S M; Martinez, O M Activation of the JAK/STAT pathway in Epstein Barr virus+-associated posttransplant lymphoproliferative disease: role of interferon-gamma. *American Journal Of Transplantation*. 2009; 9:2292-302

Vaysberg, Maria; Balatoni, Cynthia E; Nepomuceno, Ronald R; Krams, Sheri M; Martinez, Olivia M. Rapamycin inhibits proliferation of Epstein-Barr virus-positive B-cell lymphomas through modulation of cell-cycle protein expression. *Transplantation*. 2007; 83 (8):1114-21

Wiederkehr JC, Coelho IM, Avilla SG, e Silva EM, Schuller S, Ouno DD, Wiederkehr BA, Polimeni M. Prevalence of posttransplantation lymphoproliferative disease in pediatric liver transplant recipients. *Transplant Proc*. 2010 Mar;42 (2):521-2.

Wu L, Rappaport DC, Hanbidge A, et al. Lymphoproliferative disorders after liver transplantation: imaging features. *Abdom Imaging* 2001;26:200–6.

16

Metabolic Syndrome After Liver Transplantation

Rocío González Grande, Miguel Jiménez Pérez,
Ana Belen Sáez Gómez and Juan Miguel Rodrigo López
Departament of Gastroenterology and Hepatology,
Liver Transplantation Unit. University Hospital Carlos Haya, Málaga,
Spain

1. Introduction

The survival of patients who undergo liver transplantation has improved over recent years, due to the perfectioning of the surgical technique, the optimization of immunosuppressive therapy and the prevention of infection, and is estimated to be 90% at one year and 70% at five years (Pagadala et al., 2009). However, at the same time the incidence of metabolic complications has increased, and they now constitute one of the main causes of mortality unrelated to the graft (Muñoz & ElGenaidi, 2005; Watt et al., 2010). The metabolic syndrome (MS), which associates overweight, dyslipidaemia, hyperglycaemia and hypertension, has a greater prevalence in patients who have a liver transplant as compared with the general population (Francioso et al., 2008; Sorice et al., 2011). Though the impact of the MS on post-transplant mortality is controversial, its diagnosis or the presence of certain of its components increases the risk of cardiovascular complications, renal failure or fatty liver disease in the graft, and it has also been related with a greater risk for infections and rejection. The MS has special relevance in patients with hepatitis C, as the development of the MS in general, and diabetes in particular, can affect the natural history of the hepatitis C in the graft (Vedt et al., 2009). The identification of modifiable predisposing factors and early treatment of hypertension, hyperglycaemia and dyslipidaemia, together with the prevention of overweight during the peri-transplant period, can all help to reduce the morbidity and mortality in this population.

2. Diagnosis and prevalence of the metabolic syndrome in liver transplant patients

Many definitions for the MS can be found in the literature. The criteria defined by the National Cholesterol Education Program, Adult Treatment Panel III (NCEP/ATPIII) adapted by the National Heart, Lung and Blood Institute/American Heart Association (NHLBI/AHA) and International Diabetes Federation (IDF) are detailed in Table 1(Grundy et al., 2004; Alberti et al., 2006).

These criteria all have in common insulin resistance (IR) as the physiological basis of the MS. IR is defined as the reduction of sensitivity of tissues to the action of insulin, which implies a compensating hyperinsulinaemia that in the end exhausts the capacity of the pancreatic beta cells to produce insulin. Secondary to this is produced hyperglycaemia and diabetes. IR is measured using the HOMA (Homeostatic Model Assessment) index, though its measurement is not necessary for the diagnosis of the MS (Matthews et al., 1985).

$$HOMA = \text{fasting insulin (mU/ml)} \times \text{fasting glucose (mmol/L)}/22.5$$

American Heart Association	**International Diabetes Federation**
At least 3 of the following criteria: • Waist circumference >88 cm for women and >102 cm for men • Fasting glucose >100 mg/dl • Systolic blood pressure> 130mmHg and/or diastolic blood pressure >85 mmHg or on antihypertensive treatment in a patient with history of hypertension • HDL <50 mg/dl for women and <40 mg/dl for men • Triglycerides >150 mg/dl or on drug treatment for elevated TG	Abdominal obesity according to gender and ethnicity specific values (i.e. waist circumference >80 cm for women and >90 cm for men if they are American or European) and at least 2 the following criteria: • Fasting glucose>100 mg/dl • Systolic blood pressure >130 mmHg and/or diastolic blood pressure >85 mmHg or on antihypertensive treatment • HDL <50 mg/dl for women and <40 mg/dl for men • Triglycerides >150 mg/dl

Table 1. Definition of the metabolic syndrome by NHLBI/AHA and IDF 2005

The prevalence of the MS in the general population is approximately 30% (Ford et al., 2004). However, in liver transplant patients it is considerably higher, approximately 40-50% (Laryea et al., 2007; Bianchi et al, 2008), though these percentages can vary according to geographical area, and are slightly lower, for example, in the Spanish population, both transplanted and non-transplanted (Ruiz-Rebollo et al., 2010).

Independent analysis of each of the components of the MS also shows a greater incidence in the transplanted population; 40-85% develop hypertension, 13-61% diabetes, 40-66% dyslipidaemia, mainly hypertriglyceridaemia, and up to 40% obesity, which can reach 70% three years post-transplant (Laish et al., 2011).

3. Risk factors for post-transplant metabolic syndrome

Different studies have evaluated possible risk factors for the development of post-transplant metabolic syndrome (PTMS) in an attempt to identify them early and treat them as far as possible.

In general, considering that IR triggers the MS, the situations that predispose to this condition are applicable, in addition to the underlying aetiology of the liver disease and the use of immunosuppressive drugs.

Of the causes leading to the liver transplant, HCV infection (Bigam et al., 2000) and cryptogenic cirrhosis are significantly associated with PTMS (Ong et al., 2001), versus other factors such as autoimmune disorders or hepatitis B. Biliary diseases are not related with PTMS, perhaps because of the later hepatocyte involvement, which is, after all, responsible for glucose metabolism (Laryea et al., 2007). Review of all the publications available confirms the two-way relation of the hepatitis C virus, insulin-resistance and the development of diabetes (Hanouneh et al., 2008).

Immunosuppressive drugs, particularly steroids and calcineurin inhibitors, are associated with the appearance of cardiovascular risk factors, though tacrolimus is more diabetogenic and cyclosporine predisposes more to hypertension and dyslipidaemia (Marchetti & Navalesi, 2000). In fact, most of the metabolic complications appear during the first months after the transplant, when the immunosuppressive treatment is greater. Nevertheless, no clear relation exists between the MS and a particular immunosuppressive regimen, probably because of its multifactorial origin (Bianchi et al., 2008).

The characteristics of the donor and the recipient also influence the development of PTMS; mainly the age of both, the presence of any of the components of the MS prior to the transplant, and the existence and degree of graft steatosis are considered risk factors.

4. Components of PTMS

4.1 Obesity

Overweight is defined as a body mass index (BMI) of 25-30 and obesity as a BMI >30, with the latter being classified into class I (BMI of 30-35), class II (BMI of 35-40) and class III (BMI>40). Obesity can also be differentiated between peripheral or central obesity, with the latter having more implication in the metabolism (Watt, 2010).

Pre-transplant obesity is associated with greater peri-operative morbidity and mortality, with a longer hospital stay and reduced patient and graft survival. An analysis by the Scientific Registry of Transplant Recipients showed that five-year post-transplant mortality was greater in recipients with class II and III obesity (Nair et al., 2002), though no consideration was given to the influence of ascites on overweight. Studies that corrected obesity for ascites found no significant differences regarding morbidity or survival between obese and non-obese recipients, though ascites was found to be indicative of a worse postoperative course (Leonard et al., 2008). These studies could, however, be influenced by the fact that the obese patients were studied more closely from the cardiological aspect, with more exhaustive screening for pre-transplant cardiovascular risk.

Post-transplant obesity is very usual. Patients who are overweight prior to the transplant usually remain so, and up to one third develop de novo obesity (Wawrzynonowicz-Syczewska et al., 2009). The main triggering factor is the return to dietary habits but not to physical activity (Painter et al., 2001), which leads to a progressive weight gain, generally greater during the first post-transplant months. The immunosuppressive medication has traditionally been considered a trigger of overweight, though the association is in fact controversial and it has only been shown with the long-term use of steroids (Everhart et al., 1998).

Whilst not associated with greater mortality, post-transplant obesity, particularly central obesity, causes an imbalance in the production of adipokines, favouring those that produce peripheral insulin resistance, and thus PTMS (Fox et al., 2007). In addition, obesity is related with osteoarthritis, sleep apnoea syndrome, and alterations in the distribution volume of drugs. The toxicity of non-lipophylic drugs that are adjusted to weight may be increased, and the blood levels of lipophylic drugs reduced (Watt & Charlton, 2010). Obesity can also affect the activity of the cytochrome P450 (Kotlyar & Carson, 1999).

The management of pre-transplant overweight is mainly based on dietary measures and lifestyle recommendations. Though there is currently no BMI that is an absolute contraindication for liver transplantation, obesity is considered a surgical and post-operative risk factor. The recommendations after the transplant are similar to those for the general population. Weight should be controlled, and the patient instructed about the prevention of obesity, with a suitable diet and physical exercise. Immunosuppression, especially corticosteroids, should be minimized as far as possible.

Bariatric surgery has been considered as a treatment option in patients with morbid obesity (Takata et al., 2008). However, performing it before the transplant operation is associated with technical difficulties, and after transplantation it may affect the absorption of the immunosuppressive medication, with repercussions on graft viability, and may also make treatment of any biliary problems more difficult (Butte et al., 2007).

Concerning pharmacological measures, pancreatic lipase inhibitors like tetrahydrolipstatin (orlistat), which can be used in the general population with morbid obesity, present important interactions with the immunosuppressive agents, and thus have to be limited in the transplant population (Desai et al., 2010).

4.2 Diabetes

Candidate patients for a liver transplant may have diabetes or, more likely, glucose intolerance due to the IR present in many patients with hepatic cirrhosis. In this context, IR can be related with the hyperglucagonaemia found in many cirrhotic patients, as well as with the lower insulin degradation by a diseased liver or by the leakage phenomena from a portosystemic shunt. After the transplant, the insulin levels and glucose metabolism become normal in up to 6% of these patients (Watt & Charlton, 2010). However, from 20% to 60% remain diabetic or develop post-transplant diabetes mellitus (PTDM). The main risk factors for the development of PTDM are prior diabetes, obesity, hepatitis C and a family history of diabetes (Anastáscio et al., 2010).

After the transplant, the immunosuppressive drugs are the main trigger for de novo DM. Steroids induce IR in a dose-dependent manner, by reducing the pancreatic production of insulin and increasing hepatic gluconeogenesis (Schake et al., 2002). Calcineurin inhibitors can also reduce insulin production via a direct toxic effect and/or reduction in the peripheral use of insulin. Tacrolimus seems to have a greater diabetogenic effect than cyclosporine (Haddad et al., 2006). The effect of mTOR inhibitors on the development of IR is unclear; on one hand they may favour the response to insulin and thus reduce the risk of diabetes, though on the other hand they can also block the proliferation of pancreatic beta cells, thereby predisposing to PTDM (Vodenik et al., 2009).

PTDM is associated with cardiovascular complications, increased and accelerated progression of fibrosis in patients with hepatitis C, and a reduction in the response to antiviral therapy (Veldt et al., 2009). It is also associated with a greater incidence of chronic rejection and late hepatic artery thrombosis. The survival of transplant patients who develop diabetes is lower than that for those without diabetes. In addition, these patients can present the same microvascular complications as in the general population, including retinopathy, nephropathy and infections (Desai et al., 2010).

The aims of treatment in the transplant patient with diabetes are similar to those in the general population: fasting blood glucose levels of 80-130 mg/dl, post-prandial levels of 140-180 mg/dl and glycosylated haemoglobin <6.5-7% (Bilbao et al., 2010)..

The treatment of PTDM includes dietary measures, limiting the intake of carbohydrates, and physical activity. A reduction in steroids or their complete withdrawal, plus dose optimization of calcineurin inhibitors or their minimization, adding other immunosuppressive drugs (mycophenolate or mTOR inhibitors) may suffice, thereby avoiding pharmacological therapy (Dumortier et al., 2006; Herrero el at., 2006).

Hyperglycaemia during the early post-transplant period requires treatment with insulin, which can later be reduced or even stopped. The drugs of choice for maintenance therapy are oral antidiabetic agents (Marchetti, 2005). The choice of oral antidiabetic agent to be used should be based on the advantages and possible side effects of each drug group in general or each drug in particular. The sulphonylureas can favour overweight and hypoglycaemia and should be avoided in patients with advanced kidney failure; the alpha glucosidase inhibitors can produce adverse side effects in the digestive system; the thiazolidinediones, which have a greater glucose lowering action, have been shown to increase the cardiovascular risk in the general population and are not therefore advised (Watt & Charlton, 2010). Metformin may be the most suitable oral antidiabetic agent because it lacks hepatic metabolism and is the recommended first line drug of choice, though it should be remembered that it can produce lactic acidosis in patients with kidney failure (Sharif, 2011).

4.3 Dyslipidaemia

Prior to the transplant, most cirrhotic patients do not have dyslipidaemia, due to the lower liver production of lipids and the malnutrition experienced by most of them. An exception, though, is patients with cholestatic liver disease, but in these cases the pattern of dyslipidaemia is not associated with a greater risk of arteriosclerosis (Muñoz & ElGenaidi, 2005).

After the transplant, however, dyslipidaemia, both hypertriglyceridaemia and hypercholesterolaemia, is very frequent, occurring in up to 70% of transplant patients within one year (Bianchi et al., 2008). Some authors consider dyslipidaemia to be the main cardiovascular risk factor (Reuben, 2001).

As with the other components of the PTMS, the aetiology of dyslipidaemia involves many factors, though the immunosuppressive agents are the main triggering factor. Steroids are associated with hyperlipidaemia as they stimulate the activity of acetyl-CoA carboxylase and the synthesis of fatty acids, thus raising concentrations of total cholesterol and triglycerides (Ballantyne et al., 1992). M-TOR inhibitors increase lipoprotein-lipase activity, increasing the hepatic synthesis of triglycerides (Morrisett et al., 2003). Calcineurin inhibitors reduce the excretion of cholesterol to the bile and the peripheral LDL-cholesterol receptors, thereby raising circulating levels of cholesterol (Chan et al., 1998).

Treatment of the hypercholesterolaemia starts with dietary measures, including supplements of omega 3 fatty acid. In most cases, though, this is insufficient and it is necessary to initiate pharmacological treatment. The recommendations for this are the same as for the general population. In patients with no cardiovascular events, the LDL cholesterol should be maintained <130 mg/dl, though for secondary prevention this level should be <100 mg/dl. Statins are the drugs of choice in both the general and the transplant populations, reducing cardiovascular disease as well as having a certain immunosuppressive effect that has been related with a lower incidence of rejection (Martin et al., 2008). Most statins use the same metabolic pathways as calcineurin inhibitors (P450 cytochrome), which explains the pharmacological interactions and the greater risk for myositis and rhabdomyolysis (Desai et al., 2010). It is therefore recommended to start with low doses and gradually increase them according to needs. In particular, pravastatin is eliminated via the kidneys and fluvastatin uses a different cytochrome, so that these two may be the statins of choice (Watt & Charlton, 2010). Treatment with ion exchange resins, whilst it may help normalize cholesterol levels, interrupts the enterohepatic circulation and may, secondarily, alter levels of calcineurin inhibitors, particularly cyclosporine.

Hypertriglyceridaemia is better treated with dietary restriction, with drugs generally being reserved for patients with severe hypertriglyceridaemia. Fibrates, such as gemfibrozil, are indicated in these cases, but with caution if associated with statins due to the greater muscular toxicity.

Ezetimibe, an inhibitor of the enterohepatic recirculation of lipids, has been show to be well-tolerated and effective when used in combination with statin, but interacts with immunosuppressive drugs and can produce hepatotoxicity (Almutairi et al., 2009).

In all cases the use of steroids should be kept to a minimum and calcineurin inhibitors optimized.

4.4 Hypertension

The incidence of hypertension before transplant is very low. However, after transplantation, the hyperdynamic circulation of the cirrhotic patient is reverted, with an increase in blood pressure that can reach values considered normal. Once again, the immunosuppressive drugs, whether or not in the presence of other risk factors, are related with the onset of hypertension, considered as a systolic pressure ≥140 mmHg and a diastolic pressure ≥90 mmHg; this occurs in around 60-70% of all patients (Watt et al., 2010). The pathophysiology of post-transplant hypertension does not reside in alterations of the renin-angiotensin-aldosterone system, as occurs in the non-transplanted population. The fundamental mechanism is related to the systemic and renal haemodynamic changes produced by the immunosuppressive drug. Calcineurin inhibitors, particularly cyclosporine, produce renal vasoconstriction of the afferent arteriole, with secondary renal hypoperfusion leading to reabsorption of sodium and water (Textor et al., 2000). Steroids potentiate this latter situation through their mineralocorticoid effect and mTOR inhibitors can produce hypertension if associated with calcineurin inhibitors.

The aims of treatment are to maintain blood pressure figures <140/90 mmHg (or lower in the presence of other risk factors), and the first step is restriction of dietary salt, coupled with control of other risk factors and the undertaking of physical activity.

As far as drugs are concerned, calcium antagonists are considered the first choice as they can reverse renal vasoconstriction. Within this group of drugs, diltiazem, verapamil or nicardipine interfere in the hepatic metabolism of calcineurin whilst amlodipine does not, and this latter is thus the most used (Watt, 2010). Angiotensin converting enzyme (ACE) inhibitors or angiotensin receptor blockers (ARB) produce vasodilation of the efferent arteriole, reducing glomerular pressure and hyperfiltration (Desai et al., 2010). They are the choice group for patients with proteinuria and renal failure because they slow its progress.

Beta blockers are not first-line drugs, but they can be used in selected cases. Finally, diuretics in association with other antihypertensive drugs are beneficial in cases that are difficult to control, but should not be used as a single therapy and also require strict electrolyte control. The reduction of calcineurin inhibitors favours blood pressure control.

5. Consequences of the metabolic syndrome

5.1 Major cardiovascular complications

Major cardiovascular complications or events mainly include ischaemic heart disease, stroke or peripheral ischaemia phenomena. Transplant patients who develop PTMS have an accumulated incidence of cardiovascular disease around twice that of transplant patients without PTMS (12.9% vs. 4.9%, respectively; Figure 1, Laish et al 2011). Cardiovascular mortality can reach 40% (Laish et al., 2011; Laryea et al., 2007; Anastáscio et al., 2010).

5.2 Fatty liver graft disease

Up to 60% of patients transplanted due to nonalcoholic steatohepatitis (NASH) relapse at one year and 100% at five years. In cases of cryptogenic cirrhosis, the presence of different degrees of steatosis in the graft is 50% at two years post-transplant. Although no exact study has been undertaken on the repercussion of steatosis on graft function, between 2.5% and 15% of relapses of NASH are estimated to end in cirrhosis. The main independent risk factor for fatty liver graft disease is a 10% increase in body mass index (Charlton, 2009; Dureja et al., 2011).

5.3 Influence of HCV recurrence

A bidirectional relation exists between HCV and IR, with 21% of HCV-positive patients being diabetic, and the presence of HCV multiplies the long-term risk of developing diabetes by 2-3 times. A recent analysis of cardiovascular risk after liver transplantation according to HCV status showed higher incidence of DM among HCV-positive patients (Pérez et al., 2011). Inversely, IR or the presence of established diabetes is associated with greater viral replication, a higher degree of steatosis and fibrosis and worse response to antiviral therapy (Arase et al., 2009). The main reason for this association is that not only does HCV block the intracellular signals that trigger insulin after binding to the receptor, but also IR stimulates hepatic lipogenesis and stellate cells, thus increasing steatosis and fibrosis. IR and hyperinsulinaemia induce resistance to interferon, such that patients with a HOMA >2 have a lower percentage of sustained viral response (SVR). In parallel, those patients who achieve a SVR have a lower risk of developing diabetes because, in the absence of viral replication, the IR almost disappears (Romero et al., 2009)

5.4 Renal failure

In both the general population and in persons who have a transplant, patients with the MS present a greater incidence of renal failure. The reduction in glomerular filtration and the presence of microalbuminuria are associated with the number of components of the MS present. IR, and secondary hyperinsulinaemia and hyperglycaemia, cause an imbalance between vasodilatating and vasoconstricting substances, in favour of the latter; they favour oxidative stress and endothelial damage; stimulate the renin-angiotensin-aldosterone axis and release of growth factors. This all leads to structural damage in the kidney, mainly tubular atrophy, glomerulosclerosis and tubulointerstitial fibrosis, damage that eventually produces a reduction in glomerular filtration, proteinuria and a rise in creatinine. If added to this there is renal damage caused by the immunosuppressive drugs, transplant patients with PTMS thus have a greater incidence of chronic transplant nephropathy (Morales et al., 2006).

6. Prevention and treatment of PTMS

It is necessary to identify patients with risk factors for PTMS as obesity, pretransplant diabetes, older age, and transplantation due to HCV infection or cryptogenic cirrhosis, which in many cases is in fact an unrecognized steatohepatitis. Usual check-ups should include a search for the early detection of components of PTMS and, if found, they should be treated as per the recommendations above. In all cases good dietary advice is recommended as well as the promotion of physical activity. Concerning immunosuppression, the use of steroids and calcineurin inhibitors should be reduced as much as is possible. This generally means the early introduction of other immunosuppressive drugs, mainly mycophenolate and mTOR inhibitors, which permits calcineurin inhibitors to be spared. In patients presenting with several cardiovascular risk factors or in those who have had a cardiovascular event, antiaggregation therapy should be considered.

7. Conclusions

The MS and each of its individual components are more prevalent in transplant patients than in the general population. The presence of PTMS is associated with a grater incidence of cardiovascular diseases and chronic transplant nephropathy. It is related with a worse course of HCV recurrence and favours the onset of fatty liver graft disease. Immunosuppressive drugs are the main factor related with PTMS. Strict vigilance should be exercised at the regular clinic visits for the appearance of any of the components of MS and treatment started accordingly. The immunosuppression should be individualised, recommending the early introduction of calcineurin inhibitor sparing drugs, with fewer metabolic and renal side effects.

8. References

Alberti KG, Zimmet P, & Shaw J. Metabolic syndrome a new world-wide definition. A consensus statement from the international diabetes federation. Diabet 2006; 23: 469-480.

Almutairi F, Peterson TC, Molinari M, Walsh MJ, Alwayn I, & Peltekian KM. Safety and effectiveness of ezetimibe in liver transplant recipients with hypercholesterñemia. Liver transplantation 2009; 15: 504-508.

Anastácio LR, Lima AS, & Toulson Davisson Correia MI. Metabolic syndrome and its components after liver transplantation: incidence, prevalence, risk factors, and implications. Clinical nutrition 2010; 29: 175-179.

Arase Y, Suzuki F, Suzuki Y, Akuta N, Kobayasi M, Kawamura Y, et al. Sustained virological response reduces incidence of onset of type 2 diabetes in chronic hepatitis C. Hepatology 2009; 49: 739-744.

Ballantyne CM, Radovancevic B, Farmer JA, et al. Hyperlipedaemia after heart transplantation: report of a 6 year experience with treatment recommendations. J Am Coll Cardiol 1992; 19: 1315-1321.

Bianchi G, Marchesini G, Marzicchi R, Pinna A & Zoli M. Metabolic syndrome in liver transplantation relation to etiology and immunosuppression. Liver transplantation 2008; 14: 1648-1654.

Bigam Dl, Pennington JJ, Carpentier A, Wanless IR, Hemming AW, Crosford R, et al. Hepatitis C-related cirrhosis: a predictor of diabetes mellitus after liver transplantation. Hepatology 2000; 32: 87-90.

Bilbao I, Castells Ll, Lázaro JL, Campos I, Rodriguez R, Charco R. Sindrome metabólico postrasplante. Cir Esp 2010; 88: 71.

Butte J, Devaud N, Jarufe NP, Boza C, Perez G, Torres J, et al. Sleeve gastrectomy as treatment for severe obesity after orthotopic liver transplantation. Obes Surg 2007; 17: 1517- 1519.

Chan FK, Zhang Y Lee SS, Shaffer EA. The effects of liver transplantation and cyclosporine on bile formation and lipid composition: an experimental study in the rat. J Hepatol 1998; 28: 329-336.

Charlton M. Obesity, Hyperlipidemia, and metabolic syndrome. Liver Transplantation 2009; 15: S83-S89.

Desai S, Hong J, & Saab S. Cardiovascular risk factors following orthotopic liver transplantation: predisposing factors, incidence and management. Liver International 2010; 10: 948-957.

Dumortier J, Bernard S, Bouffard Y, & Boillot O. Conversion from tacrolimus to cyclosporine in liver transplanted patients with diabetes mellitus. Liver transplantation 2006; 12: 659-664.

Dureja P, Mellinger J, Agni RA, Chang F, Avey G, Lucey M, & Said A. NAFLD recurrence in liver transplant recipients. Transplantation 2011; 91: 684-689.

Everhart JE, Lombardero M, Lake JR, Wiesnwr RH, Zetterman RK, & Hoofnagle JH. Weight change and obesity after liver transplantation: incidence and risk factors. Liver Transpl Surg 1998; 4: 285-296.

Ford ES, Giles WH, Mokdad AH. Increasing prevalence of the metabolic syndrome among U.S. adults. Diabetes Care 2004; 27: 2444-2449

Fox C, Massaro JM; Hoffmann U, Pou KM, Maurosvish-Horvat O, Liu CY, et al. Abdominal visceral and subcutaneous adipose tissue compartments: association with metabolic risk factors in the Framingham heart study. Circulation 2007, 116: 39-48.

Grundy SM, Brewer Jr HB, Cleeman JI, Smith Jr SC, & Lenfant C. Definition of metabolic syndrome. Report of the national heart, lung, and blood Institute/American heart association conference on scientific issues related to definition. Circulation 2004; 109: 433-438.

Haddad E, McAlister VC, Renoug E, Malthaner R, Kjaer MS, Gluud LL. Cyclopsporin versus Tacrolimus for liver transplanted patients. Cochrane database syst rev 2006; 18.

Hanouneh IA; Feldstein AE, McCullough AJ, Miller C, Aucejo F, Yerian L, et al. The significance of metabolic syndrome in the setting of recurrent hepatitis C after liver transplantation. Liver transplantation 2008; 14: 1287-1293.

Herrero JI, Quiroga J, Sangro B et al. Conversion from calcineurin inhibitors to mycophenolate Mofetilo in liver transplanted patients with diabetes mellitus. Liver transplantation 2006; 35:1877-1879.

Kotlyar M, & Carson S. Effects of obesity on the cytochrome P450 enzyme system. Int J Clin Pharmacol Ther 1999; 37: 8-19.

Laish I, Braun M, Mor E, Sulkes J, Harif Y, & Ben Ari, Z. Metabolic syndrome in liver transplant recipients: prevalence, risk factors, and association with cardiovascular events. Liver transplantation 2011; 17: 15-22.

Laryea M, Watt KD, Molinari M, Walsh M, McAlister V, Marotta P et al. Metabolic syndrome in liver transplant recipients: prevalence and association with major vascular events. Liver transplantation 2007; 13: 1109-1114.

Leonard J, Heimbach J, Malinchoc M, Watt K, & Charlton M. The impact of obesity on long-term outcomes in liver transplant recipients-results of the NIDDK liver transplant database. Am J Transpant 2008; 8: 667-672.

Marchetti P, & Navelesi R. The metabolic effects of cyclosporine and tacrolimus. J endocrinol Invest 2000; 23: 482-490.

Marchetti P. New-onset diabetes after liver transplantation: from pathogenesis to management. Liver transplantation 2005; 11: 612-620.

Martin J, Cavanaugh TM; Trumbull L, Bass M, Weber Jr F, Aranda-Michel, et al. Incidence of adverse events with HMG-CoA reductase inhibitors in liver transplant patients. Clin Transplant 2008; 22: 113-119.

Matthews DR, Hosker JP, Rudenski AS, Naylos BA, Treacher DF, & Turner RC. Homeostasis model assessment: insulin resistance and B-cell function from fasting plasma glucose and insulin concentrations in man. Diabetologia 1985; 28: 412-419.

Morales JM, Domnguez-Gil B, Gutierrez MªJ. Impacto de la inmunosupresi6n en el perfil cardiovascular después del trasplante renal. Nefrología 2006; 26: 181-194.

Morrisett JD, Abdel-Fattah G, & Kahan BD. Sirolimus changes lipid concentrations and lipoprotein metabolism in kidney transplant recipients. Transplant Proc 2003; 35: S143-S150.

Muñoz SJ, ElGenaidi H. Cardiovascular risk factors after liver transplantation. Liver transplantation 2005; 11 (suppl 2): S52-S56.

Nair S, Verma S, & Thuluvath RJ. Obesity and its effect on survival in patients undergoing orhotopic liver transplantation in the United States. Hepatology 2002; 35: 105-109.

Ong J, Younossi ZM, Reddy V, Price LL, Gramilich T, Mayes J & Bopari N. Cryptogenic cirrhosis and posttransplantation nonalcoholic fatty liver disease. Liver Transplantation 2001; 7: 797-801.

Pagadala M, Dasarathy S, Eghtesad B & McCullough A.J. Posttransplant metabolic syndrome: an epidemic waiting to happen. Liver transplantation 2009; 15: 1662-1670

Painter P, Krasnoff J, Paul SM, & Ascher NL. Physical activity and health -related quality of life in liver transplant recipients. Liver transplantation 2001; 7: 213-219.

Pérez MJ, García DM; Taybi BJ, Daga JAP, Rey JML, Grande RG, Lombardo JdlC, & López JMR. Cardiovascular risk factors after liver transplantation: Analysis of related factors. Transplant Proc 2011; 43,739-741.

Reuben A. Long-term management of the liver transplant patient: diabetes, hyperlipemia, and obsesity. Liver transplantation 2001; 7: S13-S21.

Romero-Gómez M, Diago M, Andrade RJ, Calleja JL; Salmerón J, Fernández-Rodriguez CM; et al. Spanish treatment of resistence to insulin in hepatitis C genotype 1 group. Treatment of insulin resistance with metformin in naïve genotype 1 chronic hepatitis C patients receiving peginterferon alfa-2a plus ribavirin. Hepatology 2009; 50: 1702-1708.

Ruiz-Rebollo ML, Sanchez-Antolin G, García-Pajares F, Fernandez-Orcajo P, González-Sagrado, Cítores-Pascual et al. Transplantation proceedings 2010¸42: 663-665.

Schake H. Döcke W, Asadullah K. Mechanisms involved in the side effects of glucocorticoids. Pharmacol Ther 2002; 96: 23-43.

Sharif A. Should metfomin be our antiglycemic agent of choice post-traplantation?. Am J Transplant 2011; 11: 1376-1381.

Sorice GP; Muscogiuri G, Mezza T, Prioletta A & Giaccari A. Metabolic syndrome in transplant patients: an academic or a health burden?. Transplantation proceedings 2011; 43: 313-317.

Takata M, Campos GM, Ciovica R, Rabi C, Rogers SJ, Cello JP, et al. Laparoscopic bariatric surgery improves candidacy in morbidly obese patients awaiting transplantation. Sur Obes relat Dis 2008; 4: 159-164.

Textor SC, Taler SJ, Canzanello VJ, Chwartz L, & Augustine JE. Posttransplantation hypertension related to calcineurin inhibitors. Liver transplantation 2000; 6: 521-530.

Veldt BJ, Poterucha JJ, Watt KD, Wiesner RH, Hay JE, Rosen CB et al. Insulin resistance, serum adipokines and risk of fibrosis progression in patients transplanted for hepatitis C. Am J Transplant 2009; 9: 1406-1413.

Vodenik B, Rovira J, & Campistol JM. Mammalian target of rapamycin and diabetes: what does the current evidence tell us? Transplant Proc 2009; 41: S31-S38.

Watt KD, Pedersen RA, Kremers WK, Heimbach JK & Charlton MR. Evolution of causes and risk factors for mortality post-liver transplant: results of the NIDDK long-term follow-up study. Am J Transplant 2010; 10: 1420-1427.

Watt KD. Obesity and metabolic complications of liver transplantation. Liver transplantation 2010; 16 (suppl 2): S65-S71.

Watt KD & Charlton MR. Metabolic syndrome and liver transplantation: a review and guide to management. J Hepatol 2010; 53: 199-206.

Wawrzynonowicz-Syczewska M, Karpińska E, Jurczyk K, Laurans L, & Boroń-Kaczmarska A. Risk factors and dynamics of weight gain in patients after liver transplantation. Ann Transplant 2009; 14: 45-50.

17

Autoimmune Hepatitis After Liver Transplantation

Pierpaolo Di Cocco et al.*,
Renal Failure and Transplant Surgery, Department of Surgery, University of L'Aquila, Italy

1. Introduction

Autoimmune hepatitis (AIH) is a progressive, chronic inflammatory liver disease of unknown etiology that occurs in children and adults with a prevalence of female. This clinical syndrome is caused by an immune response that is misdirected against self or foreign antigens that resemble self-antigens, leading to a progressive inflammatory and fibrotic process of the liver (Krawitt, 2006; Czaja, 2001, 2007a, 2007b; Vergani et al, 2002; Manns & Vogel, 2006, Vergani & Mieli-Vergani, 2008). The complications of AIH are the same as any other progressive liver disease. Primary hepatocellular carcinoma is a known consequence; in some patients, chronic hepatitis progresses to cirrhosis and, ultimately, to carcinoma. Liver transplantation is required when end stage liver disease develops (Krawitt, 2006).

AIH has been widely described in liver transplant recipients with and without AIH before transplantation. In the first scenario the term of recurrent AIH has been proposed, while de novo AIH implies the development of AIH in the graft of a recipient who did not have the disease before. De novo and recurrent AIH develop in the clinical context of immune suppression. Consequently the diagnosis may depend more heavily on the exclusion of other causes for allograft dysfunction rather than on the presence of criteria for the diagnosis of classic AIH codified by the international scoring system. The careful analysis of these cases provides exiting and exceptional opportunities to study the pathogenesis of AIH in a human model. To understand the bases for recurrent and de novo AIH after liver transplantation, it is necessary to apply current hypotheses of pathogenesis for classic disease.

2. Pathogenic mechanism of AIH

The pathogenesis of AIH remains uncertain, but conditions that favor its emergence are becoming clearer. Environmental agents like viruses, toxins or drugs (Krawitt, 2006, Czaja et

* Giuseppe Orlando[2], Katia Clemente[1], Lauren Corona[3], Vinicio Rizza[1], Linda De Luca[1], Maurizio DAngelo[1], Federica Delreno[1], Francesco Pisani[1] and Antonio Famulari[1]
[1]*Renal Failure and Transplant Surgery, Department of Surgery, University of L'Aquila, Italy*
[2]*Transplant Surgery and Regenerative Medicine, Wake Forest University, Winston-Salem, North Carolina, USA*
[3]*Wayne State University School of Medicine, USA*

al, 1992, Czaja, 1999a) may trigger a cascade of T-cell mediated events against liver antigens in a context of genetic predisposition (Czaja & Manns, 1995; Alvarez, 1999, Molmenti et al, 2002; Sanchez-Urdazpal et al, 1992), leading to a progressive necroinflammatory liver disease.

Although multiple genes are probably involved in a predisposition to AIH, human leukocyte antigen (HLA) genes appear to play the dominant role (Donaldson et al 1998, Donaldson, 2002). Type 1 AIH, characterized by circulating antinuclear antibodies, smooth muscle antibodies, antiactin antibodies, atypical perinuclear antineutrophilic cytoplasmic antibodies and autoantibodies against soluble liver antigen and liver-pancreas antigen is associated with the HLA DR3 serotype, particularly among white patients. In Japan the most common associated HLA locus is HLA DR4; among white North Americans and northern Europeans, susceptibility relates to the alleles DRB1-0301 and DRB1-0401 (Hytiroglou et al, 2009; Hennes et al, 2008). Type 2 AIH, a rare disorder characterized by antibodies against liver-kidney microsome 1 and liver cytosol 1 has been associated with the HLA DRB1 and HLA DQB1 alleles (Djilali-Saiah et al 2004).

Loss of self tolerance is the requisite for autoimmune disease, and it distinguishes autoimmune conditions from disorders associated with immunologic reactions to foreign antigens. The most promising considerations are defects in the negative selection of autoreactive immunocytes (Czaja, 2007c; Czaja & Carpenter, 2006) and clonal expansion of immunocytes cross-reactive to homologous antigens (molecular mimicry) (Hubscher, 2001; Prados et al, 1998; Ayata et al, 2000). The negative selection removes thymocytes that are capable of strongly binding with self peptides presented by major histocompatibility complex (MHC). This process is an important component of immunological tolerance and serves to prevent the formation of self reactive T cells. According to experimental evidences the risk of autoimmune disease probably relates to actions of genes that limit this process (Czaja & Carpenter, 2006; Banff Working Group, 2006). Molecular mimicry has been proposed as pathogenetic mechanism for AIH. This hypothesis has been substantiated in experimental models by showing that the immunocytes can be activated by diverse but similar epitopes, and they can be clonally expanded to show a broad cross-reactivity. Such cells then can be directed against self-antigens that mimic foreign antigens (Hubscher, 2001; Prados et al, 1998; Ayata et al, 2000). Molecular mimicry is a useful concept to explain how different viruses, drugs or unknown environmental agents might produce a self-perpetuating hepatic injury with the same clinical expression. It also may explain how AIH recurs or develops de novo after liver transplantation. In addition, experimental evidences suggest that genetic polymorphisms affecting the cytokine microenvironment (Gonzales-Koch et al, 2001; Donaldson et al, 1991), immune regulators (Czaja et al, 1993a) and the mechanism of apoptosis (Czaja et al, 1997) could influence the immunocyte activation and perpetuate the immune response.

The identification of CD4+ regulatory T cells has reinvoked the concept that failure of or escape from normal suppression of reactivity against the self has an essential role in the development of autoimmune disease. Recent experimental evidence suggests that immunoregulatory dysfunction characterized by decreased numbers of CD4+CD25+ regulatory T cells may occur in AIH (Longhi et al, 2004).

2.1 Pathogenesis of recurrent AIH

AIH recurs after liver transplantation in 11% to 83% of cases with considerable variation between studies depending on the diagnostic criteria applied. Many studies suggest that the risk of recurrence increases with the time after transplantation (Birnabaum et al, 1997; Campsen et al, 2008; Prados et al, 1998; Sempoux et al, 1997). In an interesting study, Duclos-Vallee et al. suggest that the histological recurrence of AIH may develop 1-5 years before the laboratory manifestations (Duclos-Vallee et al, 2003).

The pathogenesis of recurrent AIH is uncertain, although it is widely accepted that a strong genetic predisposition may affect its occurrence, behavior and outcome (Czaja, 2008a), as well as its risk of recurrence (Czaja, 1999b, 2002, 2009). HLA mismatching between donor and recipient has been proposed as a factor in recurrent disease (Wright, 1992), but its importance continues to be disputed (Gonzales-Koch et al, 2001; Ayata et al, 2000; Milkiewicz, 1999, Reich, 2000, Devlin, 1995). Some authors suggest that matched rather than mismatched HLA may be a factor influencing the development and severity of the disease (Neumann et al, 2003; Futagawa & Terasaki, 2004). In this instance, it seems that similar class II MHC molecules between donor and recipient can intensity the autoreactive response.

HLA DRB1*03 is present in over 70% of the recipients who experience recurrence (Gonzales-Koch et al, 2001), and the DRB1*0301 allele may be a factor in promoting disease severity before transplantation (Czaja, et al, 1997) and disease recurrence after transplantation (Gonzales-Koch et al, 2001, Czaja, 2008b, Devlin et al, 1995). Other autoimmune promoters might include gene polymorphisms that alter the cytokine microenvironment (Czaja et al, 1999a) or involve polymorphisms of genes affecting immunocyte activation, such as those encoding cytotoxic T lymphocyte antigen-4 (Agarwal, 2000). Furthermore, the female predisposition for recurrent AIH suggests that an acquired preferential X chromosome inactivation (that has been described in primary biliary cirrhosis) may also be important (Miozzo et al, 2007). Potential associations with loci in other chromosomes are under investigation (Fukagawa et al, 2001; Vogel et al, 2002).

The donor liver may contain antigenic substrates against which the recipient-derived immunocytes can react, and these substrates could be normal components that share homologies with other self-antigens within the recipient (Czaja, 2002). The structural and conformational homologies between antigenic targets within the donor liver and those within the recipient might provoke a promiscuous T cell response through molecular mimicry.

Knowledge concerning antigenic targets responsible for initiating the cascades of events in recurrent AIH is still rudimentary. A leading candidate has been the asialoglycoprotein receptor, a surface membrane protein. Hepatocytic microsomal enzymes, such as CYP2D6, and cytosolic components, such as transfer ribonucleoprotein complexes, are also under investigation (Czaja, 2002). Professional antigen presenting cells exist outside the liver, and antigenic peptides can be presented and subsequently processed independently of the graft (Obhrai, 2006; Bell & Westermann, 2008; Vierling, 1999). T cell subsets, cross-reactive to homologous hepatic antigens, could be expanded by the presentation of donor antigens on recipient-derived antigen-presenting cells that replace those of the donor liver (Vierling, 1999). The rapidity of this replacement and the number of antigen-presenting cells in the recipient lymph nodes and spleen might affect the timing and severity of the recurrence (Czaja, 2002).

Promiscuous T cells that have been primed to react to molecular homologies are probably already present within the recipient (Sprent, 1993; Vierling, 1999), and the appearance and severity of recurrent AIH simply reflect the dose of antigenic targets within the donor liver (Czaja, 2002). Alternatively, the immunological response may be newly created by protracted exposure to donor-derived hepatic antigens (Czaja 2002, 2009). This hypothesis suggests that recurrent AIH could reflect an immune response against donor liver antigens that is not HLA-restricted (Czaja, 2002). The class II MHC molecules within the donor liver could directly activate the immunocytes of the recipient and generate a response that is not dependent on the presentation of antigenic peptide or HLA matching (Vierling, 1999). In this instance, the MHC molecules of the donor liver would be the antigenic targets and HLA restrictions on immunocyte activation would be overridden.

Components of the Autoreactive Response	**Putative Mechanisms**
Class II MHC molecules	Present autoantigen to T helper lymphocyte Initiate immunocyte activation
HLA susceptibility alleles	Encode structure of the antigen binding groove of the class II MHC molecule Determine optimal autoantigen for presentation *DRB1*03* in white North Americans
Professional antigen presenting cells	Macrophages and dendritic cells Exist outside the liver within the recipient Re-populate the donor liver after transplantation
Donor liver autoantigens	Promote promiscuous T cell response against homologous targets in the donor liver, such as microsomal antigens (CYP2D6, UDGT), cytosolic components (ribonucleoprotein complexes), surface membrane receptors (asialoglyoprotein receptor), class II MHC molecules, or superimposed viral antigens
Promiscuous T lymphocytes	Target multiple antigens in the donor liver that resemble the original activating epitope Retain long memories for the antigenic target Re-invigorate after long dormancy
Counter-regulatory cytokines or regulatory T cell populations	Facilitate autoreactivity by reduced suppressive actions

Abbreviations: CYP2D6, cytochrome 2D6; HLA, human leukocyte antigen; MHC, major histocompatibility complex; UDGT, uridine diphosphate glucuronosyltransferase

Table 1. Pathogenic Mechanisms of Recurrent Autoimmune Hepatitis

Viral infections are another source of antigenic homologies that may activate promiscuous T cells (Czaja, 2002) (Table 1). The genomic sequences of hepatitis C virus, herpes simplex virus, and cytomegalovirus have homologies with CYP2D6 (Manns et al, 1991; Ma et al, 2006), and other mimicries between viral and self-antigens undoubtedly exist that can trigger recurrent AIH (Vergani et al, 2002; Bogdanos et al, 2001). Viruses may also produce an inflammatory process within the graft that may resemble the recurrent AIH. An anti-graft response against a viral antigen may be indistinguishable from an autoimmune response, and the recurrent AIH in this instance could represent a normal immune response against an unsuspected viral agent in an immunosuppressed host (Vierling, 1999). The complexity and inner connectivity of the counter-regulatory mechanisms that must be disrupted to cause recurrent AIH allows broad speculation about the triggering events and the factors which perpetuate the disease (Czaja 2002, 2008b).

Another factor related to the recurrence of AIH is represented by the net state of immunosuppression. Corticosteroid withdrawal, adjustments in the dose and nature of the immunosuppressive drugs (cyclosporine, tacrolimus, and mycophenolate mofetil), acute and chronic rejection, superimposed infection, and drug toxicities are post-transplantation events that have all been implicated in the recurrence of AIH (Hubscher, 2001; Neuberger, 2002; Schreuder et al, 2009). Recurrence has been associated with reduction in the doses of immunosuppressive medication, especially corticosteroids (Neuberger et al, 1984; Gonzalez-Koch et al, 2001; Prados et al, 1998; Khalaf et al, 2007). These observations indicate that the pathogenic mechanisms of AIH are perpetuated after liver transplantation and that they can be suppressed but not eradicated by treatment schedules that are properly dosed (Czaja, 1999b). Recent studies, however, have indicated that the requirement for corticosteroid suppression may not be permanent after liver transplantation and that corticosteroid therapy can be successfully withdrawn in 50-68% of patients (Campsen et al, 2008; Trouillot et al, 1999). There is evidence that AIH recurs in 35% of individuals withdrawn from corticosteroids, but the recurrence has not been associated with discontinuation of the medication by multivariate analysis (Campsen et al, 2008). These findings do not discount the earlier observations that corticosteroid withdrawal or dose reduction contributes to disease recurrence, but they suggest that successful withdrawal is possible if the effort is persistent, individualized and well-timed (Czaja, 1999b).

Patients transplanted for AIH have a higher frequency of acute and chronic rejection (81% versus 47%, $p<0.001$) and corticosteroid-resistant rejection (38% versus 13%, $p=0.003$) than patients transplanted for other conditions (Vogel et al, 2004; Hayashi et al, 1998), and in one series, the frequency of acute cellular rejection was higher (33% versus 14%) than in other transplanted patients from the same institution and from other institutions (33% versus 4%) (Czaja, 1999b; Trouillot et al, 1999). The propensity for acute and chronic cellular rejection may reflect an intrinsic immune hyper-reactivity within the patient with AIH (Czaja, 1999b). Alternatively, rejection may be the basis for releasing hepatic antigens that sensitize the susceptible individual and trigger the recurrence (Czaja, 2009). Patients with recurrent AIH have a higher frequency of rejection during the first 3, 6 and 12 months after transplantation than patients without recurrent disease, but previous rejection is not a requisite for recurrence (Molmenti et al, 2002). Another factor that has been implicated in recurrence has been the calcineurin inhibitors used in the immunosuppressive regimen after transplantation (Schreuder et al, 2009; Gautam et al, 2006). Cyclosporine and tacrolimus may have paradoxical effects which can promote the autoreactive response. Cyclosporine inhibits signal transduction from the engaged T cell antigen receptor (Hess et al, 2001), and it may also have a direct toxic effect on the thymic stroma (Beschorner et al, 1988). These actions may alter the editing of T lymphocytes within the thymus and impair the negative selection of autoreactive cells. Furthermore, the impairment of T cell antigen receptor signaling can prevent the apoptosis of autoreactive lymphocytes which can in turn extend their survival (Lotem et al, 1999; Wang et al, 1999). Tacrolimus affects the thymic microenvironment in a fashion like cyclosporine, and it might also paradoxically enhance immune reactivity (Cooper et al, 1991). These theoretical considerations have not been established in human disease (Gautam et al, 2006), and both medications have been used successfully in the treatment of recurrent AIH (Hubscher, 2001). Nevertheless, the failure of recurrent AIH to respond to one calcineurin inhibitor might warrant institution of the other (Hurtova et al, 2001).

Risk Factor	**Theoretical Consequences**
Long duration after transplantation	Activated "memory immunocytes" re-charge Corticosteroids are withdrawn Immunosuppressive regimens are reduced Acute or chronic cellular rejection occurs Drug toxicity develops Viral infection superimposed
Corticosteroid withdrawal	Facilitates autoimmune response
Reduced immunosuppression	Facilitates autoimmune response
Acute or chronic rejection	Releases hepatic antigens Invigorates promiscuous lymphocytes
Calcineurin inhibitor	Reduces thymic negative selection of immunocytes Impairs apoptosis of activated immunocytes Provokes paradoxical autoreactive response
HLA matching or mismatching	Intensifies autoreactive response
Female gender	Acquired preferential X chromosome inactivation Impairs mechanisms that protect self-tolerance
Severity of original disease	Immune reactivity persists post-transplant Genetic predisposition for severe disease facilitates recurrence

Table 2. Risk Factors Associated with Recurrent Autoimmune Hepatitis After Transplantation

The severity of the original liver disease may also be a factor in disease recurrence after liver transplantation. Patients with recurrent AIH have higher serum levels of immunoglobulin G and histological findings of plasma cell infiltration and severe inflammatory activity more often immediately prior to transplantation than patients without recurrence (Montano-Loza et al, 2009). These observations suggest that recurrent AIH is a continuum of the original disease or a newly created process in a susceptible host with a propensity for severe immune reactivity (Czaja, 2009). They imply that aggressive disease suppression immediately prior to transplantation might alter the consequences after transplantation (Montano-Loza et al, 2009) or that an vulnerable individual may be identified early who warrants close surveillance after transplantation (Czaja, 2009). Most likely, the intrinsic bases for recurrent AIH interact with the extrinsic factors to define the true risk.

2.2 Pathogenesis of de novo AIH

De novo AIH is a late complication that develops in patients undergoing transplantation for nonautoimmune liver disease (Czaja, 2002, 2007b). Since its first description by the King's College group (Kerkar et al, 1998), it has been widely reported in both adult and child recipients after deceased or living liver donor (Hernandez et al, 2001; Gupta et al, 2001; Henegan et al, 2001; Salcedo et al, 2002; Aguilera et al, 2001; Miyagawa et al, 2004; Inui et al, 2005; Venick et al, 2007; Di Cocco et al, 2008). The frequency of de novo disease may be increased because the population at risk is exposed to a great number of risk factors. Children seem to have a predilection for the syndrome (Birnbaum et al, 1997; Campsen et al, 2008; Duclos-Valle et al, 2003; Yao et al, 2007; Czaja & Freese, 2002) and immunosuppression with cyclosporine is a common feature (Birnbaum et al, 1997; Pappo et al, 1995; Czaja & Freese, 2002).

Pathogenic mechanisms involved in the de novo AIH probably are the same as those responsible for the disease before transplantation. Impaired negative selection of autoreactive immunocytes and molecular mimicry are still the principal pathogenic considerations, but their emergence as initiators of disease must be analyzed within the context of the clinical setting. Immunosuppressive therapy and exposure to diverse pathogens after transplantation may severely compromise the ability of an immune system already weakened by chronic illness and/or immaturity to preserve self tolerance.

Cyclosporine inhibits signal transduction from the engaged T-cell antigen receptor (Ayata et al, 2002) and also may have a direct toxic effect on the thymic stroma (Seyam et al, 2007). These actions may alter the editing of T lymphocytes within the thymus and impair the negative selection of autoreactive cells. Impairment of T cell antigen-receptor signaling can prevent the apoptosis of class II MHC-restricted autoreactive lymphocytes, which in turn may leak into the peripheral compartment and be intolerant of self. Cyclosporine inhibits the calcineurin-mediated pathway in the signaling of the apoptosis, and in this fashion, it may extend the survival of autoreactive cells (Czaja, 1999b, 2007b; Khalaf et al, 2007). Active immune mediated lesions within the colon, liver, stomach, and pancreas have been described in an animal model treated with cyclosporine, and the findings constitute cyclosporine-induced autoimmune disease (Trouillot et al, 1999).

A T-cell-dependent autoaggressive disease also has been reported after syngenic and/or autologous bone marrow transplantation in recipients treated with cyclosporine (Hayashi et al, 1998), and it may reflect cyclosporine-induced failure of T-lymphocytes to recognize class II MHC antigens as self (Gautam et al, 2006; Hess et al, 2001). Pretreatment of animal models of bone marrow transplantation with monoclonal antibodies against class II MHC determinants prevents adoptive transfer of syngenic graft-versus-host disease, whereas antibodies against class I MHC antigens are unable to prevent this outcome (Beschorner et al, 1988; Lotem et al, 1999). Tacrolimus affects the thymic microenvironment in a fashion like cyclosporine, and it also can induce a graft-versus-host-like reaction after syngenic bone marrow transplantation in rats (Cooper et al, 1991). These observations suggest that such immunosuppressive drugs (cyclosporine and tacrolimus) may have paradoxical effects in some liver transplant patients. Immunosuppression is the desired primary action, but enhanced autoreactivity may be a secondary consequence in some individuals. Young patients with immature immune system would logically be most vulnerable for the autoimmune response and most instances of de novo AIH have been reported in the pediatric group. An active thymus, immature T-cell-antigen receptor repertoire and repeated exposure to multiple homologous infectious and/or drug-related antigens would be likely additional requisites for de novo disease.

Importantly, no conclusive data show that cyclosporine or tacrolimus induce AIH in humans, and both medications have been used successfully to treat classic AIH in adults and children (Cooper et al, 1991; Hurtova et al, 2001; Czaja, 2008; Wright et al, 1992; Reich et al, 2000; Devlin et al, 1995). Furthermore, animal models of cyclosporine-induced AIH have been highly perturbed models that may have no clinical relevance (Trouillot et al, 1999).

3. Clinical features and diagnostic criteria

AIH is an inflammatory process of unknown cause that is characterized by increased serum aspartate (AST) and alanine (ALT) aminotransferase levels, hypergammaglobinemia, autoantibodies, and interface hepatitis on histological examination (Krawitt, 2006; Czaja & Freese, 2002). Immunoglobulin G is the predominant serum γ-globulin component that is abnormally increased, and the typical autoantibodies associated with the disease are antinuclear antibodies (ANA), smooth muscle antibodies (SMA), and antibodies to liver kidney microsome type 1 (anti-LKM1) (Czaja, 2007b).

Antinuclear antibodies and SMA tend to cluster together, and they are not commonly expressed in association with anti-LKM1 (Homberg et al, 1987; Czaja et al, 1992; Czaja, 1999a). This mutual exclusivity has justified the designations of type 1 AIH to identify the disease associated with ANA and SMA and type 2 AIH to identify the disease associated with anti-LKM1 (Czaja & Manns, 1995). These terms have not been endorsed by the International Autoimmune Hepatitis Group (IAIHG) since the serological types may not be distinct pathological entities (Alvarez et al, 1999). Nevertheless, the designations have been useful descriptors in clinical practice and in research studies, and they have become entrenched in the terminology of the disease. The same basic features of AIH in the native liver have characterized recurrent AIH in the transplanted liver.

Transplant recipients with AIH are younger and more commonly women than other transplant recipients (Molmenti et al, 2002), and they have HLA DRB1*03 more frequently (Sanchez-Urdazpal et al, 1992; Gonzalez-Koch et al, 2001). HLA DRB1*03 and DRB1*04 are the principal susceptibility factors for AIH in white North American and northern European patients (Donaldson et al, 1991), and HLA DRB1*03 has been associated with early age of disease onset and a higher frequency of treatment failure than patients with other HLA (Czaja et al, 1993, 1997; Czaja & Carpenter, 2006). The same clinical phenotype that has typified AIH in native patients also characterizes the patients who develop recurrent disease after transplantation (Gonzalez-Koch et al, 2001; Hubscher, 2001). In de novo AIH, Salcedo et al. found a significant increase in the prevalence of HLA DR3 and a trend to higher frequencies for HLA-B8, -DR15, -DR51 and –Q6 (Salcedo et al, 2002). Symptoms may vary from none to severe (jaundice and hepatic failure), and the presence of disease must be actively sought in asymptomatic patients by the regular monitoring of liver indices (serum AST, ALT, bilirubin, and γ-globulin levels) and protocol liver biopsies (Pappo et al, 1995; Duclos-Vallee et al, 2003; Yao et al, 2007).

Type	**Feature**	**Frequency**
Clinical	Female	Common
	Young	Common
	Asymptomatic	Common
	Jaundice	Rare
Laboratory	Increased Serum AST/ALT	Required
	Increased Serum γ-globulin	Usual
	Increased Serum immunoglobulin G	Usual
	HLA DRB1*03	Common (ethnic dependent)
	No viral markers	Required
Serological	ANA/SMA	Common
	Anti-LKM1	Possible
Histological	Interface hepatitis	Required
	Plasma cell infiltration	Common
	Lobular hepatitis	Rare
	Acidophil bodies	Rare
	Mixed features	Possible
	Non-specific hepatitis	Possible

Abbreviations: ALT, alanine aminotransferase; AST, aspartate aminotransferase; ANA, antinuclear antibodies; anti-LKM1, antibodies to liver/kidney microsome type 1; HLA, human leukocyte antigen; SMA, smooth muscle antibodies

Table 3. Clinical Features of Recurrent Autoimmune Hepatitis After Liver Transplantation

The importance of autoantibodies in the diagnosis of recurrent and de novo AIH is still debated. The majority of patients in whom a diagnosis of recurrent AIH is made have positive autoantibodies. However, several studies have shown that autoantibodies persist in the majority of patients who undergo transplantation for AIH, generally at lower titers than before liver transplantation, irrespective of other features suggestive of disease recurrence (Ahmed et al, 1997; Prados et al, 1998; Gotz et al, 1999; Reich et al, 2000). This is analogous to the situation that exists for patients undergoing liver transplantation for primary biliary cirrhosis; most remain positive for antimitochondrial antibodies without necessarily having other features to suggest disease recurrence (Esquivel et al, 1988; Mattalia et al, 1997). One study suggested that the presence of autoantibodies in titers exceeding pretransplantation levels may be the manifestation of recurrent AIH (Reich et al, 2000) but this observation, based on small number of cases requires further confirmation. It is possible as suggested by Gonzales-Koch et al., that the formation of autoantibodies may be impaired in the setting of immunosuppression (Gonzales-Koch et al, 2001). Impaired antibody formation after liver transplantation is well recognized in hepatitis C virus (HCV)-positive patients, many of whom have high viral RNA levels without detectable anti-HCV antibodies (Poterucha et al, 1992; Hsu et al, 1994).

Autoantibodies arising de novo after liver transplantation have also been noted in association with episodes of rejection (Duclos-Valle et al, 2000). Classic autoantibodies are commonly present in the serum of these patients but atypical serum autoantibodies are characteristically observed (Alvarez et al, 1999; Hubscher, 2001). Among these atypical antibodies, one antibody type seems to be direct against the cytosolic enzyme glutathione S-transferase T1. Interestingly GSTT1 mismatch between the donor and the recipient has been reported as a prerequisite for the development of de novo AIH after liver transplantation (Aguilera et al, 2001; Inui et al, 2005). In addition the early detection of anti-GSTT1 antibodies may help to identify a subset of patients at risk of developing de novo AIH (Salcedo et al, 2009).

Several studies have shown the important role of the routine liver biopsies in the diagnosis of AIH without biochemical evidence of hepatitis (Ahmed et al, 1997; Prados et al, 1998; Gotz et al, 1999). Interface hepatitis is the histological hallmark of recurrent AIH after transplantation, and plasma cell infiltration is a feature of the disease (Gonzalez-Koch et al, 2001; Hubscher, 2001; Ayata et al, 2000; Banff Working Group et al, 2006) Concurrent immunosuppressive therapy can modify the nature and severity of the inflammatory infiltrate, and the histological diagnosis may be based on more subtle changes than those observed in the native disease (Gonzalez-Koch et al, 2001; Hubscher, 2001). Plasma cell infiltration is neither specific nor required for the diagnosis of recurrent AIH (Banff Working Group et al, 2006). Acidophil bodies in conjunction with lymphoplasmacytic infiltrates are seen in early recurrent AIH (Ayata et al, 2000), and an acute lobular hepatitis is also compatible with the diagnosis (Ayata et al, 2000; Sempoux et al, 1997). The histological changes of acute or chronic rejection may occur simultaneously with those of AIH, and concurrent pathological processes must be considered when confusing mixed and atypical histological features are present (Pappo et al, 1995; Hytiroglou et al, 2009).

The histological findings of de novo AIH may differ from the interface hepatitis usually found in the classic AIH (Gupta et al, 2001). In de novo AIH there is histological evidence of portal and periportal hepatitis with or without centrilobular necrosis and lymphoplasmacytic portal tract infiltrate with a variable degree of plasma cells. Histological features of bile ductular proliferation and markedly increased serum concentrations of gamma glutamyl transpeptidase suggest the likelihood of treatment failure and probably indicate a variant syndrome of AIH (Campsen et al, 2008; Berg et al, 2002). De novo disease in some adults has been associated with severe centrilobular necrosis that may confound diagnosis and adult patients have been reported to express an atypical antiliver/kidney cytosolic antibody of uncertain pathogenic significance (Czaja, 2007b). This antibody reacts to rat hepatocyte cytoplasm, chiefly in the centrilobular area, and also shows indirect immunofluorescence in distal and proximal tubules of rat kidney (Czaja, 2007b).

The diagnostic guidelines (Alvarez et al, 1999), not tested in patients receiving immunosuppressive therapy, cannot be used with confidence in the post-transplantation setting (Hubscher, 2001; Li & Neuberger, 2009; Neuberger, 2002; Duclos-Valle, 2005; Schreuder et al, 2009). As stated before, the diagnosis of recurrent and de novo AIH requires the presence of compatible clinical, laboratory and histological findings, and it depends mainly on the exclusion of other conditions that can resemble it (Milkiewicz et al, 1999).

Acute or chronic cellular rejection is the main diagnosis that must be excluded (Banff Working Group et al, 2006; Lefkowitch, 2002). The key clinical distinctions between AIH after liver transplantation and acute cellular rejection are time to disease onset, HLA DRB1*03 status, and autoantibody production. Recurrent autoimmune hepatitis develops after a median interval of 2 years (Czaja, 2002, 2009; Gonzalez-Koch et al, 2001), whereas acute cellular rejection typically develops within 6 weeks after transplantation with a median interval of 8 days (Wiesner et al, 1998). Patients with recurrent AIH commonly have HLA DRB1*03, and they have autoantibodies of substantial titer (Sanchez-Urdazpal et al, 1992; Gonzalez-Koch et al, 2001). The major histological distinctions between recurrent AIH and acute cellular rejection are the moderate-severe interface hepatitis and plasma cell infiltration that characterize AIH, and the eosinophils, endotheliitis, and cholangitis that characterize acute cellular rejection (Lefkowitch, 2002).

Autoimmune hepatitis and chronic rejection each occur months after transplantation, but this is their only point of resemblance. Each condition should be easily distinguished from the other as cholestasis, portal ductopenia, centrilobular fibrosis, and foam cell arteriopathy characterize chronic rejection (Banff Working Group et al, 2006; Lefkowitch, 2002). The principal pathogenic distinctions between the recurrent AIH and the rejection responses probably relate to the origin of the antigen-presenting cells that initiate the immune response and the nature of the antigens that are targeted by the activated immunocytes. The autoimmune response requires re-population of the donor liver with antigen-presenting cells (such as dendritic cells and macrophages) from the recipient. The presentation of self-antigens common to both the donor and recipient can initiate the autoimmune response in the donor liver. In contrast, the rejection response is based on the reactivity of promiscuous cytotoxic T lymphocytes from the recipient against foreign antigens presented by the donor liver, including class II MHC molecules, viral proteins, and novel donor organ antigens (Czaja, 2002; Vierling, 1999).

Plasma cell hepatitis and isolated central perivenulitis can also confuse the diagnosis of recurrent AIH. Each condition is probably a variant of rejection. Plasma cell hepatitis does not improve with corticosteroid treatment; it may develop as immunosuppressive therapy is reduced; and it improves as the immunosuppressive regimen is intensified (Demetris & Sebagh, 2008; Fiel et al, 2008). Isolated central perivenulitis can be found in 28% of allografts, and it can lead to de novo autoimmune hepatitis or chronic liver injury, especially if it occurs late after transplantation (Krasinskas et al, 2008). Typically, perivenulitis is untreated, but this approach is debated and anti-rejection therapy has been proposed.

Diagnosis	Distinctive Features
Recurrent autoimmune hepatitis	Late onset (median, 2 years) Interface hepatitis Plasma cell infiltration Autoantibodies (serum titer ≥1:320) HLA DRB1*03 (ethnic dependent)
Acute cellular rejection	Early onset (median, 8 days) Endotheliitis Cholangitis (histological finding) Eosinophilic infiltrates
Chronic cellular rejection	Late onset (range, 3-8 months) Cholestasis (histological finding) Portal ductopenia Centrilobular fibrosis Foam cell arteriopathy
Plasma cell hepatitis	Rejection variant Associated with reduced immunosuppression Unresponsive to corticosteroids Improves with increased immunosuppression
Isolated central perivenulitis	Rejection variant Progressive if late occurrence May result in autoimmune hepatitis
Hepatitis C virus infection	Portal lymphoplasmacytic response possible Serological markers of active viremia
De novo AIH	Late onset (median, 2 years) Children predilection Interface hepatitis Portal and periportal hepatitis with or without centrilobular necrosis and lymphoplasmacytic portal tract infiltrate Autoantibodies (classic and atypical) Response to prednisone and azathioprine

Table 4. Differential Diagnosis of Recurrent and De Novo AIH After Transplantation

Superimposed viral infections, especially HCV, must always be excluded in patients with graft disruption after transplantation because may elicit a pronounced lymphoplasmacytic response within the portal tract that can be difficult to distinguish from recurrent AIH (Banff Working Group et al, 2006; Demetris & Sebagh, 2008). Furthermore, recurrent AIH and HCV infection may occur together in the same allograft (Pappo et al, 1995). A comprehensive virological assessment is warranted to exclude infection in all patients with features of recurrent AIH after transplantation.

The absence of reliable diagnostic markers for recurrent AIH has compelled reliance on the histological findings to support the diagnosis, and the features of nonspecific chronic hepatitis have been the minimal bases for the diagnosis in some cases (Hubscher, 2001). Seronegative AIH has been described in native patients (Czaja et al, 1993; Gassert et al, 2007; Heringlake et al, 2009), and there is an emerging experience that suggests that it may be a relevant consideration in patients with graft dysfunction after liver transplantation (Nakhleh et al, 2005; Berg et al, 2002; Ayata et al, 2002; Seyam et al, 2007). Most patients who undergo liver transplantation for cryptogenic chronic hepatitis can be classified into conventional diagnostic categories after review of their liver tissue specimens before and after liver transplantation, but 15% remain cryptogenic and at risk for disease recurrence and progression (Ayata et al, 2002).

Cirrhosis may develop after transplantation in seronegative patients with recurrent histological features of chronic hepatitis, especially in those patients transplanted for seronegative fulminant hepatitis, and the possibility of recurrent seronegative AIH cannot be excluded in these individuals (Seyam et al, 2007). Consequently, recurrent AIH should be considered in all patients with acute and chronic graft dysfunction after liver transplantation. The diagnostic criteria must accommodate the atypical manifestations encountered after transplantation that may reflect superimposed medication effects and diverse other diseases associated with the transplantation.

4. Outcome

Recurrent AIH is typically a mild inflammatory process in an asymptomatic individual who has been inadequately immunosuppressed after transplantation or prematurely withdrawn from corticosteroids (Gonzalez-Koch et al, 2001; Prados et al, 1998; Neuberger, 2002; Khalaf, 2007). Recurrent disease usually responds to the re-introduction of corticosteroid therapy or adjustments in the doses of the original immunosuppressive agents (Gonzalez-Koch et al, 2001; Faust, 2000, 2001). The frequency of recurrence does not correlate with the frequency of graft loss, and patient and graft survivals after recurrence have been similar to those of other transplanted diseases (Li &Neuberger, 2009; Schreuder, 2009). Survival in patients with recurrent disease has ranged from 78-89% (Vogel et al, 2004; Yusoff et al, 2002).

Progression to cirrhosis and graft loss can occur (Milkiewicz et al, 1999; Ratziu et al, 1999; Rowe et al, 2008), and recurrent AIH with graft loss after the second transplantation has been reported (Reich et al, 2000). Furthermore, not all patients with recurrent AIH are inadequately immunosuppressed at the time of presentation (Ratziu et al, 1999) or responsive to the re-institution of corticosteroid therapy (Prados et al, 1998; Neuberger, 2002). Patients with severe, aggressive recurrent AIH have not been fully characterized, and the individuals at risk for a dire outcome cannot be reliably identified. The serological type of the original disease may affect the need for transplantation (Cattan et al, 2002), but it does not correlate with prognosis after transplantation (Vogel et al, 2004). Similarly, the severity of the disease at transplantation does not predict outcome after the procedure (Montano-Loza et al, 2009). Patients transplanted for fulminant AIH have lower frequencies of recurrence after transplantation and better survivals than patients transplanted for chronic AIH (Reich et al, 2000; Nunez-Martinez et al, 2003), but most patients who develop recurrent AIH do not have fulminant presentations. The outcome of de novo AIH remains largely unknown, but several cases with severe liver damage and hepatic failure leading to death have been described (Hernandez et al, 2001), indicating the needing for specific management of this complication.

5. Treatment

The first course of action is to establish the correct diagnosis, reassess the adequacy of the immunosuppressive regimen, and determine the compliance of the patient. Measurement of the drug metabolites in blood may be necessary to ensure the adequacy of dosing and the compliance of the individual (Rumbo et al, 2004). The second course of action is to optimize the doses of the conventional immunosuppressive medication and to re-introduce corticosteroids if they have been withdrawn (Neuberger, 2002). Treatment with prednisone and azathioprine is typically effective in recurrent (Birnbaum et al, 1997; Pappo et al, 1995; Duclos-Vallee et al, 203; Czaja & Freese, 2002; Czaja, 2007b) and de novo AIH (Salcedo et al, 2002). Failure to respond or disease progression despite compliance with therapy justifies a closely monitored empiric trial with alternative immunosuppressive agents. The calcineurin inhibitor could be changed to another drug in this same category (Hurtova et al, 2001); a purine antagonist (azathioprine or mycophenolate mofetil) could be added or its dose optimized (Rumbo et al, 2004); or rapamycin, which is a mTOR (mammalian target of rapamycin) inhibitor, could be introduced (Kerkar et al, 2005). These agents have been reported as effective salvage therapies in small single-center case reports, but none have been established by large multicenter experiences or organized clinical trials. Patients in whom therapy fails have worsening fibrosis and possible graft loss (Vogel et al, 2004; Campsen et al, 2008) and those not administered corticosteroids progress to cirrhosis, require re-transplantation or die of liver failure (Czaja, 2007b). Re-transplantation must be considered if the disease continues to progress with the understanding that the disease could recur in the second graft and again jeopardize its survival (Reich et al, 2000).

6. Summary

AIH commonly recurs after liver transplantation, and asymptomatic histological recurrence may precede clinical recurrence by 1-5 years. Acute and chronic cellular rejection, drug toxicity, and viral infection must be confidently excluded, and treatment typically requires adjustment in the doses of immunosuppressive medication or the re-institution of corticosteroid therapy. Empiric treatments with another calcineurin inhibitor, purine antagonist (azathioprine or mycophenolate mofetil), or mTOR inhibitor (rapamycin) are available for refractory disease, and re-transplantation may be necessary.

Future studies are needed to codify diagnostic criteria, define risk factors that are predictive of recurrence and its progression, standardize surveillance schedules after transplantation, develop a uniform management algorithm, and elucidate mechanisms of disease.

Insights into the pathogenesis of recurrent and de novo AIH may elucidate a similar behavior in the native disease. Native AIH also exacerbates frequently after corticosteroid withdrawal, and this flare may occur after long intervals of quiescence. The concepts that activated immunocytes can trigger the same disease after a long dormancy or that a susceptible host with a genetic predisposition can develop newly created episodes of the same disease may apply to both conditions. The experiences in liver transplantation have much to teach about AIH, and future investigations that clarify the mechanisms of recurrent and of de novo AIH will have broad implications for autoimmune diseases in general, not only for classical AIH. Future investigations must continue to utilize the human transplantation experience to elucidate the key mechanisms of the autoimmune response in the native liver.

7. References

Agarwal, K; Czaja, AJ; Jones, DEJ & Donaldson, PT. CTLA-4 gene polymorphism and susceptibility to type 1 autoimmune hepatitis. Hepatology. 2000;31:49-53

Aguilera, J; Wichmann, I; Sousa, JM; Bernardos, A; Franco, E et al. Antibodies against glutathione-S transferase T1 (GSTT1) in patients with de novo autoimmune hepatitis following liver transplantation. Clin Exp Immunol. 2001;126:535-39

Ahmed, M; Mutimer, D; Hathaway, M; Hubscher, S; McMaster, P & Elias, E. Liver transplantation for autoimmune hepatitis: a 12-year experience. Transplant Proc. 1997;29:496

Alvarez, F; Berg, PA; Bianchi, FB; Bianchi, L; Burroughs, AK; Cancado, EL; et al. International Autoimmune Hepatitis Group Report: review of criteria for diagnosis of autoimmune hepatitis. J Hepatol. 1999;31(5):929-38

Ayata, G; Gordon, FD; Lewis, WD; Pomfret, E; Pomposelli, JJ; Jenkins, RL; et al. Cryptogenic cirrhosis: clinicopathologic findings at and after liver transplantation. Hum Pathol. 2002;33(11):1098-104

Ayata, G; Gordon, FD; Lewis, WD; Pomfret, E; Pomposelli, JJ; Jenkins, RL; et al. Liver transplantation for autoimmune hepatitis: a long-term pathologic study. Hepatology. 2000;32(2):185-92

Banff Working Group, Demetris AJ, Adeyi O, Bellamy CO, Clouston A, Charlotte F, et al. Liver biopsy interpretation for causes of late liver allograft dysfunction. Hepatology. 2006;44(2):489-501

Bell, EB & Westermann, J. CD4 memory T cells on trial: immunological memory without a memory T cell. Trends Immunol. 2008;29(9):405-11

Berg, T; Neuhaus, R; Klein, R; Leder, K; Lobeck, H; Bechstein, WO; et al. Distinct enzyme profiles in patients with cryptogenic cirrhosis reflect heterogeneous causes with different outcomes after liver transplantation (OLT): a long-term documentation before and after OLT. Transplantation. 2002;74(6):792-8

Beschorner, WE; Suresch, DL; Shinozawa, T; Santos, GW & Hess, AD. Thymic immunopathology after cyclosporine: effect of irradiation and age on medullary involution and recovery. Transplant Proc. 1988;20(3 Suppl 3):1072-8

Bethoux, F; Miller, DM & Kinkel, RP. Recovery following acute exacerbations of multiple sclerosis: from impairment to quality of life. Mult Scler. 2001;7(2):137-42

Birnbaum, AH; Benkov, KJ; Pittman, NS; McFarlane-Ferreira, Y; Rosh, JR & LeLeiko, NS. Recurrence of autoimmune hepatitis in children after liver transplantation. J Pediatr Gastroenterol Nutr. 1997;25(1):20-5

Bogdanos, DP; Choudhuri, K & Vergani, D. Molecular mimicry and autoimmune liver disease: virtuous intentions, malign consequences. Liver. 2001;21(4):225-32

Campsen, J; Zimmerman, MA; Trotter, JF; Wachs, M; Bak, T; Steinberg, T; et al. Liver transplantation for autoimmune hepatitis and the success of aggressive corticosteroid withdrawal. Liver Transpl. 2008;14(9):1281-6

Cattan, P; Berney, T; Conti, F; Calmus, Y; Homberg, JC; Houssin, D; et al. Outcome of orthotopic liver transplantation in autoimmune hepatitis according to subtypes. Transpl Int. 2002;15(1):34-8

Ciruelo, E; de la Cruz, J; Lopez, I & Gomez-Reino, JJ. Cumulative rate of relapse of lupus nephritis after successful treatment with cyclophosphamide. Arthritis Rheum. 1996;39(12):2028-34

Cooper, MH; Hartman, GG; Starzl, TE & Fung, JJ. The induction of pseudo-graft-versus-host disease following syngeneic bone marrow transplantation using FK 506. Transplant Proc. 1991;23(6):3234-5

Czaja, AJ. Recurrent autoimmune hepatitis after liver transplantation: a disease continuum or a fresh start? Liver Transpl. 2009;15(10):1169-71

Czaja, AJ. Performance parameters of the diagnostic scoring systems for autoimmune hepatitis. Hepatology. 2008;48(5):1540-8 (a)

Czaja, AJ. Genetic factors affecting the occurrence, clinical phenotype, and outcome of autoimmune hepatitis. Clin Gastroenterol Hepatol. 2008;6(4):379-88 (b)

Czaja AJ. Autoimmune hepatitis. Part A: pathogenesis. Expert Rev Gastroenterol Hepatol. 2007;1(1):113-128 (a)

Czaja, AJ. Autoimmune hepatitis. Part B: diagnosis. Expert Rev Gastroenterol Hepatol. 2007;1(1):129-43 (b)

Czaja AJ. Evolving concepts in the diagnosis, pathogenesis and treatment of autoimmune hepatitis. Minerva Gastroenterol Dietol. 2007;53(1):43-78 (c)

Czaja, AJ & Carpenter, HA. Distinctive clinical phenotype and treatment outcome of type 1 autoimmune hepatitis in the elderly. Hepatology. 2006;43(3):532-8

Czaja, AJ. Autoimmune hepatitis after liver transplantation and other lessons of self-intolerance. Liver Transpl. 2002;8(6):505-13

Czaja, AJ & Freese DK. Diagnosis and treatment of autoimmune hepatitis. Hepatology. 2002;36(2):479-97

Czaja, AJ; Menon, KV & Carpenter, HA. Sustained remission after corticosteroid therapy for type 1 autoimmune hepatitis: a retrospective analysis. Hepatology. 2002;35(4):890-7

Czaja, AJ. Understanding the pathogenesis of autoimmune hepatitis. Am J Gastroenterol. 2001;96(4):1224-1231

Czaja, AJ. Behavior and significance of autoantibodies in type 1 autoimmune hepatitis. J Hepatol. 1999;30(3):394-401 (a)

Czaja, AJ. The immunoreactive propensity of autoimmune hepatitis: is it corticosteroid-dependent after liver transplantation? Liver Transpl Surg. 1999;5(5):460-3 (b)

Czaja, AJ; Strettell, MD; Thomson, LJ; Santrach, PJ; Moore, SB; Donaldson, PT; et al. Associations between alleles of the major histocompatibility complex and type 1 autoimmune hepatitis. Hepatology. 1997;25(2):317-23

Czaja, AJ & Manns, MP. The validity and importance of subtypes in autoimmune hepatitis: a point of view. Am J Gastroenterol. 1995;90(8):1206-11

Czaja, AJ; Carpenter, HA; Santrach, PJ & Moore, SB. Significance of HLA DR4 in type 1 autoimmune hepatitis. Gastroenterology. 1993;105(5):1502-7 (a)

Czaja, AJ; Carpenter, HA; Santrach, PJ; Moore, SB & Homburger, HA. The nature and prognosis of severe cryptogenic chronic active hepatitis. Gastroenterology. 1993;104(6):1755-61 (b)

Czaja, AJ; Manns, MP & Homburger HA. Frequency and significance of antibodies to liver/kidney microsome type 1 in adults with chronic active hepatitis. Gastroenterology. 1992;103(4):1290-5

Demetris, AJ & Sebagh, M. Plasma cell hepatitis in liver allografts: Variant of rejection or autoimmune hepatitis? Liver Transpl. 2008;14(6):750-5

Devlin, J; Donaldson, P; Portmann, B; Heaton, N; Tan, KC & Williams, R. Recurrence of autoimmune hepatitis following liver transplantation. Liver Transpl Surg. 1995;1(3):162-5

Di Cocco, P; Barletta, A; Clemente, K; D'Angelo, M; Greco, S; et al. De novo autoimmune hepatitis following liver transplantation: a case report. Transplant Proc. 2008;40:2073-74

Djilali-Saiah, I; Renous, R; Caillat-Zucman, S; Debray, D & Alvarez, F. Linkage disequilibrium between HLA class II region and autoimmune hepatitis in pediatric patients. J Hepatol. 2004;40:904-9

Donaldson, PT. Genetics in autoimmune hepatitis. Semin Liver Dis 2002; 22: 353-64

Donaldson, PT; Albertini, RJ & Krawitt, EL. Immunogenetic studies of autoimmune hepatitis and primary sclerosing cholangitis. In: Krawitt, EL; Wiesner, RH; Nishioka, M eds. Autoimmune liver diseases. 2nd ed. Amsterdam: Elsevier, 1998:141-65

Donaldson, PT; Doherty, DG; Hayllar, KM; McFarlane, IG; Johnson, PJ & Williams, R. Susceptibility to autoimmune chronic active hepatitis: human leukocyte antigens DR4 and A1-B8-DR3 are independent risk factors. Hepatology. 1991;13(4):701-6

Duclos-Vallee, JC. Recurrence of autoimmune hepatitis, primary biliary cirrhosis and primary sclerosing cholangitis after liver transplantation. Acta Gastroenterol Belg. 2005;68(3):331-6

Duclos-Valle, JC; Johanet, C; Bach, JF & Yamamoto, AM. Autoantibodies associated with acute rejection after liver transplantation for type 2 autoimmune hepatitis. J Hepatol. 2000;33:163-166

Duclos-Vallee, JC; Sebagh, M; Rifai, K; Johanet, C; Ballot, E; Guettier, C; et al. A 10 year follow up study of patients transplanted for autoimmune hepatitis: histological recurrence precedes clinical and biochemical recurrence. Gut. 2003;52(6):893-7

Esquivel, CO; Van Thiel, DG; Demetris, AJ; Bernardos, A; Iwatsuki, S; et al. Transplantation for primary biliary cirrhosis. Gastroenterology. 1988;94:1207-16

Faust, TW. Recurrent primary biliary cirrhosis, primary sclerosing cholangitis, and autoimmune hepatitis after transplantation. Liver Transpl. 2001;7(11 Suppl 1):S99-108

Faust, TW. Recurrent primary biliary cirrhosis, primary sclerosing cholangitis, and autoimmune hepatitis after transplantation. Semin Liver Dis. 2000;20(4):481-95

Fiel, MI; Agarwal, K; Stanca, C; Elhajj, N; Kontorinis, N; Thung, SN; et al. Posttransplant plasma cell hepatitis (de novo autoimmune hepatitis) is a variant of rejection and may lead to a negative outcome in patients with hepatitis C virus. Liver Transpl. 2008;14(6):861-71

Fukagawa, NK; Liang, P; Li, M; Ashikaga, T; Reddy, KR & Krawitt, EL. Glutathione S-transferase M1 null genotype in autoimmune hepatitis. Dig Dis Sci. 2001;46:2080-3

Futagawa, Y & Terasaki, PI. An analysis of the OPTN/UNOS Liver Transplant Registry. Clin Transpl. 2004:315-29

Gassert, DJ; Garcia, H; Tanaka, K & Reinus, JF. Corticosteroid-responsive cryptogenic chronic hepatitis: evidence for seronegative autoimmune hepatitis. Dig Dis Sci. 2007;52(9):2433-7

Gautam, M; Cheruvattath, R & Balan, V. Recurrence of autoimmune liver disease after liver transplantation: a systematic review. Liver Transpl. 2006;12(12):1813-24

Gonzalez-Koch, A; Czaja, AJ; Carpenter, HA; Roberts, SK; Charlton, MR; Porayko, MK; et al. Recurrent autoimmune hepatitis after orthotopic liver transplantation. Liver Transpl. 2001;7(4):302-10

Gotz, G; Heuhas, R; Bechstein, WO; Lobeck, H; Berg, T; et al. Recurrence of autoimmune hepatitis after liver transplantation. Transplant Proc. 1999;31:430-1

Gray, D & Skarvall, H. B-cell memory is short-lived in the absence of antigen. Nature. 1988;336(6194):70-73

Gupta, P; Hart, J; Millis, JM; Cronin, D & Brady, L. De novo hepatitis with autoimmune antibodies and atypical histology: a rare cause of late graft dysfunction after pediatric liver transplantation. Transplantation. 2001;71:664-68

Hayashi, M; Keeffe, EB; Krams, SM; Martinez, OM; Ojogho, ON; So, SK; et al. Allograft rejection after liver transplantation for autoimmune liver diseases. Liver Transpl Surg. 1998;4(3):208-14

Henegan, MA; Portmann, BC; Norris, SM; Williams, R; Muiesan, P et al. Graft dysfunction mimicking autoimmune hepatitis following liver transplantation in adults. Hepatology. 2001;34:464-70

Hennes, EM; Zeniya, M; Czaja, AJ; Pares, A; Dalekos, GN; Krawitt, EL; et al. Simplified criteria for the diagnosis of autoimmune hepatitis. Hepatology. 2008;48(1):169-76

Heringlake, S; Schutte, A; Flemming, P; Schmiegel, W; Manns, MP & Tillmann, HL. Presumed cryptogenic liver disease in Germany: High prevalence of autoantibody-negative autoimmune hepatitis, low prevalence of NASH, no evidence for occult viral etiology. Z Gastroenterol. 2009;47(5):417-23

Hernandez, HM; Kowarik, P; Whitinton, PF & Alonso, EM. Autoimmune hepatitis as a late complication of liver transplantation. J Pediatr Gastroenterol Nutr. 2001;32:131-36

Hess, DA; O'Leary, EF; Lee, JT; Almawi, WY; Madrenas, J & Rieder, MJ. Inhibition of cytokine production and interference in IL-2 receptor-mediated Jak-Stat signaling by the hydroxylamine metabolite of sulfamethoxazole. FASEB J. 2001;15(10):1855-7

Homberg, JC; Abuaf, N; Bernard, O; Islam, S; Alvarez, F; Khalil, SH; et al. Chronic active hepatitis associated with antiliver/kidney microsome antibody type 1: a second type of "autoimmune" hepatitis. Hepatology. 1987;7(6):1333-9

Hsu, HH; Wright, TL; Tsao, SC; Combs, C; Donets, M; et al. Antibody response to hepatitis C infection after liver transplantation. Am J Gastroenterol. 1994;89:1169-74

Hubscher, SG. Recurrent autoimmune hepatitis after liver transplantation: diagnostic criteria, risk factors, and outcome. Liver Transpl. 2001;7(4):285-91

Hurtova, M; Duclos-Vallee, JC; Johanet, C; Emile, JF; Roque-Afonso, AM; Feray, C; et al. Successful tacrolimus therapy for a severe recurrence of type 1 autoimmune hepatitis in a liver graft recipient. Liver Transpl. 2001;7(6):556-8

Hytiroglou P, Gutierrez JA, Freni M, Odin JA, Stanca CM, Merati S, et al. Recurrence of primary biliary cirrhosis and development of autoimmune hepatitis after liver transplant: A blind histologic study. Hepatol Res. 2009;39(6):577-84

Inui, A; Sogo, T; Komatsu, H; Miyakawa, H & Fujisawa, T. Antibodies against cytokeratin 8/18 in a patient with de novo autoimmune hepatitis after living-donor liver transplantation. Liver Transpl. 2005;11: 504-7

Kerkar, N; Dugan, C; Rumbo, C; Morotti, RA; Gondolesi, G; Shneider, BL; et al. Rapamycin successfully treats post-transplant autoimmune hepatitis. Am J Transplant. 2005;5(5):1085-9

Kerkar, H; Hadzic, N; Davies, ET; Portmann, B; Donaldson, PT; et al. De novo autoimmune hepatitis after liver transplantation. Lancet. 1998;35:409-13

Khalaf, H; Mourad, W; El-Sheikh, Y; Abdo, A; Helmy, A; Medhat, Y; et al. Liver transplantation for autoimmune hepatitis: a single-center experience. Transplant Proc. 2007;39(4):1166-70

Krawitt, EL. Autoimmune Hepatitis. N Engl J Med. 2006; 354:54-66

Krasinskas, AM; Demetris, AJ; Poterucha, JJ & Abraham, SC. The prevalence and natural history of untreated isolated central perivenulitis in adult allograft livers. Liver Transpl. 2008;14(5):625-32

Lefkowitch, JH. Diagnostic issues in liver transplantation pathology. Clin Liver Dis. 2002;6(2):555-70

Li, KK & Neuberger, J. Recurrent nonviral liver disease following liver transplantation. Expert Rev Gastroenterol Hepatol. 2009;3(3):257-68

Longhi, MS; Ma, Y; Bogdanos, DP; Cheeseman, P; Mieli-Vergani, G & Vergani, D. Impairment of CD4+CD25+ regulatory T cells in autoimmune liver disease. J Hepatol. 2004;41:31-7

Lotem, J; Kama, R & Sachs, L. Suppression or induction of apoptosis by opposing pathways downstream from calcium-activated calcineurin. Proc Natl Acad Sci U S A. 1999;96(21):12016-20

Ma, Y; Bogdanos, DP; Hussain, MJ; Underhill, J; Bansal, S; Longhi, MS; et al. Polyclonal T-cell responses to cytochrome P450IID6 are associated with disease activity in autoimmune hepatitis type 2. Gastroenterology. 2006;130(3):868-82

Manns, MP & Vogel A. Autoimmune hepatitis, from mechanisms to therapy. Hepatology. 2006;43(2 Suppl 1):S132-144

Manns, MP; Griffin, KJ; Sullivan, KF & Johnson, EF. LKM-1 autoantibodies recognize a short linear sequence in P450IID6, a cytochrome P-450 monooxygenase. J Clin Invest. 1991;88(4):1370-8

Mattalia, A; Lurtig, B; Rosina, F; Leung, PS; Van de Water, J; et al. Persistence of autoantibodies against recombinant mitochondrial and nuclear pore proteins after orthotopic liver transplantation for primary biliary cirrhosis. J Autoimmun. 1997;10:491-497

McLean, AR & Michie, CA. In vivo estimates of division and death rates of human T lymphocytes. Proc Natl Acad Sci U S A. 1995;92(9):3707-11

Milkiewicz, P; Hubscher, SG; Skiba, G; Hathaway, M & Elias, E. Recurrence of autoimmune hepatitis after liver transplantation. Transplantation. 1999;68(2):253-6

Miozzo, M; Selmi, C; Gentilin, B; Grati, FR; Sirchia, S; Oertelt, S; et al. Preferential X chromosome loss but random inactivation characterize primary biliary cirrhosis. Hepatology. 2007;46(2):456-62

Miyagawa-Hayashino, A; Haga, H; Egawa, H; Hayashimo, Y; Sakurai, T; et al. Outcome and risk factors of de novo autoimmune hepatitis in living donor liver transplantation. Transplantation. 2004;78:128-35

Molmenti, EP; Netto, GJ; Murray, NG; Smith, DM; Molmenti, H; Crippin, JS; et al. Incidence and recurrence of autoimmune/alloimmune hepatitis in liver transplant recipients. Liver Transpl. 2002;8(6):519-26

Montano-Loza, AJ; Mason, AL; Ma, M; Bastiampillai, RJ; Bain, VG & Tandon, P. Risk factors for recurrence of autoimmune hepatitis after liver transplantation. Liver Transpl. 2009;15(10):1254-61

Nakhleh, RE; Krishna, M; Keaveny, AP; Dickson, RC; Rosser, B; Nguyen, JH; et al. Review of 31 cases of morphologic hepatitis in liver transplant patients not related to disease recurrence. Transplant Proc. 2005;37(2):1240-2

Neuberger, J. Transplantation for autoimmune hepatitis. Semin Liver Dis. 2002;22(4):379-86

Neuberger, J; Portmann, B; Calne, R & Williams, R. Recurrence of autoimmune chronic active hepatitis following orthotopic liver grafting. Transplantation. 1984;37(4):363-5

Neumann, UP; Guckelberger, O; Langrehr, JM; Lang, M; Schmitz, V; Theruvath, T; et al. Impact of human leukocyte antigen matching in liver transplantation. Transplantation. 2003;75(1):132-7

Nunez-Martinez, O; De la Cruz, G; Salcedo, M; Molina, J; De Diego, A; Ripoll, C; et al. Liver transplantation for autoimmune hepatitis: fulminant versus chronic hepatitis presentation. Transplant Proc. 2003;35(5):1857-8

Obhrai, JS; Oberbarnscheidt, MH; Hand, TW; Diggs, L; Chalasani, G & Lakkis, FG. Effector T cell differentiation and memory T cell maintenance outside secondary lymphoid organs. J Immunol. 2006;176(7):4051-8

Pappo, O; Ramos, H; Starzl, TE; Fung, JJ & Demetris AJ. Structural integrity and identification of causes of liver allograft dysfunction occurring more than 5 years after transplantation. Am J Surg Pathol. 1995;19(2):192-206

Poterucha, JJ; Rakela, J; Lumeng, L; Lee, CH; Taswell, HF; et al. Diagnosis of chronic hepatitis C after liver transplantation by the detection of viral sequences with polymerase chain reaction. Hepatology. 1992;14:42-45

Prados, E; Cuervas-Mons, V; de la Mata, M; Fraga, E; Rimola ,A; Prieto, M; et al. Outcome of autoimmune hepatitis after liver transplantation. Transplantation. 1998;66(12):1645-50

Ratziu, V; Samuel, D; Sebagh, M; Farges, O; Saliba, F; Ichai, P; et al. Long-term follow-up after liver transplantation for autoimmune hepatitis: evidence of recurrence of primary disease. J Hepatol. 1999;30(1):131-41

Reich, DJ; Fiel, I; Guarrera, JV; Emre, S; Guy, SR; Schwartz, ME; et al. Liver transplantation for autoimmune hepatitis. Hepatology. 2000;32(4 Pt 1):693-700

Rowe, IA; Webb, K; Gunson, BK; Mehta, N; Haque, S & Neuberger, J. The impact of disease recurrence on graft survival following liver transplantation: a single centre experience. Transpl Int. 2008;21(5):459-65

Rumbo, C; Shneider, BL & Emre, SH. Utility of azathioprine metabolite measurements in post-transplant recurrent autoimmune and immune-mediated hepatitis. Pediatr Transplant. 2004;8(6):571-5

Salcedo, M; Rodriguez-Mahou, M; Rodriguez-Sainz, C Rincon, D; Alvarez, E; et al. Risk factors for developing de novo autoimmune hepatitis associated with anti-glutathione S-transferase T1 antibodies after liver transplantation. Liver Transpl. 2009;15:530-9

Salcedo, M; Vaquero, J; Banares, R; Rodriguez-Mahou, M; Alvarez, E et al. Response to steroids in de novo autoimmune epatiti after liver transplantation. Hepatology. 2002;35:349-55

Sanchez-Urdazpal, L; Czaja, AJ; van Hoek, B; Krom, RA & Wiesner, RH. Prognostic features and role of liver transplantation in severe corticosteroid-treated autoimmune chronic active hepatitis. Hepatology. 1992;15(2):215-21

Schreuder, TC; Hubscher, SG & Neuberger, J. Autoimmune liver diseases and recurrence after orthotopic liver transplantation: what have we learned so far? Transpl Int. 2009;22(2):144-52

Sempoux, C; Horsmans, Y; Lerut, J; Rahier, J & Geubel, A. Acute lobular hepatitis as the first manifestation of recurrent autoimmune hepatitis after orthotopic liver transplantation. Liver. 1997;17(6):311-5

Seyam, M; Neuberger, JM; Gunson, BK & Hubscher, SG. Cirrhosis after orthotopic liver transplantation in the absence of primary disease recurrence. Liver Transpl. 2007;13(7):966-74

Sprent, J. Lifespans of naive, memory and effector lymphocytes. Curr Opin Immunol. 1993;5(3):433-8

Trouillot, TE; Shrestha, R; Kam, I; Wachs, M & Everson, GT. Successful withdrawal of prednisone after adult liver transplantation for autoimmune hepatitis. Liver Transpl Surg. 1999;5(5):375-80

Venick, RS; McDiarmid, SV; Farmer, DG; Gornbein, J; Martin, MG; et al. Rejection and steroid dependence: unique risk factors in the development of pediatric posttransplant de novo autoimmune hepatitis. Am J Transplant. 2007;7:955-63

Vergani, D & Mieli-Vergani G. Aetiopathogenesis of autoimmune hepatitis. World J Gastroenterol. 2008;14(21):3306-12

Vergani, D; Choudhuri, K; Bogdanos, DP & Mieli-Vergani, G. Pathogenesis of autoimmune hepatitis. Clin Liver Dis. 2002;6(3):727-737

Vierling, JM. Immunology of acute and chronic hepatic allograft rejection. Liver Transpl Surg. 1999;5(4 Suppl 1):S1-S20

Vogel, A; Heinrich, E; Bahr, MJ; Rifai, K; Flemming, P; Melter, M; et al. Long-term outcome of liver transplantation for autoimmune hepatitis. Clin Transplant. 2004;18(1):62-9

Vogel, A; Strassburg, CP & Manns, MP. Genetic association of vitamin D receptor polymorphisms with primary biliary cirrhosis and autoimmune hepatitis. Hepatology. 2002;35:126-31

Wang, HG; Pathan, N; Ethell, IM; Krajewski, S; Yamaguchi, Y; Shibasaki, F; et al. Ca2+-induced apoptosis through calcineurin dephosphorylation of BAD. Science. 1999;284(5412):339-43

Wiesner, RH; Demetris, AJ; Belle, SH; Seaberg, EC; Lake, JR; Zetterman, RK; et al. Acute hepatic allograft rejection: incidence, risk factors, and impact on outcome. Hepatology. 1998;28(3):638-45

Wright, HL; Bou-Abboud, CF; Hassanein, T; Block, GD; Demetris, AJ; Starzl, TE; et al. Disease recurrence and rejection following liver transplantation for autoimmune chronic active liver disease. Transplantation. 1992;53(1):136-9

Yao, H; Michitaka, K; Tokumoto, Y; Murata, Y; Mashiba, T; Abe, M; et al. Recurrence of autoimmune hepatitis after liver transplantation without elevation of alanine aminotransferase. World J Gastroenterol. 2007;13(10):1618-21

Yusoff, IF; House, AK; De Boer, WB; Ferguson, J; Garas, G; Heath, D; et al. Disease recurrence after liver transplantation in Western Australia. J Gastroenterol Hepatol. 2002;17(2):203-7

18

Bone Disease After Organ Transplantation with Special Regard of Post Transplantation-Osteoporosis After Liver Transplantation

Daniel Kaemmerer[1] and Gabriele Lehmann[2]
[1]*Zentralklinik Bad Berka,*
[2]*Department of Internal Medicine III, University Hospital Jena*
Germany

1. Introduction

The frequency of disorders of bone metabolism (osteopenia, osteoporosis) after liver transplantation is stated up to 50%. The first three to six months after transplantation are linked to the greatest bone density loss. The probability for sustaining a fracture in the post-transplantation phase is indicated with up to 65%. Most fractures are sustained still within the first two years after the transplantation and the most common site is the spine followed by costal fractures and femoral neck fractures. Vertebral body fractures and femoral fractures in particular cause a dramatic limitation of the patients' mobility and quality of life; in addition, an increase of mortality occurs.

2. Definition of osteoporosis

Osteoporosis is a systematic skeletal disease; its course is characterized by a reduction of bone mass, a microarchitectural deterioration of bone and thus an increase of bone fragility and a susceptibility to fracture. The reference standard of the WHO allows quantifying the extent of bone mineral density reduction with DXA method. A T-score - the standard deviations of the measurement from the average of 30-year-old healthy Caucasians - between -1 and -2.5 indicates osteopenia whereas scores below -2.5 indicate osteoporosis. After occurrence of one or several fractures due to low-energy trauma an apparent osteoporosis is existent.

3. Pathophysiology

Genesis of post-transplantation bone disease after liver transplantation (LT) is multifactorial, it comprises among others the pre-existent bone density loss in case of chronic liver disease, hypogonadism, deficit of vitamin D and increase of parathyroid hormone, malnutrition, nicotine and alcohol abuse. These factors will be potentiated by postoperative immobility, the medical substitution of immunosuppressives, glucocorticoids and of heparins.

3.1 Hepatic osteodystrophia

Osteoporosis in combination with chronic liver diseases is based on the imbalance between bone formation and degradation. The existing cirrhosis is often a result of alcohol abuse. Bone biopsies from patients with ethyl toxic liver cirrhosis show a lower trabecular bone volume. At the same time, a clear reduction of osteoblast activity and a lower bone formation rate occur.

Patients with primary biliary cirrhosis (PBC) often show lower vitamin K levels. Vitamin K is linked to the synthesis of osteocalcin and has an anti-apoptotic effect on osteoblasts; lowered vitamin K levels thus can favour an osteopenia in case of PBC.

A hyperbilirubinemia is associated with proliferation-inhibiting effects on osteoblasts. However, a direct link to lower bone mineral density is not proven. Bone resorptive components play an important pathophysiologic role for the hepatic osteodystrophia. In the course of the inflammatory process and the fibrosis in the liver, there is an increase of IL-1, IL-6 and TNFα. These inflammatory mediators lead to a release of RANKL from osteoblasts. Due to the linking to RANK, which is expressed by osteoclasts, there is an increase in the genesis of osteoclasts from progenitor cells and in osteoclast activity. This leads to an acceleration of bone resorption. A hypogonadism often occurs in patients with chronic liver disease. The reasons are the reduction of releasing hormones of the hypothalamus and the reduction of gonad function. That leads in women to low levels of oestrogens which induce the activation of bone resorption and thus a bone density loss. In men that leads to lowered testosterone levels and elevated levels of oestrogens due to the increased aromatase reaction with augmented transformation of testosterone to oestrogen.

The growth factor IGF-1 is produced to a large extent by liver cells; the decreased liver function due to chronic liver disease thus causes lowered IGF-1 levels. Glucocorticoids are applied within the therapy of autoimmune hepatitis and immediately after liver transplantation; they influence the bone metabolism in many ways.

3.2 Immunosuppressive therapy

The immunosuppressive therapy is indicated as another important factor for the development of post transplantation bone disease after liver transplantation. Especially the effect of glucocorticoids on the bone metabolism must be pointed out. Particularly in the first six months after liver transplantation, high dosage glucocorticoids are used. Because an indirect link between the applied amount of cortisone and the bone mineral density after transplantation is assumed, cortisone has a quite important effect on the bone metabolism in liver transplanted patients.

The effects of corticosteroids on the bone metabolism after liver transplantation can be divided into two stages. In the first six months after the transplantation, glucocorticoids provoke a decoupling between bone formation and resorption due to a decrease of osteoblast activity and a simultaneous increase of osteoclast activity. This decoupling is marked by a rapid loss of bone mineral density and accumulated occurrence of fractures. In the ensuing period and thus the reduction of applied cortisone doses, the bone density loss is firstly slowed down and finally, due to the reoccurring of coupling of bone formation and resorption, it comes to the recovery of bone metabolism.

Steroids have many direct and indirect effects on the bone metabolism. Indirect effects do not concern single cell lines, their targets are in the field of endocrinologic processes which are linked to the bone metabolism.

Glucocorticoids conduct to a lowered expression of calcium channels in the intestine and thus to lowered calcium absorption and they increase the kidney's excretion of calcium. The consequence is a calcium loss which can lead to a secondary hyperparathyroidism and to a higher osteoclast activity.

Glucocorticoids influence the hypothalamo-hypophyseal axis. They induce an inhibition of growth hormone production and of testosterone or oestrogen production. The consequence is a higher osteoclast activity and a lower osteoblast activity.

In combination with the occurrence of a steroid myopathy, the limitation of musculoskeletal interaction due to glucocorticoids leads to a further decrease in osteoblast activity. The consequence is a higher osteoclast activity and a lower osteoblast activity.

A direct effect on bone resorption originates from changes in the RANK Ligand/osteoprotegerin system. Under treatment with glucocorticoids, an increased synthesis of RANK Ligand from osteoblasts can be observed, whereas osteoprotegerin synthesis is inhibited.

RANK Ligand binds to the RANK receptor on osteoclasts and thus increases the osteoclast activity. At the same time, the lowered expression of osteoprotegerin facilitates the docking of RANK Ligand on RANK because osteoprotegerin is unable to neutralize RANK Ligand.

M-CSF is essential for osteoclast maturation and its production is increased by the glucocorticoids. The inhibition of caspase 3 leads to a decreased apoptosis rate of osteoclasts and results in longer survival time of osteoclasts. Moreover, glucocorticoids cause a higher production of collagenase 3 so that the synthesis of type I collagen is inhibited. The result of liver transplantation is an elevated resorption of bone matrix.

The effects that have glucocorticoids on osteoblasts are closely linked to the increased expression of caspase 3 and the formation of the dickkopf-related protein. Caspase 3 causes an increase of the osteoblast apoptosis rate whereas the dickkopf-related protein inhibits the genesis of osteoblasts. In course of a glucocorticoid therapy, the apoptosis of osteocytes is increased and due to a feedback mechanism, there is an increase of osteoblast activity. The glucocorticoids also influence the differentiation of mesenchymal stem cells. Due to stimulation of the PPARγ2, the mesenchymal stamm cells differenciate increasingly to adipozytes instead of osteoblasts.

In addition, in course of a glucocorticoid therapy less Runx2 is generated and in consequence, the osteoblast genesis is increased additionally.

Apart from steroids, other immunosuppressive drugs are applied in course of liver transplantation. Cyclosporin A, tacrolimus and azathioprine are applied as traditional immunosuppressive drugs; but also more recent substances as sirolimus and mycophenolate mofetil (MMF) are applied more and more frequently at present.

Cyclosporin A, tacrolimus and mycophenolate mofetil have very different effects on the bone metabolism. Osteopenia occurred more often by appliance of cyclosporine than by tacrolimus (whereas mycophenolate mofetil seems not to have negative effects on the bone mineral density).

The bone status before transplantation functions as predictive factor for the bone density loss after liver transplantation. Low bone density data before transplantation thus increase the risk to suffer after the liver transplantation from bone density loss. The extended immobilisation in course of the hospitalization and an inadequate low-calcium diet are still linked to post-transplantation bone disease.

3.3 Vitamin D and parathyroid hormone deficiency

Patients suffering from chronic liver disease often present after liver transplantation a lowered vitamin D status and increased parathyroid hormone levels. The parathyroid hormone level seems to correlate negatively with the patients' bone mineral density.

Disorders of bone metabolism already develop during the progression of chronic liver disease and are closely linked with its pathogenesis. Analysis of the lowered bone density prevalence are available for cholestatic liver diseases, for viral hepatitis, for alcohol-related liver diseases and for hereditary haemochromatosis.

By interpretation of bone density loss, it has to be considered that obesity and ascites may lead to measurement errors. It is thus indispensable to consider other risk factors (hypogonadism, immobility, low body mass index) to evaluate the risk of fracture.

Because the extent of the bone metabolism disorder at the time of liver transplantation has an important effect on the further progression, an evaluation of bone turnover and skeletal status prior to transplantation is needed. Among bone mineral density measurement, spinal radiographs are used to detect vertebral body deformations. Blood tests include calcium and phosphate levels, alkaline phosphatase, parathyroid hormone levels and 25-hydroxycholecalciferol as indicator of vitamin D status.

4. Therapy

To date, no evidence-based recommendations exist for the prophylaxis and therapy of bone metabolism disorders by chronic liver diseases and after liver transplantation. The need for compensation of the deficiency in 25-hydroxycholecalciferol, for a daily calcium supply of 1-2 gram and for a reduction in glucocorticoid dosage with the aim of a glucocorticoid-free immunosuppression is consensus.

To avoid bone mass loss, several antiresorptive agents are applied. But most of these studies demonstrate considerable deficiencies and do not comply with the requirements of evidence-based medicine.

The database to the application of biophosphonates after liver transplantation is limited. It refers to the application of pamidronate, zoledronate, ibandronate intravenously and etidronate and alendronate per os.

A therapy with calcitonin (40 IU/d by 17 patients) started after liver transplantation showed, compared to etidronate (400 mg p.o. for 15 days every 3 months, 23 patients), a significant increase in bone mineral density after one year of 6.4 vs. 8.2%. The examined bone formation markers osteocalcin and procollagen I propetid have been unaltered high in both groups during time of treatment. Because of the absence of a control group a conclusion about the efficiency is not possible.

Against that, Hay has been unable to prove in a controlled 12 months study effects on bone mineral density and fracture incidence in patients with primary sclerosing cholangitis (n=37) and with primary biliary cirrhosis (n=26) by application of calcitonin (100 IU daily for 6 months after transplantation).

In a survey with 53 patients was observed that application of alfacalcidol in combination with calcium and cyclic etidronate after liver transplantation does not influence bone density loss and fracture incidence. Against that, Neuhaus has proven an increase in bone mineral density on lumbar spine for all treatment groups by a therapy started six months after liver transplantation with calcitriol with or without calcium and sodium fluoride.

4.1 Alendronate

The effect of alendronate in comparison with etidronate has been examined in 2003 in 32 women with PBC. 16 patients each received either 10 mg alendronate/day or etidronate 400 mg/day for 14 days every 3 months. 26 patients have completed the two-year study. There were no changes in lumbar and femoral BMD in the etidronate group. After 2 years, lumbar spine BMD increased by 5.8±1.4% in patients on alendronate vs.1.9±1.1% in patients on etidronate; femoral neck BMD increased by 3.5±0.9% vs. 0.4±1.3%. No new vertebral fractures occurred.

A prospective uncontrolled study examined in 136 patients awaiting liver transplantation the effect of a prophylactic alendronate therapy in case of densitometric detection of osteoporosis and osteopenia and in patients whose initial normal BMD decreases after liver transplantation. It was possible to prove not only the prohibition of bone density loss post transplantationem in patients with initial osteoporosis diagnosis but an increase of bone mineral density after two years.

This result is consistent with the one for a therapy with alendronate, calcium and calcitriol by 59 patients post liver transplantation who had in comparison with an historic control group without an antiosteoporotic therapy a significant increase in mineral density after 12 months and no fractures [22].

In a prospective, controlled, open study with 98 patients with liver cirrhosis for over 24 months, the same authors have shown a significant increase in mineral bone density on lumbar spine, femoral neck and femur total by therapy with 70 mg alendronate weekly in the first three months after liver transplantation compared to a control group with patients receiving only calcium and calcitriol. Vertebral body fractures emerged in both treatment groups (18.8% by calcium and calcitriol and 6.8% by alendronate added). Osteocalcin and urinary DPD decreased in the alendronate group according to baseline values by -35.6% and -63% and increased in the control group by 30% and 15%.

4.2 Pamidronate

A not-randomised study reports on a reduction of fracture risk due to monthly infusion with pamidronate three months before and up to nine months after liver transplantation. However, only 13 patients have been treated with pamidronate, so a generalization is out of question.

In a prospective examination with 99 patients, it was not possible to prove after a singular infusion of pamidronate pre-liver transplantation any effects on the development of bone mineral density and the fracture rate in the first year post liver transplantation.

A histomorphometric examination describes the bone remodeling at tissue level in paired biopsies before and three months after successful liver transplantation in seven patients after a single infusion of pamidronate before liver transplantation in comparison to five untreated patients. In contrast to the untreated patients, those with pamindronate treatment did not show an increased bone formation rate but a significant reduction in the size of resorption lacunae. The data suggest a reduction of postoperative high turnover due to preoperative pamidronate therapy.

Recently, the results of a randomised, double-blind, placebo-controlled study with 79 patients have shown that the application of 90 mg pamidronate (38 pat.) two weeks before and three months after liver transplantation leads to a significant increase of lumbar BMD after 12 months with an increase in density of 2.9% vs.1%. There was no difference in the density loss of femoral neck and the fracture incidence.

4.3 Zoledronate

The ability to prevent bone loss after infusion of zoledronate within 7 days of transplantation and 1, 3, 6 and 9 months after liver transplantation in 32 patients compared to 30 placebo-treated ones could be demonstrated.

Moreover, in a controlled, prospective, open study after eight infusions each of 4 mg zoledronate in the first 12 months after liver transplantation in 47 patients has shown a reduction in serological and histological bone turnover markers and a reduction of fracture incidence.

4.4 Ibandronate

In an open, prospective, placebo-controlled study, 34 patients have been treated for over one year with 2 mg ibandronate every 12 weeks intravenously, calcium and cholecalciferol starting on the day of liver transplantation. The control group received exclusively calcium and cholecalciferol. BMD measurements were carried out after 3, 6, 12 and 24 months. Fractures have been detected constantly.

A further reduction of BMD at all measured sites in the first few months after liver transplantation has been shown for all patients. However, after 12 and 24 months ibandronate treated patients demonstrated significant higher BMD and lower prevalence of fractures.

5. Conclusion

In summarising, a great variability can be observed in the available data about the extent of the impact on BMD and on the risk of fracture due to application of bisphosphonates or other osteotropic agents in course of a liver transplantation. The capability to reduce the BMD loss in the early stages after liver transplantation due to bisphosphonates is reported consistently. Despite this ambiguity, it has to be recommended to evaluate the bone status before liver transplantation and to start a bisphosphonate therapy in case of osteoporosis. For differential therapeutic outcomes, randomised, double-blind, prospective and controlled studies are necessary. Informing and guiding patients to a bone-healthier lifestyle and the elimination of avoidable risk factors remains unaffected.

6. References

Atamaz, F., S. Hepguler, M. Akyildiz, Z. Karasu, and M. Kilic. "Effects of Alendronate on Bone Mineral Density and Bone Metabolic Markers in Patients with Liver Transplantation." [In eng]. *Osteoporosis international: a journal established as result of cooperation between the European Foundation for Osteoporosis and the National Osteoporosis Foundation of the USA* 17, no. 6 (2006): 942-9.

Bell, H., N. Raknerud, J. A. Falch, and E. Haug. "Inappropriately Low Levels of Gonadotrophins in Amenorrhoeic Women with Alcoholic and Non-Alcoholic Cirrhosis." [In eng]. *Eur J Endocrinol* 132, no. 4 (Apr 1995): 444-9.

Bernstein, C. N., W. D. Leslie, and M. S. Leboff. "Aga Technical Review on Osteoporosis in Gastrointestinal Diseases." [In eng]. *Gastroenterology* 124, no. 3 (Mar 2003): 795-841.

Beuers, U., K. H. Wiedmann, G. Kleber, and W. E. Fleig. "[Therapy of Autoimmune Hepatitis, Primary Biliary Cirrhosis and Primary Sclerosing Cholangitis. Consensus of the German Society of Digestive System and Metabolic Diseases]." [In ger]. *Z Gastroenterol* 35, no. 12 (Dec 1997): 1041-9.

Canalis, E. "Mechanisms of Glucocorticoid-Induced Osteoporosis." [In eng]. *Curr Opin Rheumatol* 15, no. 4 (Jul 2003): 454-7.

Canalis, E., G. Mazziotti, A. Giustina, and J. P. Bilezikian. "Glucocorticoid-Induced Osteoporosis: Pathophysiology and Therapy." [In eng]. *Osteoporos Int* 18, no. 10 (Oct 2007): 1319-28.

Chappard, D., B. Plantard, H. Fraisse, S. Palle, C. Alexandre, and G. Riffat. "Bone Changes in Alcoholic Cirrhosis of the Liver. A Histomorphometric Study." [In eng]. *Pathol Res Pract* 184, no. 5 (May 1989): 480-5.

Cohen, A., P. Sambrook, and E. Shane. "Management of Bone Loss after Organ Transplantation." *J Bone Miner Res* 19, no. 12 (Dec 2004): 1919-32.

Collier, J. "Bone Disorders in Chronic Liver Disease." [In eng]. *Hepatology* 46, no. 4 (Oct 2007): 1271-8.

Compston, J. E. "Osteoporosis after Liver Transplantation." *Liver Transpl* 9, no. 4 (Apr 2003): 321-30.

Crawford, B. A., C. Kam, J. Pavlovic, K. Byth, D. J. Handelsman, P. W. Angus, and G. W. McCaughan. "Zoledronic Acid Prevents Bone Loss after Liver Transplantation: A Randomized, Double-Blind, Placebo-Controlled Trial." [In eng]. *Annals of internal medicine* 144, no. 4 (Feb 21 2006): 239-48.

de Kroon, L., G. Drent, A. P. van den Berg, and E. B. Haagsma. "Current Health Status of Patients Who Have Survived for More Than 15 Years after Liver Transplantation." [In eng]. *Neth J Med* 65, no. 7 (Jul-Aug 2007): 252-8.

Eastell, R., E. R. Dickson, S. F. Hodgson, R. H. Wiesner, M. K. Porayko, H. W. Wahner, S. L. Cedel, B. L. Riggs, and R. A. Krom. "Rates of Vertebral Bone Loss before and after Liver Transplantation in Women with Primary Biliary Cirrhosis." *Hepatology* 14, no. 2 (Aug 1991): 296-300.

Encke, J., W. Uhl, W. Stremmel, and P. Sauer. "Immunosuppression and Modulation in Liver Transplantation." [In eng]. *Nephrol Dial Transplant* 19 Suppl 4 (Jul 2004): iv22-5.

Gallagher, J. C. "Advances in Bone Biology and New Treatments for Bone Loss." [In eng]. *Maturitas* 60, no. 1 (May 20 2008): 65-9.

Garcia-Valdecasas-Campelo, E., E. Gonzalez-Reimers, F. Santolaria-Fernandez, M. J. De la Vega-Prieto, A. Milena-Abril, M. J. Sanchez-Perez, A. Martinez-Riera, and L. Gomez-Rodriguez Mde. "Serum Osteoprotegerin and Rankl Levels in Chronic Alcoholic Liver Disease." [In eng]. *Alcohol Alcohol* 41, no. 3 (May-Jun 2006): 261-6.

Guanabens, N., A. Pares, I. Ros, L. Alvarez, F. Pons, L. Caballeria, A. Monegal, *et al.* "Alendronate Is More Effective Than Etidronate for Increasing Bone Mass in Osteopenic Patients with Primary Biliary Cirrhosis." [In eng]. *The American journal of gastroenterology* 98, no. 10 (Oct 2003): 2268-74.

Guichelaar, M. M., R. Kendall, M. Malinchoc, and J. E. Hay. "Bone Mineral Density before and after Olt: Long-Term Follow-up and Predictive Factors." *Liver Transpl* 12, no. 9 (Sep 2006): 1390-402.

Guichelaar, M. M., J. Schmoll, M. Malinchoc, and J. E. Hay. "Fractures and Avascular Necrosis before and after Orthotopic Liver Transplantation: Long-Term Follow-up and Predictive Factors." [In eng]. *Hepatology* 46, no. 4 (Oct 2007): 1198-207.

Hay, J. E., M. Malinchoc, and E. R. Dickson. "A Controlled Trial of Calcitonin Therapy for the Prevention of Post-Liver Transplantation Atraumatic Fractures in Patients with Primary Biliary Cirrhosis and Primary Sclerosing Cholangitis." [In eng]. *J Hepatol* 34, no. 2 (Feb 2001): 292-8.

Hofbauer, L. C., and M. Rauner. "Minireview: Live and Let Die: Molecular Effects of Glucocorticoids on Bone Cells." [In eng]. *Mol Endocrinol* 23, no. 10 (Oct 2009): 1525-31.

Hommann, M., D. Kammerer, G. Lehmann, A. Kornberg, B. Kupper, W. Daffner, G. Wolf, and U. Settmacher. "Prevention of Early Loss of Bone Mineral Density after Liver Transplantation by Prostaglandin E1." [In eng]. *Transplant Proc* 39, no. 2 (Mar 2007): 540-3.

Janes, C. H., E. R. Dickson, R. Okazaki, S. Bonde, A. F. McDonagh, and B. L. Riggs. "Role of Hyperbilirubinemia in the Impairment of Osteoblast Proliferation Associated with Cholestatic Jaundice." *J Clin Invest* 95, no. 6 (Jun 1995): 2581-6.

Jia, D., C. A. O'Brien, S. A. Stewart, S. C. Manolagas, and R. S. Weinstein. "Glucocorticoids Act Directly on Osteoclasts to Increase Their Life Span and Reduce Bone Density." [In eng]. *Endocrinology* 147, no. 12 (Dec 2006): 5592-9.

Kaemmerer, D., G. Lehmann, G. Wolf, U. Settmacher, and M. Hommann. "Treatment of Osteoporosis after Liver Transplantation with Ibandronate." [In eng]. *Transpl Int* 23, no. 7 (Jul: 753-9.

Kanis, J. A. "Assessment of Fracture Risk and Its Application to Screening for Postmenopausal Osteoporosis: Synopsis of a Who Report. Who Study Group." [In eng]. *Osteoporos Int* 4, no. 6 (Nov 1994): 368-81.

Kanis, J. A., N. Burlet, C. Cooper, P. D. Delmas, J. Y. Reginster, F. Borgstrom, and R. Rizzoli. "European Guidance for the Diagnosis and Management of Osteoporosis in Postmenopausal Women." [In eng]. *Osteoporos Int* 19, no. 4 (Apr 2008): 399-428.

Kanis, J. A., P. Delmas, P. Burckhardt, C. Cooper, and D. Torgerson. "Guidelines for Diagnosis and Management of Osteoporosis. The European Foundation for Osteoporosis and Bone Disease." [In eng]. *Osteoporos Int* 7, no. 4 (1997): 390-406.

Kanis, J. A., and C. C. Gluer. "An Update on the Diagnosis and Assessment of Osteoporosis with Densitometry. Committee of Scientific Advisors, International Osteoporosis Foundation." [In eng]. *Osteoporos Int* 11, no. 3 (2000): 192-202.

Kanis, J. A., E. V. McCloskey, H. Johansson, A. Oden, L. J. Melton, 3rd, and N. Khaltaev. "A Reference Standard for the Description of Osteoporosis." [In eng]. *Bone* 42, no. 3 (Mar 2008): 467-75.

Khan, K. M., S. Mulia, R. Kaul, and S. Raatz. "Effect of Nutrition and Body Composition on Bone Density after Liver Transplantation." [In eng]. *Transplant Proc* 39, no. 10 (Dec 2007): 3292-4.

Khan, M. A., and S. L. Morgan. "Tone the Bones of Your Chronic Liver Disease Patients." [In eng]. *Clin Gastroenterol Hepatol* 7, no. 8 (Aug 2009): 814-5.

Kim, H. J., H. Zhao, H. Kitaura, S. Bhattacharyya, J. A. Brewer, L. J. Muglia, F. P. Ross, and S. L. Teitelbaum. "Glucocorticoids Suppress Bone Formation Via the Osteoclast." [In eng]. *J Clin Invest* 116, no. 8 (Aug 2006): 2152-60.

Kowdley, K. V., M. J. Emond, J. A. Sadowski, and M. M. Kaplan. "Plasma Vitamin K1 Level Is Decreased in Primary Biliary Cirrhosis." [In eng]. *Am J Gastroenterol* 92, no. 11 (Nov 1997): 2059-61.

Kulak, C. A., V. Z. Borba, J. Kulak Junior, and E. Shane. "Transplantation Osteoporosis." [In eng]. *Arq Bras Endocrinol Metabol* 50, no. 4 (Aug 2006): 783-92.

Leslie, W. D., C. N. Bernstein, and M. S. Leboff. "Aga Technical Review on Osteoporosis in Hepatic Disorders." *Gastroenterology* 125, no. 3 (Sep 2003): 941-66.

Maalouf, N. M., and E. Shane. "Osteoporosis after Solid Organ Transplantation." [In eng]. *J Clin Endocrinol Metab* 90, no. 4 (Apr 2005): 2456-65.

Millonig, G., I. W. Graziadei, D. Eichler, K. P. Pfeiffer, G. Finkenstedt, P. Muehllechner, A. Koenigsrainer, R. Margreiter, and W. Vogel. "Alendronate in Combination with Calcium and Vitamin D Prevents Bone Loss after Orthotopic Liver Transplantation: A Prospective Single-Center Study." *Liver Transpl* 11, no. 8 (Aug 2005): 960-6.

Monegal, A., N. Guanabens, M. J. Suarez, F. Suarez, G. Clemente, M. Garcia-Gonzalez, M. De la Mata, *et al.* "Pamidronate in the Prevention of Bone Loss after Liver Transplantation: A Randomized Controlled Trial." [In eng]. *Transpl Int* 22, no. 2 (Feb 2009): 198-206.

Neuhaus, R., R. Lohmann, K. P. Platz, O. Guckelberger, M. Schon, M. Lang, J. Hierholzer, and P. Neuhaus. "Treatment of Osteoporosis after Liver Transplantation." [In eng]. *Transplant Proc* 27, no. 1 (Feb 1995): 1226-7.

Ninkovic, M., S. Love, B. D. Tom, P. W. Bearcroft, G. J. Alexander, and J. E. Compston. "Lack of Effect of Intravenous Pamidronate on Fracture Incidence and Bone Mineral Density after Orthotopic Liver Transplantation." *J Hepatol* 37, no. 1 (Jul 2002): 93-100.

Papatheodoridis, G. V., and S. Manolakopoulos. "Easl Clinical Practice Guidelines on the Management of Chronic Hepatitis B: The Need for Liver Biopsy." [In eng]. *J Hepatol* 51, no. 1 (Jul 2009): 226-7.

Pares, A., and N. Guanabens. "Treatment of Bone Disorders in Liver Disease." [In eng]. *J Hepatol* 45, no. 3 (Sep 2006): 445-53.

Pignata, S., B. Daniele, M. G. Galati, G. Esposito, P. Vallone, F. Fiore, P. Ricchi, and M. Pergola. "Oestradiol and Testosterone Blood Levels in Patients with Viral Cirrhosis and Hepatocellular Carcinoma." [In eng]. *Eur J Gastroenterol Hepatol* 9, no. 3 (Mar 1997): 283-6.

Reeves, H. L., R. M. Francis, D. M. Manas, M. Hudson, and C. P. Day. "Intravenous Bisphosphonate Prevents Symptomatic Osteoporotic Vertebral Collapse in Patients after Liver Transplantation." *Liver Transpl Surg* 4, no. 5 (Sep 1998): 404-9.

Riemens, S. C., A. Oostdijk, J. J. van Doormaal, C. J. Thijn, G. Drent, D. A. Piers, E. W. Groen, *et al.* "Bone Loss after Liver Transplantation Is Not Prevented by Cyclical Etidronate, Calcium and Alphacalcidol. The Liver Transplant Group, Groningen." [In eng]. *Osteoporos Int* 6, no. 3 (1996): 213-8.

Sambrook, P. N., P. J. Kelly, A. M. Keogh, P. Macdonald, P. Spratt, J. Freund, and J. A. Eisman. "Bone Loss after Heart Transplantation: A Prospective Study." *J Heart Lung Transplant* 13, no. 1 Pt 1 (Jan-Feb 1994): 116-20; discussion 21.

Sanchez, A. J., and J. Aranda-Michel. "Liver Disease and Osteoporosis." *Nutr Clin Pract* 21, no. 3 (Jun 2006): 273-8.

Segal, E., Y. Baruch, R. Kramsky, B. Raz, A. Tamir, and S. Ish-Shalom. "Predominant Factors Associated with Bone Loss in Liver Transplant Patients - after Prolonged Post-Transplantation Period." *Clin Transplant* 17, no. 1 (Feb 2003): 13-9.

Shah, S. H., T. D. Johnston, H. Jeon, and D. Ranjan. "Effect of Chronic Glucocorticoid Therapy and the Gender Difference on Bone Mineral Density in Liver Transplant Patients." *J Surg Res* 135, no. 2 (Oct 2006): 238-41.

Shi, X. M., H. C. Blair, X. Yang, J. M. McDonald, and X. Cao. "Tandem Repeat of C/Ebp Binding Sites Mediates Ppargamma2 Gene Transcription in Glucocorticoid-Induced Adipocyte Differentiation." [In eng]. *J Cell Biochem* 76, no. 3 (Jan 2000): 518-27.

Smallwood, G. A., J. M. Wickman, E. Martinez, A. C. Stieber, and T. G. Heffron. "Osteoporosis Screening in an Outpatient Liver Transplant Clinic: Impact of Primary Immunosuppression." *Transplant Proc* 34, no. 5 (Aug 2002): 1569-70.

Smith, D. L., N. J. Shire, N. B. Watts, T. Schmitter, G. Szabo, and S. D. Zucker. "Hyperbilirubinemia Is Not a Major Contributing Factor to Altered Bone Mineral Density in Patients with Chronic Liver Disease." [In eng]. *J Clin Densitom* 9, no. 1 (Jan-Mar 2006): 105-13.

Stein, E., P. Ebeling, and E. Shane. "Post-Transplantation Osteoporosis." [In eng]. *Endocrinol Metab Clin North Am* 36, no. 4 (Dec 2007): 937-63; viii.

Valero, M. A., C. Loinaz, L. Larrodera, M. Leon, E. Moreno, and F. Hawkins. "Calcitonin and Bisphosphonates Treatment in Bone Loss after Liver Transplantation." *Calcif Tissue Int* 57, no. 1 (Jul 1995): 15-9.

Vedi, S., M. Ninkovic, N. J. Garrahan, G. J. Alexander, and J. E. Compston. "Effects of a Single Infusion of Pamidronate Prior to Liver Transplantation: A Bone Histomorphometric Study." *Transpl Int* 15, no. 6 (Jun 2002): 290-5.

Wang, F. S., J. Y. Ko, D. W. Yeh, H. C. Ke, and H. L. Wu. "Modulation of Dickkopf-1 Attenuates Glucocorticoid Induction of Osteoblast Apoptosis, Adipocytic Differentiation, and Bone Mass Loss." [In eng]. *Endocrinology* 149, no. 4 (Apr 2008): 1793-801.

Willenberg, H. S., and H. Lehnert. "[Basics and Management of Glucocorticoid-Induced Osteoporosis]." [In ger]. *Internist (Berl)* 49, no. 10 (Oct 2008): 1186-90, 92, 94-6.

Wu, Y. L., J. Ye, S. Zhang, J. Zhong, and R. P. Xi. "Clinical Significance of Serum Igf-I, Igf-Ii and Igfbp-3 in Liver Cirrhosis." [In eng]. *World J Gastroenterol* 10, no. 18 (Sep 15 2004): 2740-3.

19

Betaherpesviruses in Adult Liver Transplant Recipients

Ronaldo Luis Thomasini et al.*
Department of Clinical Medicine – State University of Campinas
Laboratory of Clinical Pathology – Hermínio Ometto Foundation – University Center
Brazil

1. Introduction

Liver transplantation similar to other allograft transplants requires the use of immunossupressive therapy to avoid graft rejection in the host. Immunossupressive drugs can also decrease the capacity of the host immune system to response against infectious agents which would not be a problem to immunocompetent persons. Many infectious agents such as bacteria, fungus, protozoa and viruses can cause serious complication in the post-transplant course (Blair & Shimon, 2005).

Several different viruses have been studied at long of the time and these studies have demonstrated that herpesviruses can be important infectious agents and affects the management of the liver transplant recipients (Kotton, 2010).

Herpesviruses belong to the *Herpesviridae* family (Hudnall et al., 2008), and have been isolated eight different types of these viruses (Table 1). The human herpesvirus simples type I and type II (HSV-1 and HSV-2), are usually associated with labial and genital herpes, respectively. However, genital herpes can be a consequence of HSV-1 infection and labial herpes can also be caused by HSV-2. The human herpesvirus type 3 (varicella-zoster) causes chickenpox, especially in children, and re-infection or reactivation, may be the cause of the appearance of zoster. Human herpesvirus type 4 (Epstein-Barr virus) is associated with infectious mononucleosis syndrome, Burkitt's lymphoma and nasopharyngeal carcinoma. The human herpesvirus type 8 is associated with Kaposi's sarcoma, and can cause death in immunosuppressed individuals, especially in acquired immunodeficiency syndrome (HIV/AIDS).

Cytomegalovirus (CMV), Human Herpesvirus 6 (HHV-6) and Human Herpesvirus 7 (HHV-7) are DNA viruses, members of the *betaherpesvirinae* subfamily of the *Betaherpesviridae* (Tong et al., 2000). Cytomegalovirus primary infection causes 'mononucleosis like syndrome' and

---

* Fernanda Costa[1], Ana Maria Sampaio[2], Sandra Helena Alves Bonon[1], Paula Durante[1], Ilka de Fátima Santana Ferreira Boin[2], Fabiana Souza Maximo Pereira[3] and Sandra Cecília Botelho Costa[1]
[1]*Department of Clinical Medicine – State University of Campinas; Brazil*
[2]*Liver Transplant Unit - State University of Campinas; Brazil*
[3]*Department of Clinical Medicine – Hospital da Baleia; Brazil*

HHV-6 and HHV-7 primary infections cause common febrile infectious syndromes in early childhood, known as *exanthem subitum* and roseola.

Virus	Synonymous	Sub-family	Abbreviation
Human herpesvirus -1	Herpes simplex-1	α	HSV-1/HHV-1
Human herpesvirus -2	Herpes simplex-2	α	HSV-2/HHV-2
Human herpesvirus -3	Varicella-zoster	α	VZV/HHV-3
Human herpesvirus -4	Epstein-Barr	γ	EBV/HSV-4
Human herpesvirus -5	Cytomegalovirus	β	CMV/HHV-5
Human herpesvirus -6	None	β	HHV-6
Human herpesvirus -7	None	β	HHV-7
Human herpesvirus -8	None	γ	KSHV/HHV-8

Table 1. Complete list of the human herpesviruses

Betaherpesviruses are ubiquitous and seropositivity for these viruses can differ dependently of geographical region and other characteristics of the studied cohort. CMV seroprevalence is largely known around the world while HHV-6 and HHV-7 seroprevalences remain less studied. However, is estimated that HHV-6 and HHV-7 prevalences would also be high in the majority of the places.

In immunocompetent individuals, beteherpesviral primary infections are usually self-limiting although some cases of neurological manifestations have been described especially regarding HHV-6 in children (Donati et al., 2003; Matsumoto et al., 2011). It is not clear whether the neurological manifestation is caused by herpesviral brain tissue invasion or is an indirect effect of the infection.

After primary infection, betaherpesviruses remain latent in the host and could reactivate sporadically leading to a transient viremia. Although some syndromes (e.g. chronic fatigue syndrome and multiple sclerosis) have been related to herpesviral reactivation, the role of the viruses in these syndromes remains unclear (Dewhurst, 2004).

CMV, HHV-6 and HHV-7 can more frequently reactivate during immunosuppression following organ transplantation (Tong et al., 2000). CMV infection is known as major infectious complications after transplantation and has been considered an important cause of morbidity and mortality in bone marrow transplantation and solid organ transplant recipients. Although the role and impact of CMV infection on the post-transplant course is well characterized, the other two members of the betaherpesviruses family have been acknowledged only recently.

1.1 Cytomegalovirus

The diseases caused by CMV occur in underdeveloped and developing countries and the prevalence varies from 40 to 60% in the northern hemisphere countries, while in Africa and Latin America rates from 80 to 100% were observed (Suassuna et al., 1995; Costa et al., 1999). About 80% of the population between the late childhood and early adolescence is already infected by CMV (Almeida et al., 2001) and can harbor the virus in several body sites, especially in the salivary glands and different types of leukocytes. The peripheral blood mononuclear cells appear to be the most important site for CMV latency.

There are different variants or genetically distinct strains of CMV and therefore the cross-protective immunity is considered partial (Ishibashi et al., 2006). The possibilities for the occurrence of a new exposure to another CMV strain are numerous. Immunosuppressed patients can be submitted to transfusions of blood components containing latent viruses, they may receive bone marrow or solid organs containing CMV and, in some cases, undergoing dialysis in equipment contaminated with viruses. It is for this reason that has been verified that the rate of cytomegalovirus infection/reinfection in these circumstances can be high (approximately 50%).

In healthy adults, CMV is usually asymptomatic. Some individuals may have symptoms similar to infectious mononucleosis syndrome, such as lymphadenopathy, fever, rash, malaise, arthralgia, hepatomegaly and splenomegaly. In immunocompromised patients, CMV may modulate the immune response and leads to more complex clinical presentation including death, dependently of the situation involved.

The American Society of Transplantation classified the presence of CMV in the body into two situations (Kotton et al., 2010).

- CMV infection: evidence of CMV replication regardless of symptoms (different from latent CMV).
- CMV disease: evidence of CMV infection associated with symptoms. CMV disease can be further categorized as a viral syndrome with fever, malaise, leukopenia, thrombocytopenia or as a tissue invasive disease.

Whereas liver transplantation, epidemiological studies demonstrate a high incidence of CMV active infection. Some facts should be considered, for example, the previously infected patients who receive organs from donors with genotypically distinct latent viruses may develop a new infection. In addition, the surgical stress generated by the transplantation procedure may lead to a reactivation of latent CMV (Kotton et al., 2010).

CMV disease is considered one of the most common complications after liver transplant recipients, with significant morbidity and mortality (Thomasini et al., 2007). Studies in the transplant series have shown that higher viral load values correlate with increased risk for development of disease.

Thus, sensitive techniques were described in an attempt to identify earlier individuals who have higher risk to development of CMV disease with the goal to reduce the severity of the cases. The direct detection of the virus by conventional techniques, urine or saliva, is a procedure with limited clinical value. Moreover, it is technically difficult, expensive and provides results only after 3-5 weeks. Culture of CMV in blood or urine has low sensitivity.

Culture of tissue samples is an option for confirmatory diagnosis of invasive diseases, especially in the case of gastrointestinal manifestations, in which, generally molecular and antigen-based diagnosis are negatives (Kotton et al., 2010).

Before liver transplantation, serology for CMV can be used in both the organ donor and the recipient. A quantitative test for anti-CMV IgG should be used in combination with IgM test due to IgG serological tests are more specific than IgM tests. The serology of donor and recipient is the key to predicting the risk of infection. In the case of donor and recipient were sero-negative during the pre transplant, serology should be repeated at the time of transplantation, if there is a significant time between screening and transplantation.

However, recent blood transfusion could present false results in the serological tests. In patients after liver transplantation, serology has no role in diagnosis of active CMV disease.

The detection of CMV antigen matrix (pp65) –antigenemia is a technique highly sensitive, rapid, quantitative, and with significant clinical correlation (van der Bij et al., 1988; Bonon et al., 2005). Patients who present positive results can be submitted to antiviral therapy and the response can be monitored periodically to demonstrate the efficacy of the treatment and the possibility of drug resistance. The limitation may be the definition of a limit of positivity ('cut-off') to start the treatment. Moreover, neutropenia can raise difficulties to perform this technique due to the fact that antigenemia requires a sufficient number of neutrophils to detect CMV viral antigen. CMV causes an abortive replication within neutrophils and leads to uptake of antigen in perinuclear area (Kas-Deelen et al., 2001) which can be detected by use of monoclonal antibodies against pp65-antigen. Either fluorescent or enzyme labelled conjugate can be used to reveal the reaction. However, enzyme labelled conjugate can be revealed by coloured reaction and dispenses the use of ultraviolet microscope. Figure 1 shows positive pp65-antigenemia using enzyme labelled conjugate.

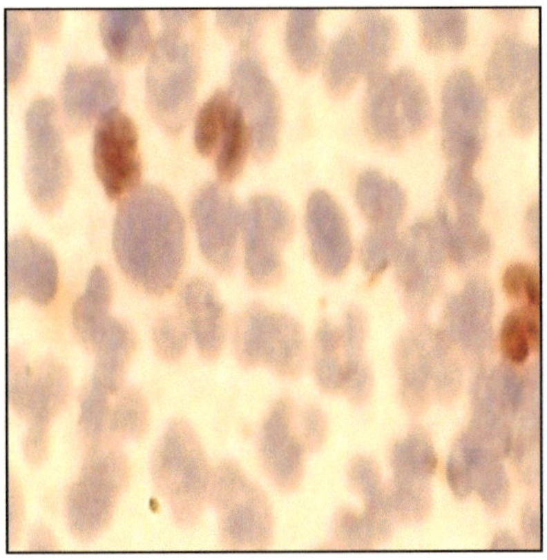

Fig. 1. Nuclei of neutrophils stained in brown indicating positive pp65-atigenemia (counterstained with Harris´s hematoxylin). Mouse C10 and C11 monoclonals atibody against pp65-matrix CMV antigen and rabitt anti-mouse Ig horseradish peroxidase conjugate. The reaction was revealed by hydrogen peroxide and amino-ethyl-carbazole (Sampaio et al., 2011)

Molecular techniques such as Polymerase Chain Reaction (PCR) and Nucleic Acid Sequence Based Amplification (NASBA) had gradually been incorporated in the laboratorial diagnosis of CMV.

Whereas the viral biology, it is necessary to demonstrate the presence of viral mRNA, or portions of the viral genome expressed only in the replicative phase and not in latency. Using PCR the sensitivity of the PCR should be adjusted to detect only significant viral loads which could not easily performed. Unfortunately, due to very high sensitivity, molecular techniques may reveal positive results without relevant clinical features (Thomasini et al., 2007). In patients with higher risk level to progression of the CMV disease, such as liver transplantation, positive results in molecular tests can be an indicative to introduction to the preemptive therapy despite some of these patients not have clinical manifestation.

Antigenemia has been considered to be less sensitive than molecular tests although has significant clinical correlation. In other hand, the molecular techniques are more sensitive, but may be dissociated of clinical manifestation in some situations. Thus, in patients at high risk (liver transplant recipients, CMV sero-negative patients who received organs from sero-positive patients, patients who used mycophenolate or anti-OKT 3) would be benefited whether monitored by molecular techniques or by antigenemia relying on lower 'cut-off' levels.

More recently, real-time PCR has been considered faster, very sensitive and provides more accurate discrimination than other molecular techniques. However, the establishment of the 'cut-off' levels to discriminate between significant viral load and transient viremia is also necessary. Moreover, real-time PCR has been considered expensive and requires specialized staff. Either plasma or whole blood specimens can provide diagnosis and prognostic information regarding CMV disease. Qualitative PCR is an option for surveillance if this technique is the unique available option. The diagnosis of tissue invasive CMV disease, should be confirmed by immunohistochemistry or *in situ* DNA hybridization The decision regarding which test to use will depend on many factors including available resources, technical staff, patient population, volume of samples tested and cost (Kotton et al., 2010).

The gold standard for treatment of CMV is intravenous ganciclovir, although oral valganciclovir is non inferior in nonlife-threatening disease. In patients with life-threatening CMV disease and in children, intravenous ganciclovir still the preferred drug, because data on the effect of oral treatment are limited. The treatment should be monitored weekly by viral loads and treating must continue until one or two consecutive negative samples are obtained, but not shorter than 2 weeks (Kotton et al., 2010).

Universal prophylaxis involves the administration of antiviral drugs to overall of patients or a subset of "at risk" patients. Antiviral administration are usually started in the immediate or very early post transplant period and continued about 3 to 6 months. Several antivirals have been used, including acyclovir, valacyclovir intravenous ganciclovir, oral ganciclovir and valganciclovir. In the preemptive therapy, laboratory monitoring detects asymptomatic viral replication and antiviral therapy is initiated to prevent the progression to clinical disease. One of the major concerns with preemptive therapy is that it may not prevent the indirect effects on graft and patient survival.

Dosing of antiviral medications should be based on standard recommended dosing algorithms (for patients with normal creatinine clearance: valganciclovir 900 mg once a day, intravenous ganciclovir 5 mg/kg once a day, or oral ganciclovir 1,000 mg three times a day) and carefully adjusted for renal function.

Drug resistance in some CMV strain had been reported and this fact must be considered in non-responsive patients. Some studies have focused in genotyping of CMV which could indicate strains presenting resistance to conventional treatment.

1.2 Human Herpesvirus 6

In Brazil serological prevalence surveys conducted in North and Southeast regions show that antibodies against HHV-6 were present in 90% of the individuals among the studied population (0-40 years-old) with occurrence of the primary infection in the first years of life

(Freitas et al., 1997; Linhares et al., 1991). Reactivation of latent HHV-6 is common after liver transplantation, possibly induced and facilitated by allograft rejection and immunosuppressive therapy (Abdel et al., 2009; Griffths et al., 2000). HHV-6 may affect the success of the transplant procedure which is observed clinical findings as: fever, neutropenia, nervous central system manifestations or other visceral involvements (DesJardin et al., 2001). In addition, HHV-6 viremia is an independently significant predictive factor for invasive fungal infections and is associated with late mortality in liver transplantation recipients (Rogers et al., 2000). On the other hand, the rejection of the transplanted organ can also be enhanced when the patient is co-infected with CMV (Lautenschlager et al., 2000; Humar et al., 2000).

The expression of different cellular antigens can be dramatically altered in HHV-6-infected tissues which the viral infection can induce to CD4 up regulation and CD3 down modulation in the T cells. HHV-6 can severely affect the physiology of secondary lymphoid organs through direct infection of T lymphocytes and modulation of key membrane receptors and chemokines (Grivel et al., 2003). Since the effects of HHV-6 in cellular immune system it could be affect the response against other infectious agents or facilitate the mechanism of graft rejection in the host.

The diagnosis of reactivation or new infection by HHV-6 is not made easily. Serological techniques are available but the contribution of a positive result is limited by the high prevalence of infection in adults, as mentioned above (Freitas et al., 1997; Linhares et al., 1991). The report of specific HHV-6 IgM in sera or a four-fold rise in IgG antibodies can be used as diagnostic criteria, but is not as sensitive as desired. Moreover, the interpretation of serological results is complicated by the fact that both primary and secondary infections with other herpes viruses may be associated with a concurrent antibody response to HHV-6 (Osman et al., 1997). In addition, the presence of residual IgM against HHV-6 in the bloodstream can complicate the interpretation of the serological tests (Peigo et al., 2009).

Antigenemia techniques to detect HHV-6 in blood have been described in the literature (Sampaio et al., 2011; Lautenschlager et al., 2002). Similar to pp65-atigenemia used for CMV, monoclonals antibodies against specific HHV-6 protein could be use with the purpose to detect only active infections. The antigenemia could be an alternative to molecular techniques because is a quantitative method and requires relatively few apparatus. HHV-6 antigenemia, different from CMV, requires the use of purified lymphocytes to detect antigen. Positivity in peripheral monocytes occurs occasionally although lymphocytes are more frequently positive.

Although the use of HHV-6 antigenemia could be promissory, the technique still needs improvements and establishment of 'cut-off' values to clinical use. Moreover, the sensitivity and specificity to detect HHV-6 active infection have been not completely studied.

The techniques based on nuclei acid amplification are also available for the diagnosis of HHV-6 (Secchiero et al., 1995). However, the results obtained are controversial, because it depends on the PCR's method employed (Shibata et al., 1992; Demmler et al., 1998).

Since HHV-6 disease can be established, infection can be treated with intravenous ganciclovir, foscarnet, or cidofovir and this should be complemented by a reduction in immunosuppression (Razonable & Lautenschlager, 2010). The efficacy of acyclovir against HHV-6 infection seems to be lower than others. Moreover, foscarnet and cidofovir could be more effective than ganciclovir against HHV-6 infection of astroglioma cells. Although ganciclovir and cidofovir are therapeutic options, on the basis of *in vitro* data and limited clinical experience reported in the literature, foscarnet is probably the preferred treatment for HHV-6 associated encephalitis.

Patients could be treated with intravenous ganciclovir (2.5 mg/kg daily) for 3-6 weeks, cidofovir 5mg/kg once weekly for 2 consecutive weeks or intravenous foscarnet (40 mg/kg every 12 hours) for 3-4 weeks (Vinnard et al., 2009). However, in patients with renal failure, dose must be adjusted to avoid toxicity in the patients. In addition, viral monitoring is necessary (by PCR or antigenemia) to avoid interruption of the treatment prior disappearance of viremia.

Similar to CMV, some strains of HHV-6 can present drug resistance and the strategies described above could also not have efficacy.

1.3 Human Herpesvirus 7

HHV-7 has been isolated from T-CD4^{+} cells purified from peripheral blood mononuclear cells of a healthy individual by Frenkel et al. (1990). HHV-7 like other betaherpesviruses remains latent or at low level of viral replication after primary infection or can reactivate during immunosuppressed states (Ihira et al., 2001). HHV-7 shares many properties of HHV-6, suggesting that the factors that control their reactivation or increased viral replication in immunosuppressed patients may be similar (Mendez et al., 2001).

HHV-7 infects most specifically, T-CD4^{+} cells, which could result in cytotoxicity and mmunomodulatory activities (Secchiero et al., 2001). It has also been demonstrated that the down modulation of human leukocyte antigen (HLA) and beta-2-microglobulin expression by HHV-7 is linked to viral replication and is not merely the consequence of the interaction of virions with the cell surface. Infected cells can therefore efficiently escape from host immune pressure that might explain the persistence of HHV-7–positive cells in several types of tumors and chronic infectious diseases (Mirandola, 2006). Although HHV-7 has restricted tropism to CD4^{+} cells, it should be noted that HHV-7–infected T-CD4^{+} cells kill uninfected T-CD8^{+} cells *in vitro*. Moreover, HLA class I and beta-2-microglobulin are also down modulated in the T-CD8^{+} cells on the presence of HHV-7–infected leukocytes *in vitro* (Secchiero et al., 2001). Similar to HHV-6, HHV-7 infection could modulate the host immune system enhancing the risk to graft rejection and other type of infections.

Although in liver transplant recipients HHV-6 has been related to clinical consequences (Feldstein et al., 2003), the specific clinical syndrome spectrum of HHV-7 remains not clear (Ihira et al., 2001; Mendez et al., 2001). Several methods and different biological materials have been proposed to detect HHV-7 infection. Serological assays presents the same problems reported to HHV-6 and interpretation of these test are frequently difficult. Nested polymerase chain reaction (nested-PCR) using DNA extracted from either serum or plasma could detect only HHV-7 active infection (Ihira et al., 2001; Feldstein et al., 2003).

In our center, we found that nested-PCR carried out in DNA extracted from sera did not detect latent HHV-7 in a healthy cohort (Thomasini et al., 2008). In addition, positive IgM anti-HHV-7 and/or significant increase in IgG anti-HHV-7 titers were correlated with positive nested-PCR for HHV-7 in adult liver transplant recipients (Peigo et al., 2009). However, many technical and clinical aspects remain to be clarified regarding these tests.

Antigenemia can be performed to detected HHV-7 antigen in peripheral lymphocytes using similar technique describe to HHV-6 (Sampaio et al., 2011; Lautenschlager et al., 2002). HHV-7 antigen can be detected mainly in lymphocytes probably in T-CD4+ lymphocytes.

The majority of HHV-7 infections do not require antiviral medication, but the severe complications could be treated with ganciclovir and its derivates or foscarnet and cidofovir (Ongrádi et al., 2010).

There a few reports in the literature regarding treatment against HHV-7 infection probably due to fact that HHV-7 commonly causes not remarkable clinical outcomes. However, studies have demonstrated that treatment based on ganclclovir or valganciclovir following the same protocol used to CMV can be effective against concomitant HHV-6 and HHV-7 infection after lung and heart-lung transplantation (Lehto et al., 2007). Thus, the same protocol could hypothetically be used against HHV-7 in liver transplant patients.

2. Experience of the State University of Campinas regarding betaherpesviruses in liver transplantation

The aim of this study was to detect and to monitor CMV, HHV-6 and HHV-7 active infections in adult liver transplant recipients using nested-PCR and to describe the clinical aspects related to betaherpesviruses in these patients.

2.1 Materials and methods

Twenty-nine adult liver transplant patients (20 man and 9 woman), median age of 47 years (range 18 to 66), transplanted at the Liver Transplant Unit (University Hospital, State University of Campinas - Sao Paulo - Brazil) were included in this study.

The basic immunosuppressive therapy consisted of cyclosporine (0.4 mg/kg/d), methylpredinisolone (1.0 g first month, 20 mg at 30 days decreasing to 5 mg/mo to 90 days), azathioprine (100mg/d). Mycophenolate mofetil (100 mg/d) and tracolimus (FK) (0.1 mg/kg/d) were prescribed based on selected patient's characteristics and specific protocol studies. Acyclovir (5 mg/kg per day for 2 months) was employed as antiviral prophylaxis to *Herpes simplex*.

No routine CMV prophylaxis was used and ganciclovir (5mg/kg/d) for 6 weeks was administrated as treatment for symptomatic CMV patients. High doses of methylpredinisolone were used as antirejection treatment. Patient's characteristics related to age, sex and underlying liver disease were summarized in Table 2.

Peripheral blood was obtained from patients at the time of transplantation, as well as weekly for the first month and once a month to 180 days. Ethylenediamine tetraacetic acid (EDTA)-treated blood samples were used to DNA extraction from peripheral blood leukocytes (PBL) and serum (from without anticoagulant tube) of each blood sample was also separated by centrifugation. The obtained sera were then frozen (-20°C) until testing. The protocol was designed on accordance with the requirements for research involving human subjects in Brazil, and it was approved by the Institutional Ethics Committee.

2.1.1 CMV serological assay

Anti-CMV IgG and IgM were tested in sera of the donors and patients before transplantation. Assays were carried out using ELISA-Commercial Kits (Sorin Diagnostics, Saluggia, Italy) following manufacture's instructions.

Patient´s Characteristics	
Median age (years)	47 (range: 18-66)
Sex (male/female)	20/9
Diagnosis of underlying liver disease	
Hepatitis C	15
Alcoholic liver disease	3
Hepatitis B	2
Hepatitis C and alcohol	2
Cryptogenic cirrhosis	2
Hepatitis B and alcohol	1
Primary biliary cirrhosis	1
Autoimmune hepatitis	1
Primary sclerosing cholangitis	1
Hemochromatosis and alcohol	1

Table 2. Demographic characteristics of the patients studied

2.1.2 HHV-6 and -7 serological assays

IgG and IgM antibodies against HHV-6 and HHV-7 were tested in sera of the donors and patients before transplantation by an indirect immunofluorescent assay. The standard HHV-6 and HHV-7 antigens were prepared from viral culture of each virus (cord blood mononuclear cells infected by only one virus) and absence of cross-infectivity was confirmed by immunological or molecular methods. Infected cells were coated onto wells of immunofluorescence slides, air dried, and then fixed (cold methanol-acetone). The wells were covered with serial dilutions of patients' sera (starting from a 1:10 dilution) and incubated for 1 h at 37°C. For IgM detection, a single dilution of 1:20 of each sample was carried out. Slides were washed 3 times with PBS, wells were covered with anti-human IgG or IgM fluorescent conjugate diluted PBS/Evans's blue (Biomerieux Inc., Lyon, France), and then incubated for 1 h at 37°C.The slides were washed 3 times with PBS, buffered glycerin mounted, and immediately observed under an ultraviolet (UV) photo microscope (Leica DM2000,Wetzlar, Germany). All the samples were pre-treated with RFAb-sorbant (Hoescht-Behring, Kanata, Ontario, Canada) to avoid interference of IgG and rheumatoid factor in the IgM immunofuorescent assay (Ihira et al., 2001; Ablashi et al., 1998). The antibody titer was defined as the reciprocal of the serum dilution showing specific fluorescence.

2.1.3 Peripheral blood leukocyte (PBL) DNA extraction

Briefly, PBL were lysed after separation following protocol previously described (Bonon et al., 2005). PBL DNA was precipitated with cold ethanol and then eluted in 50μL of TE-buffer (10mM Tris, 1mM EDTA) and stored frozen (-20°C) until PCR analysis.

2.1.4 Serum DNA extraction

Briefly, DNA was extracted from 200 µL of serum using a phenol-chloroform protocol after incubation overnight in lysis buffer (10mM Tris-HCl pH 8.0, 10 mM EDTA, 10 mM NaCl, 0.2% dodecyl sodium sulfate and 100 µg proteinase K) at 56°C followed by DNA precipitation with cold ethanol. The resulting DNA pellet was eluted in 50µL of TE-buffer (10mM Tris, 1mM EDTA) and stored frozen (-20°C) until PCR analysis.

2.1.5 CMV nested-PCR

Five microliters of DNA extracted from PBL, as described above, were used in the nested-PCR using reaction mixture containing specific primers to CMV following protocol previously described (Shibata et al.,1992; Demmler et al.,1998).

2.1.6 HHV-6 and HHV-7 nested-PCR

Nested-PCR was carried out for each virus using 5 µL of DNA, extracted from serum as described above. Primers and protocol used to HHV-6 nested-PCR were previously described by Secchiero et al. (1995). Primers and protocol used to HHV-7 nested-PCR were previously described by Pozo et al. (1999) with some modifications (originally a multiplex-PCR).

Amplifications were carried out on a Peltier Thermal Cycler - MJ Research (Watertown–MA-USA).This The nested-PCR product was analyzed under UV light after electrophoresis in 2% agarose (Gibco-BRL) stained with ethidium bromide. All nested-PCR was carried out in duplicate using a second fresh aliquot. Polymerase chain reaction for beta-globin gene was carried out to detect contamination of serum with leukocytes and false negative results from incorrect DNA extraction from PBL.

Positive and negative controls for each virus were included systematically. Genomes amplifications using the referred primers results in DNA fragments containing 159, 258 and 122 base pairs of CMV, HHV-6 and HHV-7, respectively. Some nested-PCR products of each virus were sequenced analyzed and compared to the GenBank database using Software ChromasPro® (Thecnelysium Pty Ltd).

2.1.7 Definitions

CMV active infection was defined based on detection of CMV DNA in PBL by nested-PCR. HHV-6 and HHV-7 active infections were also defined based on detection of virus DNA in serum by nested-PCR. Transient viremia was defined when virus DNA was detectable only once or in no-consecutive samples.

Latent infection, reinfection and reactivation were defined base on criteria proposed by Ljungman et al., 2002. Co-infections were defined when two or more viruses were detected in the same sample.

Symptomatic CMV infection ('CMV disease') was divided into two situations: Tissue-invasive disease and "CMV viral syndrome" (Kotton et al., 2010).

Briefly, Tissue-invasive disease was defined based on symptoms consistent with CMV disease including fever, malaise, myalgia, anorexia and leukopenia accompanied of CMV active infection and when biopsy proven CMV identification (Taber et al. 2004, Ljungman et al., 2002). "CMV hepatitis" and "CMV gastrointestinal disease" was diagnosed based on criteria proposed by Ljungman *et al.* (2002). "CMV viral syndrome" was defined based on unexplained fever (>37.5ºC) for at least 3 days, in combination with at least one of the following features: arthralgia, leukopenia (<3 x10^9/l), thrombocytopenia (<150x10^9/l), liver enzymes elevation (ALT>50 U/l). Asymptomatic CMV infection was defined when CMV active infection occurs without signs, symptoms, or laboratory abnormalities described above.

Clinical symptoms such as fever, encephalitis, interstitial pneumonitis, hepatitis and laboratorial findings as leukopenia and thrombocytopenia were taken into account and CMV, HHV-6 and HHV-7 active infections were compared to these episodes. The laboratorial monitoring of graft function was based on elevation of serum alanine aminotransferase, alkaline phosphatase, gamma-glutamyl transpeptidase and bilirrubins. Rejection episodes were documented based on histopathological analysis of the liver biopsies (Banffs schema).

2.1.8 Statistical analysis

The comparison of categorical variables was performed using Fisher's exact test or chi-squired test and Mann-Withney-U test for continuous variables. A $p<0.05$ was considered statistically significant.

3. Results

All patients and donors had positives anti-CMV, anti-HHV-6 and anti-HHV-7 IgG before transplantation (D+/R+), indicating that all of them patients were virus reactivations/reinfections. CMV DNA was detected in 20 (68.9%) of 29 patients, median time to first CMV detection was of 50 days (range 7 to181). HHV-6 DNA was detected in 13 (44.8%) of 29 patients, median time to first HHV-6 detection was of 27 days (range 0 to 143). HHV-7 DNA was detected in 14 (48.2%) of 29 patients, median time to first HHV-7 detection was of 19 days (range 0 to 170). Six patients had HHV-7 DNA detectable already at the time of transplantation contrasting with two cases of HHV-6 and none of CMV. IgM against HHV-7 was detected in 100% of these patients who had detectable DNA already at the time of transplantation (P=0.002). Neither patient nor donor had positive IgM against CMV and HHV-6.

The three viruses together were found in 6/29 (20.7%) patients but in none sample at the same time. Co-infections by CMV/HHV-6, CMV/HHV-7 and HHV6/HHV-7 occurred in 5 (17.2%), 2 (6.9%) and 2 (6.9%) of the patients, respectively. Kinetic of the detection for three viruses was shown in Figure 2.

The statistical analysis showed that the detection of CMV, HHV-6 and HHV-7 was independent of one another (P>0.05). Diagrams illustrating positive nested-PCR for any combination of betaherpesviruses were shown in Figure 3.

Among the 20 patients with detectable CMV DNA, 10 (34.4% of total of the patients enrolled in this study) developed symptomatic CMV infections including "CMV viral syndrome" (n=5), CMV hepatitis (n=4) and CMV gastrointestinal disease (n=1). The symptoms have occurred 16 days (average) after first CMV DNA detection. Considering the patients with no detectable CMV DNA in their blood, none had CMV disease. The relationship between the detection of CMV DNA and symptomatic CMV infection was considered statistically significant (P=0.009). HHV-6 was detected in 50% of the patients with symptomatic CMV infection and in 30% of the patients without symptoms (P=0.32). HHV-7 was also detected in 60% of the symptomatic CMV infection and in 70% of the patients with asymptomatic infection (P=0.50). Of 10 patients who had liver dysfunction, 7 (70%, P=0.006) had symptomatic CMV infection and 2 (20%) had only HHV-6 active infection at the time of dysfunction.

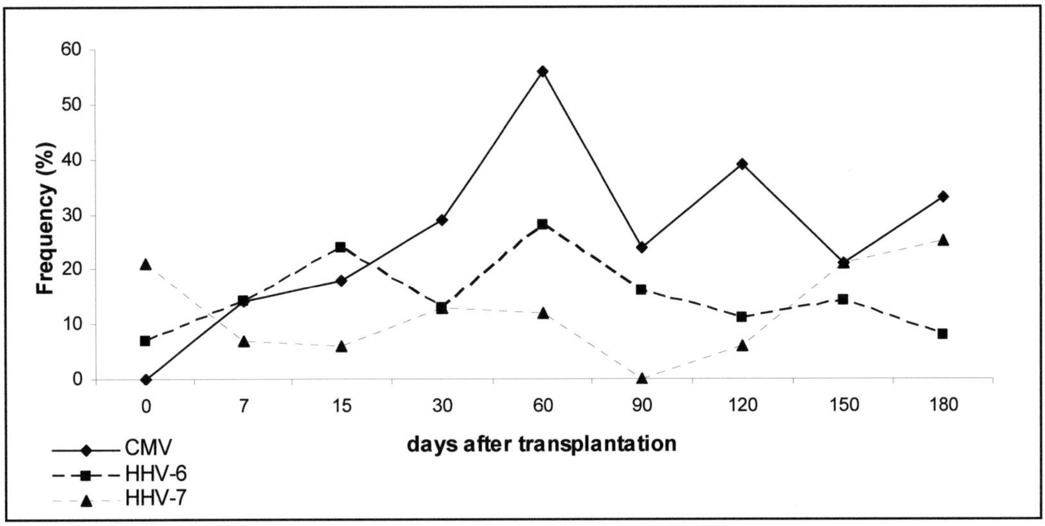

Fig. 2. Kinetic of detection for CMV, HHV-6 and HHV-7 in liver transplant recipients by nested-PCR

Of 10 patients that had liver dysfunction, five presented episodes of graft rejection graded as mild. One was related to CMV hepatitis. One had symptomatic CMV/HHV-6 co-infection (CMV hepatitis) 36 days prior rejection and one other had symptomatic CMV/HHV-7 co-infection ("CMV viral syndrome") 45 days prior rejection. Two patients that had co-infection before graft rejection were accompanied with persistent liver dysfunction until rejection episode. Another two patients had only HHV-6 infection accompanied with thrombocytopenia and leukopenia were related with rejection episodes. Unfortunately, we were not able to perform viral antigens detection in liver biopsies. In patients who had liver dysfunction and/or graft rejection, no underlying liver disease (HCV or HBV) were relapsed until end of the monitoring (180 days) and no other infectious agent was found. Only one case of "CMV viral syndrome" was recurrent and occurred after graft rejection.

Two episodes of pneumonitis were related with HHV-6/HHV-7 co-infection. One case of pneumonitis and two of encephalitis were also related with only HHV-6 infection and no others infectious agents were found. However, other tests to detect HHV-6 and HHV-7 in tissue samples might not be performed. In CMV and HHV-6 free patients no symptoms or significant laboratorial findings could be related to HHV-7.

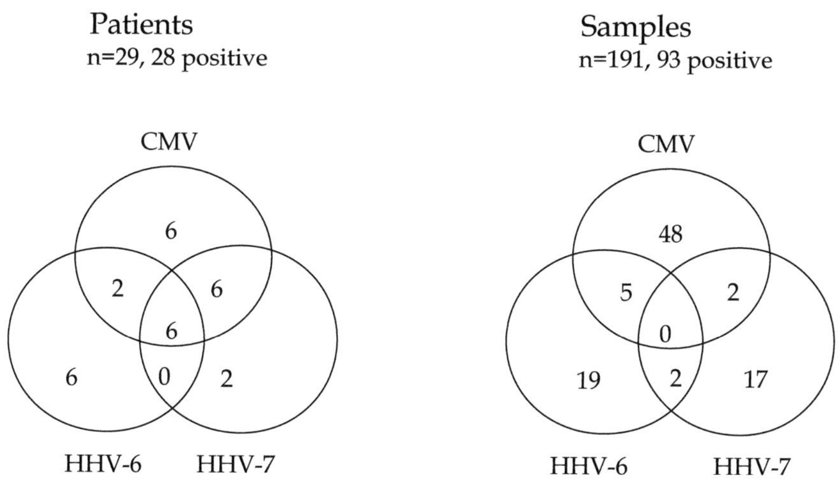

Fig. 3. Venn diagrams illustrating the number of patients (n=29) or number of positive samples (n=198) that were positive nested-PCR for any combination of betaherpesviruses

4. Discussion

The high frequency of positive IgG test against CMV observed agrees with previously data indicating a prevalence of 90 to 100% anti-CMV antibodies in Brazilian population (Suassuna et al., 1995; Costa et al., 1999). Previously studies in Brazilian population have also demonstrated high prevalence of HHV-6 and HHV-7 (90 and 84%, respectively).

CMV, HHV-6 and HHV-7 were frequently detected in patients after liver transplant (68.9%, 44.8% and 48.2%, respectively). Ihira et al. (2001) and Feldstein et al. (2003) suggested that the detection of virus DNA in serum by PCR is a useful marker of HHV-6 and HHV-7 active infection. In adult liver transplant recipients, Griffths et al. (1999) found CMV DNA in 47%, HHV-6 DNA in 32% and HHV-7 DNA in 48% of the patients. Ihira et al. (2001) found HHV-6 DNA in 38% and HHV-7 DNA in 40% of the patients until 8 weeks after liver transplantation. Humar et al. (2000) found CMV DNA in 63.6% and HHV-6 DNA in 54.5% of the liver transplant recipients.

The rate difference in each report depends of the sensitivity of PCR, type of transplantation, immunosuppressive protocol, the size of samples used and differences among subjects. However, the rate found in this study was relatively similar with others reports. Interesting, 6/29 (20.7%) patients had positive detectable HHV-7 DNA at the time of transplantation without symptoms. In addition, IgM against HHV-7 was found in all samples contributing to the hypothesis of true active infection had occurred. Since that this method did not detect latent infection in previously study (Thomasini et al., 2008) and blood was collected before surgery, it could be explained by reactivation caused by underlying liver disease or by transient viremia. Although some syndromes related to HHV-7 in immunocompetent patients have been described (Ward et al., 2005), studies in pre-transplant time should be performed to evaluate each hypothesis.

Ten of twelve (50%) patients who had detectable CMV DNA developed symptomatic CMV infection. The remaining 10 patients without symptoms could be explained by the high sensibility of the PCR, that can detect lower viral load (Tokimatsu et al.,1995), and they were not treated. However, the statistical analysis showed correlation between detection of CMV DNA and symptomatic CMV infection. Our symptomatic CMV incidence (34.4%) was higher (1.54-fold) than incidence reported by Humar et al. (2000) that reported symptomatic CMV infection in 21.6% of the patients. Similar to this study, Härmä et al. (2006) found 30% of symptomatic CMV infection during 3 first months after transplantation.

We have considered that this higher incidence of CMV infection and symptomatic CMV infection due to high prevalence of CMV in Brazilian population, no routine or preemptive ganciclovir therapy and use of cyclosporine. Humar et al. (2000) have found an independently increasing risk factor for development of CMV disease when patient had D+/R+ CMV serostatus and all patients enrolled in this study were D+/R+. It is conflicting with most reports that suggest higher risk factor when CMV serostatus is D+/R-. Hoppe et al. (2004) had suggests a higher probability of CMV infection among patients treated with cyclosporine compared to tracolimus.

Some cases of pneumonitis and encephalitis were related to HHV-6 active infection or with co-infections HHV-6/HHV-7. Previously reports had suggested association an increase risk of graft rejection associated with CMV (Lautenschlager et al., 1997). Although we have found that symptomatic CMV infection was present in most cases of liver dysfunction and graft rejection, CMV co-infection with HHV-6 or HHV-7 and HHV-6 alone were more likely related with graft rejection than CMV alone. Härmä et al. (2006) had suggested a role of HHV-6 in liver dysfunction and graft rejection (with HHV-6 antigens detected in liver biopsies in same patients). Griffiths et al. (1999) found also association between liver dysfunction and graft rejection with HHV-6 and dysfunction with HHV-7. HHV-6 could either be participating directly in the rejection process or potentially exacerbating the inflammatory response characteristic of rejection (Emery, 2001). However, the fact that the most of patients with HHV-6 active infection were asymptomatic in this study (probably due to transient viremia) turned difficult to establish a relation between liver dysfunction/graft rejections with HHV-6 active infection. In addition, all of the positive patients included in this study have betaherpesviruses reactivation/reinfection and not primary infection. Betaherpesviruses primary infections could have more significant clinical outcomes and this hypothesis should be considered in pediatric liver transplantation which primary infections could be more frequent.

In CMV and HHV-6 free patients no symptoms or significant laboratorial findings could be related to HHV-7. However, the role of the HHV-7 in down regulation of CD4 expression in lymphocytes has been described (Secchiero et al., 1997; Secchiero et al., 1998) and a possible immnunomodulatory effects do not be discarded. Studies regarding CMV, HHV-6 and HHV-7 including determination of viral load with 'cut-off' values for clinical manifestation and detection of viral antigens in liver biopsies as well as evaluation of cellular and humoral immune response could be performed. In this study we have considered qualitative nested-PCR which had limited value for clinical monitoring of the betaherpesvirus.

5. Conclusion

The results described above show that few patients remain free of betaherpesviruses after liver transplantation. Most of the patients with active infection with more than one virus were infected sequentially and not concurrently. Active infection with HHV-6, HHV-7 or CMV might develop independently of one another. Most patients with HHV-6 or HHV-7 active infections were asymptomatic. In few patients, HHV-6 could be associated with some clinical manifestations and episodes of graft dysfunction and rejection. Qualitative nested-PCR was considered of limited value to clinical monitoring of betaherpesviruses.

6. References

Abdel Massih, R.C. & Razonable, R.R. (2009), Human herpesvirus 6 infections after liver transplantation. *World Journal of Gastroenterology,* Vol. 15, (February 2009), pp. (2561-2569) ISSN 1007-9327

Almeida, L.N.B., Azevedo, R.S., Amaku, M. & Massad, E. (2001) Cytomegalovirus seroepidemiology in an urban community of São Paulo, Brazil. *Revista Saúde Pública,* Vol. 35, (February 2001), pp. (124-129) ISSN 0034-8910

Blair, J.E. & Shimon, K. (2005). Bacterial, Mycobacterial, and Protozoal Infections After Liver Transplantation—Part I. *Liver Transplantation,* Vol. 11, No. 12, (December 2005), pp. (1452-1459), ISSN 1527-6465

Bonon, S.H., Menoni, S.M., Rossi, C.L., De Souza, C.A., Vigorito, A.C. & Costa S.C.B. (2005), Surveillance of cytomegalovirus infection in haematopoietic stem cell transplantation patients. *Journal of Infectious Disease,* Vol. 50, (February 2005), pp. (130-137) ISSN 0022-1899

Costa, S.C.B., Miranda, S.R.P., Alves, G. (1999), Detection of cytomegalovirus infection by PCR in renal transplant patients. *Brazilian Journal of Medical and Biological Research,* Vol. 32, (1999), pp. (953-959) ISSN 1678-4510

Demmler, G.J., Buffone, C.J. & Schimbor C.M. (1988), Detection of cytomegalovirus in urine newbornes by using polymerase chain reaction DNA amplication. *Journal of Infectious Disease,* Vol. 158, (1988), pp. (1177-1184) ISSN 0022-1899

DesJardin, J.A., Cho, E., Supran, S., Gibbons, L., Werner, B.G., Snydman, D.R. (2001) Association of human herpesvirus 6 reactivation with severe cytomegalovirus-associated disease in orthotopic liver transplant recipients. *Clinical Infectious Disease,* Vol. 33, (August 2001), pp. (1358-1362) ISSN 1058-4838

Dewhurst, S. (2004), Human herpesvirus type 6 and human herpesvirus type 7 infections of the central nervous system. *Herpes,* Vol. 11, (June 2004), pp. (105-111) ISSN 0969-7667

Donati, D., Akhyani, N., Fogdell-Hahn, A., Cermelli, C., Cassiani-Ingoni, R., Vortmeyer, A., Heiss, J.D., Cogen, P., Gaillard, W.D., Sato, S., Theodore, W.H. & Jacobson, S. (2003), Detection of Human Herpesvirus-6 in Mesial Temporal Lobe Epilepsy Surgical Brain Resections. *Neurology,* Vol. 61, (October 2003), pp. (1405–1411), ISSN 10158618

EMERY, V.C. (2001), Human Herpesvirus 6 and 7 in solid organ transplant recipients. *Clinical Infectious Disease,* Vol. 32, (2001), pp. (1357-1360) ISSN 1058-4838

Feldstein, A.E., Razonable, R.R. & Boyce, T.G. (2003), Prevalence and clinical significance of human herpesvirus 6 and 7 active infection in pediatric liver transplant patients. *Pediatric Transplantation,* Vol. 7, (2003), pp. (25-129) ISSN 1397-3142

Freitas, R.B. & Linhares, A.C. (1997), Prevalence of human herpesvirus 6 antibody in the population of Belem, Para, northern Brazil. *Transactions of the Royal Society of Tropical Medicine and Hygiene,* Vol. 91, (May 1997), pp. (538-540) ISSN 0035-9203

Frenkel, N., Schirmer, E.C. & Wyatt I.S. (1990), Isolation of a new herpervirus from human CD4 T cells. *Proceedings of the National Academy of Science of United States of America,* Vol. 87, pp. (748) ISSN 0027-8424

Griffits, P.D., Clark, D.A. & Emery, V.C. (2000), Betaherpevirus in transplant recipients. *Journal of Antimicrobial Chemotherapy,* Vol. 45, (March 2000), pp. (29-34) ISSN 1460-2091

Griffiths, P.D., Ait-khaled, M. & Beatcroft, C.P. (1999), Human herpesvirus 6 and 7 as potential pathogens after liver transplant: prospective comparison with the effect of cytomegalovirus. *Journal of Medical Virology*, Vol. 59, (1999), pp. (496-501) ISSN 0146-6615

Grivel, J.C., Santoro, F., Chen, S., Fagá, G., Malnati, M.S. & Ito Y. (2003), Pathogenic effects of human herpesvirus 6 in human lymphoid tissue ex vivo. *Journal of Virology*, Vol. 77, (2003), pp. (8280-8289) ISSN 1098-5514

Härmä, M., Höckrstedt, K. & Lyytikäinen. (2006), HHV-6 and HHV-7 antigenemia related to CMV infection after liver transplantation. *Journal of Medical Virology*, Vol. 78, (2006), pp. (800-805) ISSN 0146-6615

Hoppe, L., Bressane, R. & Lago, L.S. (2004), Risk factors associated with cytomegalovirus–positive antigenemia in orthotopic liver transplant patients. *Transplantation Proceedings*, Vol. 26, (April 2004), pp. (961-963) ISSN 0041-1345

Hudnall, S.D., Chen, T., Allison, P., Tyring, S.K. & Ashley Heath, A. (2008), Herpesvirus prevalence and viral load in healthy blood donors by quantitative real-time polymerase chain reaction. *Transfusion*, Vol. 48, No. 6, (June 2008), pp. (1180-1187), ISSN 0041-1132

Humar, A., Malkan, G. & Moussa, G. (2000), Human Herpesvirus-6 is associated with cytomegalovirus reactivation in liver transplant recipients. *Journal of Infectious Diseases*, Vol. 181, (2000), pp. (1450-1453) ISSN 0022-1899

Ihira, A.M., Yoshikawa, T. & Suzuki, K. (2001), Correlation between human herpesvirus 6 and 7 infections after living related liver transplantation. *Microbiology and Immunology*, Vol. 45, (March 2001), pp. (225-232) ISSN 1348-0421

Ishibashi, K., Tokumoto, T., Tanabe, K., Shirakawa, H., Hashimoto, K., Kushida, N., Yanagida, T., Inoue, N., amaguchi, O., Toma, H., & Suzutani, T. (2007), Association of the Outcome of Renal Transplantation with Antibody Response to Cytomegalovirus Strain—Specific Glycoprotein H Epitopes. *Clinical Infectious Disease*, Vol. 45, (January 2007), pp. (60-67) ISSN 1058-4838

Kas-Deelen, A.M., T.H., Thea, T.H., Blomb, N., van der Strated, B.W.A., De Maarc, E.F., Smitb, J., van Sonc, W.J. (2001), Uptake of pp65 in in vitro Generated pp65-Positive Polymorphonuclear Cells Mediated by Phagocytosis and Cell Fusion?. *Intervirology*, Vol. 44, (2001), pp. (8–13) ISSN 0300-5526

Kotton C.N. (2010), Management of cytomegalovirus infection in solid organ transplantation. *Nature Reviews Nephrology*, Vol. 6, No. 12, (December 2010), pp. (711-721), ISSN 1759-5061

Kotton, C.N., Kumar, D., Caliendo, A.M., Asberg, A., Chou, S., Snydman, D.R., Allen, U. & Humar, A. (2010), International consensus guidelines on the management of cytomegalovirus in solid organ transplantation. *Transplantation*, Vol. 15, (April 2010), pp. (779-795) ISSN 1534-0608

Lautenschlager, I., Linnavuori, K., Lappalainen, M., Suni, J. & Hokerstedt, K. (2000), HHV-6 reactivation is often associated with CMV infection in liver transplant patients. *Transplant International*, Vol. 13, (January 2000), pp. (351-353) ISSN 0934-0874

Lautenschlager, I., Lappalainen, M., Linnavuori, K., Suni, J. & Höckerstedt, K. (2002); CMV infection is usually associated with concurrent HHV-6 and HHV-7 antigenemia in liver transplant patients. *Journal of Clinical Virology, Vol. 25,* (August 2002), pp. (57-61) ISSN 1386-6532

Lautenschlager, I., Höckerstedt, K. & Jalanko, H. (1996), Persistent cytomegalovirus in liver allografts with chronic rejection. *Hepatology*. Vol. 25, (January 1997), pp. (190-194) ISSN 1527-3350

Lehto J.T., Halme M., Tukiainen P., Harjula A., Sipponen J. & Lautenschlager I., (2007), Human herpesvirus-6 and -7 after lung and heart-lung transplantation. *Journal of Heart and Lung Transplantation,* Vol. (26), (January), pp. 41-47, ISSN 1053-2498

Linhares, M.I., Eizuru, Y., Tateno, S. & Minamishima, Y. (1991), Seroprevalence of human herpesvirus 6 infection in Brazilian and Japanese populations in the north-east of Brazil. *Microbiology and Immunology,* Vol. 25, (November 1991), pp. (1023-1027) ISSN 1348-0421

Ljungman, P., Griffiths, P. & Paya, C. (2002), Definition of cytomegalovirus infection and disease in transplant recipients. *Clinical Infectious Diseases,* Vol. 34, (2002), pp. (1094-1097) ISSN 1058-4838

Matsumoto, H., Hatanaka, D., Ogura, Y., Chida, A., Nakamura, Y. & Nonoyama, S. (2011), Severe Human Herpesvirus 6-associated Encephalopathy in Three Children: Analysis of Cytokine Profiles and the Carnitine Palmitoyltransferase 2 Gene. *Pediatric Infectious Disease Journal,* Vol. 7, (June 2011), pp. () ISSN 0891-3668

Mendez J.C., Dockrell, D.H. & Espy, M.J. (2001), Human β-herpesvirus interactions in solid organ transplant recipients. *Journal of Infectious Diseases,* Vol. 183, (2001), pp. (179) ISSN 0022-1899

Mirandola, P., Sponzilli, I., Solenghi, E., Micheloni, C., Rinaldi, L. & Gobbi, G. (2006), Down-regulation of human leukocyte antigen class I and II and beta 2-microglobulin expression in human herpesvirus-7-infected cells. *Journal of Infectious Disease,* Vol. 1937, (2006), pp. (917-926) ISSN 0022-1899

Osman, H.K., Peiris, J.S., Taylor, C.E., Karlberg, J.P. & Madeley, C.R. (1997), Correlation between the detection of viral DNA by the polymerase chain reaction in peripheral blood leukocytes and serological responses to human herpesvirus 6, human herpesvirus 7, and cytomegalovirus in renal allograft recipients. *Journal of Medical Virology,* Vol. 53, (March 1997), pp. (288-294) ISSN 0146-6615

Pozo, F. & Tenorio, A. (1999), Dectection and typing of lymphotropic herpesvirus by multiplex polymerase chain reaction. *Journal of Virological Methods,* Vol. 79, (1999), pp. (9-19) ISSN 0166-0934

Peigo, M.F., Thomasini, R.L., Puglia, A.L.P., Costa, S.C.B., Bonon, S.H.A., Boin, I.F.S., Leonardi, M. & Mota, N.G.S. (2009), Human herpesvirus-7 in Brazilian liver transplant recipients: a follow-up comparison between molecular and immunological assays Human herpesvirus-7 in Brazilian liver transplant recipients: a follow-up comparison between molecular and immunological assays. *Transplant Infectious Disease,* Vol. 11, (December 2009), pp. (497-502) ISSN 1399-3062

Razonable, R.R., Lautenschlager, I. (2010), Impact of human herpes virus 6 in liver transplantation. *World Journal of Hepathology,* Vol. 27, (September 2010), pp. (345-353) ISSN

Ongrádi, J., Kövesdi, V. & Kováts, E. (2010), Human Herpesvirus 7. *Orsovay Hetilap,* Vol. 151, (April 2010), PP. (645-651) ISSN 1416-4841

Rogers, J., Rohal, S., Carrigan, D.R., Kusne, S., Knox, K.K., & Gayowski, T. (2000), Human herpesvirus-6 in liver transplant recipients: role in pathogenesis of fungal infections, neurological complications, and outcome. *Transplantation,* Vol. 69, (December 2000), pp. (2566-2573) ISSN 1534-0608

Sampaio, A.M., Thomasini, R.L., Guardia, A.C., Stucchi, R.S., Rossi, C.L., Costa, S.C. & Boin, I.F. (2011), Cytomegalovirus, human herpesvirus-6, and human herpesvirus-7 in adult liver transplant recipients: diagnosis based on antigenemia. *Transplantation Proceedings,* Vol. 43, (April 2011), pp. (1357-13579) ISSN 0041-1345

Sechiero, P., Carrigan, D.R., Asano, Y., Benedetti, L., Crowley, R.W. & Komaroff, A.L. (1995), Detection of Human Herpesvirus 6 in plasma of children with primary infection and immunosuppressed patients by Polymerase Chain Reaction. *The Journal of Infectious Diseases*, Vol. 171, (1995), pp. (273-280) ISSN 0022-1899

Secchiero, P., Mirandola, P., Zella, D., Celeghini, C., Gonelli, A. & Vitale, M. (2001), Human herpesvirus 7 induces the functional up-regulation of tumor necrosis factor-related apoptosis-inducing ligand (TRAIL) coupled to TRAIL-R1 down-modulation in CD41 T cells. *Blood*, Vol. 98, (2001), pp. (2474-2481) ISSN 0006-4971

Secchiero, P., Gibellini, D. & Flamand, L. (1997), Human Herpesvirus 7 induces the down-regulation of CD4 antigen in lymphoid T cells without affecting p56Ick levels. *Journal of Immunology*, Vol. 159, (July 1997), pp. (3412-3423) ISSN 0022-1767

Secchiero, P., Zella, D., Barabitskaja, O., Reitz, M.S., Capitani, S., Gallo, R., & Zauli, G. (1998), Progressive and persistent downregulation of surface CXCR4 in CD4+ T cells infected with human Herpesvirus 7, *Blood*, Vol. 92, (December 1998), pp. (4521-4528) ISSN 0006-4971

Shibata, D., Martin, W.J. & Appleman, M.D. (1992), Detecion of cytomegalovirus DNA in peripheral blood leukocytes after allogenic marrow transplantation. *Blood*, Vol. 80, (1992), pp. (1358-1364) ISSN 0006-4971

Suassuna, J.H., Leite, L.L. & Villela, L.H. (1995), Prevalence of cytomegalovirus infection in different patient groups of an urban university in Brazil. *Revista da Sociedade Brasileira de Medicina Tropical*, Vol. 28, (1995), pp. (105-108) ISSN 0037-8682

Taber, D.J., Ashcraft, E. & Baillie, G.M. (2004), Valganciclovir prophylaxis in patients at high risk for the development of cytomegalovirus disease. *Transplant Infectious Disease*, Vol. 6, (2004), pp. (101-109) ISSN 1399-3062

Tokimatsu, I., Tashiro, T. & Nasu, M. (1995), Early diagnosis and monitoring of human cytomegalovirus pnemonia in patients with adult T-cell leukemia by DNA amplication in serum. *Chest*, Vol. 107, (1995), pp. (1024-1027) ISSN 0012-3692

Tong, C.Y.W., Barkran, A., Willians, H., Cheung, C.Y. & Peiris J.S. (2000), Association of human herpesvirus 7 with cytomegalovirus disease in renal transplant recipients. *Transplantation*, Vol. 70, (July 2000), pp. (213-216), ISSN 1534-0608

Thomasini, R.L., Sampaio, A.M., Bonon, S.H.A., Boin, I.F., Leonardi, L.S. & Costa SC. (2007), Detection and monitoring of human herpesvirus 7 in adult liver transplant patients: impact on clinical course and association with cytomegalovirus. *Transplantation Proceedings*, Vol. 39, (May 2007), pp. (1537-1539) ISSN 0041-1345

Thomasini, R.L., Martins, J.M. & Parola, D.C. (2008), Detection of human herpesvirus-7 by qualitative nested-PCR: comparison between healthy individuals and liver transplant recipients. *Revista da Sociedade Brasileira de Medicina Tropical*, Vol. 41, (June 2008), pp. 556-559 ISSN 0037-8682

van der Bij, W., Schirm, J., Torensma, R., van Son, W.J., Tegzess & A.M. The TH. (1988), Comparison between viremia and antigenemia for detection of cytomegalovirus in blood. *Journal of Clinical Microbiology*, Vol. 26, (December 1988), pp. (2531-2535) ISSN 0095-1137

Vinnard C., Barton T., Jerud E. & Blumberg E. (2009), A report of human herpesvirus 6–associated encephalitis in a solid organ transplant recipient and a review of previously published cases. *Liver Transplantation*, Vol. 15 (October), pp. 1242-1246 ISSN 1527-6473

Ward, K.N. (2005), The natural history and laboratory diagnosis of human herpesvirus-6 and -7 infections in the immunocompetent. *Journal of Clinical Virology*, Vol. 32, (2005), pp. (183-193) ISSN 1386-6532

20

Donor-Derived Infectious Complications and Disease Transmission

Kun-Ming Chan and Wei-Chen Lee
Division of Liver and Organ Transplantation Surgery, Department of General Surgery, Chang Gung Memorial Hospital at Linkou, Chang Gung University College of Medicine, Taiwan, Republic of China

1. Introduction

Organ transplantation is now the treatment of choice for many end-stage diseases. However, the gap between organ demand and donor availability has progressively widened, and the severe shortage of organs for transplantation has resulted in the increasing use of expanded donor criteria, allowing the inclusion of older donors as well as donors with mild disease. Thus, organ donation may involve the risk of the transmittal of unwanted host factors, such as infections and malignancies. Infectious microbes and unexpected diseases that are present in an organ donor have the potential to be transmitted to the transplant recipient. Although the transmission of donor-derived infectious diseases was reported to occur in less than 1% of all donations from deceased donors, significant morbidity and mortality can occur following such disease transmissions. Infectious diseases remain a major complication in solid organ transplantation, and the study of donor-derived infections is an evolving field. Despite recent improvements in the microbiological screening of donors and detailed reviews of potential donors' medical records, persistent clusters of donor-derived infections in transplant recipients remain. Bacterial, viral, fungal, parasitic, and other rare infections can be transmitted through organs and tissue allografts. However, the transmission of microorganisms from allografts is not likely to cause infectious complications in every transplant recipient. The risk of infection is mostly related to the recipient's net state of immunosuppression. The balance between the recipient's state of immunosuppression and epidemiological exposures contribute to the risk of infection (Fishman, 2007; Fishman & Rubin, 1998). Immunosuppression not only increases the risk of tissue invasion, dissemination, and superinfection, but also blunts the typical inflammatory responses that alert clinicians to the presence of infection after exposure. As a result, the recognition of infection is more difficult in transplant recipients than in individuals with normal immunities. The presentations of infections are often complicated by noninfectious events, such as allograft rejection. Specifically, 40% of infections in liver transplant recipients were not associated with fever (Chang et al., 1998). Thus, intervention treatments of infections may be delayed. The goals of patient care after organ transplantation are to prevent the transmission of donor-derived infections, to recognize the presence of infections in solid-organ transplant recipients, and to intervene early when such infections occur. In addition, malignancies that are transmitted from the donor due to direct transmission of tumors or to tumors arising in cells of donor origin can also occur in organ transplantation. For example, melanoma, which is one of the most frequently reported and lethal donor-derived malignancies, has a high transmission rate. Therefore, potential organ donors should be carefully screened for histories of malignancies.

2. Potential infections of the donor

Potential infections acquired from a donor can be classified into two categories: infections that already existed in the patient prior to becoming a potential donor and nosocomial exposures of the donor after hospitalization. Preexisting infections may be present in either living or deceased donors, and the majority of such infections are viral. Some of these infections, which might be detected by donor and recipient screening, involve infection from a seropositive donor to a seronegative recipient, including the transmission of cytomegalovirus (CMV), Epstein-Barr virus (EBV), or toxoplasmosis, while others are unexpected despite routine donor screening. Unexpected clusters of donor-derived viral infections in transplant recipients have occurred, including rabies, West Nile virus (WNV), Human immunodeficiency virus (HIV), herpes simplex virus, hepatitis B virus (HBV), and hepatitis C virus (HCV) (Morris et al., 2010). Nosocomial donor infections are most commonly related to bacterial pathogens. These infections are usually caused by the same nosocomial pathogens that infect other patients with similar lengths of stay in the intensive care unit. Wu and colleagues have shown that several factors, including a longer stay in an intensive care unit, previous cardiopulmonary cerebral resuscitation, and the use of inotropic agents, contribute to the risk of infection of a potential donor (Wu et al., 2008). Additionally, infected donors may also transmit microorganisms that are resistant to formal antimicrobial treatments. The use of organs from deceased donors with potential infections is controversial, and there is a need for improved microbiological screening tools and therapies.

Opportunistic infections are generally uncommon in the first 1–4 weeks after transplantation because the impact of immunosuppression depends on prolonged exposure to suppressive therapies. Unexplained early infections in this period are generally donor-derived or associated with surgery-related complications. Thus, a thorough investigation of infectious diseases in a potential donor is mandatory. The implementation of a preventive strategy of universal prophylaxis that provides antimicrobial therapy to all at-risk potential donors may alter the incidence and severity of organism transmission as well as post-transplant infections. However, routine antimicrobial prophylaxis should be adjusted based on the organ transplanted, individual exposures, and hospital epidemiology. Prophylaxis can also be adjusted according to known colonization patterns. All active infections in the donor should be eradicated or controlled prior to transplantation, as these may be transmitted and reactivated in the transplant recipient, which may lead to significant morbidity and mortality.

3. Screening of the risks of infections of organ donors

Benjamin Franklin said that an ounce of prevention is worth a pound of cure. The pretransplantation screening of potential organ donors is essential for the prevention of disease transmission, as well as the success of solid organ transplantation. Pretransplantation infectious disease screenings of potential donors are helpful in: (1) identifying conditions that may disqualify the donor, (2) identifying and treating active infections prior to transplantation, (3) identifying the risk of infection and determining strategies for preventing and mitigating infection after transplantation, and (4) implementing preventive interventions, such as updating the recipient's vaccination status. Although there is general consensus on the major infections for which screening should be performed, there is some variation in the types of screening used in different transplantation centers. A number of publications have discussed guidelines for the pretransplant screening of organ donors (Avery, 2004; Delmonico & Snydman, 1998; Fischer & Avery, 2009). Some documented infections preclude organ donation under specific infectious conditions, including uncontrolled sepsis, HIV or human T-cell lymphotropic virus (HTLV) infection, rabies, WNV infection, and lymphocytic choriomeningitis virus (LCMV) infection. Therefore, organ donors should be screened for the risk of infection on the basis of organ-procurement standards. The screening should include the donor's medical history as well as laboratory serologic testing.

3.1 Screening the donor's medical/behavioral history

A thorough medical history and physical examination are the first steps in donor screening. An accurate medical and social history, as well as the donor's recent and remote exposures, is important in the assessment of donor eligibility. This initial evaluation may address current or active infections prior to organ procurement. Each potential donor should be screened for medical conditions that may affect the function of the donated organ, for the presence of transmissible disease or malignancies that are treated or untreated, or for any other known condition that may be transmitted by the donor organ that may reasonably affect the recipient. This history should also be used to identify whether the potential donor has factors associated with an increased risk of transmission of infection, including the blood-borne pathogens HIV, HBV, and HCV. The data that should be collected when assessing donor eligibility are summarized in Table 1.

Medical history
Previous infection
Vaccinations
Occupational exposures
Travel history
History of transfusions with blood or blood products
Any contact with people with human immunodeficiency virus (HIV), hepatitis B virus (HBV), hepatitis C virus (HCV), or other transmissible diseases
Tattooing, ear or body piercing
Use of illicit drugs
Sexual behavior
Incarceration
Contact with animals, including pets, bats, stray dogs, or rodents
Physical examination

Table 1. Suggested data to be collected for determining eligibility prior to organ donation

However, due to the limited pool of donors, it has become increasingly important to consider marginal donors, including those with infections at the time of donation. The decision to use organs from an infected donor reflects the urgency of transplantation for the recipient and the availability of alternative organs.

3.1.1 Exclusion of high-risk donors

The transmission of HIV through liver transplantation has been reported sporadically (Ahn & Cohen, 2008; Samuel et al., 1988). The Centers for Disease Control and Prevention of the United States (US) has issued guidelines for the classification of donors possessing a high risk for HIV infection (CDC, 1994). Potential donors who meet any of the criteria listed below should be excluded from the donation of organs or tissues and may be considered only if the risk to the recipient of not performing the transplant is deemed greater than the risk of HIV transmission and disease. In such a circumstance, it is recommended to inform the recipient and discuss the possibility of HIV transmission.

Behavior/history exclusionary criteria

1. Men who have had sex with another man in the preceding 5 years.
2. Persons who report nonmedical intravenous, intramuscular, or subcutaneous injection of drugs in the preceding 5 years.
3. Persons with hemophilia or related clotting disorders who have received human-derived clotting factor concentrates.
4. Men and women who have engaged in sex in exchange for money or drugs in the preceding 5 years.
5. Persons who have had sex in the preceding 12 months with any person described in items 1-4 above or with a person known or suspected to have HIV infection.
6. Persons who have been exposed in the preceding 12 months to known or suspected HIV-infected blood through percutaneous inoculation or through contact with an open wound, non-intact skin, or mucous membrane.
7. Inmates of correctional systems. (This exclusion is to address issues such as difficulties with informed consent and the increased prevalence of HIV in this population.)

Specific exclusionary criteria for pediatric donors

- Children meeting any of the exclusionary criteria listed above for adults should not be accepted as donors.
- Children born to mothers with HIV infections or mothers who meet the behavioral or laboratory exclusionary criteria for adult donors (regardless of their HIV status) should not be accepted as donors unless HIV infection can be definitely excluded in the child as follows:
  - Children greater than 18 months of age who are born to mothers with, or at risk for, HIV infection, who have not been breast fed within the last 12 months, and whose HIV antibody tests, physical examination, and review of medical records do not indicate evidence of HIV infection can be accepted as donors.
  - However, children less than or equal to 18 months of age who are born to mothers with, or at risk for, HIV infection should not be accepted as donors regardless of their HIV test results.

3.2 Laboratory screening tests

In the US, all laboratory testing of donors must be performed in an appropriately accredited laboratory utilizing nationally licensed, approved, or cleared serological screening tests. Laboratory screening of potential donors is generally performed for HIV, HBV, HCV, and syphilis. The serological tests most frequently used for donor screening are listed in Table 2.

Human immunodeficiency virus (HIV) antibody
Hepatitis B (HBV) serologic tests:
HBV surface antigen (HBsAg)
HBV core antibody (HBcAb IgM and IgG)
HBV surface antibody (HBsAb)
Hepatitis C (HCV) antibody
Venereal Disease Research Laboratory (VDRL) test or Rapid Plasma Reagin (RPR)
Cytomegalovirus (CMV) antibody IgM and IgG
Epstein-Barr virus (EBV) antibody panel
Herpes simplex virus antibody
Varicella-Zoster virus antibody
Human T cell lymphotrophic virus (HTLV-I/II) antibody (for donors originating from high-incidence areas)
Toxoplasma antibody (optional, not routinely performed for noncardiac donors)
Blood and urine cultures

Table 2. Common screening tests for potential organ donors

Serology for HTLV-I/II is routinely performed in the US, but in Europe and other areas, this assay is restricted to donors living in, or originating from, high-incidence areas. However, the risk of infection may be difficult to assess, especially if HTLV has been transmitted vertically or sexually. Toxoplasmosis is a major concern, particularly in heart transplantation, but it is rarely transmitted to liver recipients (Mayes et al., 1995). Thus, toxoplasmosis screening is not routinely performed for noncardiac donors. Donor screening for toxoplasmosis is also not advocated based on the small amount of information gained and the high rate of false-positive results. In addition, a seropositive result for toxoplasma does not contraindicate organ donation, but does provide information that determines appropriate prophylaxis and treatment options following transplantation.

3.2.1 Donors with identified infections

The use of organs from deceased donors who had fevers or viral infections remains controversial, indicating the need for improved microbiological screening tests. However, the urgent demand for organs has led to the use of organs from donors with identified infections for specific recipients based on the urgency of the need for transplantation and the availability of antimicrobial therapies. Ideally, all active bacterial or fungal infections in the donor should be treated and resolved prior to transplantation. Currently, no recommendations are available regarding the optimal duration of therapy before transplantation or the interval required between resolution of the infection and transplantation. It may not be possible to document clearance of the infection in an emergent situation of life-saving transplantation. Common infections in donors that have been treated adequately should not preclude the use of organs, and decisions must be flexible and individualized to the recipient.

Additionally, livers from donors with HBV infection (HBcAb- or HBsAg-positive) may be used in recipients who have previously been infected or are in life-threatening situations, with appropriate treatment with specific anti-HBV antiviral agents (Seehofer & Berg, 2005; Trautwein, 2004). Similarly, the use of HCV-infected organs is generally reserved for HCV-infected recipients or for selected HCV-negative recipients (Ghobrial et al., 2001; Vargas et al., 1999; Velidedeoglu et al., 2002). Suggested organ donation strategies that are based on donor screening data are summarized in Table 3 (Grossi & Fishman, 2009).

Serologic finding	Action
Antibody to human immunodeficiency virus (HIV)	Exclude from organ donation
Antibody to human T-cell lymphotropic virus (HTLV) I/II	Generally exclude from organ donation (may be used in life-threatening situations with informed consent)
Antibody to hepatitis C virus (HCV)	If used, organs are usually reserved for recipients with antibodies to HCV or severely ill recipients
Antibody to cytomegalovirus (CMV)	Use information to determine prophylaxis (in conjunction with recipient serology)
Antibody to Epstein-Barr virus (EBV)	Consider PCR monitoring if donor is seropositive and recipient is seronegative
Hepatitis B virus (HBV) surface antigen (HBsAg) + or HBV core antibody (HBcAb IgM) +	Exclude from organ donation (possible use in life-threatening situations with intensive prophylaxis)
HBV surface antibody (HBsAb) +	Generally safe for organ donation
HBV core antibody (HBcAb) IgG +	High-risk for transmission if liver is used for donation, but used at some centers with intensive prophylaxis; nonhepatic organs carry a small risk of transmission of HBV and are used for vaccinated recipients or with prophylaxis
Rapid Plasma Reagin (RPR) +	Not a contraindication to donation. Recipient should receive benzathine penicillin
Antibody to Toxoplasma	Not a contraindication to donation. Sulfa-allergic, seronegative heart transplant recipients with a seropositive donor should receive pyrimethamine prophylaxis

Table 3. Suggested strategies based on donor screening results

3.3 Additional considerations for donor screening

Despite the use of highly sensitive assays and the development of new policies, the transmission of infections to organ transplant recipients remains uncommon. However, it does occur with sufficient frequency to suggest that the current approaches to donor screening are inadequate. Many potential exposures are too nonspecific to allow appropriate decision-making regarding the risk of transmission.

3.3.1 Hemodilution of donor blood samples

All blood samples obtained and used for screening tests must be assessed for hemodilution, which is defined as the dilution of plasma that is sufficient to affect the results of communicable disease testing. Blood samples from a deceased organ donor who underwent blood loss and transfusion of blood products or infusion of colloids and crystalloids are likely to be hemodiluted, which might lead to false-negative test results. The Food and Drug Administration (FDA) of the US has published regulations to test specimens from donors who have undergone transfusion or infusion (FDA, 2007). Test results from donors who have suffered blood loss that was sufficient to require fluid replacement, certain volumes of transfusion, and/or infusions should be interpreted with caution. The donor might be ineligible unless a pretransfusion sample was available for testing or an appropriate algorithm was used to determine if plasma dilution is sufficient to affect test results.

3.3.2 The window period

The window period is the time between initial infection and when a test can reliably detect that infection, and the poor sensitivity of antibody-based tests within this period increases the risk of infection transmission through organ transplantation. As seroconversion may not occur during an acute infection, some active infections remain undetectable. For example, the period from initial HIV exposure to the development of HIV antibodies is approximately 22 days, but it can be up to 3-6 months. On average, it takes 2-8 weeks from the time of possible exposure for the development of detectable levels of HIV antibodies, leading to accurate test results. Therefore, the donor may be seronegative while potentially infected. However, recent improvements in the sensitivity of virus-detection assays using nucleic acid testing (NAT) have resulted in a significant shortening of the window period (Busch et al., 2005; Fiebig et al., 2003). The use of NAT may also detect viral replication in HBV core antigen (HBcAg)-positive donors who are HBV surface antigen (HBsAg)-negative, in addition to reducing the window period of HBV infection (Biswas et al., 2003; Kleinman & Busch, 2006). The window period of HCV infection can be reduced by the use of NAT as well (Kolk et al., 2002; Schreiber et al., 1996), suggesting the routine use of NAT in the screening of potential organ donors for HIV, HBV, and HCV.

3.3.3 Living donors versus deceased donors

The screening of living and deceased donors is largely different based on the period during which the evaluation is performed. The screening of a prospective living donor is conducted at the transplantation center, and the time between screening and transplantation is variable. The screening of living donors should include a thorough medical and behavioral history, physical examination, laboratory serological tests, radiographic imaging studies, and tests for any untreated underlying infectious diseases as needed. Repeat screening tests should be considered in the presence of newly developing clinical symptoms and signs in living donors between the time of initial screening and transplantation.

In contrast, the period for deceased donor screening is very short, typically on the order of hours. The laboratories associated with organ procurement organizations (OPOs) should operate on a 24-hour basis in order to generate the information needed to determine donor eligibility (Delmonico & Snydman, 1998; Schaffner, 2001). Because of time constraints, serologic tests are often limited to routinely available and rapid methods. In addition, the quality of testing may not be identical in each OPO, and some infections that require more sensitive testing may be difficult to detect at an early stage. Therefore, a detailed medical history of the potential deceased donor is required to identify potential infections that might not be reflected in serologic tests. If a deceased donor with a potential infection risk is to be used, the recipient should be informed of the risk of infection transmission. In the future, the development of more sensitive and rapid molecular serologic tests may allow immediate detection of viral infections, such as HBV, HCV, and HIV.

4. Transmission of specific pathogens

A variety of pathogens, including bacteria, fungi, parasites, and viruses, may be transmitted through organ transplantation (Table 4) (Gottesdiener, 1989; Ison et al., 2009).

Bacteria	*Mycobacteria*
Staphylococcus aureus	Mycobacterium tuberculosis
Klebsiella species	Nontuberculous mycobacteria
Bacteroides fragilis	
Pseudomonas aeruginosa	*Parasites/Protozoa*
Escherichia coli	Toxoplasma gondii
Salmonella species	Strongyloides stercoralis
Yersinia enterocolitica	Plasmodium species
Treponema pallidum	Trypanosoma cruzi
Brucella species	
Bartonella species	*Viruses*
Enterobacter species	Cytomegalovirus
Acinetobacter species	Epstein-Barr virus
	Herpes simplex virus
Fungi	Varicella-zoster virus
Aspergillus species	Human herpesvirus-6, 7, 8
Candida species	Hepatitis B, C
Histoplasma capsulatum	Human immunodeficiency virus
Cryptococcus neoformans	Human T cell lymphotrophic virus (HTLV)
Cocciodioides immitis	Parvovirus B19
Scedosporium apiospermum	Rabies
Prototheca species	Lymphocytic choriomeningitis virus (LCMV)
	BK virus
	West Nile virus

Table 4. Pathogens that are transmitted with solid organ transplantation

4.1 Bacteria

Bacteria are the most common cause of infections in liver transplant recipients, with a reported incidence of 35–70%. Numerous factors may be associated with recipient infection, and bacterial transmission from the donor is one of the possible sources. Deceased donors may harbor known or unsuspected bacterial infections, which should be rapidly evaluated by review of medical records, temperature charts, radiography, and cultures when available. It is desirable to obtain blood cultures prior to transplantation since occult donor bacteremia may occur. If an illness might have involved bacteremia, a thorough investigation should be performed to make sure that the target organ has not been infected. Previous studies, conducted on a small scale, have documented severely compromised initial allograft function when organs from infected donors were used for desperate recipients (Bull et al., 1995; Nery et al., 1997). Therefore, transplantation programs have been reluctant to use organs from donors known to have active bacterial infections. Occasionally, however, a bacterial or fungal blood culture taken before organ recovery is reported as positive only after life-saving organs have been transplanted into a needy recipient. A retrospective review of bacteremic donors has found no evidence that transmitting bacterial infection results in poorer outcomes after organ transplantation (Freeman et al., 1999). Moreover, organs have been successfully transplanted from donors with bacterial meningitis with no evidence of infectious complications in the recipients, who were given appropriate antimicrobial therapy (Lopez-Navidad et al., 1997; Satoi et al., 2001). Therefore, potential donors with positive blood cultures should not be totally excluded as possible donors. This may increase organ availability and help improve the organ shortage.

4.1.1 Syphilis

Syphilis is a sexually transmitted infection with a worldwide incidence that is caused by the spirochete *Treponema pallidum*. Although the transmission of syphilis by means other than sexual routes is infrequent, it can be transmitted through blood transfusion and organ transplantation. Serologic testing of potential organ donors for syphilis is recommended, but evidence of syphilis infection is not considered a contraindication to organ donation if appropriate prophylactic antibiotics, such as benzathine penicillin, are administered to the recipient (Caballero et al., 1998; Ko et al., 1998). Therefore, current guidance suggests that organ transplantation from a donor with serologic evidence of a syphilis infection is safe as long as there is appropriate treatment of recipients in the posttransplantation phase. Recommended regimens of 2-3 doses weekly of 2.4 million units of intramuscular benzathine penicillin or an equivalent early syphilis therapeutic regimen should be given as soon as possible after transplantation for appropriate prophylaxis and treatment of early syphilis acquired from transplantation.

4.2 Fungi

Any known active and invasive fungal infection in the potential donor is a contraindication to transplantation. However, endemic mycoses may be present in dormant forms and transmitted to recipients by organ transplantation. For example, histoplasmosis that was transmitted by transplantation has been described, but most cases appeared to involve the reactivation of a past infection in the recipient (Limaye et al., 2000). Nonetheless, radiographic signs of suspected previous histoplasmosis have not been considered a contraindication to donation, and a consensus regarding recommendations for donor screening for endemic mycoses has not emerged yet.

4.2.1 Candida species

The incidence of fungal infections in liver transplant recipients is higher than in recipients of other types of solid organ transplants. The reasons for this high rate of fungal infection are not completely understood, but specific risk factors, including retransplantation, prolonged or repeat surgeries, high transfusion requirements, renal failure, fungal colonization, and predisposition to fungal infections in liver transplant recipients, have been identified (Castaldo et al., 1991; Collins et al., 1994). The incidence of invasive fungal infections following liver transplantation ranges between 14% and 42%, and these infections are associated with high overall mortality rates (Briegel et al., 1995; Paya, 2002). Most fungal infections generally occur within the first 3 months following liver transplantation and are viewed as classic nosocomial infections instead of donor-derived transmissions. Infections due to Candida species are the most common invasive fungal infections among solid organ transplant recipients, accounting for over half of all fungal infections. However, the occurrence of invasive candidiasis, especially among liver and small bowel transplant recipients, is often substantially higher.

The diagnosis of invasive candidiasis is dependent on the recovery of the organism from a sterile body site, such as the bloodstream, intraabdominal fluid, pleural fluid, or abscess material. Unfortunately, cultures, especially blood cultures, are not sensitive enough to identify patients with invasive candidiasis. Even with newer blood culture techniques, the overall sensitivity of blood cultures for identifying Candida species is estimated to be 70% (Berenguer et al., 1993). Thus, the development of nonculture-based diagnostic methodologies is especially important. Presently, the 1-3, beta-d-glucan assay is probably the most reliable, with a sensitivity and specificity of 70% and 87%, respectively, among patients who have proven invasive candidiasis (Obayashi et al., 2008; Ostrosky-Zeichner et al., 2005). The treatment of invasive candidiasis in organ transplant recipients, which is similar to treatment in most other patients, is based on updated clinical practice guidelines for the management of candidiasis (Pappas et al., 2009).

4.2.2 Aspergillus species

Aspergillosis accounts for 1–9.2% of invasive fungal infections in liver transplant recipients (Brown et al., 1996; Gavalda et al., 2005; Kusne et al., 1992). It is similar to other fungal infections in that aspergillosis is likely to be a nosocomial infection after transplantation and not due to donor-derived transmission. A number of well-characterized risk factors have been shown to portend a high risk of invasive aspergillosis following liver transplantation, of which retransplantation and renal failure are among the most significant (Fortun et al., 2002; Gavalda et al., 2005; Singh et al., 2001). Historically, invasive aspergillosis in liver transplant recipients has predominantly occurred in the early posttransplant period. The mortality rate of liver transplant recipients with invasive aspergillosis has ranged from 83–88% (Denning, 1996; Singh et al., 1997; Singh et al., 2006), highlighting the need for aggressive diagnostic evaluation and treatment. A substantial delay in establishing an early diagnosis remains a major impediment to the successful treatment of invasive aspergillosis. Cultures of respiratory tract secretions are less sensitive, and fungus may only be detected in clinical samples from the late stages of the disease. However, a positive culture of Aspergillus from respiratory tract samples does not always indicate invasive disease, and the significance of a positive culture from an airway sample also varies with the type of organ transplant.

The utility of the galactomannan test for the early diagnosis of invasive aspergillosis has been assessed in solid organ transplant recipients. However, false-positive galactomannan tests have been documented in up to 13% of liver transplant recipients (Kwak et al., 2004), but the sensitivity of the assay for the diagnosis of invasive aspergillosis may be improved by testing bronchoalveolar lavage (Husain et al., 2007). The diagnosis of invasive aspergillosis using the 1-3, beta-d-glucan assay has not been fully defined, but one study has shown that the test was useful for the diagnosis of invasive aspergillosis in living-donor liver transplant recipients (Kawagishi et al., 2006).

Currently, prophylaxis against invasive aspergillosis is not routinely recommended in all solid organ transplant recipients. A more rational approach is to provide antifungal prophylaxis to high-risk liver transplant recipients (Singh & Husain, 2009). The treatment of invasive aspergillosis in liver transplant recipients remains generally the same as in other patients. Prompt initiation of antifungal therapy is crucial for achieving optimal outcomes in recipients with invasive aspergillosis. Because of their lower potential of nephrotoxicity, lipid formulations of amphotericin B have been the mainstay for the treatment of invasive aspergillosis in solid organ transplantation since the early 1990s. The availability of newer triazole agents and echinocandins that have potent anti-Aspergillus activity and better tolerability profiles have led to an expanded arsenal of antifungal agents for the treatment of invasive aspergillosis. Voriconazole is now regarded as the drug of choice for the primary treatment of invasive aspergillosis in all hosts, including solid organ transplant recipients, based on the clinical guidelines of the Infectious Diseases Society of America (IDSA) for the treatment of invasive aspergillosis (Walsh et al., 2008). For the primary treatment of invasive pulmonary aspergillosis, intravenous or oral voriconazole is recommended for most patients, while the parenteral formulation is recommended for seriously ill patients. In patients developing toxicity to or with contraindications against voriconazole, liposomal amphotericin B is considered an alternative primary therapy according to the IDSA guidelines, but higher doses are not recommended. Amphotericin B lipid complex, itraconazole, caspofungin, posaconazole, or micafungin are other rational choices for alternative therapies for invasive aspergillosis (Walsh et al., 2008).

Currently, caspofungin, which is the only echinocandin approved by the FDA for the treatment of invasive aspergillosis, has been used successfully as a single agent or in combination with other drugs for salvage therapy in invasive aspergillosis (Carby et al., 2004; Forestier et al., 2005). However, the efficacy of combination antifungal therapy for invasive aspergillosis has not been fully defined. Thus, the routine administration of a combination regimen for primary therapy is not recommended. In the context of salvage therapy, an additional antifungal agent may be added to existing therapy, or combination antifungal drugs from different classes other than those in the initial regimen may be used (Walsh et al., 2008).

4.2.3 Cryptococcus species

Cryptococcosis, which is the third most common invasive fungal infection, accounts for approximately 8% of the invasive fungal infections in solid organ transplant recipients. The overall incidence of cryptococcal disease in solid organ transplant recipients ranges from 0.3–5% (Singh & Forrest, 2009). As in most other hosts, cryptococcal disease in solid organ transplant recipients is considered a reactivation of a quiescent infection. However, rare cases of transmission from donor organ and tissue grafts have also been reported (Beyt & Waltman, 1978; Kanj et al., 1996; Ooi et al., 1971). Approximately 53–72% of solid organ transplant recipients with cryptococcosis develop disseminated disease or central nervous system (CNS) involvement. Among solid organ transplant recipients, liver transplant recipients had a 6-fold higher risk for developing disseminated disease than recipients of other types of transplants. The overall mortality of solid organ transplant recipients with cryptococcosis in the current era is 14%, but it may be higher in those with CNS involvement (Singh et al., 2007).

All patients with suspected cryptococcosis should undergo complete evaluations, including lumbar punctures, blood and urine cultures, chest X-rays, or bronchoalveolar lavages with biopsies when necessary, in order to determine the extent of the disease, as this will dictate management. Distinguishing between disseminated disease and localized pulmonary and asymptomatic disease is necessary prior to initiating therapy. In patients with neurologic and disseminated disease or severe pulmonary disease, the recommended treatment includes induction therapy with an amphotericin B product and flucytosine, followed by consolidation with fluconazole, and, finally, maintenance with fluconazole (200–400 mg/day) for 6–12 months in order to complete the regimen. The recommended treatment for focal or incidentally detected pulmonary disease in otherwise asymptomatic patients is fluconazole (400 mg/day) for 6–12 months (Dromer et al., 2008; Saag et al., 2000). Currently, the use of extended-spectrum azoles, such as voriconazole, itraconazole, and posaconazole, have not shown any extra benefits over fluconazole (Singh & Forrest, 2009).

4.3 Mycobacteria

Mycobacterium tuberculosis (TB) is a serious opportunistic infection that may affect transplant recipients. The prevalence of active TB among solid organ transplant recipients is estimated to be 1.2–6.4% in most countries, and it has been reported to be up to 15% in highly endemic areas. The mortality rate in these populations is close to 30% (Munoz et al., 2005). The incidence of active TB in adult liver transplant recipients has been reported to be 0.47–2.3% (Munoz et al., 2005; Torre-Cisneros et al., 2009). The most frequent mode of acquisition is thought to be reactivation of dormant disease; however, transmission with an allograft has been documented to occur in liver transplant recipients (Aguado et al., 2009; Kiuchi et al., 1997). Because of this risk, all potential living donors should be given a thorough history, documenting TB risk factors, exposures, and infections, and undergo a tuberculin skin test (TST) or interferon-γ release assay. If either test is positive, additional testing and a symptom review should be performed in order to rule out active infection. Prospective living donors with active TB should not be considered for transplantation, and those with latent TB infection should be given treatment (with isoniazid for 9 months or rifampin for 4 months) prior to transplantation. However, one study demonstrated no benefit to treating prospective living donors with latent TB infections prior to transplantation (Hernandez-Hernandez et al., 2006). The optimal length of therapy prior to liver donations remains unclear, and a shorter course of therapy might be feasible with the caveat that the recipients will be treated after liver transplantation. In the case of deceased donors, it is not possible to perform TSTs, but a history of previously active TB and any associated treatment should be obtained from the donor's family or relatives. Organs from potential donors, whether living or deceased, with active TB or a high suspicion of active TB should not be used. Recipients of organs from donors with latent TB should consider preventive therapy with isoniazid for up to 9 months (Yehia & Blumberg, 2010).

The initiation of posttransplant preventive treatment should begin as soon as medically possible after the recipient is stabilized in order to prevent the development of reactivated diseases. Once therapy is started, transplant recipients should be routinely monitored for drug-related hepatotoxicity. A suggested approach is to monitor liver enzymes at 2-week intervals for 6 weeks and then monthly. If significant hepatotoxicity is observed, alternative regimens, such as ethambutol plus either levofloxacin or moxifloxacin, could be considered for high-risk individuals (Aguado et al., 2009). If no alternative treatment is possible, then careful clinical follow-up with prompt diagnostic attention to pulmonary symptoms is likely the best strategy.

The standard treatment recommendation for active TB in the general population is to administer a 4-drug regimen of isoniazid, rifampin, pyrazinamide, and ethambutol for a 2-month intensive phase, followed by a continuation phase of 4–7 months (Blumberg et al., 2003). Other agents used in the treatment of TB are aminoglycosides and fluoroquinolones, which are primarily used in cases of multidrug resistance or intolerance of first-line medications. Treatment of active TB in liver transplant recipients should consider the known risks of drug-related hepatotoxicity and drug-drug interactions between antituberculosis medications and immunosuppressive agents. These considerations also have an impact on the suggested length of treatment. The ideal length of TB therapy in liver transplant recipients remains controversial, and it is affected by the extent of the disease, choice of regimen, response to therapy, and resistance profile of the organism.

4.4 Protozoa/parasites

Parasitic diseases may affect transplant recipients as a result of natural infection, recrudescence of a previous latent infection in the recipient, or transmission by organ transplantation. For the most part, only those organisms that can complete their life cycle within the human host lead to more severe infections in an immunocompromised host. The incidence of parasitic infection is expected to increase in solid organ transplant recipients due to the universal expansion of transplantation programs, and the increase in the numbers of donors or recipients who are originally from endemic areas but are currently spreading throughout the world.

4.4.1 Toxoplasma gondii

Toxoplasma gondii infection in transplant recipients can be caused by a primary infection transmitted by an allograft. Although recipients of heart transplantation have the highest incidence of this disease among solid organ transplant recipients, toxoplasmosis has been described in liver transplant recipients as well. Transplant recipients with active toxoplasmosis may present with brain abscess, chorioretinitis, pneumonitis, or disseminated disease. The diagnosis of toxoplasmosis requires the identification of tachyzoites in biopsy samples or clear seroconversion. The presence of multiple ring-enhancing lesions in a CNS imaging study, especially with the coexistence of anti-toxoplasma IgG antibodies, is suggestive of CNS toxoplasmosis and is sufficient to start presumptive treatment for CNS toxoplasmosis. Optimal treatment after solid organ transplantation has not been well-defined. The recommendations of treatment for active toxoplasmosis generally includes a prolonged course (4–6 weeks or longer) of pyrimethamine and sulfadiazine with folinic acid, followed by suppressive therapy, or trimethoprim-sulfamethoxazole treatment, followed by suppressive therapy (Kotton & Lattes, 2009).

4.4.2 Trypanosoma cruzi

Chagas disease, caused by the flagellate protozoan parasite *Trypanosoma cruzi*, has been transmitted by unscreened blood transfusion, from infected mother to fetus, by laboratory accidents, or even by organ transplantation (de Faria & Alves, 1993; Vazquez et al., 1993). Routine screening for *Trypanosoma cruzi* prior to transplantation is not yet mandatory. In countries where the disease is endemic, transplant teams do accept organs from infected donors provided no better donor is available in a reasonable life-saving situation and with informed consent. Diagnosis can be achieved by direct parasitological tests, including the examination of whole blood preparations, by a concentration method (Strout test) (Strout, 1962) in the acute phase, and by serological tests in the intermediate and chronic stages. Two drugs, nifurtimox and benznidazole, are available for treatment. Parasitic cure is achieved in 60–100% of acute cases when either drug is administered for 30–60 days (Bern et al., 2007).

4.4.3 Strongyloides stercoralis

Strongyloides stercoralis is endemic in tropical and subtropical regions. Strongyloidiasis, which has mainly been described in kidney transplant recipients, has been considered in most cases to be caused by reactivation of a latent infection (Hoy et al., 1981). More recently, a few cases have been documented in pancreatic and intestine transplant recipients and were attributed to transmission from the donated organs (Ben-Youssef et al., 2005; Patel et al., 2008). The clinical disease may present with pulmonary involvement, sepsis, meningitis with multiple gram-negative rods, and acute and severe abdominal disease, including ileus and intestinal obstruction, and gastrointestinal hemorrhage. These symptoms are caused by the damage inflicted by larvae that penetrate through the intestinal wall. A definitive diagnosis is based on the identification of larvae in clinical specimens, mainly in stool and duodenal aspirate. All recipients with confirmed diagnoses should be treated with ivermectin or albendazole. Thiabendazole is another agent that has been extensively used clinically, but it is probably the least satisfactory of all available drugs because of its high relapse rates and toxicities (Liu & Weller, 1993). Strongyloidiasis can be a devastating disease in transplant recipients despite therapy. The mortality rate approaches 50–70% in recipients with hyperinfection syndrome and disseminated infection (Patel et al., 2008).

4.5 Viruses

Solid organ transplant recipients are uniquely predisposed to develop severe clinical illnesses related to a variety of common and opportunistic viruses. Transplant recipients may acquire viral infections from the donor (donor-derived transmission), from reactivation of endogenous latent infection, or from the community. Herpes viruses, most notably CMV and EBV, are the most common opportunistic viral pathogens that cause infection after solid organ transplantation. HBV and HCV are unique challenges, particularly among liver transplant recipients. Infection by polyoma BK virus is an important cause of allograft dysfunction in kidney transplant recipients, but viremia is relatively uncommon in liver transplant recipients. Other less common viral infections, including adenoviruses, parvovirus B19, and WNV, may affect liver transplant recipients as well. Treatment of virus infections with proven effective antiviral drug therapies should be weighed against the potential reduction of immunosuppression. For viruses without proven effective therapies, reduction in the degree of immunosuppression remains the sole effective strategy for management. Therefore, the prevention of viral infections is of the utmost importance, and this may be accomplished by pretransplant screening of the donor and recipient to determine prophylactic and preventive strategies to be utilized after transplantation or posttransplant vaccinations and effective antiviral treatments.

4.5.1 Cytomegalovirus

Cytomegalovirus (CMV) infections, which have been recognized in every human population, are widely distributed in the general population with seroprevalence ranging from 30-97% (Humar & Snydman, 2009; Paya, 2001). The patterns of CMV acquisition vary greatly based on geographic and socioeconomic backgrounds of each population, and seroprevalence increases generally with age. Importantly, CMV infection is a major cause of morbidity in patients receiving solid organ transplants. CMV disease usually occurs 1-4 months after liver transplantation, and those recipients who are seronegative for CMV and receive an allograft from a seropositive donor are at highest risk. Other risk factors for CMV disease include the recipient's overall state of immunosuppression (e.g., type of drug, dose, timing, duration) and various host factors (e.g., age, comorbidity, neutropenia). The risk of CMV disease also varies with the type of transplant. This may be due to the degree of immunosuppression or the viral load present in the transplanted allograft. The lowest risk of disease occurs when both donor and recipient are seronegative for CMV. Thus, pretransplant CMV screening of donors and recipients should be performed to allow for risk stratification.

The diagnosis of CMV infection and disease has evolved considerably. Historically, the histological detection of owl's eye inclusion bodies has been used for the diagnosis of CMV disease. However, this method is limited by its invasive approach and insensitivity for detecting CMV organ involvement. For years, culture-based methods, such as shell-vial centrifugation detection or culture of the organism from clinical specimens, were used for CMV diagnosis. However, tissue culture can take weeks and the shell-vial centrifugation assay is insensitive compared with molecular assays. Newer methods for diagnosing CMV disease include detection of the pp65 antigen and a molecular diagnostic test; both methods are performed on serum and are rapid, with reasonable sensitivity and specificity. The pp65 antigen assay is a semiquantitative fluorescent assay that is based on the detection of infected cells in peripheral blood. This assay has a far higher sensitivity and specificity than culture-based methods (Mazzulli et al., 1999). Molecular diagnostic tests, which may detect CMV deoxyribonucleic acid (DNA), can be qualitative or quantitative. Quantitative measurements of CMV DNA levels have become popular at many transplantation centers. The viral loads measured are associated with the severity of CMV infection (Humar et al., 1999). Generally, both the pp65 antigen assay and quantitative CMV viral load testing can be utilized in preemptive protocols for the diagnosis of CMV infection, as well as to guide the management of CMV disease (Caliendo et al., 2000; Emery et al., 2000).

Currently, two strategies commonly used for CMV prevention include universal prophylaxis and preemptive therapy. Universal prophylaxis involves providing antiviral therapy to all at-risk patients beginning in the early posttransplant period for a defined duration of 3–6 months. Drugs that have been considered for universal prophylaxis include ganciclovir, valganciclovir, acyclovir, valacyclovir, and immunoglobulin preparations (Gane et al., 1997; Paya et al., 2004; Snydman et al., 1993). Valganciclovir, which is a valine ester prodrug of ganciclovir, has improved bioavailability over the oral form ganciclovir. In preemptive therapy, patients are monitored for early evidence of CMV replication at regular intervals (often weekly). Patients with early replication are then treated with antiviral therapy in order to prevent symptomatic disease. Each approach has advantages and disadvantages that must be considered in the context of the patient and the allograft. The major concern with CMV prophylaxis continues to be late-onset CMV disease, which is defined as disease occurring sometime after discontinuation of antiviral prophylaxis. In contrast, preemptive therapy has the potential advantage of targeting therapy to patients at highest risk and thereby decreasing drug costs and toxicity.

No consensus exists regarding the optimal treatment of CMV disease. However, intravenous ganciclovir has been used successfully in numerous therapeutic trials to treat solid organ transplant recipients with CMV disease and has been considered the mainstay for therapy. The basic principle governing CMV treatment is the clearance of viremia. Therefore, patients with evidence of CMV viremia should be maintained on therapy until viremia has dropped below the negative threshold level for a given test. This helps prevent relapse and the development of resistance to ganciclovir. The incidence of ganciclovir-resistant CMV remains generally low in most cases after solid organ transplant. In a prospective multicenter study, the overall rate of resistance was 1.9% in those who received oral ganciclovir versus 0% among those receiving valganciclovir (Boivin et al., 2004). However, resistance should be suspected if the patient develops CMV disease after prolonged courses of antiviral prophylaxis or the viral load fails to respond to standard ganciclovir treatment. Genetic resistance testing may be very helpful in managing resistant CMV. Therapeutic options for resistant CMV include reduction or discontinuance of immunosuppression and increasing the dosage of intravenous ganciclovir or switching to foscarnet alone or foscarnet in combination with low dose ganciclovir. Other unproven or untested therapeutic options, including cidofovir, compassionate release maribavir, leflunomide, and artesunate, may be considered for refractory cases (Humar & Snydman, 2009).

4.5.2 Epstein-Barr virus

EBV is also a herpes virus, and humans are the only known hosts of EBV. This virus has a worldwide distribution with seropositive rates of 90% among adults, and its transmission depends on the socioeconomic background of the population. In most nonindustrialized communities, the vast majority of individuals are EBV-seropositive before the age of 5 years. However, in the more developed affluent counties, seropositivity can be delayed until the fourth decade of life (Allen, 2005). Although EBV infection may be acquired from the community, donor-derived transmission from an EBV-seropositive donor organ is an important source of infection among solid organ transplant recipients. EBV is associated with the majority of cases of posttransplantation lymphoproliferative disorder (PTLD), which is recognized as one of the most devastating complications of organ transplantation. The development of PTLD after solid organ transplantation usually occurs in the first year after transplantation. Prolonged or extensive immunosuppression and transplantation from an EBV-seropositive donor into a seronegative recipient are the two major risk factors for the development of PTLD after solid organ transplantation. CMV infection, which may contribute to the net state of immunosuppression, is known to be another risk factor for the development of PTLD after transplantation. The incidence of PTLD also varies with the type of organ transplantation; the risk for the development of PTLD is highest after small bowel transplantation (up to 32%), followed by moderate risk (3–12%) following lung, heart, and liver transplantation, and relatively low risk (1–2%) for kidney transplantation (Gottschalk et al., 2005). The reasons for these differences are not completely understood, but the recipient's net state of immunosuppression and the amount of lymphoid tissue present in the transplanted allografts may be important.

PTLD may present with a diverse spectrum of nonspecific clinical symptoms and signs that involve other organs, including the CNS, bone marrow, kidneys, lungs, small intestine, and spleen. Because early diagnosis and treatment may result in better outcome, there is great interest in developing tests to predict the development of PTLD. Several investigations have indicated that monitoring EBV viral load and analysis of EBV-specific cytotoxic T lymphocyte responses may be helpful in assessing the risk of PTLD development in recipients (Qu et al., 2000; Rose et al., 2001; Smets et al., 2002). However, tissue biopsies with histological classifications remain the current mainstay of PTLD diagnosis.

The treatment of PTLD remains controversial because of the lack of a unifying consensus dictating the specific treatment approaches that should be undertaken for all categories of patients. The general approach to therapy involves a stepwise strategy that starts with the reduction of immunosuppression; subsequent therapies depend on the clinical situation and should be based largely on the clinical response and histopathological characteristics of the disease. Additional therapies currently used in clinical practice include antiviral agents, intravenous immune globulin, cytokine and anticytokine therapies, surgery or radiation, anti-B cell antibodies, and T cell-based cellular immunotherapies (Allen & Preiksaitis, 2009; Gottschalk et al., 2005). However, the efficacy of individual therapies is difficult to assess because they are often combined. Additional future research is needed to address several unresolved issues and to enhance the diagnosis, prevention, and treatment of PTLD.

4.5.3 Hepatitis B virus

The transmission of HBV by organ transplantation is hazardous to allograft recipients. The acquisition of HBV infection has been associated with rapidly progressive liver disease, leading to high rates of liver failure and mortality. Therefore, all prospective donors and recipients should be tested for HBV prior to liver transplantation. Although the response to vaccination in patients with end-stage organ disease may be suboptimal, it is prudent to vaccinate all seronegative transplant candidates with HBV vaccine. Donor screening usually includes, at least, HBsAg and HBV core antibody (HBcAb) assays, and it is most useful to test for IgG and IgM in the HBcAb assay. HBsAg or HBcAb-IgM positivity usually indicates active HBV infection, and HBsAg-negative and HBcAb-IgM-positive individuals may represent infection in the window period. A HBsAg-negative and HBcAb-IgG-positive result may represent either a false-positive test or persistent HBV infection (Lok et al., 1988). Isolated HBsAb positivity, which usually indicates prior vaccination or resolved infection, is not generally considered a risk for HBV transmission. Historically, prospective organ donors with either HBsAg or HBcAb positivity were not utilized because of the significant risk of HBV transmission to a liver transplant recipient. However, it has now become more common to transplant livers from HBcAb+ or HBsAg-positive donors with intensive posttransplantation prophylaxis (Dodson et al., 1999; Wachs et al., 1995).

The relative risk of HBV transmission and posttransplantation management based on the serologic test results of the donor is summarized in Table 5. A donor who is positive for HBsAg poses the greatest risk of HBV transmission after transplantation. The risk of HBV infection may be reduced in recipients who are positive for anti-HB antibodies; however, infection has been well documented after transplantation from a donor positive for HBsAg, irrespective of the recipient's immunization status. Therefore, all recipients receiving transplanted organs from HBsAg-positive donors should be prophylactically treated with hepatitis B immunoglobulin (HBIG) and antiviral therapy. The major drawback of HBIG therapy is the cost, and, therefore, diverse strategies of HBIG administration, in terms of dosage and duration, exist in different transplantation centers. However, frequent monitoring of liver function, HBsAg, anti-HB antibodies, and HBV DNA in the allograft recipient, as well as the maintenance of adequate anti-HB antibody levels, is recommended.

Antibodies against the HBcAg are only present after HBV infection, and they cannot be the result of previous HBV vaccination. Therefore, organs from any donor testing positive for anti-HBc antibodies can transmit HBV to allograft recipients. A positive result for anti-HBc antibodies should be further defined by determining whether the antibodies are of the IgM or the IgG class in order to identify donors with either recent HBV exposure or current HBV infection. If the anti-HBc antibody is of the IgM class, indicating a recent or ongoing acute HBV infection, then recipients should be treated in a manner analogous to allograft recipients from an HBsAg-positive donor. If the anti-HBc antibody is of the IgG class, then there is high risk of HBV transmission with liver transplantation. The approach to liver transplantation from an anti-HBc IgG-positive donor should be as aggressive as that from an HBsAg-positive donor. Therefore, the same regimens of HBIG in combination with oral lamivudine are recommended. However, several centers have described the successful prevention of graft HBV using lamivudine therapy alone (Malkan et al., 2000; Mutimer et al., 2000). Additionally, HBsAg, anti-HB antibody levels, and HBV DNA should be closely monitored in recipients in order to detect active infection as well (Chung et al., 2001).

Donor HBV serology	Risk of HBV transmission	Post-transplantation Prophylaxis
HBsAg +	High	HBIG and lamivudine
Anti-HBc IgM +, HBsAg -, Anti-HBs +/-	High	HBIG and lamivudine
Anti-HBc IgG +, HBsAg -, Anti-HBs +/-	High	HBIG and lamivudine or lamivudine alone
HBsAg -, Anti-HBc -, Anti-HBs +/-	Rare	Not recommended

HBsAg, hepatitis B Surface antigen; Anti-HBc, antibody of hepatitis B core antigen; Anti-HBs, antibody of hepatitis B surface antigen; HBIG, hepatitis B immunoglobulin.

Table 5. Relative risk of HBV transmission and suggested post-transplantation management of liver transplant recipients according to donor serologic status

The lowest risk of HBV transmission occurs when the donor is negative for both HBsAg and anti-HBc antibodies, a situation that is considered evidence of no active infection. However, in rare cases, HBV transmission to liver allograft recipients has been reported, even when the donors are negative for all markers of HBV, including HBsAg, anti-HBc antibodies, and anti-HB antibodies (Chazouilleres et al., 1994)

4.5.4 Hepatitis C virus

Prospective organ donors with HCV infection have traditionally posed a dilemma because of the high risk of transmission of HCV through organ transplantation. A donor positive for HCV RNA, indicating active viral replication, has a much higher risk of transmission (Pereira et al., 1992). The risks of transmission from HCV RNA-negative and HCV antibody-positive donors have not yet been fully defined. However, all recipients of organs from HCV-infected donors are indeed at risk of becoming HCV infected after liver transplantation. In recent years, the use of organs from HCV-seropositive donors for life-saving transplantations in HCV-seronegative recipients has been studied, with acceptable results. There are no increases in the 1- and 5-year mortality and morbidity rates associated with liver transplantation from HCV-positive versus HCV-negative donors (Rosengard et al., 2002).

The greatest concern of HCV infection after liver transplantation is that at least 25% of recipients progress to cirrhosis within 5 years, with a 42% annual risk of decompensation once cirrhosis has developed (Berenguer, 2002). The treatment of HCV in liver transplant recipients is complicated further by poor sustained viral response (SVR) rates and reports of progressive fibrosis with hepatic decompensation despite SVR. Combination therapy for HCV after liver transplantation is currently recommended, and the most widely used is pegylated-interferon (Peg-IFN) plus ribavirin. Treatment of HCV with Peg-IFN plus ribavirin after liver transplantation is generally only successful in achieving SVR in 20–45% of recipients and is associated with high rates (30–50%) of discontinuation due to intolerability (Ponziani et al., 2011; Wang et al., 2006). The inability to reach target RBV doses due to the high prevalence of renal insufficiency in recipients is a major limiting factor in achieving an acceptable SVR rate (Chalasani et al., 2005; Gane et al., 1998).

In contrast to HBV, there is no HCV vaccine to prevent transmission. A general concept in managing liver transplant recipients at risk for HCV infection or recurrence is to avoid precipitating factors, such as acute rejection, the use of older or extended criteria donors, and CMV infection. Additionally, slow tapering of all immunosuppressive agents and avoiding over- or under-immunosuppression is theoretically more likely to lead to a lower incidence of HCV recurrence and acute rejection.

4.5.5 Human immunodeficiency virus (HIV)

HIV-seropositive donors have traditionally not been utilized in transplantation, due to the known risk of transmission to the recipient. However, despite routine screening, transmission of HIV, which can be an uncommon complication of organ transplantation, is a public health concern. Specifically, if the donor is in the window period after infection but prior to development of anti-HIV antibodies, the recipient is at risk of HIV infection (Ahn & Cohen, 2008).

The CDC guidelines address donor screening, testing, and exclusion for prevention of HIV transmission through organ transplantation. The guidelines note that prospective donors may be considered if "the risk to the recipient of not performing the transplant is deemed to be greater than the risk of HIV transmission and disease." In this circumstance, informed consent is deemed essential. Posttransplant testing of all recipients of high-risk donors for HIV is suggested but not mandated. The treatment of recipients infected by donor-derived HIV transmission is similar to that of HIV-seropositive individuals who have undergone liver transplantation after HIV infection has been confirmed. To maintain virological control of HIV infection, it is recommended to regularly and quantitatively measure HIV RNA and CD4-positive T-cell counts. If patients have persistent HIV viremia, a phenotypic HIV drug resistance assay should be carried out to determine alternative treatment options (Blumberg & Stock, 2009).

4.5.6 Other unusual viruses

Respiratory viruses, including influenza, respiratory syncytial virus, parainfluenza virus, rhinovirus, human metapneumovirus, coronavirus, bocavirus, and polyomaviruses, have been identified as causes of significant morbidity and mortality among transplant recipients. All of these viruses cause a range of diseases, from mild congestion and rhinorrhea, to more severe tracheobronchitis, bronchiolitis, and pneumonia. Transplant recipients are at a higher risk of infectious complications than are immunocompetent hosts, and they often present with mild or atypical symptoms. Although respiratory viruses are increasingly recognized in transplant recipients, there is still much to be learned about their impact. Prospective studies are needed to define the optimal timing, duration, and treatment regimen of each of the viruses.

Parvovirus B19, which is a nonenveloped single-stranded DNA virus, is a common human pathogen that causes erythema infectiosum in children. The virus is primarily spread person-to-person by infected respiratory droplets, but transmission through organ transplantation has been reported as well (Yango et al., 2002). Parvovirus B19 infection can be either symptomatic or asymptomatic, depending on the age and immunologic status of the host. In immunocompromised hosts, this infection can cause persistent anemia and occasionally pancytopenia. Therefore, parvovirus B19 infection should be specifically suspected in solid organ transplant recipients with otherwise unexplained anemia. Currently, there is no antiviral drug available for the treatment of parvovirus infection, but intravenous immunoglobulin has been shown to be beneficial in transplant recipients with parvovirus B19 infection (Eid et al., 2006).

Adenovirus is an important viral infection in pediatric liver transplantation. The clinical presentations of infected patients range from self-limited fever, gastroenteritis, or cystitis, to devastating illness with necrotizing hepatitis or pneumonia. Symptomatic infections frequently occur early after transplantation, indicating the possibility of donor transmission (Ison, 2006). The diagnoses of adenovirus can be performed through antigen detection, culture, molecular diagnosis, or histopathology. Unfortunately, there is no definitive treatment for adenoviral infection at this time. The most important component of therapeutic strategy is supportive care along with a reduction of the degree of immunosuppression (Ison & Green, 2009).

Human T-lymphotropic virus (HTLV-I/II), which is endemic in certain areas including the Caribbean and Japan, is often asymptomatic. Infection with HTLV-I can progress to HTLV-I-associated myelopathy/tropical spastic paraparesis or adult T-cell leukemia/lymphoma after years or decades. Serology for HTLV-I/II is routinely performed in the US but not in other areas. In Europe and other areas, this assay is restricted to donors living in, or originating from, high-incidence areas. HTLV-I-seropositive donors are often not utilized and are only considered in life-threatening situations with appropriate informed consent. However, the use of HTLV-I-seropositive donors should be conducted with caution because the donor-derived transmission of HTLV-I with rapid development of myelopathy in recipients has been reported (Toro et al., 2003).

West Nile virus (WNV), a flavivirus that can cause meningoencephalitis has recently appeared in the United States. WNV transmission through blood transfusions and solid organ transplantation has been reported as well (Iwamoto et al., 2003). Organ recipients receiving immunosuppressive drugs may be at high risk for severe disease after WNV infection. The US Health Resources and Service Administration has issued a guidance statement regarding donors and WNV, which recommends testing all prospective live donors with nucleic acid amplification tests (NAAT) prior to transplant and suggests avoiding the use of organs from donors with any form of unexplained or confirmed WNV encephalitis.

Lymphocytic choriomeningitis virus (LCMV), a rodent-associated arenavirus, has been reported with donor-derived transmission to organ recipients leading to fatal infection (Fischer et al., 2006). LCMV infection in humans with normal immune systems usually causes either asymptomatic or mild, self-limited illnesses. Aseptic meningitis can occur in some patients, but the infection is rarely fatal. However, LCMV can cause serious infection in persons with impaired immune systems.

Rabies, a rhabdovirus, is another potentially fatal donor-derived infection (Srinivasan et al., 2005). The virus spreads inward from nerve endings in muscle or skin to the CNS and then disseminates outward to other organs. The majority of infected individuals develop the furious or encephalitic form of the disease, while others develop the paralytic or dumb form, mimicking Guillain-Barre syndrome. The disease is highly lethal, leading to very few survivors following infection (Willoughby et al., 2005). Therefore, clinicians are encouraged to avoid donors who pose even a small risk of rabies infection.

5. Transmission of malignancy

Malignancy after transplantation can develop in three different ways: (1) de novo occurrence, (2) recurrence of malignancy, and (3) donor-related malignancy that can be due to either direct transmission of tumors or tumors arising in cells of donor origin. Despite all efforts to secure a safe organ for transplantation, there continues to be some risk of donor-derived malignancy that can be transmitted to recipients (Ison et al., 2009). Such risks may specifically be overlooked in the emergent donation process. Therefore, the risk of unintended transmission of tumors from donors to recipients must be placed in perspective. Few reports on transmitted cancers have been published, and the risk has never been reliably quantified. One study quantified the risk using a population-based cancer registry, and they estimated a 1.3% risk of having a donor with an undetected malignancy and a 0.2%

risk of cancer transmission (Birkeland & Storm, 2002). These risks are small compared with the benefits of organ transplantation.

Melanoma is one of the most frequently reported and lethal donor-derived malignancies with a high transmission rate (Strauss & Thomas, 2010). The transmission of melanoma might be related to the biological characteristics of melanoma, including tumor dormancy, late recurrence, circulating tumor cells, and the destiny of micrometastases. Melanoma cell dormancy explains the late recurrence that can occur long after the initial treatment of melanoma. The high incidence of circulating tumor cells should be considered in the context of melanoma transmission, even in organ donors with early melanoma who present apparently disease-free following removal of a primary melanoma up to several decades previously. This scenario suggests that melanoma cells can remain dormant at distant sites for decades and possibly forever in immunocompetent patients and reactivate only after transplantation into an immunosuppressed recipient. Therefore, prospective organ donors should be carefully screened for a history of melanoma. The current recommendation for the treatment of donor-related melanoma in renal transplant recipients includes withdrawal or discontinuation of immunosuppression leading to graft rejection, followed by explantation of the allograft after rejection (Penn, 1996). However, this approach is certainly not feasible for liver transplant recipients because of the lack of alternative organ support.

Additionally, prospective organ donors with a past history of several malignancies, including choriocarcinoma, lung cancer, and advanced-stage breast or renal cancer, should be avoided, despite curative resections. Donors with an extended disease-free interval after curative breast, colon, or renal surgery may be used after a detailed review of pathology reports. The use of organs from donors with small, localized, low-grade renal cell carcinoma is acceptable, as demonstrated by the fact that kidneys with such locally excised tumors have been transplanted without evidence of malignancy transmission. Moreover, organs from donors with in situ cancers can be considered with minimal hesitation and with the recipient's informed consent. Donors with cerebral malignancies rarely transmit these tumors to recipients. The risk of malignancy transmission utilizing organs from donors with benign or low-grade astrocytoma (grade I and II) is extremely low. In contrast, the use of organs from donors with high-grade astrocytoma (grade III-IV) tumors, malignant tumors with ventriculosystemic shunts, or histories of extensive cranial surgery that disrupts the blood-brain barrier, is associated with a higher donor malignancy transmission rate (Buell et al., 2003).

Once a donor-transmitted malignancy is suspected, confirmation is essential in order to determine treatment approach. Confirmation can be made by the comparison of donor and recipient tumor histology, fluorescence in-situ hybridization (FISH), which has been utilized to identify the donor origin of tumor cells in sex-mismatched transplant recipients, or PCR-based amplification of highly polymorphic regions in the DNA. Recent reports have relied upon FISH and PCR analysis to confirm tumor origins (Gandhi & Strong, 2007). The fact that tumors in transplant recipients arise from foreign DNA can be exploited. However, there is currently no consensus in the guidelines for the management of recipients with donor-transmitted malignancies. In some cases, the reduction or cessation of immunosuppression might lead to rejection of the donor-derived tumor, which is perceived as a foreign antigen by the recovering immune system of the recipients, similar to the rejection of a transplanted organ by a nonimmunosuppressed recipient. However, a majority of the recipients also require a traditional approach to treating the malignancy, including specific antineoplastic chemotherapy, radiotherapy, or surgery.

6. Conclusion

Donor-derived disease transmission remains a rarely recognized complication of solid organ transplantation, although the reported number of potential donor-derived infections and malignancies has increased every year. This increase is most likely the result of the improved recognition and the development of a formalized reporting process. The true incidence rates are not well known but will be clarified over time through enhanced reporting systems and the improved evaluation of suspicious cases. Since there is substantial morbidity and mortality among affected recipients, a better understanding of the risk of disease transmission is important in order to better inform patients and to provide advice on how to minimize transmissions in the future.

Additionally, thorough pretransplantation screening of the donor and recipient for potential diseases is essential to the success of transplantation as well as to determine prophylactic and preventive strategies to be utilized after transplantation. Future advances will likely include more rapid diagnostic testing to refine the assessment of the risks of transmission posed by a particular donor. Moreover, clinicians should be constantly aware of the possibility of the donor-derived transmission of diseases. Earlier identification of transmission events may decrease morbidity and mortality rates through earlier intervention.

7. Acknowledgments

We thank the CONMED CO., LTD. (Taipei city, Taiwan, Republic of China) for their support in proofreading the content to ensure the accuracy and to improve the quality of the writing.

8. Reference

Aguado, JM, Torre-Cisneros, J, Fortun, J, Benito, N, Meije, Y, Doblas, A, & Munoz, P. (2009) Tuberculosis in solid-organ transplant recipients: consensus statement of the group for the study of infection in transplant recipients (GESITRA) of the Spanish Society of Infectious Diseases and Clinical Microbiology. *Clin Infect Dis* 48, 1276-1284, 1537-6591

Ahn, J, & Cohen, SM. (2008) Transmission of human immunodeficiency virus and hepatitis C virus through liver transplantation. *Liver Transpl* 14, 1603-1608, 1527-6473

Ahn, J, & Cohen, SM. (2008) Transmission of human immunodeficiency virus and hepatitis C virus through liver transplantation. *Liver Transpl* 14, 1603-1608, 1527-6473

Allen, U, & Preiksaitis, J. (2009) Epstein-barr virus and posttransplant lymphoproliferative disorder in solid organ transplant recipients. *Am J Transplant* 9 Suppl 4, S87-96, 1600-6143

Allen, UD. (2005) The ABC of Epstein-Barr virus infections. *Adv Exp Med Biol* 568, 25-39, 0065-2598

Avery, RK. (2004) Prophylactic strategies before solid-organ transplantation. *Curr Opin Infect Dis* 17, 353-356, 0951-7375

Ben-Youssef, R, Baron, P, Edson, F, Raghavan, R, & Okechukwu, O. (2005) Stronglyoides stercoralis infection from pancreas allograft: case report. *Transplantation* 80, 997-998, 0041-1337

Berenguer, J, Buck, M, Witebsky, F, Stock, F, Pizzo, PA, & Walsh, TJ. (1993) Lysis-centrifugation blood cultures in the detection of tissue-proven invasive candidiasis. Disseminated versus single-organ infection. *Diagn Microbiol Infect Dis* 17, 103-109, 0732-8893

Berenguer, M. (2002) Natural history of recurrent hepatitis C. *Liver Transpl* 8, S14-18, 1527-6465

Bern, C, Montgomery, SP, Herwaldt, BL, Rassi, A, Jr., Marin-Neto, JA, Dantas, RO, Maguire, JH, Acquatella, H, Morillo, C, Kirchhoff, LV, Gilman, RH, Reyes, PA, Salvatella, R, & Moore, AC. (2007) Evaluation and treatment of chagas disease in the United States: a systematic review. *JAMA* 298, 2171-2181, 1538-3598

Beyt, BE, Jr., & Waltman, SR. (1978) Cryptococcal endophthalmitis after corneal transplantation. *N Engl J Med* 298, 825-826, 0028-4793

Birkeland, SA, & Storm, HH. (2002) Risk for tumor and other disease transmission by transplantation: a population-based study of unrecognized malignancies and other diseases in organ donors. *Transplantation* 74, 1409-1413, 0041-1337

Biswas, R, Tabor, E, Hsia, CC, Wright, DJ, Laycock, ME, Fiebig, EW, Peddada, L, Smith, R, Schreiber, GB, Epstein, JS, Nemo, GJ, & Busch, MP. (2003) Comparative sensitivity of HBV NATs and HBsAg assays for detection of acute HBV infection. *Transfusion (Paris)* 43, 788-798, 0041-1132

Blumberg, EA, & Stock, P. (2009) Solid organ transplantation in the HIV-infected patient. *Am J Transplant* 9 Suppl 4, S131-135, 1600-6143

Blumberg, HM, Burman, WJ, Chaisson, RE, Daley, CL, Etkind, SC, Friedman, LN, Fujiwara, P, Grzemska, M, Hopewell, PC, Iseman, MD, Jasmer, RM, Koppaka, V, Menzies, RI, O'Brien, RJ, Reves, RR, Reichman, LB, Simone, PM, Starke, JR, & Vernon, AA. (2003) American Thoracic Society/Centers for Disease Control and Prevention/Infectious Diseases Society of America: treatment of tuberculosis. *Am J Respir Crit Care Med* 167, 603-662, 1073-449X

Boivin, G, Goyette, N, Gilbert, C, Roberts, N, Macey, K, Paya, C, Pescovitz, MD, Humar, A, Dominguez, E, Washburn, K, Blumberg, E, Alexander, B, Freeman, R, Heaton, N, & Covington, E. (2004) Absence of cytomegalovirus-resistance mutations after valganciclovir prophylaxis, in a prospective multicenter study of solid-organ transplant recipients. *J Infect Dis* 189, 1615-1618, 0022-1899

Briegel, J, Forst, H, Spill, B, Haas, A, Grabein, B, Haller, M, Kilger, E, Jauch, KW, Maag, K, Ruckdeschel, G, & et al. (1995) Risk factors for systemic fungal infections in liver transplant recipients. *Eur J Clin Microbiol Infect Dis* 14, 375-382, 0934-9723

Brown, RS, Jr., Lake, JR, Katzman, BA, Ascher, NL, Somberg, KA, Emond, JC, & Roberts, JP. (1996) Incidence and significance of Aspergillus cultures following liver and kidney transplantation. *Transplantation* 61, 666-669, 0041-1337

Buell, JF, Trofe, J, Sethuraman, G, Hanaway, MJ, Beebe, TM, Gross, TG, Alloway, R, First, MR, & Woodle, ES. (2003) Donors with central nervous system malignancies: are they truly safe? *Transplantation* 76, 340-343, 0041-1337

Bull, DA, Stahl, RD, McMahan, DL, Jones, KW, Hawkins, JA, Renlund, DG, Taylor, DO, & Karwande, SV. (1995) The high risk heart donor: potential pitfalls. *J Heart Lung Transplant* 14, 424-428, 1053-2498

Busch, MP, Glynn, SA, Stramer, SL, Strong, DM, Caglioti, S, Wright, DJ, Pappalardo, B, & Kleinman, SH. (2005) A new strategy for estimating risks of transfusion-transmitted viral infections based on rates of detection of recently infected donors. *Transfusion (Paris)* 45, 254-264, 0041-1132

Caballero, F, Domingo, P, Rabella, N, & Lopez-Navidad, A. (1998) Successful transplantation of organs retrieved from a donor with syphilis. *Transplantation* 65, 598-599, 0041-1337

Caliendo, AM, St George, K, Kao, SY, Allega, J, Tan, BH, LaFontaine, R, Bui, L, & Rinaldo, CR. (2000) Comparison of quantitative cytomegalovirus (CMV) PCR in plasma and CMV antigenemia assay: clinical utility of the prototype AMPLICOR CMV MONITOR test in transplant recipients. *J Clin Microbiol* 38, 2122-2127, 0095-1137

Carby, MR, Hodson, ME, & Banner, NR. (2004) Refractory pulmonary aspergillosis treated with caspofungin after heart-lung transplantation. *Transpl Int* 17, 545-548, 0934-0874

Castaldo, P, Stratta, RJ, Wood, RP, Markin, RS, Patil, KD, Shaefer, MS, Langnas, AN, Reed, EC, Li, SJ, Pillen, TJ, & et al. (1991) Clinical spectrum of fungal infections after orthotopic liver transplantation. *Arch Surg* 126, 149-156, 0004-0010

CDC. (1994) Guidelines for Preventing Transmission of Human Immunodeficiency Virus Through Transplantation of Human Tissue and Organs. *MMWR* 43(RR-8), 1-17, <http://www.cdc.gov/mmwr/preview/mmwrhtml/00031670.htm>

Chalasani, N, Manzarbeitia, C, Ferenci, P, Vogel, W, Fontana, RJ, Voigt, M, Riely, C, Martin, P, Teperman, L, Jiao, J, & Lopez-Talavera, JC. (2005) Peginterferon alfa-2a for hepatitis C after liver transplantation: two randomized, controlled trials. *Hepatology* 41, 289-298, 0270-9139

Chang, FY, Singh, N, Gayowski, T, Wagener, MM, & Marino, IR. (1998) Fever in liver transplant recipients: changing spectrum of etiologic agents. *Clin Infect Dis* 26, 59-65, 1058-4838

Chazouilleres, O, Mamish, D, Kim, M, Carey, K, Ferrell, L, Roberts, JP, Ascher, NL, & Wright, TL. (1994) "Occult" hepatitis B virus as source of infection in liver transplant recipients. *Lancet* 343, 142-146, 0140-6736

Chung, RT, Feng, S, & Delmonico, FL. (2001) Approach to the management of allograft recipients following the detection of hepatitis B virus in the prospective organ donor. *Am J Transplant* 1, 185-191, 1600-6135

Collins, LA, Samore, MH, Roberts, MS, Luzzati, R, Jenkins, RL, Lewis, WD, & Karchmer, AW. (1994) Risk factors for invasive fungal infections complicating orthotopic liver transplantation. *J Infect Dis* 170, 644-652, 0022-1899

de Faria, JB, & Alves, G. (1993) Transmission of Chagas' disease through cadaveric renal transplantation. *Transplantation* 56, 746-747, 0041-1337

Delmonico, FL, & Snydman, DR. (1998) Organ donor screening for infectious diseases: review of practice and implications for transplantation. *Transplantation* 65, 603-610, 0041-1337

Denning, DW. (1996) Therapeutic outcome in invasive aspergillosis. *Clin Infect Dis* 23, 608-615, 1058-4838

Dodson, SF, Bonham, CA, Geller, DA, Cacciarelli, TV, Rakela, J, & Fung, JJ. (1999) Prevention of de novo hepatitis B infection in recipients of hepatic allografts from anti-HBc positive donors. *Transplantation* 68, 1058-1061, 0041-1337

Dromer, F, Bernede-Bauduin, C, Guillemot, D, & Lortholary, O. (2008) Major role for amphotericin B-flucytosine combination in severe cryptococcosis. *PloS one* 3, e2870, 1932-6203

Eid, AJ, Brown, RA, Patel, R, & Razonable, RR. (2006) Parvovirus B19 infection after transplantation: a review of 98 cases. *Clin Infect Dis* 43, 40-48, 1537-6591

Emery, VC, Sabin, CA, Cope, AV, Gor, D, Hassan-Walker, AF, & Griffiths, PD. (2000) Application of viral-load kinetics to identify patients who develop cytomegalovirus disease after transplantation. *Lancet* 355, 2032-2036, 0140-6736

FDA, USA. (8/8/2007) Guidance for Industry. Eligibility Determination for Donors of Human Cells, Tissues, and Cellular and Tissue-Based Products (HCT/Ps). <http://www.fda.gov/BiologicsBloodVaccines/GuidanceComplianceRegulatoryInformation/Guidances/Tissue/ucm073964.htm>

Fiebig, EW, Wright, DJ, Rawal, BD, Garrett, PE, Schumacher, RT, Peddada, L, Heldebrant, C, Smith, R, Conrad, A, Kleinman, SH, & Busch, MP. (2003) Dynamics of HIV viremia and antibody seroconversion in plasma donors: implications for diagnosis and staging of primary HIV infection. *AIDS* 17, 1871-1879, 0269-9370

Fischer, SA, & Avery, RK. (2009) Screening of donor and recipient prior to solid organ transplantation. *Am J Transplant* 9 Suppl 4, S7-18, 1600-6143

Fischer, SA, Graham, MB, Kuehnert, MJ, Kotton, CN, Srinivasan, A, Marty, FM, Comer, JA, Guarner, J, Paddock, CD, DeMeo, DL, Shieh, WJ, Erickson, BR, Bandy, U, DeMaria, A, Jr., Davis, JP, Delmonico, FL, Pavlin, B, Likos, A, Vincent, MJ, Sealy, TK, Goldsmith, CS, Jernigan, DB, Rollin, PE, Packard, MM, Patel, M, Rowland, C, Helfand, RF, Nichol, ST, Fishman, JA, Ksiazek, T, & Zaki, SR. (2006) Transmission of lymphocytic choriomeningitis virus by organ transplantation. *N Engl J Med* 354, 2235-2249, 1533-4406

Fishman, JA. (2007) Infection in solid-organ transplant recipients. *N Engl J Med* 357, 2601-2614, 1533-4406

Fishman, JA, & Rubin, RH. (1998) Infection in organ-transplant recipients. *N Engl J Med* 338, 1741-1751, 0028-4793

Forestier, E, Remy, V, Lesens, O, Martinot, M, Hansman, Y, Eisenmann, B, & Christmann, D. (2005) A case of Aspergillus mediastinitis after heart transplantation successfully treated with liposomal amphotericin B, caspofungin and voriconazole. *Eur J Clin Microbiol Infect Dis* 24, 347-349, 0934-9723

Fortun, J, Martin-Davila, P, Moreno, S, De Vicente, E, Nuno, J, Candelas, A, Barcena, R, & Garcia, M. (2002) Risk factors for invasive aspergillosis in liver transplant recipients. *Liver Transpl* 8, 1065-1070, 1527-6465

Freeman, RB, Giatras, I, Falagas, ME, Supran, S, O'Connor, K, Bradley, J, Snydman, DR, & Delmonico, FL. (1999) Outcome of transplantation of organs procured from bacteremic donors. *Transplantation* 68, 1107-1111, 0041-1337

Gandhi, MJ, & Strong, DM. (2007) Donor derived malignancy following transplantation: a review. *Cell Tissue Bank* 8, 267-286, 1389-9333

Gane, E, Saliba, F, Valdecasas, GJ, O'Grady, J, Pescovitz, MD, Lyman, S, & Robinson, CA. (1997) Randomised trial of efficacy and safety of oral ganciclovir in the prevention of cytomegalovirus disease in liver-transplant recipients. The Oral Ganciclovir International Transplantation Study Group [corrected]. *Lancet* 350, 1729-1733, 0140-6736

Gane, EJ, Lo, SK, Riordan, SM, Portmann, BC, Lau, JY, Naoumov, NV, & Williams, R. (1998) A randomized study comparing ribavirin and interferon alfa monotherapy for hepatitis C recurrence after liver transplantation. *Hepatology* 27, 1403-1407, 0270-9139

Gavalda, J, Len, O, San Juan, R, Aguado, JM, Fortun, J, Lumbreras, C, Moreno, A, Munoz, P, Blanes, M, Ramos, A, Rufi, G, Gurgui, M, Torre-Cisneros, J, Montejo, M, Cuenca-Estrella, M, Rodriguez-Tudela, JL, & Pahissa, A. (2005) Risk factors for invasive aspergillosis in solid-organ transplant recipients: a case-control study. *Clin Infect Dis* 41, 52-59, 1537-6591

Ghobrial, RM, Steadman, R, Gornbein, J, Lassman, C, Holt, CD, Chen, P, Farmer, DG, Yersiz, H, Danino, N, Collisson, E, Baquarizo, A, Han, SS, Saab, S, Goldstein, LI, Donovan, JA, Esrason, K, & Busuttil, RW. (2001) A 10-year experience of liver transplantation for hepatitis C: analysis of factors determining outcome in over 500 patients. *Ann Surg* 234, 384-393; discussion 393-384, 0003-4932

Gottesdiener, KM. (1989) Transplanted infections: donor-to-host transmission with the allograft. *Ann Intern Med* 110, 1001-1016, 0003-4819

Gottschalk, S, Rooney, CM, & Heslop, HE. (2005) Post-transplant lymphoproliferative disorders. *Annu Rev Med* 56, 29-44, 0066-4219

Grossi, PA, & Fishman, JA. (2009) Donor-derived infections in solid organ transplant recipients. *Am J Transplant* 9 Suppl 4, S19-26, 1600-6143

Hernandez-Hernandez, E, Alberu, J, Gonzalez-Michaca, L, Bobadilla-del Valle, M, Quiroz-Mejia, RA, Baizabal-Olarte, R, Correa-Rotter, R, & Sifuentes-Osornio, J. (2006) Screening for tuberculosis in the study of the living renal donor in a developing country. *Transplantation* 81, 290-292, 0041-1337

Hoy, WE, Roberts, NJ, Jr., Bryson, MF, Bowles, C, Lee, JC, Rivero, AJ, & Ritterson, AL. (1981) Transmission of strongyloidiasis by kidney transplant? Disseminated strongyloidiasis in both recipients of kidney allografts from a single cadaver donor. *JAMA* 246, 1937-1939, 0098-7484

Humar, A, Gregson, D, Caliendo, AM, McGeer, A, Malkan, G, Krajden, M, Corey, P, Greig, P, Walmsley, S, Levy, G, & Mazzulli, T. (1999) Clinical utility of quantitative cytomegalovirus viral load determination for predicting cytomegalovirus disease in liver transplant recipients. *Transplantation* 68, 1305-1311, 0041-1337

Humar, A, & Snydman, D. (2009) Cytomegalovirus in solid organ transplant recipients. *Am J Transplant* 9 Suppl 4, S78-86, 1600-6143

Husain, S, Paterson, DL, Studer, SM, Crespo, M, Pilewski, J, Durkin, M, Wheat, JL, Johnson, B, McLaughlin, L, Bentsen, C, McCurry, KR, & Singh, N. (2007) Aspergillus galactomannan antigen in the bronchoalveolar lavage fluid for the diagnosis of invasive aspergillosis in lung transplant recipients. *Transplantation* 83, 1330-1336, 0041-1337

Ison, MG. (2006) Adenovirus infections in transplant recipients. *Clin Infect Dis* 43, 331-339, 1537-6591

Ison, MG, & Green, M. (2009) Adenovirus in solid organ transplant recipients. *Am J Transplant* 9 Suppl 4, S161-165, 1600-6143

Ison, MG, Hager, J, Blumberg, E, Burdick, J, Carney, K, Cutler, J, Dimaio, JM, Hasz, R, Kuehnert, MJ, Ortiz-Rios, E, Teperman, L, & Nalesnik, M. (2009) Donor-derived disease transmission events in the United States: data reviewed by the

OPTN/UNOS Disease Transmission Advisory Committee. *Am J Transplant* 9, 1929-1935, 1600-6143

Iwamoto, M, Jernigan, DB, Guasch, A, Trepka, MJ, Blackmore, CG, Hellinger, WC, Pham, SM, Zaki, S, Lanciotti, RS, Lance-Parker, SE, DiazGranados, CA, Winquist, AG, Perlino, CA, Wiersma, S, Hillyer, KL, Goodman, JL, Marfin, AA, Chamberland, ME, & Petersen, LR. (2003) Transmission of West Nile virus from an organ donor to four transplant recipients. *N Engl J Med* 348, 2196-2203, 1533-4406

Kanj, SS, Welty-Wolf, K, Madden, J, Tapson, V, Baz, MA, Davis, RD, & Perfect, JR. (1996) Fungal infections in lung and heart-lung transplant recipients. Report of 9 cases and review of the literature. *Medicine (Baltimore)* 75, 142-156, 0025-7974

Kawagishi, N, Satoh, K, Enomoto, Y, Akamatsu, Y, Sekiguchi, S, Fujimori, K, & Satomi, S. (2006) Risk factors and impact of beta-D glucan on invasive fungal infection for the living donor liver transplant recipients. *Tohoku J Exp Med* 209, 207-215, 0040-8727

Kiuchi, T, Inomata, Y, Uemoto, S, Satomura, K, Egawa, H, Okajima, H, Yamaoka, Y, & Tanaka, K. (1997) A hepatic graft tuberculosis transmitted from a living-related donor. *Transplantation* 63, 905-907, 0041-1337

Kleinman, SH, & Busch, MP. (2006) Assessing the impact of HBV NAT on window period reduction and residual risk. *J Clin Virol* 36 Suppl 1, S23-29, 1386-6532

Ko, WJ, Chu, SH, Lee, YH, Lee, PH, Lee, CJ, Chao, SH, & Chang, SC. (1998) Successful prevention of syphilis transmission from a multiple organ donor with serological evidence of syphilis. *Transplant Proc* 30, 3667-3668, 0041-1345

Kolk, DP, Dockter, J, Linnen, J, Ho-Sing-Loy, M, Gillotte-Taylor, K, McDonough, SH, Mimms, L, & Giachetti, C. (2002) Significant closure of the human immunodeficiency virus type 1 and hepatitis C virus preseroconversion detection windows with a transcription-mediated-amplification-driven assay. *J Clin Microbiol* 40, 1761-1766, 0095-1137

Kotton, CN, & Lattes, R. (2009) Parasitic infections in solid organ transplant recipients. *Am J Transplant* 9 Suppl 4, S234-251, 1600-6143

Kusne, S, Torre-Cisneros, J, Manez, R, Irish, W, Martin, M, Fung, J, Simmons, RL, & Starzl, TE. (1992) Factors associated with invasive lung aspergillosis and the significance of positive Aspergillus culture after liver transplantation. *J Infect Dis* 166, 1379-1383, 0022-1899

Kwak, EJ, Husain, S, Obman, A, Meinke, L, Stout, J, Kusne, S, Wagener, MM, & Singh, N. (2004) Efficacy of galactomannan antigen in the Platelia Aspergillus enzyme immunoassay for diagnosis of invasive aspergillosis in liver transplant recipients. *J Clin Microbiol* 42, 435-438, 0095-1137

Limaye, AP, Connolly, PA, Sagar, M, Fritsche, TR, Cookson, BT, Wheat, LJ, & Stamm, WE. (2000) Transmission of Histoplasma capsulatum by organ transplantation. *N Engl J Med* 343, 1163-1166, 0028-4793

Liu, LX, & Weller, PF. (1993) Strongyloidiasis and other intestinal nematode infections. *Infect Dis Clin North Am* 7, 655-682, 0891-5520

Lok, AS, Lai, CL, & Wu, PC. (1988) Prevalence of isolated antibody to hepatitis B core antigen in an area endemic for hepatitis B virus infection: implications in hepatitis B vaccination programs. *Hepatology* 8, 766-770, 0270-9139

Lopez-Navidad, A, Domingo, P, Caballero, F, Gonzalez, C, & Santiago, C. (1997) Successful transplantation of organs retrieved from donors with bacterial meningitis. *Transplantation* 64, 365-368, 0041-1337

Malkan, G, Cattral, MS, Humar, A, Al Asghar, H, Greig, PD, Hemming, AW, Levy, GA, & Lilly, LB. (2000) Lamivudine for hepatitis B in liver transplantation: a single-center experience. *Transplantation* 69, 1403-1407, 0041-1337

Mayes, JT, O'Connor, BJ, Avery, R, Castellani, W, & Carey, W. (1995) Transmission of Toxoplasma gondii infection by liver transplantation. *Clin Infect Dis* 21, 511-515, 1058-4838

Mazzulli, T, Drew, LW, Yen-Lieberman, B, Jekic-McMullen, D, Kohn, DJ, Isada, C, Moussa, G, Chua, R, & Walmsley, S. (1999) Multicenter comparison of the digene hybrid capture CMV DNA assay (version 2.0), the pp65 antigenemia assay, and cell culture for detection of cytomegalovirus viremia. *J Clin Microbiol* 37, 958-963, 0095-1137

Morris, MI, Fischer, SA, & Ison, MG. (2010) Infections transmitted by transplantation. *Infect Dis Clin North Am* 24, 497-514, 1557-9824

Munoz, P, Rodriguez, C, & Bouza, E. (2005) Mycobacterium tuberculosis infection in recipients of solid organ transplants. *Clin Infect Dis* 40, 581-587, 1537-6591

Mutimer, D, Dusheiko, G, Barrett, C, Grellier, L, Ahmed, M, Anschuetz, G, Burroughs, A, Hubscher, S, Dhillon, AP, Rolles, K, & Elias, E. (2000) Lamivudine without HBIg for prevention of graft reinfection by hepatitis B: long-term follow-up. *Transplantation* 70, 809-815, 0041-1337

Nery, JR, Weppler, D, Ketchum, P, Olson, L, Fragulidis, GP, Khan, MF, Webb, MG, Miller, J, & Tzakis, AG. (1997) Donor infection and primary nonfunction in liver transplantation. *Transplant Proc* 29, 481-483, 0041-1345

Obayashi, T, Negishi, K, Suzuki, T, & Funata, N. (2008) Reappraisal of the serum (1-->3)-beta-D-glucan assay for the diagnosis of invasive fungal infections--a study based on autopsy cases from 6 years. *Clin Infect Dis* 46, 1864-1870, 1537-6591

Ooi, BS, Chen, BT, Lim, CH, Khoo, OT, & Chan, DT. (1971) Survival of a patient transplanted with a kidney infected with Cryptococcus neoformans. *Transplantation* 11, 428-429, 0041-1337

Ostrosky-Zeichner, L, Alexander, BD, Kett, DH, Vazquez, J, Pappas, PG, Saeki, F, Ketchum, PA, Wingard, J, Schiff, R, Tamura, H, Finkelman, MA, & Rex, JH. (2005) Multicenter clinical evaluation of the (1-->3) beta-D-glucan assay as an aid to diagnosis of fungal infections in humans. *Clin Infect Dis* 41, 654-659, 1537-6591

Pappas, PG, Kauffman, CA, Andes, D, Benjamin, DK, Jr., Calandra, TF, Edwards, JE, Jr., Filler, SG, Fisher, JF, Kullberg, BJ, Ostrosky-Zeichner, L, Reboli, AC, Rex, JH, Walsh, TJ, & Sobel, JD. (2009) Clinical practice guidelines for the management of candidiasis: 2009 update by the Infectious Diseases Society of America. *Clin Infect Dis* 48, 503-535, 1537-6591

Patel, G, Arvelakis, A, Sauter, BV, Gondolesi, GE, Caplivski, D, & Huprikar, S. (2008) Strongyloides hyperinfection syndrome after intestinal transplantation. *Transpl Infect Dis* 10, 137-141, 1399-3062

Paya, C, Humar, A, Dominguez, E, Washburn, K, Blumberg, E, Alexander, B, Freeman, R, Heaton, N, & Pescovitz, MD. (2004) Efficacy and safety of valganciclovir vs. oral ganciclovir for prevention of cytomegalovirus disease in solid organ transplant recipients. *Am J Transplant* 4, 611-620, 1600-6135

Paya, CV. (2001) Prevention of cytomegalovirus disease in recipients of solid-organ transplants. *Clin Infect Dis* 32, 596-603, 1058-4838

Paya, CV. (2002) Prevention of fungal infection in transplantation. *Transpl Infect Dis* 4 Suppl 3, 46-51, 1398-2273

Penn, I. (1996) Malignant melanoma in organ allograft recipients. *Transplantation* 61, 274-278, 0041-1337

Pereira, BJ, Milford, EL, Kirkman, RL, Quan, S, Sayre, KR, Johnson, PJ, Wilber, JC, & Levey, AS. (1992) Prevalence of hepatitis C virus RNA in organ donors positive for hepatitis C antibody and in the recipients of their organs. *N Engl J Med* 327, 910-915, 0028-4793

Ponziani, FR, Gasbarrini, A, Pompili, M, Burra, P, & Fagiuoli, S. (2011) Management of hepatitis C virus infection recurrence after liver transplantation: an overview. *Transplant Proc* 43, 291-295, 1873-2623

Qu, L, Green, M, Webber, S, Reyes, J, Ellis, D, & Rowe, D. (2000) Epstein-Barr virus gene expression in the peripheral blood of transplant recipients with persistent circulating virus loads. *J Infect Dis* 182, 1013-1021, 0022-1899

Rose, C, Green, M, Webber, S, Ellis, D, Reyes, J, & Rowe, D. (2001) Pediatric solid-organ transplant recipients carry chronic loads of Epstein-Barr virus exclusively in the immunoglobulin D-negative B-cell compartment. *J Clin Microbiol* 39, 1407-1415, 0095-1137

Rosengard, BR, Feng, S, Alfrey, EJ, Zaroff, JG, Emond, JC, Henry, ML, Garrity, ER, Roberts, JP, Wynn, JJ, Metzger, RA, Freeman, RB, Port, FK, Merion, RM, Love, RB, Busuttil, RW, & Delmonico, FL. (2002) Report of the Crystal City meeting to maximize the use of organs recovered from the cadaver donor. *Am J Transplant* 2, 701-711, 1600-6135

Saag, MS, Graybill, RJ, Larsen, RA, Pappas, PG, Perfect, JR, Powderly, WG, Sobel, JD, & Dismukes, WE. (2000) Practice guidelines for the management of cryptococcal disease. Infectious Diseases Society of America. *Clin Infect Dis* 30, 710-718, 1058-4838

Samuel, D, Castaing, D, Adam, R, Saliba, F, Chamaret, S, Misset, JL, Montagnier, L, & Bismuth, H. (1988) Fatal acute HIV infection with aplastic anaemia, transmitted by liver graft. *Lancet* 1, 1221-1222, 0140-6736

Satoi, S, Bramhall, SR, Solomon, M, Hastings, M, Mayer, AD, de Goyet, JV, Buckels, JA, McMaster, P, & Mirza, DF. (2001) The use of liver grafts from donors with bacterial meningitis. *Transplantation* 72, 1108-1113, 0041-1337

Schaffner, A. (2001) Pretransplant evaluation for infections in donors and recipients of solid organs. *Clin Infect Dis* 33 Suppl 1, S9-14, 1058-4838

Schreiber, GB, Busch, MP, Kleinman, SH, & Korelitz, JJ. (1996) The risk of transfusion-transmitted viral infections. The Retrovirus Epidemiology Donor Study. *N Engl J Med* 334, 1685-1690, 0028-4793

Seehofer, D, & Berg, T. (2005) Prevention of hepatitis B recurrence after liver transplantation. *Transplantation* 80, S120-124, 0041-1337

Singh, N, Alexander, BD, Lortholary, O, Dromer, F, Gupta, KL, John, GT, del Busto, R, Klintmalm, GB, Somani, J, Lyon, GM, Pursell, K, Stosor, V, Munoz, P, Limaye, AP, Kalil, AC, Pruett, TL, Garcia-Diaz, J, Humar, A, Houston, S, House, AA, Wray, D, Orloff, S, Dowdy, LA, Fisher, RA, Heitman, J, Wagener, MM, & Husain, S. (2007) Cryptococcus neoformans in organ transplant recipients: impact of calcineurin-inhibitor agents on mortality. *J Infect Dis* 195, 756-764, 0022-1899

Singh, N, Arnow, PM, Bonham, A, Dominguez, E, Paterson, DL, Pankey, GA, Wagener, MM, & Yu, VL. (1997) Invasive aspergillosis in liver transplant recipients in the 1990s. *Transplantation* 64, 716-720, 0041-1337

Singh, N, & Forrest, G. (2009) Cryptococcosis in solid organ transplant recipients. *Am J Transplant* 9 Suppl 4, S192-198, 1600-6143

Singh, N, & Husain, S. (2009) Invasive aspergillosis in solid organ transplant recipients. *Am J Transplant* 9 Suppl 4, S180-191, 1600-6143

Singh, N, Limaye, AP, Forrest, G, Safdar, N, Munoz, P, Pursell, K, Houston, S, Rosso, F, Montoya, JG, Patton, P, Del Busto, R, Aguado, JM, Fisher, RA, Klintmalm, GB, Miller, R, Wagener, MM, Lewis, RE, Kontoyiannis, DP, & Husain, S. (2006) Combination of voriconazole and caspofungin as primary therapy for invasive aspergillosis in solid organ transplant recipients: a prospective, multicenter, observational study. *Transplantation* 81, 320-326, 0041-1337

Singh, N, Paterson, DL, Gayowski, T, Wagener, MM, & Marino, IR. (2001) Preemptive prophylaxis with a lipid preparation of amphotericin B for invasive fungal infections in liver transplant recipients requiring renal replacement therapy. *Transplantation* 71, 910-913, 0041-1337

Smets, F, Latinne, D, Bazin, H, Reding, R, Otte, JB, Buts, JP, & Sokal, EM. (2002) Ratio between Epstein-Barr viral load and anti-Epstein-Barr virus specific T-cell response as a predictive marker of posttransplant lymphoproliferative disease. *Transplantation* 73, 1603-1610, 0041-1337

Snydman, DR, Werner, BG, Dougherty, NN, Griffith, J, Rubin, RH, Dienstag, JL, Rohrer, RH, Freeman, R, Jenkins, R, Lewis, WD, Hammer, S, O'Rourke, E, Grady, GF, Fawaz, K, Kaplan, MM, Hoffman, MA, Katz, AT, & Doran, M. (1993) Cytomegalovirus immune globulin prophylaxis in liver transplantation. A randomized, double-blind, placebo-controlled trial. *Ann Intern Med* 119, 984-991, 0003-4819

Srinivasan, A, Burton, EC, Kuehnert, MJ, Rupprecht, C, Sutker, WL, Ksiazek, TG, Paddock, CD, Guarner, J, Shieh, WJ, Goldsmith, C, Hanlon, CA, Zoretic, J, Fischbach, B, Niezgoda, M, El-Feky, WH, Orciari, L, Sanchez, EQ, Likos, A, Klintmalm, GB, Cardo, D, LeDuc, J, Chamberland, ME, Jernigan, DB, & Zaki, SR. (2005) Transmission of rabies virus from an organ donor to four transplant recipients. *N Engl J Med* 352, 1103-1111, 1533-4406

Strauss, DC, & Thomas, JM. (2010) Transmission of donor melanoma by organ transplantation. *Lancet Oncol* 11, 790-796, 1474-5488

Strout, RG. (1962) A method for concentrating hemoflagellates. *J Parasitol* 48, 100, 0022-3395

Toro, C, Rodes, B, Poveda, E, & Soriano, V. (2003) Rapid development of subacute myelopathy in three organ transplant recipients after transmission of human T-cell lymphotropic virus type I from a single donor. *Transplantation* 75, 102-104, 0041-1337

Torre-Cisneros, J, Doblas, A, Aguado, JM, San Juan, R, Blanes, M, Montejo, M, Cervera, C, Len, O, Carratala, J, Cisneros, JM, Bou, G, Munoz, P, Ramos, A, Gurgui, M, Borrell, N, Fortun, J, Moreno, A, & Gavalda, J. (2009) Tuberculosis after solid-organ transplant: incidence, risk factors, and clinical characteristics in the RESITRA (Spanish Network of Infection in Transplantation) cohort. *Clin Infect Dis* 48, 1657-1665, 1537-6591

Trautwein, C. (2004) Mechanisms of hepatitis B virus graft reinfection and graft damage after liver transplantation. *J Hepatol* 41, 362-369, 0168-8278

Vargas, HE, Laskus, T, Wang, LF, Lee, R, Radkowski, M, Dodson, F, Fung, JJ, & Rakela, J. (1999) Outcome of liver transplantation in hepatitis C virus-infected patients who received hepatitis C virus-infected grafts. *Gastroenterology* 117, 149-153, 0016-5085

Vazquez, MC, Riarte, A, Pattin, M, & Lauricella, M. (1993) Chagas' disease can be transmitted through kidney transplantation. *Transplant Proc* 25, 3259-3260, 0041-1345

Velidedeoglu, E, Desai, NM, Campos, L, Olthoff, KM, Shaked, A, Nunes, F, Zeldin, G, Stewart, C, Blumberg, E, Abrams, J, & Markmann, JF. (2002) The outcome of liver grafts procured from hepatitis C-positive donors. *Transplantation* 73, 582-587, 0041-1337

Wachs, ME, Amend, WJ, Ascher, NL, Bretan, PN, Emond, J, Lake, JR, Melzer, JS, Roberts, JP, Tomlanovich, SJ, Vincenti, F, & et al. (1995) The risk of transmission of hepatitis B from HBsAg(-), HBcAb(+), HBIgM(-) organ donors. *Transplantation* 59, 230-234, 0041-1337

Walsh, TJ, Anaissie, EJ, Denning, DW, Herbrecht, R, Kontoyiannis, DP, Marr, KA, Morrison, VA, Segal, BH, Steinbach, WJ, Stevens, DA, van Burik, JA, Wingard, JR, & Patterson, TF. (2008) Treatment of aspergillosis: clinical practice guidelines of the Infectious Diseases Society of America. *Clin Infect Dis* 46, 327-360, 1537-6591

Wang, CS, Ko, HH, Yoshida, EM, Marra, CA, & Richardson, K. (2006) Interferon-based combination anti-viral therapy for hepatitis C virus after liver transplantation: a review and quantitative analysis. *Am J Transplant* 6, 1586-1599, 1600-6135

MJ, Chusid, MJ, & Rupprecht, CE. (2005) Survival after treatment of rabies with induction of coma. *N Engl J Med* 352, 2508-2514, 1533-4406

Wu, TJ, Lee, CF, Chou, HS, Yu, MC, & Lee, WC. (2008) Suspect the donor with potential infection in the adult deceased donor liver transplantation. *Transplant Proc* 40, 2486-2488, 0041-1345

Yango, A, Jr., Morrissey, P, Gohh, R, & Wahbeh, A. (2002) Donor-transmitted parvovirus infection in a kidney transplant recipient presenting as pancytopenia and allograft dysfunction. *Transpl Infect Dis* 4, 163-166, 1398-2273

Yehia, BR, & Blumberg, EA. (2010) Mycobacterium tuberculosis infection in liver transplantation. *Liver Transpl* 16, 1129-1135, 1527-6473

Part 6

Miscellaneous

21

Physiotherapy in Liver Transplantation

Meriç Şenduran[1] and S. Ufuk Yurdalan[2]
[1]*Dokuz Eylul University / School of PTR*
[2]*Marmara University/ Health Sciences Faculty / Department of PTR*
Turkey

1. Introduction

Liver transplantation is the definite surgical treatment for patients with end-stage liver disease and acute liver failure that improves liver functions and survival. In recent years health-related quality of life has been accepted to be in relation with surgical success and has become to be used as an important assessment parameter not only after transplantation but also during the disease process.

The most limited sub-group of quality of life is probably the physical activity level that is reduced due to low physical performance status both before and after liver transplantation. This limitation is multi-factorial depending on the stage of the disease and post-transplant period.

Rehabilitative approaches may help patients with liver disease and transplant recipients to improve quality of life by increasing muscle strength, prevent excessive fatigue, enhance aerobic capacity and increase physical activity level. In accordance with this purpose, specific physiotherapeutic interventions structured according to patients' needs in any phase of the disease process should be properly defined by the professions working in related fields.

Physiotherapy in patients with liver disease and liver transplant recipients could mainly be divided into three periods: Pre-operative physiotherapy, early post-operative physiotherapy and late post-operative physiotherapy. A similar rehabilitation process including six different periods after orthotopic liver transplantation has been previously defined as follows: pre-operative period, early and late post-operative periods, early and late ambulatory care periods and motor rehabilitation (Rongies et al., 2005).

In any period of physiotherapy, indications and contraindications for participation in this long rehabilitation process should be well-clarified. Any sign of acute rejection of the transplanted organ, acute hemorrhage, electrolyte imbalance, physiological instability, severe neurologic complications and severe cardiovascular co-morbidities may further effect the implementation of specific techniques and exercises. Therefore phase-dependent specialized assessment procedures should be carried out before planning the exercise programs. Physiotherapeutic evaluation should include the assessment of muscle strength and endurance, aerobic capacity, physical activity level, independency in daily life activities and health-related quality of life. Neurologic, metabolic or musculoskeletal co-morbidities, level of pain and fatigue, smoking and alcohol habits should also be recorded within the context of the assessment procedure.

2. Pre-operative physiotherapy

Patients waiting on transplantation list with end-stage liver disease usually show loss of muscle mass, low bone mineral density, reduced muscle strength, increased levels of fatigue and decreased aerobic capacity. Malnutrition, cardiopulmonary dysfunction, altered metabolism and corticosteroid treatment are thought to be responsible for the factors that play a role in impaired physical performance.

Diminished exercise capacity is correlated with disease severity in patients with end stage liver disease and is mainly the result of muscle wasting called "cirrhotic myopathy" and cardiac dysfunction called as "cirrhotic cardiomyopathy" (Scott et al., 1998).

Malnutrition is another important factor affecting muscle mass and the activity level. Dysfunctions of glycogen storage and gluconeogenesis in end-stage liver disease lead to a break down of muscle protein and fat for energy usage resulting in weight loss and muscle weakness (Vintro et al., 2002). Poor dietary intake, loss of appetite and medical dietary restrictions may aggravate the secondary effects of malnutrition. In addition to decreased muscle strength and fatigue, severe edema and ascites accompanying the disease negatively affect the ambulation leading to decreases in physical activity and performance level.

Stage dependent reduction in aerobic physical fitness, isokinetic muscle strength and health-related quality of life were found in patients with cirrhosis waiting on the transplantation list (Wiesinger et al., 2001). Similarly, two thirds of cirrhotics, without cardiopulmonary disease or other confounding factors displayed significantly reduced aerobic capacity measured by maximal cardiopulmonary exercise testing (Epstein et al., 1998).

All the data revealed from the published papers emphasize the reasonable needs for specific exercise and rehabilitation programs with the objectives of increasing muscle strength and endurance, aerobic capacity and optimizing daily life independency and health-related quality of life by improving physical functioning for the patients waiting on the liver transplantation list. Longer waiting times make the process more difficult. Therefore, strategies for avoiding prolonged bed rest and increasing activity level are recommended as the disease progresses. To start physiotherapeutic interventions before the transplantation will no doubtfully help the patient to overcome post-operative complications and further deconditioning due to inactivity.

3. Early post-operative physiotherapy

3.1 Physiotherapy in the Intensive Care Unit

Bed rest is a common prescription in the intensive care unit (ICU) because of drainage tubes, arterial lines, urinary and naso-gastric catheters and sometimes as a result of prolonged mechanical ventilation. Although bed rest can be considered as a part of the treatment in the ICU, immobilization may further affect the overall health status as a consequence of muscle atrophy, diminished bronchial drainage and decreased lung expansion. Physiotherapy in the ICU aims to avoid complications of immobilization, provide respiratory support in order to prevent post-operative pulmonary complications and restore functional independency (Stiller, 2000). Post-operative pulmonary complications are common in patients who have undergone open abdominal surgery (Pasquina et al., 2006; Browning et al., 2007). Decreased mucociliary activity due to anesthesia and relatively longer surgery durations and immobilization during the operation may lead to dysfunction of the respiratory system and an increase in bronchial secretion. Post-operative pain resulting from an extensive surgical incision on the upper abdominal region negatively affects coughing by inhibiting the required contraction of abdominal muscles. Pain may also inhibit the physical activities of the patient not only for mobilization but also in bed during supine position. Therefore, it is important to implement effective analgesic treatment in order to overcome post-operative pain and provide bronchial clearance by facilitating coughing mechanism and promoting activity. Diaphragmatic dysfunction is another important factor in the development of pulmonary complications resulting from both pain due to incision and phrenic nerve irritation or paralysis in rare cases.

Early post-transplant physiotherapy including interventions of pulmonary physiotherapy and early mobilization starts on the first post-operative day as soon as the patient is physiologically stabilized and lasts till the patient is discharged from the ICU. Pulmonary physiotherapy including lung expansion and diaphragmatic breathing exercises, forced expiratory technique and coughing techniques and incentive spirometry aims to provide airway clearance, increase lung expansion, restore respiratory function and prevent post-operative pulmonary complications (Clini & Ambrosino, 2005). Manual techniques including chest percussion and vibration may also be alternative treatment approaches if airway clearance is not accomplished enough although they are not much preferable after a major surgery in the presence of numerous drains. They may also cause the patient to experience more pain and anxiety. Pulmonary physiotherapy should start on the first post-operative day if the patient is already extubated just after the surgery. Unless the patient is extubated in the ICU, a physiotherapist can help to speed the weaning period up as long as the patient is cooperative enough to follow the instructions and participate in the exercises.

Activity after surgery should start as early as possible as the physiological and hemodynamic stabilities are provided. It is important to consider the cardiac and respiratory reserves of the patient and hemoglobin level as well before planning the mobilization session. Mobilization should be implemented gradually as follows in order to be well-tolerated by the patient: Limb exercises in supine position, sitting in bed, sitting on the edge of the bed, standing, preparatory walking exercises and ambulation (Senduran et al., 2010). Active-assistive or active limb exercises performed in bed and in sitting position on the edge of the bed stimulate circulation and respiration and should be implemented under supervision during the ICU admission. Lower limb exercises should not cause abdominal pain by increasing the tension on the abdominal region. Therefore, hip movements, especially flexion, should be performed in limited angles. Avoiding abdominal tension during all the activities including sitting and ambulation is necessary to motivate the patient to be more active. In order to prepare the patient for mobilization in the ICU, the surgical area should be bandaged tightly and drains, urine catheter, naso-gastric catheter should be fixed to the body of the patient with a plaster. Additionally, oxygen tube and catheter lines should be lengthened, if necessary.

Mechanical ventilation and ICU admission are standard post-operative care after liver transplantation improving post-operative outcomes by reducing physiological stress triggered by awakening and spontaneous ventilation (Mandell et al., 2002). However, early extubation is the key element to reduce health care costs by decreasing ICU stay and speed up the patients' recovery. The importance of early extubation, aggressive chest physiotherapy and early ambulation for shortening ICU stay and preventing septic complications and mortality after liver transplantation was highlighted (Mor et al., 2001). Similarly, the vitality of physiotherapy in the ICU after liver transplantation in order to recover muscle waste due to metabolic and nutritional deficits, peripheral neuropathies depending on postural components and respiratory complications was emphasized in another study (Faenza et al., 2005).

The time of physiotherapy initiation after liver transplantation and affecting factors were studied before. A significant correlation between the time of physiotherapy initiation and primary cause of liver transplantation was revealed. Patients with acute liver failure were the latest group that was enrolled in early post-operative physiotherapy suggesting the influence of compensation theory for the healing process rather than a rapid disease progression. A strong relationship between the time of initiation and the ability to take fully upright position was also detected in the same study (Rongies et al., 2005).

Hemodynamic instability is common early after liver transplantation due to cardiac abnormalities characterized by cirrhosis per se. It is well documented that end stage liver disease is characterized by hyperdynamic circulation leading to higher resting heart rate, increased cardiac output and decreased systemic vascular resistance (Wong et al., 2001). Therefore, ongoing monitoring of vital signs, especially arterial pressures, heart rate, respiratory rate and peripheral oxygen saturation is recommended during the physiotherapy interventions in the ICU in order to observe physiological responses in case of any adverse effects.

3.2 Physiotherapy in the clinical setting

Similar interventions should also continue after discharge from the ICU ward and progress according to the patient's health and physical status. Inpatient rehabilitation after liver transplantation also includes chest physiotherapy and active-assisted and active limb exercises in order to overcome post-surgical fatigue and improve physical performance level.

Pulmonary physiotherapy including lung expansion and diaphragmatic breathing exercises, forced expiratory technique and coughing techniques and incentive spirometry should continue until the discharge from the hospital whether significant pulmonary complications exist or not.

Muscular strengthening exercises, stretching exercises and posture exercises should be included in the inpatient exercise program. Strengthening exercises using elastic bands or free weights for upper and lower limbs help to prevent muscle loss and restore decreased muscle strength and endurance. Intensity of the exercises can be set according to 1 maximum repetition protocol. Stretching exercises are used to provide normal muscle elongation, especially in patients suffering from prolonged immobilization that may further affect daily activities and even ambulation. Stretching and posture exercises also help to prepare the patient for the exercise session and may stimulate relaxation and anxiety reduction.

It is important to increase the independency of self-care activities during the hospital stay. Fatigue is one of the major problems in patients with liver diseases which may be exacerbated in the early post-operative period. Exercises should progress gradually by increasing the number of repetitions, frequency during the day or the intensity according to the patient's general condition.

Studies related to inpatient physiotherapy after liver transplantation is limited in the literature. In a retrospective study, significant functional gains were achieved by acute inpatient rehabilitation in 55 liver transplant recipients. Nevertheless, the details and the content of inpatient rehabilitation that the patients participated in during their hospital stay were not mentioned (Cortazzo et al., 2005).

In another study indicating the long rehabilitation process after liver transplantation early mobilization and exercises with graded intensity were implemented to 38 liver transplant recipients during post-operative three weeks and progressed to strengthening, balance, flexibility and aerobic exercises after the third post-transplant week. Exercise treatment continued as one hour in two weeks after the discharge and lasted for 8-24 weeks. As a result of the rehabilitation process significant improvements in aerobic capacity, muscle strength and physical performance were reported (Beyer et al., 1999).

Patient education is another important part of inpatient rehabilitation especially during the first six weeks. Patients should be warned about not driving, not lifting, pushing or pullling heavy objects and not attempting sit-ups, push-ups or pull-ups.

Inpatient physiotherapy should continue until the patient is discharged from the hospital. Structured, systematic and individualized home exercise programs should be well-planned according to the patients' needs and be followed by regular controls. If there is a possibility for the patients to continue rehabilitation process in a clinical setting, they can enroll in an outpatient rehabilitation process under the supervision of physiotherapists. If outpatient rehabilitation service is not available telerehabilitation may be an alternative choice which is popular in recent days in the rehabilitation field. A simple connection from the patient's house to the clinical setting is required in order to be supervised by the professions.

4. Late post-operative physiotherapy

4.1 Early phase interventions

Early phase interventions involve the first three months after the discharge from the hospital. A home exercise program which is tailored to the individual patient should be prescribed. A handbook containing simple instructions and illustrations for exercises, suggestions for a more active life style and dietary requirements may help the patient after discharge.

The first aim of this period is to maintain the possible highest level of physical activity. Pedometers and accelerometers may be used for not only monitoring but also defining a target daily activity level and will help to motivate the patient to be more active. Patients may develop a fear of damaging the newly transplanted organ and the protective attitudes of the family members may lead to restriction of the activity. Patients should be encouraged to stay more active by the multidisciplinary team including physicians, physiotherapists, dieticians, psychologists, social workers and family members as well.

During this period the patient may experience anxiety and irritability, sleep disturbances, stress and depression. Optimum level of physical activity and continuing inpatient exercises early after the discharge period will also help the patient to overcome these symptoms.

4.2 Late phase interventions

The late post-operative period, that starts mainly three months after liver transplantation aims to provide maximum capacity for daily life independency and optimize health-related quality of life. Returning to job, social life and leisure activities and even returning to sports participation are the objectives of this life-long process. Flexibility, balance, resistance and aerobic exercises are paramount in this period.

Although liver transplantation is the only definite treatment for end-stage liver disease in order to regulate liver functions and maintain survival, it is not a solution per se for restoring the overall health status which is impaired due to loss of muscle mass, excessive fatigue, reduced physical performance and diminished aerobic capacity. Supervised rehabilitation programs are required to improve functional capacity after liver transplantation as surgery alone has a very modest and inconsistent effect on aerobic capacity (Lemzye et al., 2010). Studies investigating the level of aerobic capacity by measuring maximal oxygen uptake after liver transplantation found significant improvements in the long term process. In a related study functional capacity improved 12 months after transplantation compared to the pre-operative period whereas no significant difference existed on the 3rd month-measurements (Iscar et al., 2009). In another similar investigation no significant difference was found in terms of isokinetic muscle strength and aerobic capacity before and 1-2 months after orthotopic liver transplantation without any post-operative rehabilitative approaches (Pieber et al., 2006).

Resistance exercises help to restore muscle strength and prevent osteoporosis which may occur due to immunosuppressant therapy. Osteoporosis has been reported as a common cause of morbidity after liver transplantation leading to bone fractures especially in the first six months after the surgery (Atamaz et al., 2006). Aerobic training consisted of walking; jogging or cycling should also be planned in accordance with cardiac and pulmonary reserve of each patient. Physical activity level, co-morbidities, level of fatigue, and any complication should be considered while planning the exercise regimens. Treadmill and cycle ergometers can be alternative training methods to increase aerobic capacity. It was documented that transplant recipients experienced a positive perception of self esteem, body image and well-being after an 8-week structured aerobic exercise program (Surgit et al., 2001).

It is well-known that life-long immunosuppressive therapy has long-term consequences including not only muscle and bone loss but also cardiovascular risks due to hyperlipidemia and hypertension. Patients will benefit from regular exercise programs to delay the cardiovascular complications. Weight control is another problem during the late post-operative phase as a result of corticosteroids. Combined aerobic and resistance exercise trainings will no doubtfully help the patient to control excessive weight gain. A home-based exercise and nutrition behavior modifications initiated early after transplantation including regular follow-ups resulted in significant gains in exercise capacity, quality of life and body composition (Krasnoff et al., 2006).

Post-transplant rehabilitation programs are also suggested for reducing the complaint of physical fatigue which remains as one of the most distressing symptoms even one year after the surgery leading to a sedentary lifestyle (Van der Ber-Emons et al., 2006). Muscle energy techniques and interval trainings will provide energy saving and avoid excessive fatigue.

4.3 Sports participation

Sports participation after solid organ transplantation is the final objection of the long term rehabilitation process for maximizing quality of life. It is recommended to encourage the patients to participate in a sports activity three months after the surgery. This time is required to achieve optimal flexibility, muscular strength, muscular endurance and aerobic capacity and to provide proper post-operative wound healing and graft stabilization so that the patient can do sports without any deterioration. Patients should start with light activities such as walking, stair climbing, golf, bowling, darts, archery and fishing. Table tennis and volleyball can be suggested as medium intensity activities. Swimming, athletics, badminton, cycling, rowing, squashes, tennis, mini-marathon are recommended after getting used to light and moderate activities. However, swimming in community pools or lakes is not recommended because of high risk of infectious organisms. High impact and contact sports such as football, basketball, horse riding and bungee jumping are not preferable as they may cause a serious trauma and lead to organ damage. Patients usually have a fear of organ damage or severe pain avoiding them to participate in sports. Contact sports also have an additional fracture risk for weight bearing bones due to long term osteoporotic effects of corticosteroids. As liver transplantation surgery induces a denervation of the liver and intrahepatic vascular system strenuous exercises may carry a high risk for reduction in portal blood flow due to increased demands of contracting muscles (Ersoz&Ersoz, 2003). Besides, selected and well-prepared liver transplant recipients were able to participate in mountain trek and tolerate exposure to high altitude similar to healthy subjects after a 6-month aerobic training and a hypercaloric diet including sugars, proteins and abundant hydration (Pirenne et al., 2004).

Feeling of distress, muscle and joint pain, incisional pain and fatigue are the complaints of transplant recipients during or after exercises. Running, skiing, bike riding and tennis, shot-put and body-building were reported as the most popular sports among a group of patients with liver and kidney transplantation (Pupkal et al., 2008).

Patients may participate in a sport not only for a leisure time activity but also for professional competitions. The World Transplant Games Federation, officially recognized by the International Olympic Committee, is a world-wide organization staging international sporting events for transplant athletes for over 20 years in order to demonstrate the ability of sports participation after organ transplantation and to raise awareness of the vitality of organ donation.

5. Conclusion

In summary structured, specific and well-planned physiotherapeutic interventions tailored to individual needs of each patient are required before and after liver transplantation in order to prevent muscle and bone loss, delay cardiovascular complications and compete with excessive physical fatigue. Specific exercise programs will increase muscle strength and endurance, enhance aerobic capacity, maximize physical activity level and optimize health-related quality of life. Exercise programs accompanying dietary counseling will also help the patient to control excessive weight gain. Secondary positive effects of regular exercise on sleep disturbances, depression and anxiety may also be beneficial for liver transplant recipients.

It is possible to divide physiotherapeutic interventions mainly into three periods: pre-operative, early post-operative and late post-operative periods. These interventions should be initiated according to individual functional status while the patient is on the waiting list in order to speed up the patient's recovery during the post-transplant period.

An active style should be promoted during the whole life of the transplant recipient. Patients should also be encouraged to participate in sports activity, even on a professional level.

6. References

Atamaz, F; Hepguler, S; Karasu, Z; Kilic, M & Tokat, Y. (2006). The prevention of bone fractures after liver transplantation: Experience with Alendronate treatment. *Transpl Proc* Vol.38:1448-1452.

Beyer, N; Aadahl, M; Strange, B; Kirkegaard, P; Hansen, BA; Mohr, T & Kjaer, M. (1999). Improved physical performance after orthotopic liver transplantation. *Liver Transpl Surg* Vol.5, No. 4 (July):301-309.

Browning, L; Denehy, L & Scholes, RL. (2007). The quantity of early upright mobilization performed following upper abdominal surgery is low: an observational study. *Aust J Physiother* Vol 53:47-52.

Clini, E & Ambrosino, N. (2005). Early physiotherapy in the respiratory intensive care unit. *Resp Med* Vol.99:1096-1104.

Cortazzo, MH; Helkowski, W; Pippin, B; Boninger, ML & Zafonte, R. (2005). Acute inpatient rehabilitation of 55 patients after liver transplantation. *Am J Phys Med Rehabil* Vol.84:880-884.

Epstein, SK; Ciubotaru, RL; Zilberberg, MD; Kaplan, LM; Jacoby, C; Freeman, R & Kaplan, MM. (1998). Analysis of impaired exercise capacity in patients with cirrhosis. *Dig Dis Sci* Vol.43, No.8 (August):1701-1707.

Ersoz, G & Ersoz, S. (2003). Changes in portal blood flow following acute exercise in liver transplant recipients. *Transpl Proc* Vol.35:1456-1457.

Faenza, S; Bernardi, E; Cuppini, F; Gatta, A; Lauro, A; Mancini, E; Petrini, F; Pierucci, E; Sangiorgi, G; Santoro, A; Varotti, G & Pinna, A. (2005). Intensive care complications in liver and multivisceral transplantation. *Transpl Proc* Vol.37:2618–2621.

Iscar, M; Montoliu, MA; Ortega, T; Rodriguez, M; Glez-Pinto, I & Alonso, P. (2009). Functional capacity before and after liver transplantation. *Transpl Proc* Vol.41:1014-1015.

Krasnoff, JB; Vintro, AQ; Ascher, NL; Bass, NM; Paul, SM; Dodd, MJ & Painter, PL. (2006). A randomized trial of exercise and dietary counseling after liver transplantation. *Am J of Transpl* Vol.6:1896–1905.

Lemzye, M; Dharancy, S; Neviere, R; Pruvot, FR; Declerck, N & Wallaert, B. (2010). Aerobic capacity in patients with chronic liver disease: Very modest effect of liver transplantation. *Presse Med* Vol.39:174-181.

Mandell, MS; Lezotte, D; Kam, I & Zamudio, S. (2002). Reduced use of intensive care after liver transplantation: Influence of early extubation. *Liver Transpl* Vol.8, No.8 (August):676-681.

Mor, E; Cohen, J; Erez, E; Grozovsky, A; Shaharabani, E; Bar- Nathan, N; Yussim, A; Micowiz, R; Shapira, Z & Zinger, P. (2001). Short intensive care unit stay reduces septic complications and improves outcome after liver transplantation. *Transpl Proc* Vol.33:2939–2940.

Pasquina, WP; Tramer, MR; Grainer, J & Bernhard, W. (2006). Respiratory physiotherapy to prevent pulmonary complications after abdominal surgery. *Chest* Vol.130, No.6 (December):1887-1899.

Pieber, K; Crevenna, R; Nuhr, MJ; Quittan, M; Peck-Radosavljevic, M; Fialka-Moser, V & Wiesinger, GF. (2006). Aerobic capacity, muscle strength and health-related quality of life before and after orthotopic liver transplantation: Preliminary data of an Austrian transplantation centre. *J Rehabil Med* Vol.38:322-328.

Pirenne, J; Gelder, VF; Kharkevitch, T; Nevens, F; Verslype, C; Peetermans, WE; Kitade, H; Vanhees, L; Devos, Y; Hauser, M; Hamoir, E; Noizat-Pirenne, F & Pirotte, B. (2004). Tolerance of liver transplant patients to strenuous physical activity in high-altitude. *Am J Transpl* Vol.4:554–560.

Pupka, A; Płonek, T; Lewicki, K & Maroszyk, J. (2008). Influence of physical activity on the health condition of people after organ transplantation. *Med Sport* Vol.12, No.4:142-145.

Rongies, W; Stepniewska, S; Perzynska, EP; Dolecki, W; Wojtaszek, M; Oldakowska-Jedynak, U; Pawlak, J & Krawczyk, M. (2005). Rehabilitation principles in patients after orthotopic liver transplantation. *E&C Hepatology* Vol.1, No.1:41-44.

Rongies, W; Stepniewska, S; Golinska, B; Wojtazsek, M; Dolecki, W; Lewandowska, M; Bialoszewski, D & Krawczyk, M. (2008). An attempt to assess the influence of primary disease on the results of therapeutic rehabilitation in an early post-operative period in orthotopic liver transplant recipients. *Ann Transplant* Vol.13, No.1:40-43.

Senduran, M; Yurdalan, SU; Karadibak, D & Günerli, A. (2010). Haemodynamic effects of physiotherapy programme in intensive care unit after liver transplantation. *Disabil Rehabil* Vol.32, No.17:1461-6.

Stiller, K. (2000). Physiotherapy in intensive care. Towards an evidence-based practice. *Chest* Vol.118:1801-13.

Surgit, O; Ersoz, G; Gursel, Y & Ersoz, S. (2001). Effects of exercise training on specific immune parameters in transplant recipients. *Transpl Proc* Vol.33:3298.

Van den Berg-Emons, R; Van Ginneken, B; Wijffels, M; Tilanus, H; Metselaar, H; Stam, H & Kazemier, G. (2006). Fatigue is a major problem after liver transplantation. *Liver Transpl* Vol.12:928–933.

Van den Berg-Emons, R; Kazemier, G; Van Ginneken, B; Nieuwenhuijsen, C; Tilanus, H & Stam, H. (2006). Fatigue, level of everyday physical activity and quality of life after liver transplantation. *J Rehabil Med* Vol.38:124–129.

Vintro, AQ; Krasnoff, JB & Painter, P. (2002). Roles of nutrition and physical activity in musculoskeletal complications before and after liver transplantation. *AACN Clin Issues* Vol.13, No.2:333-47.

Wiesinger, GF; Quittan, M; Zimmermann, K; Nuhr, M; Wichlas, M; Bodingbauer, M; Asari, R; Berlakovich, G; Crevenna, R; Fialka-Moser, V & Peck-Radosavljevic, M. (2001). Physical performance and health-related quality of life in men on a liver transplantation waiting list. *J Rehabil Med* Vol.33:260–265.

Wong, F; Girgrah, N; Graba, J; Allidina, Y; Liu, P & Blendis, L. (2001). The cardiac response to exercise in cirrhosis. *Gut* Vol.49:268-275.